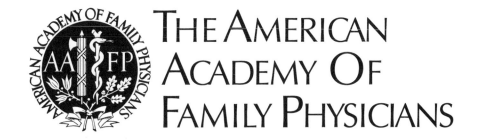

# THE AMERICAN ACADEMY OF FAMILY PHYSICIANS

# Family Health & Medical Guide

*Robert B. Kelly, M.D., M.S., Medical Editor*

*Gregg Albers, M.D., Principal Contributing Writer*
*Sarah J. West, Editor*
*David L. Baker, M.A., Medical Illustrator*

WORD PUBLISHING
Dallas·London·Vancouver·Melbourne

*The information in this book provides a general overview of health-related topics and may not apply to everyone. To find out if this information applies to you and to get more information about any health-related issue, talk to your family doctor.*

This health education material has been favorably reviewed by the American Academy of Family Physicians Foundation.

LIBRARY OF CONGRESS CATALOGING-IN-PUBLICATION DATA
Family health and medical guide / The American Academy of
Family Physicians; Robert B. Kelly, medical editor.
p. cm.
Includes index.
ISBN 0-8499-0839-6
1. Medicine, Popular. I. Kelly, Robert B. (Robert Boland), 1954-. II. American
Academy of Family Physicians.
RC81.F2352 1996                                                              95-46003
616—dc20                                                                          CIP

Printed in the United States of America
6 7 8 9   RRD 9 8 7 6 5 4 3 2 1

# FOREWORD

Health has been an important concern throughout human history. Good health can be liberating. Bad health can be limiting. However, it is easy to take good health for granted when we are healthy. It is often only when we are sick that we appreciate our good health.

Through new discoveries and new technology, we learn more every day about health and disease, and how our bodies work. As we struggle to make sense of it all, one thing that is proven time and again is the important role we each play in our own health care. That is why the American Academy of Family Physicians (AAFP) wanted to publish this book.

One of AAFP's primary roles is to educate family doctors, and make sure they have access to the educational resources and support they need to stay on top of the ever-changing world of medicine. But another of our primary goals is to educate patients. Because that is where health care really begins. With you.

You are the one who takes care of your body every day. You are the one who makes decisions about what you do about your health—what you eat, whether you exercise, whether you get your health screening exams, whether you go to your doctor when you need to, and whether you are able to do what he or she suggests.

By reading this book, you are taking the opportunity to learn more about your body and how it works. You will learn about:

- Your body's systems and the diseases and disorders that can affect them.

- Some of the emotional issues we as individuals often face.

- Important information about how to prevent many illnesses that plague our society.

- Screening tests that can save lives.

What you read can help you better communicate with your family doctor. It can help broaden your understanding of your body so that you can ask your doctor more detailed questions and learn even more.

Educated doctors. Educated patients. That is a great step toward improving the health of our society.

**Robert Graham, M.D.**
Executive Vice President
American Academy of Family Physicians

# DEFINITIONS

## The American Academy of Family Physicians

The American Academy of Family Physicians is the national association of family physicians. It's one of the largest national medical specialty organizations. The Academy was founded in 1947 as the American Academy of General Practice. In 1971 it officially became the American Academy of Family Physicians and now has more than 82,000 members. The Academy's headquarters is in Kansas City, Missouri. The AAFP:

- Promotes and maintains high quality standards for family doctors providing continuing, complete health care to the public.

- Helps make sure patients and the public are educated about health-related matters.

- Preserves and promotes quality, cost-effective health care.

- Promotes the science and the art of family medicine.

- Promotes and keeps high professional standards for family doctors.

- Preserves the right of family doctors to do the medical and surgical procedures for which they're qualified by training and experience.

- Represents and leads the specialty of family practice.

## Family Physician

The Family Physician is a doctor who is educated and trained to take care of the whole family. Family doctors are trained to provide continuing and complete health care for the entire family. Family practice focuses on prevention: maintaining a family's lifelong health all the way from care for the youngest members of the family, through adulthood, to the oldest. Special training enables family physicians to treat a patient within the context of his or her family, bringing an understanding of the family's overall health and history to better care for the patient. Your family doctor can provide health maintenance and preventive services—as well as care for diseases and disorders—to individuals regardless of sex, age or the type of problem. Family doctors are highly qualified to serve as each patient's guide in all health-related matters, including the appropriate use of consultants, health services and community resources.

# Editorial Staff

**MEDICAL EDITOR**

Robert B. Kelly, M.D., M.S., *Chair, Department of Family Practice, MetroHealth Medical Center Campus, Case Western Reserve University School of Medicine, Cleveland, Ohio*

**PRINCIPAL CONTRIBUTING WRITER**

Gregg Albers, M.D., *Lynchburg, Virginia*

**EDITOR**

Sarah J. West, *Special Projects Department Manager, American Academy of Family Physicians*

**SECTION EDITORS**

Ann Carter, M.D., *Patient Education Materials Author, CRS, Denver, Colorado; and Cancer Program Surveyor, American College of Surgeons, Chicago, Illinois*

Jason Chao, M.D., *Medical Director, Family Practice Residency Program, University Hospitals of Cleveland, Case Western Reserve University, Cleveland, Ohio*

Michael Crouch, M.D., *Associate Professor of Family Medicine, Baylor Family Practice Center, Houston, Texas*

Mary Alice Gillispie, M.D., *private practice, Fargo, North Dakota*

Penny Tippy, M.D., *Associate Chair and Director, Family Practice Residency Program, Southern Illinois University School of Medicine, Carbondale, Illinois*

Barbara P. Yawn, M.D., M.S., *Olmsted Medical Group, Rochester, Minnesota*

## AAFP Staff

**EXECUTIVE VICE PRESIDENT**

Robert Graham, M.D.

**VICE PRESIDENT FOR PUBLICATIONS AND COMMUNICATIONS**

Clayton Raker Hasser

**PUBLICATIONS DIVISION DIRECTOR**

Joetta K. Melton

## Word Publishing Staff

**PUBLISHER**

Charles Kip Jordon

**MANAGING EDITOR**

Laura Kendall

## Design and Illustration

**ART DIRECTOR**

Dennis Davidson

**MEDICAL ILLUSTRATOR**

David L. Baker, M.A., *MediVisuals, Inc., Dallas, Texas, and Richmond, Virginia*

# CONTENTS

## PART 1

## PREVENTION: REACHING YOUR FULL HEALTH POTENTIAL 1

| | |
|---|---|
| Exercise | 2 |
| Health Exams | 6 |
| Immunizations | 11 |
| Nutrition | 13 |
| Sleep | 27 |
| Safety | 28 |
| Smoking Cessation | 31 |
| STD Prevention | 32 |

## ATLAS OF THE BODY 33

## PART 2

## THE BODY 41

| | | |
|---|---|---|
| 1 | Brain and Nervous System | 42 |
| 2 | Eyes | 62 |
| 3 | Ears | 76 |
| 4 | Nose and Sinuses | 86 |
| 5 | Mouth | 91 |
| 6 | Throat | 102 |
| 7 | Heart and Blood Vessels | 107 |
| 8 | Blood | 131 |
| 9 | Lungs | 141 |
| 10 | Urinary System | 158 |
| 11 | Gastrointestinal System | 169 |
| 12 | Liver and Gallbladder | 201 |
| 13 | Hormones and Glands | 207 |
| 14 | Immune System | 220 |
| 15 | Bones, Joints and Muscles | 227 |
| 16 | Hands and Feet | 255 |

## PHOTOGRAPHIC GUIDE TO SYMPTOMS 265

| | | |
|---|---|---|
| 17 | Skin and Hair | 273 |

## PART 3

## INFECTIONS 296

| | |
|---|---|
| Bacteria | 298 |
| Fungal Infections | 308 |
| Parasitic Infestations and Infections | 310 |
| Sexually Transmitted Diseases | 316 |
| Viruses | 320 |

## PART 4

### SPECIAL GROUPS                                      333

| 1 | Newborns | 334 |
| 2 | Infants and Children | 357 |
| 3 | Adolescents | 373 |
| 4 | Women | 380 |
| 5 | Men | 423 |
| 6 | Elderly | 433 |

## PART 5

### A CHILD'S GUIDE TO HEALTH                           441

## PART 6

### SELF-CARE FLOWCHARTS                                465

## PART 7

### FAMILY AND RELATIONSHIP ISSUES                      542

| Planning Your Family | 542 |
| Teaching Children About Sexuality | 554 |

### EMOTIONS, BEHAVIOR AND THE FAMILY                   559

| Addictions | 560 |
| Emotions and Feelings | 566 |
| Family Violence | 573 |
| Psychiatric Problems | 578 |

## PART 8

### FIRST AID                                           592

### APPENDICES                                          613

#### MEDICINE CABINET                                   613

| Over-the-Counter Medicines | 615 |
| Prescription Medicines | 618 |

#### TESTS                                              627

#### DICTIONARY                                         645

#### INDEX                                              664

# HOW TO USE THIS BOOK

This book is meant to serve as a resource of information for you. It's meant to help you better understand your body, your health and the role you play in staying healthy. The book is also meant to explain some of the disorders and diseases that you or your loved ones may face.

It's divided into eight parts to help make it easy to use.

**Part 1** addresses *prevention* and many of the ways you can help yourself be healthy. It covers exercise, nutrition, health exams and safety. The information is meant to give you tools to prevent diseases and accidents. It also contains an *atlas of the body*—a colorful map of the body that shows you some of the key ways the body functions.

**Part 2** is a *technical* section about your body. It also contains information on the body systems. The whole body is considered—from head to foot to skin and hair. Many of the diseases and disorders that can affect the different body systems are discussed. A photographic guide is included in this section—where you can find pictures of some of the different problems that can affect the body, particularly the skin and eyes.

**Part 3** provides information on different types of *infections*. It covers bacteria, fungi, viruses and parasites. This section also addresses how you can prevent some infections, how you get them and how they may be treated.

**Part 4** is called *Special Groups*. This section covers the life cycle, beginning with newborns, then infants and children, adolescents, women and men, and the elderly. It discusses the particular health issues that can affect these groups.

**Part 5** is a special section written for *children*. It talks about some of the main concerns they may have about health. You may want to show this section to your children. You can use it to help open up an opportunity to talk to them about health issues, including what to expect when they go to the doctor, how to respond to an accident, and reasons to avoid drugs, alcohol and cigarettes.

**Part 6** is a series of *self-care flowcharts*. They can help you figure out what certain symptoms may mean. The charts start with symptoms and "flow" through other symptoms as you answer "yes" or "no" to questions. The charts then flow to possible causes of symptoms. The charts aren't meant to serve as a "diagnostician." You'll need to see your family doctor to make certain what is causing your symptoms.

**Part 7** discusses *family planning* and how to teach children about sex. It also covers *emotional and behavior issues*, including many of the emotions we experience day to day, and also family violence and psychiatric problems. It may increase your understanding about your own behavior or that of people you know.

**Part 8** serves as a series of *appendices*. The first section provides some tips on *first aid* and what to do in certain *emergencies*. The second covers *medicines*—some of those you buy at the store and some that may be prescribed for you by your doctor. The third describes some of the *tests* that may be done to help your doctor make diagnoses. The fourth is a *dictionary*, where you can find some key terms defined. If you can't find something in the dictionary, try looking in the index, which is the final part of the book.

The *index* may well be the most important part of the book, because it's what will guide you to specific things you want to read about. Look in the index for key words to find the pages where they are discussed.

The discussions of diseases, tests, diagnoses and treatments aren't meant to replace a visit to your doctor. These descriptions represent general information about these issues. They won't describe everything in exactly the way they may be experienced by everyone. Everyone is different. How your body works and how a disease or disorder may affect you is unique. That's why it's so important to see your family doctor regularly. Because he or she knows *you*.

## PART 1

# PREVENTION: REACHING YOUR FULL HEALTH POTENTIAL

# PREVENTION: REACHING YOUR FULL HEALTH POTENTIAL

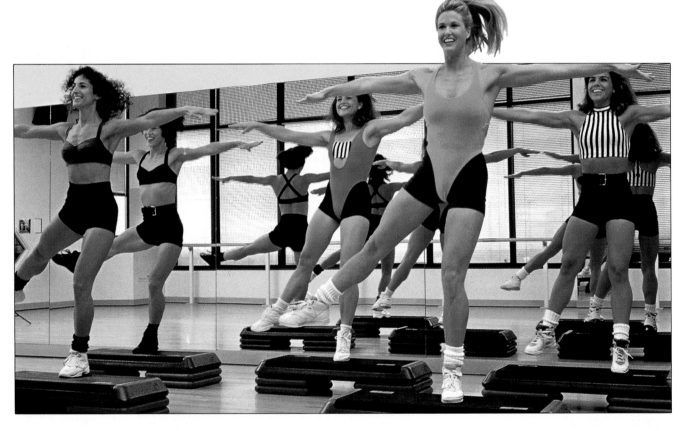

It's up to you to reach your full health potential. Your habits—how often you exercise, what you eat, how much you sleep and whether you smoke—can greatly affect your health. So can your attitude toward safety and accident prevention. Whether you take advantage of health screening tests can also influence your health. Health screening tests can detect many conditions early, when they're most easily treated. What you do can help prevent all five of the major causes of death—cancer, heart disease, stroke, lung disease and injury.

## Exercise

Regular, moderate exercise can help reduce your risk for heart disease, high blood pressure, osteoporosis, non-insulin-dependent diabetes, and colon and breast cancer. It can help you lose weight or maintain a healthy weight.

Exercise can make you feel more energetic, help you sleep better, reduce stress or anxiety and suppress your appetite. It can help relieve depression and, in women, reduce the symptoms of premenstrual syndrome. When you exercise regularly, you improve your muscle tone and bone strength. Good muscle tone and strong bones protect your tendons and ligaments from damage. Through regular exercise, your muscles become better able to use oxygen delivered through the bloodstream. Your heart and lungs become more efficient at taking in oxygen and getting rid of carbon dioxide.

## Types of Exercise

The most important type of exercise is *aerobic,* or *endurance training,* which builds cardiovascular fitness. Aerobic exercise moves large muscle groups in a rhythmic, continuous fashion over a period of time. During this type of exercise, your heart works harder to pump blood and your lungs to breathe deeply. Examples of aerobic exercises include running, bicycling, walking, aerobic dance, swimming and cross-country skiing.

The term *weight-bearing exercise* is used to describe exercises that involve working against the forces of gravity. Weight-bearing exercises build *bone density,* which helps prevent osteoporosis (p. 244) and broken bones later in life. Many aerobic exercises, such as walking, jogging, climbing stairs and dancing, are also weight bearing. Others, such as swimming, cycling and rowing, aren't. Weight-training exercises are also weight bearing.

*Weight training,* or *strength training,* builds strength and makes muscles larger. It may also increase flexibility because it involves motion. With this type of exercise, the muscle is developed as it tenses and relaxes, tenses and relaxes. Weight-training activities include exercises with free weights, some calisthenics, such as push-ups, and working out with weight machines.

*Isometric exercises* are a type of weight-training exercise. They build muscle strength by pushing against an object that doesn't move. Isometric exercises can also be done by tensing a muscle and holding it tense for 10 seconds.

Weight-training exercises, especially isometric and heavy weight lifting, can raise blood pressure. Frequent repetitions with lighter weights are less likely to increase blood pressure. If you have high blood pressure, talk to your doctor before you begin a weight-training program.

A balanced exercise program includes both aerobic (endurance) and weight (strength) training.

## Starting an Exercise Program

The ideal exercise program includes 20 to 60 minutes of vigorous activity three to five times a week.

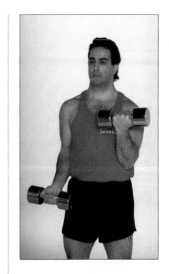

Even if you can't exercise three to five times a week, any increase you can make in your activity may benefit you. Try to do something active for a total of at least 30 minutes each day. The activity can include everyday activities, such as gardening, housecleaning or climbing stairs.

Health problems may affect your choice of activity. If you have healthy joints, you can do weight-bearing activities, such as walking, running, stair climbing, basketball or tennis.

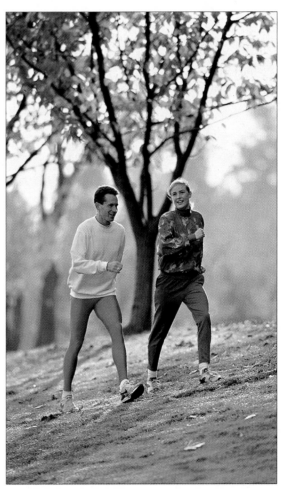

## Should I see a doctor before I start an exercise program?

*A simple walking program is safe for nearly anyone at any age, unless you have arthritis or heart disease. Talk to your doctor before starting a more strenuous exercise program if you:*

- Are a man over 40.
- Are a woman over 50.
- Have heart disease, diabetes, high blood pressure, lung disease, arthritis or any other condition that might be worsened by exercise.
- Are a heavy smoker.
- Are overweight.
- Haven't exercised for many years.
- Get breathless after simple activities such as climbing a few stairs.

## Do I need an exercise stress test?

*You may need an exercise stress test (p. 635) before you begin an exercise regimen if you:*

- Smoke.
- Are older than 45.
- Have a family history of heart problems and are older than 35.
- Have other health problems, such as diabetes, lung disease or a thyroid problem.
- Are overweight, have an elevated cholesterol count and are 40 or older.
- Have any unexplained chest pain or shortness of breath.

If you have back, hip, knee or ankle problems, choose activities that aren't weight bearing, such as swimming, cycling, rowing or exercises that can be done in a sitting or lying position. You may want to ask your doctor if you need to restrict your activities to those that aren't weight bearing.

Don't overlook brisk walking as an aerobic exercise. Walking doesn't require any fancy equipment or complicated training. All you need is a good pair of shoes and a safe place to walk, such as your local shopping mall, the high school track or a community fitness trail. Walking isn't as likely to cause injuries as some other activities, like running. Just be sure to maintain a brisk pace so you get the aerobic benefit.

When you decide to start your exercise program, follow these guidelines to make it easier and more effective.

1. Choose something you like doing. Is there an aerobic sport you've enjoyed in the past? If you can't get excited about any sport, consider riding a stationary bike or walking on a treadmill while reading or watching TV. Listen to music on headphones while walking or running. Walking with a partner may make exercise more fun.

2. Try to pick two or three different activities. Doing the same exercise day after day may become boring. Plus, different activities will work different muscles and parts of your body.

3. Start slowly, at your own level of ability. Don't overdo it. Many would-be exercisers do too much too quickly and experience too much fatigue and pain to continue.

4. Rest when you get tired or if you are injured.

5. Keep your routine simple. You don't need a lot of fancy equipment or training to walk or run. A stationary bicycle in front of the TV allows you to work out in the comfort of your home.

6. Figure out what time of day you prefer to exercise. Don't exercise too soon after eating.

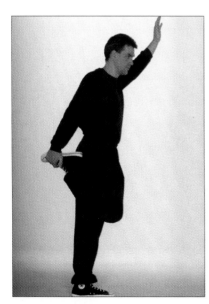 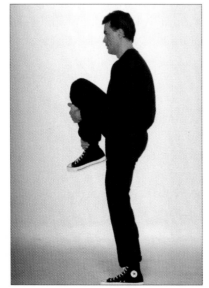

*Stretching exercises, like these for your legs, help prevent injuries by warming the muscles and strengthening the ligaments and tendons.*

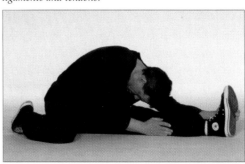

7. Make sure your program includes activities you can do indoors when rain, snow, or too hot or too cold weather keeps you from going outside. Walking in a shopping mall, using home equipment (a jump rope or aerobics video isn't expensive) or working out at the local "Y" or health club can fill in the gap when the weather doesn't cooperate.

8. If you're a senior citizen, it may be best not to exercise alone because of the risk of falling.

Make stretching a part of your routine. Each exercise session should include at least a five-minute stretching and warm-up phase, followed by 15 to 20 minutes of activity. End each exercise session with a five- to 10-minute stretching and cool-down phase.

Note your progress. Keep a graph or chart of the time you spend exercising and the activity performed. Setting a goal for how long you will exercise or how far you will go can encourage you. Be careful about being overly competitive, even with yourself. Trying to do too much too soon increases your risk of injury.

Exercise can become a family activity. Swimming, bicycling, skiing, tennis, walking, bowling, golf and even housework may be activities you can do with your family. You could do aerobic exercises with your family while watching a video in the TV room. Family exercise can also help family members improve their communication with each other.

## How to Avoid Injuries When You Exercise

- Wear supportive shoes that fit properly.
- Use safe, well-designed equipment.
- Use proper techniques.
- Stretch before and after activity.
- Don't overwork your body.
- Don't ignore aches and pains during or after exercise.

## Your Target Heart Rate

For aerobic exercise to be as beneficial as possible, you want to reach your *target heart rate* while exercising. To find your target rate, subtract your age from 220 and multiply your answer by 0.6 and 0.8. The smaller number is the lower end of your target zone, and the larger number is the upper end of your target zone. If you're in good shape, you can probably go as high as a 0.9 multiplier.

To determine your heart rate—or pulse—during exercise, it's easiest to check your pulse in the carotid artery in your neck. Place your fingers lightly on the side of your neck while exercising. Count your pulse for six seconds and then multiply that number by 10. The

## Training Curve

Set a goal to exercise five times a week for 20 to 60 minutes. Try to keep your heart rate in the target zone for 15 to 30 minutes so you get a training effect. The heart rate should increase during a warm-up and stay within the target zone during active exercise, then slow down as you cool down.

### Target Heart Rates

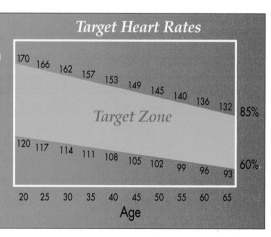

## Calories Burned by Activity

The chart below shows estimates of how many calories an average, 150-pound person burns per minute of the specified activity. Most estimates represent an average, since most of the activities can be done at different levels of intensity.

| Activity | Calories burned per minute |
|---|---|
| **Sedentary** | 1-1.25 |
| Reading | |
| Sewing | |
| Sitting | |
| Sleeping | |
| Typing | |
| Watching TV | |
| Writing | |
| **Light** | 1.25-1.50 |
| Cooking | |
| Dusting | |
| Ironing | |
| Washing dishes | |
| Walking slowly (2.5 to 3 mph) | |
| Shopping | |
| **Moderate** | 3-4 |
| Walking at 3.5 to 4 mph | |
| Sweeping floors | |
| Table tennis | |
| Fishing | |
| **Vigorous** | 4-6 |
| Gardening | |
| Bowling | |
| Golfing | |
| Other heavy work | |
| **Strenuous (low)** | 6-10 |
| Aerobic dancing | |
| Basketball | |
| Cycling, leisure | |
| Skiing | |
| Tennis | |
| **Strenuous (medium)** | 8-11 |
| Swimming | |
| **Strenuous (high)** | 11-17 |
| Running | |
| Soccer | |
| Vigorous cross-country skiing | |

Adapted from: "Food." Home and Garden Bulletin no. 228, United States Department of Agriculture, 1979.

number you get should fall within the target zone.

## Health Exams

The annual physical is no longer advocated. Instead of an annual physical, *periodic health exams* are recommended. These medical check-ups can help in the prevention, detection or treatment of conditions, such as high blood pressure or high cholesterol, and other treatable problems before they lead to more serious health problems.

When you should have these exams—and exactly what will be included in the exam—depends on the state of your health, your family history of disease and other risk factors for disease you may have. Be sure to let your doctor know about any unusual symptoms you have or any concerns you have about your health. Follow your doctor's recommendation about how often to plan a visit.

If you're seeing your doctor for the first time, he or she will review your health history and ask about any

---

# PERIODIC HEALTH EXAMS

## First Week of Life

- ❏ Antibiotic eyedrops at birth to prevent bacterial infection (gonorrhea, p. 318)
- ❏ T4/TSH to check for overactive thyroid gland (hyperthyroidism, p. 215) or an underactive thyroid gland (hypothyroidism, p. 217)
- ❏ Phenylalanine test to check for a rare inherited metabolic disorder called phenylketonuria (p. 354)

## Birth to 18 Months of Age

- ❏ Height and weight
- ❏ Hemoglobin or hematocrit test to check for anemia

*Schedule exams for two, four, six, 12, 15 and 18 months of age.*

## 19 Months to Six Years

- ❏ Height and weight
- ❏ Blood pressure
- ❏ Eye exam to check for amblyopia and strabismus (p. 65)
- ❏ Urine test to check for bacteria in the urine

*An exam should be done during this time at least once for vaccinations (p. 11) and again on the advice of your doctor.*

## Seven to 12 Years

- ❏ Height and weight
- ❏ Blood pressure
- ❏ Tanner staging to check for signs of normal sexual development

*Tanner staging should be done at least once in this age group. An exam to check whether the child has been immunized is recommended between ages 11 and 12. Other exams should be done on the advice of your doctor.*

## 13 to 18 Years

- ❏ Height and weight
- ❏ Blood pressure
- ❏ Tanner staging

*Schedule at least one visit during this time so your doctor can provide preventive services as needed based on risk factors. Then schedule visits on the advice of your doctor.*

## 19 to 39 Years

- ❏ Height and weight
- ❏ Blood pressure
- ❏ Pelvic exam in women to check for vaginal and yeast infections
- ❏ Pap smear in women to check for changes in the cervix that could be cancer (annually)
- ❏ Blood cholesterol test

*Schedule visits about every one to three years based on the advice of your doctor.*

## 40 to 64 Years

- ❏ Height and weight
- ❏ Blood pressure
- ❏ Physician exam of breasts in women to check for lumps that could be cancer (every one to two years after age 50)
- ❏ Pelvic exam in women

- ❏ Pap smear in women to check for changes in the cervix that could be cancer (every three years)
- ❏ Fecal occult blood test or sigmoidoscopy (annually beginning at age 50)
- ❏ Total blood cholesterol test
- ❏ Mammogram in women to check for signs of breast cancer (every one to two years after age 50)

*Schedule visits about every one to three years based on the advice of your doctor. An exam to check the status of immunizations, especially tetanus, is recommended at age 50.*

## 65 Years and Older

- ❏ Height and weight
- ❏ Blood pressure
- ❏ Vision test
- ❏ Hearing test
- ❏ Physician exam of breasts in women to check for lumps that could be cancer (every one to two years until age 70)
- ❏ Pelvic exam in women
- ❏ Listen to heart sounds
- ❏ Total blood cholesterol test
- ❏ Urine test to check for bacterial infection, traces of bleeding from bladder or kidney cancer
- ❏ Mammogram in women to check for signs of breast cancer (every one to two years until age 70)

*Schedule a visit every year based on the advice of your doctor.*

recent changes in your health, medicines you're taking, your family and work situation, diseases that are common in your family, your allergies to medicines, and other questions. This part of the exam will help inform your doctor about the diseases or health problems you may be at risk for. It's important to be very straightforward in answering questions and talking with your doctor, even about things that embarrass you.

The exam may also include a physical exam and some routine tests. The usual tests are outlined, by age group, in the accompanying charts. Your doctor may also want to do other tests, depending on your health history and your risk factors for certain problems or diseases. See the Tests section, beginning on page 627, for more information.

Many doctors also provide health interventions during an exam. These may include counseling, for example, to help you stop smoking if you smoke or to help you lose weight if you're overweight. Immunizations are also an example of a health intervention.

Other tests may need to be done—or done sooner than listed in the box—if you or your child is at special risk for a health problem.

**Blood tests.** Blood tests for lead may be needed in children who are at risk for lead poisoning. Your child may be at risk if he or she lives in or regularly visits a home that was built before 1960. Your child may also be at risk if a sibling, housemate or playmate is being treated for lead poisoning, or if an adult who is exposed to lead through a job or hobby lives in the same household. Your child may also be at risk of lead poisoning if an active lead smelter, battery recycling plant or other industry that involves lead is near your home.

Total cholesterol blood tests may be advisable at earlier ages than those

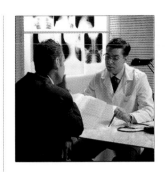

listed in the box in children who have a parent whose blood cholesterol level is 240 or higher. Total cholesterol blood tests may also be advisable for children who have a parent or grandparent with a history of heart disease before age 55.

A blood test for rubella antibodies is advisable in women of childbearing age who haven't had rubella (p. 330) or the rubella vaccine. Rubella can cause serious problems for a baby if the mother is exposed to it during her pregnancy.

A blood test for syphilis (p. 319) is advisable in people at risk of sexually transmitted diseases (STDs, p. 316), including people who have sex with many partners or who have sex with someone who has many partners or who has an STD.

Blood tests for HIV (p. 325) may be recommended in people at risk of HIV infection (p. 325).

Blood glucose tests may be recommended in obese people who have a family history of diabetes (p. 211) or for women who have a history of diabetes during pregnancy (p. 393).

**Bone mineral content tests.** These tests may be done to check for osteoporosis (p. 244). They may be recommended in women who are about to go through menopause and who are at increased risk of osteoporosis. Risk factors include being white, having had both ovaries removed before menopause, being inactive or having a slender build.

**Colonoscopy.** This test may be suggested for people who have a family history of familial polyposis (p. 175), cancer family syndrome or a personal history of previous adenomatous polyps (p. 175) or colorectal cancer (p. 175).

**Carotid artery exam.** A check of the carotid arteries in the neck may be recommended in people who have risk factors for cerebrovascular or cardiovascular disease, such as high blood pressure (p. 123), smoking or diabetes. This exam is also important in people who have signs of neurologic problems, such as transient ischemic attacks, or in people who have a history of problems with the blood vessels of the brain. In this exam, your doctor will listen to the blood flow through the carotid arteries with a stethoscope.

**Electrocardiograms.** Electrocardiograms aren't generally done for screening. They may be performed for people who would endanger public safety if they had a sudden heart attack or other cardiac problem. An example would be an airline pilot.

**Fecal occult blood test and sigmoidoscopy.** These two tests may be recommended for people age 50 and older.

**Hearing tests.** Hearing tests may be needed if you or your child is at risk of hearing problems. Risk factors for hearing problems in a child include a history of hearing problems in the family or a personal history before or right after birth of infection with herpes (p. 325), syphilis, rubella, cytomegalovirus or toxoplasmosis (p. 388). Deformities that involve the head or neck also may increase the risk of hearing problems. Infants with a low birth weight or other problems that require a transfusion are also at risk. A history of bacterial meningitis (p. 302) or a severe lack of oxygen during birth increases the risk. Another risk factor is being around loud noises for long periods of time.

**Mammograms.** Mammograms may be recommended earlier in women who have a family history of breast cancer.

**Oral cavity exam.** An exam of the oral cavity to check for cancer in the mouth may be recommended in people who smoke and in people who drink excessive amounts of alcohol or who have any unusual sores in the mouth.

**Pap smear.** Pap smears to check for cervical cancer may be recommended in women younger than 18 years old who are sexually active.

**Skin exam.** An exam of the skin may be wise for people who are at increased risk of skin cancer. Risk factors include being exposed to the sun through hobbies or your job, having a family or personal history of skin cancer and having early signs of skin cancer.

**Testicular exam.** A physician exam of the testicles may need to be done in males who have a history of problems with the testicles.

**Thyroid exam.** An exam for thyroid nodules may be advisable in people who have had radiation treatment of the upper body. Thyroid function testing may also be recommended in the elderly, particularly in women who have gone through menopause and in people who have Down syndrome (p. 348).

**Tuberculin skin test.** A tuberculin skin test may be needed in people who live with someone who has tuberculosis (p. 307) or who are at risk of having close contact with a person who has the disease, or who are at risk of having the disease. People at high risk of tuberculosis include recent immigrants or refugees from countries where tuberculosis is common, such as Asia, Africa, Central and South America, and the Pacific Islands. Family members of migrant workers, people who live in homeless shelters, and people who have certain underlying medical disorders, such as AIDS, also are at high risk for tuberculosis.

## Screening Tests You Can Do at Home

Any time you or your doctor can find a health problem early, treatment can start early. With early diagnosis and treatment, the outcome is often better than when treatment is delayed. For this reason, it's wise to check for problems yourself. You can find problems in their early stages through self-exams of the breasts, testicles, skin and lymph nodes, and just by paying attention to your body and talking to your doctor about any changes that concern you.

## Cancer Screening

Cancer is often curable, especially if it's found at an early stage. Better screening and treatments have produced many cures for what was once considered a hopeless disease. Some cancers have extremely high cure rates, while others are still very difficult to detect early and cure.

Warning signs of cancer include any slow-healing sore, unexplained lump, change in bowel habits, unusual discharge, persistent bleeding or bruising, and trouble swallowing. Some people fear cancer will be found and wait until a warning sign can no longer be ignored. Then it may be too late for effective treatment.

Your doctor may routinely do the simple screening exams when you have your periodic exam. These tests may include fecal occult blood testing and sigmoidoscopy to look for cancer of the colon and, in women, mammography and a Pap smear.

When cancer is suspected, more extensive cancer-screening tests are also available and may be recommended by your doctor. Your doctor's recommendations will be based on symptoms you have, your personal health habits, family history of disease and other factors. Talk to your doctor about the test, the cost, the benefit and the discomfort, if any, associated with cancer-screening tests.

### Signs of Cancer

- A sore that won't heal
- An unexplained lump
- A change in your bowel habits
- Unusual discharge from any site on your body
- Persistent bleeding
- Bruising easily
- Trouble swallowing
- Persistent hoarseness

### Screening Tests You Can Do at Home

| Health problem | Test | Further action |
|---|---|---|
| Breast cancer | Self-exam of breasts (p. 408) | Physician exam and mammography if lump is detected |
| Colon cancer | Blood in bowel movement | Sigmoidoscopy by your doctor if blood is present |
| Lymph node cancer | Self-exam of the lymph nodes under the arm, in the groin and neck | Physician exam and further testing if lump is found |
| Oral cancer | Self-exam of the mouth | Physician exam if a mouth sore is seen |
| Skin cancer | Self-exam of skin (p. 291) | Physician exam and biopsy if a skin lesion is found |
| Testicular cancer | Self-exam of the testicles (p. 429) | Physician exam and further testing if a lump is found |

## KEEPING TRACK OF YOUR HEALTH

| Test/prevention | Date | Result |
|---|---|---|
| Weight | | |
| | | |
| | | |
| Blood pressure | | |
| | | |
| | | |
| Cholesterol level | | |
| | | |
| | | |
| Breast exam by your doctor (for women) | | |
| | | |
| | | |
| Mammogram (for women) | | |
| | | |
| | | |
| Testicular exam by your doctor (for men) | | |
| | | |
| | | |
| Pap smear (for women) | | |
| | | |
| | | |
| Other blood tests | | |
| | | |
| | | |
| Dental visits (at least once a year) | | |
| | | |
| Other tests as advised by your doctor | | |
| | | |
| | | |
| | | |
| | | |
| | | |

## Immunizations

Immunizations, or vaccines, can help prevent many diseases in both children and adults. Immunizations work by helping the body produce *antibodies* against the disease. These antibodies work to fight infections.

## Childhood Immunizations

Diseases like polio, measles and pertussis (whooping cough) once killed or crippled many infants. Now, immunizations can prevent these and other childhood diseases. It's important that your child be vaccinated. If you can't afford the cost, call your local public health office. Many programs offer free immunizations.

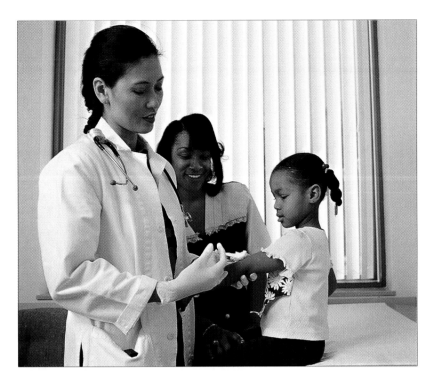

Recommendations about when to have your child immunized change occasionally. Some shots are given earlier to children who live in areas where certain diseases are more common. Keep a record of when you have your child immunized and bring the record with you when you take your child to the doctor. Use the accompanying list to help keep track of your child's immunizations.

**Polio.** The oral poliovirus vaccine (OPV) helps prevent *poliomyelitis,* or polio (p. 329). Your child should receive the OPV four times. It comes as drops that are placed in the mouth. Polio isn't common in the United States anymore. But it used to be very common, causing pain and paralysis in many children and even leading to death. Although polio is no longer common in the United States, it's still common in other parts of the world. Because it could become more common in the United States again, it's important to have your child immunized.

**Diphtheria, tetanus, pertussis.** The diphtheria, tetanus, pertussis (DTP) vaccine works to protect your child against three infections: diphtheria (p. 299), tetanus (p. 306) and pertussis (p. 303). The vaccine is given in a series of five shots. After the DTP vaccine, the spot where your child received the shot may be swollen and red. Your child may have a fever for a day or two and may be fussy and sleepy. Occasionally, DTP vaccination can cause serious problems, such as a seizure. This is rare, but if you have any concerns, talk to your doctor.

After the series of DTP vaccinations, people need to receive booster shots of the tetanus vaccine (Td). A tetanus vaccine should be obtained every 10 years throughout life. It can cause a fever and slight soreness at the site of vaccination. Serious reactions aren't common.

**Measles, mumps, rubella.** The measles, mumps, rubella (MMR) vaccine protects against measles (p. 327), mumps (p. 329) and rubella (p. 330). It's given as two shots. Typical side effects of the MMR vaccine are a rash or fever beginning one to two weeks after vaccination. The side effects last only a few days. Less frequently, the MMR vaccine can cause swelling of the glands in the neck. It can also cause aching of the joints, occurring one to three weeks after the vaccination.

***Haemophilus influenzae* type b.** This vaccine protects against *Haemophilus influenzae* type b infection. The vaccine, called Hib vaccine, is given in a series of three or four shots, depending on the type of vaccine used. It isn't associated with serious side effects, but the site of vaccination may be sore. Your child may also run a slight fever and be a little fussy after receiving the vaccine.

**Hepatitis B.** The hepatitis B virus (HBV) vaccine helps prevent a type of hepatitis. The vaccine is given in three shots and has no known serious side effects.

**Chickenpox (varicella).** This vaccine is now available for children and for adults who have never had chickenpox (p. 321). Side effects of the vaccine are uncommon.

Sometimes, there are reasons a child shouldn't be vaccinated. Some vaccines are made from live viruses and shouldn't be given if your child's immune system is compromised, which can occur with cancer or with medicines that lower immunity, such as taking daily corticosteroids (p. 622). The mumps and measles vaccines shouldn't be given to children who are seriously allergic to eggs. Also, if your child has ever had a serious reaction to an earlier shot in a series of shots, you may want to talk with your doctor about benefits and risks of completing the series of vaccinations.

## KEEPING TRACK OF YOUR CHILD'S IMMUNIZATIONS

| Immunization | Date scheduled | Date given |
|---|---|---|
| Polio | Two months | |
| | Four months | |
| | Six months | |
| | Between four and six years | |
| Diphtheria, tetanus, pertussis | Two months/DTP | |
| | Four months/DTP | |
| | Six months/DTP | |
| | 15 months/DTaP or DTP | |
| | Four to six years/DTaP or DTP | |
| | 14 to 16 years/Td | |
| Measles, mumps, rubella | Between 12 and 15 months | |
| | Between four and six years or between 11 and 12 years | |
| *Haemophilus influenzae* type b | Two months/type: | |
| | Four months/type: | |
| | Six months/type: (not PRP-OMP) | |
| | Between 12 and 15 months/type: | |
| Hepatitis B | At birth or between one and two months | |
| | Between one and two months or four months | |
| | Between six and 18 months | |
| Chickenpox | Between 12 and 18 months | |

## Immunizations for Adults

Children aren't the only ones who need immunizations. For example, adolescents and adults should get a tetanus booster every 10 years. Flu shots can be very helpful in preventing the flu (p. 326), especially for certain people, such as the elderly, who are at risk of complications from the flu or for people who are around people at risk of complications from the flu.

October and November are usually the best months to get a flu shot. Amantadine (p. 621), which can be given by your doctor, can also help prevent some types of flu viruses or ease the symptoms if it's taken within 48 hours of getting sick.

A pneumococcal vaccine should be given at 65 years of age to help prevent pneumonia (p. 154).

Hepatitis B vaccination may also be advisable if you haven't been vaccinated and are at risk for being exposed to someone who has hepatitis, such as if you're a health care worker or your sex partner has hepatitis.

## Travel Immunizations

Numerous vaccinations are available to help you avoid catching a disease that may be more common in a country you're traveling to. The Centers for Disease Control and

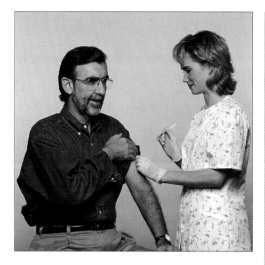

Prevention can give you information about the immunizations you may need, depending on your travel destination. The phone number is 404-332-4559. You can also call your local health department for information on vaccinations needed for travel to a foreign country.

## Nutrition

The adage, "You are what you eat" is true to some extent. Bad eating habits can increase your risk for heart disease, stroke, high blood pressure, obesity and many types of cancer. Eating right can help lower your chances of developing certain health problems. But don't believe claims that certain foods or special diets provide a "fountain of youth" or cure conditions like cancer or arthritis.

---

### People Who Should Get Flu Shots

- People who live in nursing homes or other long-term care facilities
- Adults and children with chronic heart or lung disease
- Adults and children who have diabetes, kidney disease, anemia or immune system problems, including AIDS
- Pregnant women with high-risk conditions
- Children on long-term aspirin therapy
- People over 65 years of age
- Health care workers or family members who take care of people who could have problems if they get the flu

*Note: Don't get a flu shot if you're allergic to eggs.*

---

### KEEPING TRACK OF YOUR IMMUNIZATIONS

| Immunization | Date scheduled | Date given |
| --- | --- | --- |
| Tetanus shot | Every 10 years | |
| Influenza shot | Every year starting at age 65 | |
| Pneumococcal shot | At age 65 | |

*If you missed any of your vaccinations when you were a child, talk to your doctor about whether you need them. Also talk to your doctor about whether you need a hepatitis B vaccination.*

Many people in the United States don't eat properly. They eat too much fat or cholesterol, and too many calories. If you don't eat a balanced diet, you may not be giving your body the nutrients it needs.

Nutrition is complex. Nutrients depend on each other. For example, vitamin C makes it easier to absorb the iron in foods. Long-term use of large amounts of the mineral zinc can cause a deficiency in copper and iron because zinc interferes with absorption of copper and iron. Large doses of vitamin A and iron can be toxic. That's why self-diagnosis and mega-dosing with specific vitamins or minerals can end up doing harm instead of good.

So what can you do when it comes to good nutrition? In a nutshell: Eat a well-balanced diet, with moderate amounts of a variety of foods. Get plenty of fresh fruits and vegetables, and avoid fat and sugary sweets.

## Nutrition Basics

Fiber, complex carbohydrates, saturated fats. What do all of these terms mean? Here's a guide to some nutrition basics.

**Caffeine.** Caffeine is a mild stimulant used by more than 80% of American adults who begin their day with a cola or a cup of coffee or tea. Almost all studies have shown that caffeine has physical effects. When use of caffeine is stopped abruptly, withdrawal symptoms, such as headaches and irritability, occur for up to a few weeks.

No studies have conclusively demonstrated that large amounts of caffeine produce cancer or heart disease. Caffeine has, however, been linked to a type of harmless, but painful, breast cyst.

**Calories.** This is a unit of measurement. It's used to describe the amount of energy provided by food. How many calories you need to maintain your weight depends on your size, your metabolism (how fast your body burns calories), your age and your level of physical activity. The average inactive person's daily caloric need is about 16 calories per pound of body weight. An active person needs about 20 calories per pound of body weight. And there are 3,500 calories in one pound of fat.

**Carbohydrates.** Carbohydrates—sometimes called starches—are easily converted into energy. *Complex carbohydrates* are found in breads, pastas, cereals, potatoes and other vegetables and fruits. Complex carbohydrates take longer for the digestive system to break down. *Simple carbohydrates* are sugars. Cookies and candy, for example, contain simple carbohydrates. Simple carbohydrates are digested very quickly. Unfortunately, foods such as cookies and candy don't contain a lot of nutrients besides sugars, so they're often referred to as "empty calories" or "junk food."

**Cholesterol.** *Cholesterol* is a waxy substance found in the cells of the body. Some cholesterol is in foods such as meat, milk and eggs. The liver also makes cholesterol. Saturated fats from food increase the liver's production of cholesterol. The body needs some cholesterol to function. But high levels of cholesterol in the blood can damage the arteries, such as damage from atherosclerosis (p. 111), and put you at risk for heart disease and stroke (p. 59).

You can do many things to reduce the level of cholesterol in your blood. If your cholesterol level is high (see box on p. 16), try a one- to six-month trial of diet and lifestyle changes. Lifestyle changes include exercising regularly, losing weight if you're overweight and stopping smoking if you smoke.

You can reduce your blood cholesterol level by reducing the amount of cholesterol-containing foods in your diet and by lowering the amount of saturated fats you eat (*a low-fat diet*). Eating more foods high in soluble fiber will also help.

In about one to six months, have your cholesterol level rechecked. Following a healthy diet, for example, usually lowers cholesterol levels within a couple of months.

Regular cholesterol checks are important. Early discovery and treatment of high cholesterol levels can reduce your risk of atherosclerosis, heart disease and stroke. Cholesterol levels should be checked beginning at about 20 years of age. Get your cholesterol checked at least every five years, or more often if you have other risk factors for heart disease (see box).

Cholesterol should be checked in children over two years old who have a family history of heart disease—that is, someone in their immediate family has had heart disease before age 55 or has cholesterol levels of 240 or above. Some experts recommend that cholesterol levels be checked at least once in all children.

In some people, diet and exercise alone won't lower cholesterol levels enough. In these people, medicine may help reduce the levels. Whether medicine should be used and the type of medicine needed depend on the person's age, sex and other risk factors for heart disease (see box). The advisability and cost-effectiveness of using medicine to lower cholesterol is debatable in women who haven't gone through menopause yet, in the elderly (because of troublesome side effects) and in people who have no other risk factors for heart disease.

Taking medicine to lower cholesterol levels may be a lifelong decision. The cost, inconvenience and side effects need to be balanced against the possible benefits. Remember that taking medicine to reduce cholesterol levels doesn't mean that healthy habits can be abandoned. It's still important to eat right and exercise.

**Fats.** Fats in food provide energy. But they can also be stored by the body as fat. Some fat is needed for the growth and repair of various tissues, including the nervous system. They also help in the absorption of the fat-soluble vitamins A, D, E and K.

Fats contain *saturated, monounsaturated* and *polyunsaturated fatty acids.* You can tell whether a fat is mostly saturated or unsaturated by whether it's hard (saturated) or soft (unsaturated) at room temperature. Palm and coconut

---

### Risk Factors for Heart Disease

*Your risk for heart disease is increased if you:*

- Have already had a stroke or heart attack.
- Are a man 45 years or older.
- Have a father or brother who had heart disease before age 55.
- Are a woman 55 or older or a woman under 40 who has gone through menopause and doesn't take estrogen.
- Have a mother or sister who had heart disease before 65.

### Behaviors That Increase Your Risk for Heart Disease

*Your risk for heart disease is increased if you:*

- Are inactive.
- Smoke tobacco.
- Have high blood pressure or diabetes.
- Have an HDL cholesterol level below 35.
- Are very overweight.

---

### Testing for Cholesterol Levels

Cholesterol is bound to protein molecules (called *lipoproteins*) as it travels through the bloodstream. *Low-density lipoproteins* (LDL) and *very-low-density lipoproteins* (VLDL) deliver cholesterol to the body. *High-density lipoproteins* (HDL) remove cholesterol from the bloodstream. This is why HDL cholesterol is often termed "good" cholesterol. LDL and VLDL cholesterol are more likely to damage the blood vessels if the levels are high.

*Total cholesterol* is a combination of HDL, LDL and VLDL cholesterol. A blood test will show whether your total cholesterol level is high. If the total level is high, special blood tests to determine the HDL and LDL levels may be done.

Eating less fat and cholesterol and more foods high in soluble fiber, such as the oat bran found in oatmeal, can help lower your LDL cholesterol level and may protect you from the damaging effects of cholesterol. You can raise your HDL cholesterol level by not smoking if you smoke, exercising regularly and losing weight if you're overweight.

## Cholesterol Levels for Adults

**Total Cholesterol Levels**
- Less than 200 is best.
- 200 to 239 is borderline high.
- 240 or more means you're at higher risk for artery damage, heart disease and stroke.

**LDL Cholesterol Levels**
- Less than 130 is best.
- 130 to 159 is borderline high.
- 160 or more means you're at increased risk for heart disease.

**HDL Cholesterol Levels**
- 60 or higher reduces your risk of heart disease.
- Less than 35 means you're at increased risk for heart disease.

oils, which are saturated fats, are exceptions to this rule.

Saturated fats may increase the body's production of cholesterol, which can lead to atherosclerosis (p. 111) and heart disease.

Monounsaturated fats don't increase cholesterol. They're liquid at room temperature and either semi-solid or solid when they're cold. Monounsaturated fats are olive and peanut oils.

Polyunsaturated fats also don't increase cholesterol. In fact, they lower it slightly. They're liquid at

**FATTY FOODS**

both room temperature and when cold. Fish, corn and soybean oils are polyunsaturated fats.

Hydrogenated fats, which are chemically modified to last longer, may be as unhealthy as saturated fats. They're in most margarines and are most often referred to as "partially hydrogenated oil" in the list of ingredients.

Less than 65 grams of fat a day are recommended for people on a 2,000-calorie diet.

**Fiber.** Also called roughage, fiber is the indigestible element in your diet. Dietary fiber is the part of foods that can't be digested and converted into energy.

Fiber adds bulk to the bowel movement and draws water into the large intestines, helping to move waste products through your intestines more quickly. Fiber relieves constipation and thus reduces the strain on hemorrhoids. A fiber-rich diet may help reduce your risk of colon cancer as well. Oat bran fiber has been shown to reduce cholesterol levels.

There are two main types of fiber: soluble fiber and insoluble fiber. *Soluble fiber* dissolves in water. It helps bulk your stools so that they can move better through your system to relieve constipation. It may also help lower cholesterol levels and may help stabilize or even lower blood sugar levels. Soluble fiber is found in grains, beans, oats and wheat. *Insoluble fiber* doesn't dissolve in water. It also adds some bulk to the stool and stimulates colon activity. The increased colon activity shortens the time it takes for food to pass through the colon, which may reduce the risk of colon cancer and relieve constipation. Insoluble fiber is found in raw fruits and vegetables.

If you suddenly start eating large amounts of fiber you may suffer from

---

### Fish Oils

Fish oils, or omega-3s, have made headlines as the latest way to reduce your risk of heart disease. Researchers have discovered that Greenland Eskimos who eat large quantities of cold-water fish, which are high in a form of polyunsaturated fats called omega-3, are unlikely to die of heart disease.

The health-food industry has jumped on this claim. Omega-3 fish oil capsules are available over the counter. But most doctors don't recommend taking them. The research studies are inconclusive as to whether another substance in the fish could be responsible for reducing heart disease. Instead, doctors suggest adding fish to your diet on a regular basis.

---

### Margarine vs. Butter

Margarine or butter? Both contain around 100 calories a tablespoon. Some margarines may contain fewer calories—that's because water or air has been added.

Butter has gotten a bad reputation because it contains saturated fat and cholesterol. But some researchers question whether margarine is any better. That's because of a chemical process called *hydrogenation.* If cottonseed oil is used in the margarine, hydrogenation may convert it to a cholesterol-raising fatty acid. If the margarine is made from liquid corn, safflower or soybean oil, it won't raise cholesterol.

Your best bet? Use margarine and butter sparingly. Try using other seasonings like herbs and spices instead. These don't add fat or cholesterol to your diet.

---

bloating, gas and general discomfort. Add fiber gradually to your diet.

**Proteins.** Proteins are needed for the body to grow and to repair any damage. A diet low in protein can slow your growth and inhibit the working of your immune system. Proteins contain a combination of some or all of 20 different amino acids.

Meats like beef and pork, chicken, seafood and eggs contain complete proteins that have all the essential amino acids your body needs to make protein. *Incomplete proteins* don't have all of the essential amino acids. Incomplete proteins are found in beans, rice, whole grains, nuts and dairy products. You can combine foods that contain incomplete proteins so you get all the essential amino acids. Some possible combinations: beans and tortillas, beans and rice, baked beans and cornbread, and peanut butter and bread.

**Salt.** Salty snacks, animal products, canned soups and vegetables, processed meats and snack foods generally contain large amounts of sodium. Most people with high blood pressure can lower their blood pressure by lowering their sodium intake.

The balance between sodium, calcium and potassium may be more important than how much sodium is eaten. It's best to keep your daily sodium intake under 2,400 milligrams. This can be done by not adding salt to your foods and by avoiding foods high in sodium. If you have high blood pressure, talk to your doctor about a low-sodium diet.

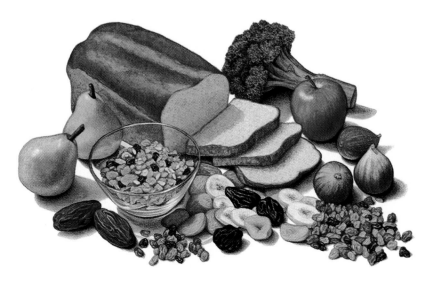

**FIBER-RICH FOODS**

**Vitamins and minerals.** Vitamins and minerals are known as "micronutrients" because only very tiny amounts are needed for good health. Vitamins come from plant or animal foods. Thirteen vitamins have been identified. The four *fat-soluble vitamins* are A, D, E and K. They need fat or bile to be absorbed by your body. Vitamin C and the eight B vitamins are *water-soluble vitamins* because they don't need fat to be absorbed.

Minerals come from soil or water. They are absorbed by plants and animals. The major minerals are calcium, phosphorus and magnesium. They are called *macro minerals* because you need larger amounts of them. The others are *trace*, or *micro*, minerals and include iron, copper, chromium, fluoride, zinc, iodine, manganese, selenium and molybdenum.

Vitamins and minerals are used in molecular reactions in your body to break down fats, carbohydrates and proteins into energy you can use.

Recommended Dietary Allowances, or RDAs, have been established to tell how much of specific vitamins and minerals is needed in a healthy diet. Don't try to calculate how many vitamins and minerals you're getting from each meal. Good nutrition isn't a matter of what you eat at a specific meal, but what you eat over the course of several days. Your body can store some vitamins and minerals for 12 months or longer, while others are needed on a daily basis.

The best way to protect against the lack of a certain vitamin or mineral (a vitamin or mineral *deficiency*) is to eat a wide variety of foods, especially fresh fruits and vegetables.

---

### High-Fiber Foods

**Soluble fiber**
- Psyllium powder
- Unprocessed wheat bran
- Unrefined breakfast cereals
- Whole wheat and rye flours
- Grainy breads, such as whole wheat, rye or pumpernickel
- Dried fruits, such as prunes, apricots and figs
- Legumes, such as chickpeas, baked beans, lima beans and soybeans

**Insoluble fiber**
- Unprocessed vegetables
- Unprocessed fruits

---

### What about supplements?

Many people take a multivitamin and mineral supplement every day. Most doctors agree there's nothing wrong with this. But if you're healthy and usually eat a balanced diet, you don't need supplements.

If you're pregnant or breast-feeding, your doctor will probably recommend that you take vitamins. Women who are considering pregnancy are advised to take 0.4 mg of folic acid each day, which may help prevent certain birth defects. But be sure to talk to your doctor before you take anything if you're pregnant.

Women who are at risk for osteoporosis (p. 244) may want to ask their doctors about taking calcium supplements to build up their bone density.

Vitamin and mineral supplements can become dangerous if you decide to take "mega-doses," or large amounts, of specific vitamins and minerals. Vitamin A, for example, can be toxic or even fatal if large doses are taken over time. Other vitamins and minerals can have unpleasant side effects if too much is taken. For example, too much vitamin C can cause diarrhea.

Although vitamin and mineral deficiencies can cause a wide variety of symptoms, most people in the United States don't suffer from such deficiencies. If you think you may be at risk, talk to your doctor.

## Vitamins, Minerals and What They Do

**Vitamins**

**Vitamin A (retinal or beta carotene).** Actions: good for vision, healthy skin and mucous membranes; enhances immune system and helps repair tissue; required for normal bone growth and tooth development. Sources: green, orange and yellow fruits and vegetables, milk, cheese, egg yolk and liver.

**Vitamin $B_1$ (thiamine).** Actions: good for nervous system; aids in carbohydrate metabolism (energy release). Sources: pork, beef, liver, legumes, nuts and grains.

**Vitamin $B_2$ (riboflavin).** Actions: maintains healthy skin; aids in carbohydrate, protein and fat metabolism. Sources: same as $B_1$ and also in milk, cheese, eggs and organ meats, such as liver and kidney.

**Vitamin $B_3$ (niacin).** Actions: needed for healthy nervous system, skin and digestion; aids in protein and fat metabolism. Sources: milk, cheese, poultry, fish, beans and grains (except corn and rice).

**Vitamin $B_5$ (pantothenic acid).** Actions: required to metabolize nutrients and for red blood cell production. Sources: legumes, whole wheat, milk, eggs, fresh vegetables, beef and saltwater fish.

**Vitamin $B_6$ (pyridoxine).** Actions: required for red blood cell formation, breakdown of copper and iron; aids in protein and fat metabolism. Sources: liver, kidney, cereal grains (wheat and corn), yeast, soybeans and peanuts.

**Vitamin $B_{12}$ (cobalamin).** Actions: good for nervous system and growth; aids in red blood cell production. Sources: fish, milk, eggs, cheese, liver, kidney and various other meats.

**Biotin.** Actions: good for the nervous system and the formation of red blood cells. Sources: liver, kidney, egg yolk, cereals, tomatoes, legumes, nuts and yeast.

**Vitamin C (ascorbic acid).** Actions: good for the immune system. Sources: citrus fruits, berries, melon, tomatoes, potatoes, cabbage and green and yellow vegetables.

**Vitamin D (calciferol).** Actions: helps prevent and treat osteoporosis; required for calcium and phosphorus absorption; enhances the immune system and may help reduce blood pressure; needed for the normal growth of bones and teeth. Sources: fortified milk, cereals, enriched breads, saltwater fish and sunlight.

**Vitamin E (tocopherol).** Actions: prevents damage to cells and tissues from oxidants; aids in circulation and in tissue repair. Sources: vegetable oils, wheat germ oil, milk, egg yolk, muscle meats, fish, whole grains, nuts, legumes, spinach and broccoli.

**Folacin (folic acid).** Actions: helps prevent certain birth defects when consumed by pregnant women and helps red blood cell production. Sources: liver, legumes, dark green leafy vegetables, oranges, whole-grain breads and cereals.

**Vitamin K.** Actions: required for blood clotting. Sources: pork, liver, green leafy vegetables (spinach, kale, cabbage), tomatoes, egg yolk and cheese.

*(continued on next page)*

**Antioxidant vitamins.** Some scientists believe that including antioxidant vitamins (vitamin A, beta carotene, vitamin C and vitamin E) in your diet can reduce your risk of cancer. Antioxidant vitamins can slow cell destruction. This may help decrease the wear and tear on body parts brought on by aging and also reduce the likelihood of cancer. But studies to prove this theory will take many years and may never be fully conclusive.

Eat a diet that's rich in fresh fruits and vegetables (excellent sources of antioxidant vitamins). Such a diet gives you the benefit of the many other nutrients plus the fiber contained in these foods.

**Minerals**

**Calcium.** Actions: aids bone and tooth formation, nerve and muscle function. Sources: milk, cheese, yogurt, salmon, seafood, sardines and leafy vegetables.

**Chloride.** Actions: maintains fluid and electrolyte balance. Sources: salt and processed foods.

**Chromium.** Actions: required for glucose metabolism (release of energy). Sources: whole grains, cheese, various meats and brewer's yeast.

**Copper.** Actions: required for absorption and metabolism of iron; necessary for blood and nerve fiber production. Sources: liver, kidney, seafood, nuts, seeds and tap water from copper pipes.

**Fluoride.** Actions: helps maintain bones and teeth. Sources: fluoridated tap water, tea and sardines.

**Iodine.** Actions: required to form thyroid hormones. Sources: iodized salt, seafood, saltwater fish and kelp.

**Iron.** Actions: required for energy production, blood production and immune system health. Sources: liver, various other meats, fish, eggs, green leafy vegetables, enriched breads and cereals.

**Magnesium.** Actions: required for growth of bones and teeth; aids in nerve and muscle functions; necessary for energy production. Sources: milk, cheese, yogurt, seafood, fish, various meats and dark green leafy vegetables.

**Manganese.** Actions: required for bone growth, blood sugar regulation and energy production; needed for energy production and for healthy immune and nervous systems. Sources: fruits, vegetables, legumes, nuts and whole grains.

**Molybdenum.** Actions: needed for metabolism. Sources: milk, legumes, whole-grain breads and cereals.

**Phosphorus.** Actions: required for healthy bones, energy production and metabolism. Sources: milk, cheese, eggs, various meats, fish, whole grains and legumes.

**Potassium.** Actions: required for nerve function, muscle contractions, hormone release; helps maintain healthy blood pressure. Sources: vegetables, legumes, fruits, milk, cheese, various meats and whole grains.

**Selenium.** Actions: may help prevent cancer and heart disease. Sources: liver, kidney, various other meats, seafood and whole grains.

**Sodium.** Actions: helps balance fluids. Sources: salt and processed foods.

**Sulfur.** Actions: required for hair, cartilage and nail development. Sources: various meats, fish, eggs and legumes.

**Zinc.** Actions: required for digestion, metabolism, wound healing, tissue repair and reproductive health. Sources: liver, various other meats, seafood, eggs and whole-grain cereals.

**Water.** This nutrient is often overlooked, yet you couldn't survive for more than a few days without it. Water is needed for just about every process of your body. In addition, your body is made up of at least half water.

The feeling of being thirsty helps you know when to drink more fluids. But it's not exact. That's why you should drink six to eight eight-ounce glasses of water or other liquid every day. (If you're watching your weight, remember that soft drinks and other sweetened drinks contain around 100 calories per eight ounces.)

## Eating Healthy

Once you understand the basics of what's in your diet, the next step is figuring out which foods make a healthy diet. There are several methods you can use: the component-percentage method of food selection, the Eating Right Pyramid and the four basic food groups.

## Diet-Component-by-Percentage

This way of looking at the daily diet has become increasingly popular. This method uses the percentage of carbohydrates, proteins and fats in the diet as the measure of nutrition. With this method, a healthy diet consists of the following:

- 20% to 30% of the calories you consume each day should come from fat.
- 50% to 65% should come from carbohydrates.
- 10% to 20% should come from protein.

You can figure these percentages by using calories or grams. Food labels on processed foods tell the number of grams of each of these components. See page 23 for information on how to read a food label. Each gram of fat contains nine calories, while each gram of protein or carbohydrate has only four calories.

Very-low-fat diets are not recommended except under your doctor's supervision because they may not provide sufficient amounts of essential nutrients in fat-soluble vitamins A, D, E and K.

## The Eating Right Pyramid

The Eating Right Pyramid helps show how more servings should come from certain types of foods.

At the base of the pyramid is the food group that includes *breads, grains, cereals and pasta*. These foods contain mostly carbohydrates and have little fat. They are often high in fiber. People who are striving for a healthy diet should eat between six and 11 servings of these foods a day, depending on the size of serving, your body size and the desired weight to be lost or maintained.

The next level includes *fruits and vegetables*. Experts recommend eating

---

### Servings

**Grains, breads, cereal, rice and pasta.** A serving equals one slice of bread or a small roll; half a bagel or half an English muffin; one ounce of cold cereal; half a cup of cooked cereal, rice or pasta; or three or four small crackers or two large crackers.

**Fruits.** A serving equals one medium-size piece of fresh fruit, one-half cup of chopped or canned fruit, or three-fourths cup of fruit juice.

**Vegetables.** A serving equals one cup of raw, leafy vegetables, one-half cup of other vegetables (cooked or raw) or three-fourths cup of vegetable juice.

**Meat.** (beef, pork, poultry, fish), dried beans, eggs or nuts. A serving equals two to three ounces of cooked meat or one-half cup of cooked dried beans. One egg or two tablespoons of peanut butter equals one ounce of meat.

**Dairy.** A serving equals one cup of milk or yogurt, one and a half ounces of natural cheese or two ounces of processed cheese.

---

five to eight servings a day. They suggest you choose the freshest, least processed fruits and vegetables possible. These foods are also high in fiber. They contain carbohydrates and natural sugars but are very low in fat.

On top of fruits and vegetables in the pyramid is the *milk and meat group*. Four to six servings a day are recommended to obtain adequate protein, again depending on the size of the serving and the amount or percentage of fat in each serving. These foods are the best sources of protein, but they also may be high in fat. Animal products often contain cholesterol. When possible, choose low-fat, low-cholesterol forms of these foods.

The smallest group on the pyramid includes *fats, oils, butter, salad dressings, sweets and desserts*. Many snack foods, such as potato chips and candy bars, cakes and pies, are included in this

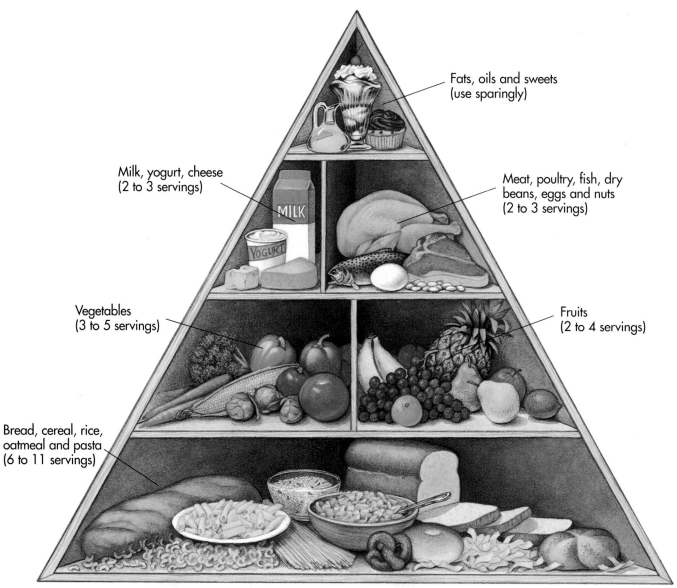

Fats, oils and sweets
(use sparingly)

Milk, yogurt, cheese
(2 to 3 servings)

Meat, poultry, fish, dry
beans, eggs and nuts
(2 to 3 servings)

Vegetables
(3 to 5 servings)

Fruits
(2 to 4 servings)

Bread, cereal, rice,
oatmeal and pasta
(6 to 11 servings)

**THE EATING RIGHT FOOD PYRAMID**

group. No specific number of servings is suggested because these foods don't have any significant nutritional value. Use the foods in this group sparingly.

## The Four Basic Food Groups

With this method, you choose a certain number of servings from each food group every day:

**Bread, cereal, rice and pasta.** Whole grains are often high in fiber. These foods contain more vitamin $B_1$, vitamin E, chromium, selenium and sodium than other food groups. Eat six to 11 servings a day.

**Fruits and vegetables.** Most fruits and vegetables are high in vitamins, minerals and fiber. They may contain some carbohydrates. They contain almost no fat. Eat two to four servings of fruits a day and three to five servings of vegetables.

**Meat, poultry, fish, dry beans, eggs or nuts.** These foods contain protein along with fat. Animal products are the only source of vitamin $B_{12}$. Eat two to three servings every day.

**Milk and dairy products.** These foods are good sources of calcium and vitamin D. They also contain protein.

Have two to three servings a day. Choose low-fat dairy products to reduce the fat content. Pregnant and breast-feeding women need four servings a day.

## How to Read a Food Label

Food labels show nutritional information as percentages of "daily values," based on a 2,000-calorie-a-day diet and also on a 2,500-calorie-a-day diet. You'll find the following information on the labels:

**Serving size.** It's important to check this. The serving size of ice cream may be one-half cup. If you're eating several scoops, you need to remember that a serving is a half cup. Several scoops of ice cream may amount to more than one serving.

**Number of servings per container.** This will help you get a truer sense of the amount that equals a serving of that food.

The rest of the information is given as *amounts per serving*.

**Calories.** Counting calories can be a useful part of watching your weight.

**Calories from fat.** Labels are often misleading. The important issue isn't the number of calories from fat. It's the *percentage* of calories from fat. A desirable percentage is 20% to 30%. To calculate the percentage of calories

| What's in condiments? | | | |
|---|---|---|---|
| Product | Calories (per serving) | Sodium (mg) | Fat (g) |
| Barbecue sauce | 60 | 220 | 0 |
| Dijon-style mustard | 24 | 465 | 1 |
| Horseradish | 4 | 50 | 0 |
| Ketchup | 16 | 156 | 1 |
| Mayonnaise | 100 | 80 | 11 |
| Mustard | 11 | 188 | 1 |
| Pickle relish | 21 | 107 | 0 |
| Salsa | 5 | 81 | 0 |
| Taco sauce | 4 | 110 | 0 |
| Steak sauce | 12 | 275 | 1 |
| Worcestershire | 12 | 147 | 0 |

from fat, look at the nutrition label and follow the formula below.

Calories from fat ÷ calories per serving X 100 = percentage of calories from fat. For example, 25 calories from fat ÷ 100 calories per serving = .25 X 100 = 25%.

**Total fat.** The number of grams of fat are listed on the label. This information is helpful for anyone counting fat grams in their diet. The percentage of the daily value is also given. The number of grams of fat is also given for saturated fat, polyunsaturated fat and monounsaturated fat. Saturated fat is more harmful than unsaturated and monounsaturated fats.

**Cholesterol.** Cholesterol is also given as an amount and a percentage. The daily intake of cholesterol should be less than 300 mg.

---

### Ten Rules for Healthy Eating

*Most people don't want to count calories or grams or figure out percentages. The following guidelines can make healthy eating a little easier.*

1. Eat a variety of foods.
2. Eat only enough to maintain a healthy weight for your height and frame.
3. Choose foods low in fat, saturated fat and cholesterol.
4. Eat or drink no-fat or low-fat dairy products, except young children, who should have whole milk until about age two and then whole milk or 2% milk.
5. Choose lean cuts of beef, pork, fish, chicken and turkey.
6. Eat many fruits and vegetables, especially those that are fresh or frozen instead of canned.
7. Choose fiber-rich foods like whole-grain breads and cereals, oat bran and beans.
8. Use sugars only in moderation.
9. Use salt and sodium only in moderation.
10. Drink alcoholic beverages only in moderation. That means no more than one drink a day for women and two for men.

## Nutrition Facts

Serving Size 1/2 cup (114g)
Serving Per Container 4

**Amount Per Serving**

**Calories** 90        Calories from Fat 30

| | % Daily Value* |
|---|---|
| **Total Fat** 3g | **5%** |
| Saturated Fat 0g | **0%** |
| **Cholesterol** 0mg | **0%** |
| **Sodium** 300mg | **13%** |
| **Total Carbohydrate** 13g | **4%** |
| Dietary Fiber 3g | **12%** |
| Sugars 3g | |
| **Protein** 3g | |

| | | | |
|---|---|---|---|
| Vitamin A | 80% | Vitamin C | 60% |
| Calcium | 4% | Iron | 4% |

*Percent Daily Values are based on a 2,000 calorie diet. Your daily values may be higher or lower depending on your calorie needs:

| | | Calories | 2,000 | 2,500 |
|---|---|---|---|---|
| Total Fat | Less than | | 65g | 80g |
| Sat Fat | Less than | | 20g | 25g |
| Cholesterol | Less than | | 300mg | 300mg |
| Sodium | Less than | | 2,400mg | 2,400mg |
| Total Carbohydrate | | | 300g | 375g |
| Fiber | | | 25g | 30g |

Calories per gram:

Fat 9   •   Carbohydrate 4   •   Protein 4

**Sodium.** Sodium is also given in two numbers—the amount and the percentage.

**Total carbohydrate.** Carbohydrates are listed as an amount and a percentage. Within this category, dietary fiber, soluble fiber and sugars are listed.

**Protein.** Protein is listed as an amount.

Vitamins and minerals are listed as a percentage of the recommended daily allowance.

If something isn't listed on the label, the food doesn't provide a significant amount of that nutrient.

## Maintaining a Healthy Weight

Maintaining a normal weight can help you stay healthy. Being overweight increases your risk for heart disease, high blood pressure, arthritis, stroke, diabetes mellitus, gallstones and back problems. Being underweight can increase your risk for osteoporosis and for bone fractures if you fall. Maintaining a healthy weight goes beyond good nutrition, although what you eat plays a major role in what you weigh. Your weight is also closely related to how active you are and how much exercise you get.

Each person has his or her own calorie needs and expenditures. Reasons vary as to why someone is overweight or underweight. Some people simply eat too much food, and some people don't eat enough food. Some go on starvation diets because of eating disorders (p. 582). Some eat a near-normal diet but don't burn many calories or burn a lot of calories. Differences in the rate that calories are used can be the result of a person's natural metabolism rate or the amount of exercise that person is getting.

Two measurements are important in understanding obesity. The first is a weight/height measurement, which

---

### Professional Help for Nutrition

Watch out if you decide to see a professional nutritionist. Some people call themselves nutritionists but have no training in the subject and are more interested in selling their products than in helping you.

Who is qualified to give nutritional advice? A registered dietitian, someone who has a Ph.D. in nutrition from a university's accredited nutrition program or a medical doctor. To find a qualified person, ask your doctor, the dietetics department at your local hospital or a university nutrition department.

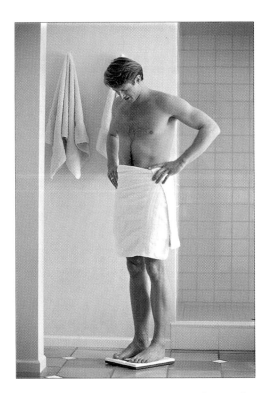

Sudden, unexplained weight loss can be the result of a serious underlying medical condition, including depression. Weight loss can be caused by diabetes (p. 211), hyperthyroidism (p. 215), infections such as tuberculosis (p. 307) or AIDS (p. 325), changes in the way the intestines absorb food, or cancer.

## Losing Weight the Right Way

Gaining weight—and attempting to lose it—seems to be the norm in our society. At any given time, at least a third of women and a fifth of men are trying to lose weight.

compares your size to normal weight ranges for your body build (see box). If you're more than about 20% over your desired weight, you're considered *obese*.

Another measurement is your body-fat content, which can be figured in a number of ways. This must be done by a health professional.

Gaining weight becomes easier as you get older, even if you don't change your eating habits. As you age, your metabolism slows down. Your body doesn't burn as much energy as it did when you were younger.

Most people are overweight because of their diet and inadequate exercise. But some may suffer from depression (p. 587), which can cause overeating and which can be treated. Other people overeat in response to stress. A few people who are overweight suffer from a medical condition known as hypothyroidism (p. 217), which is a hormone deficiency. In some cases, hypothyroidism can result in weight gain.

If you have difficulty losing weight or if you suddenly gain weight for no obvious reason, talk to your doctor.

### Weight-Height Chart

| Height* | Weight in pounds** | |
| | 19 to 34 years old | 35 and older |
| --- | --- | --- |
| 5'0" | 97-128 | 108-138 |
| 5'1" | 101-132 | 111-143 |
| 5'2" | 104-137 | 115-148 |
| 5'3" | 107-141 | 119-152 |
| 5'4" | 111-146 | 122-157 |
| 5'5" | 114-150 | 126-162 |
| 5'6" | 118-155 | 130-167 |
| 5'7" | 121-160 | 134-172 |
| 5'8" | 125-164 | 138-178 |
| 5'9" | 129-169 | 142-183 |
| 5'10" | 132-174 | 146-188 |
| 5'11" | 136-179 | 151-194 |
| 6'0" | 140-184 | 155-199 |
| 6'1" | 144-189 | 159-205 |
| 6'2" | 148-195 | 164-210 |
| 6'3" | 152-200 | 168-216 |
| 6'4" | 156-205 | 173-222 |
| 6'5" | 160-211 | 177-228 |
| 6'6" | 164-216 | 182-234 |

*Without shoes.
**Without shoes and clothes.
Source: "Suggested Weights for Adults," Dietary Guidelines for Americans, U.S. Departments of Agriculture and Health and Human Services, 1990. Note that the lower end of each range applies to women while the upper end of the range applies to men.

## Watch Out for Quick-and-Easy Weight-Loss Claims

Beware of dieting fads that promise big weight losses with no effort, no willpower and no exercise. There is no "trick" to losing weight. Successfully losing weight—and keeping it off—depends on modifying your diet with sensible choices and designing an exercise program you can stick with.

Most people simply try to cut down on how much they eat. Some may follow extreme low-calorie or fad diets that may be dangerous. Researchers are convinced that temporary diets don't really work.

Fad diets have little to no long-lasting value. In fact, they can increase your ability to gain fat. What happens? You may lose some of your muscle along with the fat, especially if the weight is lost quickly. Yet muscle helps you burn more calories. Losing muscle makes it easier to gain back the fat.

The secret to weight loss is to eat less and exercise more. You have to change your behavior concerning food and exercise. Learning how to eat a well-balanced, moderate diet and exercising regularly will help you maintain a normal and healthy weight.

Exercise is extremely important. Regular exercise can help increase the rate at which you burn calories, and it can help convert fat into muscle.

While eating less and exercising more sounds easy, it's often a difficult approach to carry out. Counting calories and using prearranged menus to eat a balanced diet is one common do-it-yourself method of losing weight.

If counting calories is too tedious, try counting fat grams. Some people find that reducing the amount of fat while increasing their exercise helps them lose weight.

Losing weight can be particularly hard to do alone. If you need help, look for support groups and weight-loss programs. Check out their credentials with your doctor or a registered dietitian. Some weight-loss programs offer fad diets, and some can be expensive. They may require that you purchase special foods. Using these special foods can help you lose weight initially. But once you go back to eating normal food again, you may return to your old habits.

Whatever approach you use for weight loss, discuss your options with your doctor, a registered dietitian or other health-care professional trained in nutrition and eating behaviors. Remember that weight should come off slowly. It took you a long time to gain weight; it won't melt off overnight. In general, a slow weight loss is the easiest to maintain. For most

## Tips for Weight Loss

- Keep a food diary. Write down everything you eat. It may be enlightening. Write down, too, when you eat—and why. Are you hungry? Bored? Upset?

- Measure your foods for a few days so you can get used to portion sizes. You may not realize just how much food you are eating.

- Get rid of fattening foods. Fattening foods pack a lot of calories. Don't keep chocolate chip cookies or potato chips in the pantry if you're going to eat them. Learn to substitute low-calorie snacks like rice cakes and raw vegetables. Stop eating foods rich in fat and fill up on less fattening foods.

- Eat three meals a day. Eating regular meals will help discourage the urge to snack. Skipping meals can make you so hungry that you end up binge eating.

- Don't count calories. It's better to learn how to change your eating habits in general.

- Don't get discouraged. If you give in and eat a slice of chocolate cream pie for lunch, the battle with the bulge doesn't have to be over. Just return to your new eating habits right away, that very day.

people, it's wise to set a goal of no more than two pounds per week while eating a balanced diet.

If you are extremely overweight or unable to exercise, talk to your doctor. Other measures can be used, under a doctor's supervision, to get the weight off. These can include very-low-calorie liquid diets, counseling and behavior modification, and appetite suppressants. Gastric stapling, stomach-bypass surgery and even wiring the jaws shut are procedures that have been used to help very obese people lose weight. These procedures have risks, and only about 50% of the people who undergo these treatments maintain their weight loss.

Some weight-loss programs should be done only under a doctor's care and only if you're extremely overweight. One of the most common systems, for example, is the physician-based program that uses a low-calorie, high-protein diet. The diet includes a total of 500 to 1,000 calories a day and six to eight 10-ounce glasses of water each day. For continued success, such a program must be coupled with a good maintenance program after the weight is lost.

## Sleep

The exact reason we need sleep isn't known. But people can't get along without it. Not getting enough sleep can affect your mind, emotions and physical health.

Sleep is divided into different stages according to patterns of brain activity. These patterns can be measured by an electroencephalogram (p. 634). Stages 3 and 4 are the deepest stages of sleep. Rapid eye movement (REM) sleep is the stage during which you dream.

Your sleep patterns change as you age. Newborn babies sleep an average of 16 hours throughout every 24 hours. The average adult sleeps for seven to eight hours at night, although some people can get along on four hours of sleep and others need 10 or more. As you get older, you sleep more, but it takes longer to fall asleep, you may wake more often during the night and you'll probably take more naps during the day.

## Sleep Problems

If you have trouble waking up in the morning and feel tired during the day, you may not be getting enough sleep at night. Waking up four, five or six times a night reduces your sleep time and causes you to feel tired, groggy and unable to concentrate during the day.

If you have *insomnia*, you may either have trouble falling asleep or trouble staying asleep. Insomnia is usually a temporary condition that lasts less than two weeks and is often caused by worries or illness, for example. If insomnia lasts longer, talk to your doctor.

## Getting a Good Night's Sleep

You can help yourself get a good night's sleep. Discipline is sometimes needed to maintain a healthy sleep regimen.

• Don't drink extra coffee or soft drinks with caffeine to keep awake if you're drowsy during the day. The extra caffeine may keep you from sleeping well that night, so the bad sleep cycle continues.

• Finish exercising about one to two hours before going to bed. This gets your body slightly tired and helps you relax. But exercising too close to bedtime may wake you up.

• Use your bedroom for sleeping and sexual activity only. Save stimulating activities like watching TV and talking on the phone for other rooms.

• Try to go to bed at the same time each night and get up at the same time each morning.

• Make sure the room is a comfortable temperature. Often a slightly cool room is best for sound sleep.

• Relax before bedtime. Spend at least 30 minutes winding down. Some people find that reading, listening to relaxing music or taking a warm bath calms them and makes them sleepy. Sexual intimacy before sleeping also has a relaxing effect, as long as it doesn't steal too much time from your normal sleep period.

• Don't use sleep medicines or alcohol at night to help you become sleepy. Such measures may help you fall asleep the first night, but they can interfere with your sleep cycles.

• Get out of bed if you can't fall asleep in 30 minutes.

• Add an extra 30 to 60 minutes of sleep time for a few weeks and see if you feel more energetic and alert.

Interestingly, worrying about your sleep often produces enough anxiety to keep you from relaxing and falling asleep. If you can quit worrying about not sleeping, your sleep pattern will often return to normal.

Some people believe they're only sleeping a few hours a night, when sleep studies prove they're actually getting more sleep than they realize. A comforting (and sometimes sleep-inducing) thought is that by just lying still, relaxing and closing your eyes, you'll get 70% of the rest you would get by sleeping.

## Safety

Learn the rules of safety and practice them. Accidents in the home, on

---

### Causes of Insomnia

**Alcohol.** A nightcap can actually interfere with sleep patterns and stop you from getting a good night's sleep.

**Caffeine.** A cup of coffee in the evening or even late in the afternoon may keep you from falling asleep hours later.

**Circadian rhythm disturbance.** If you work different shifts or travel a lot by plane, your circadian rhythm, or internal clock, may be upset.

**Depression.** This is a common reason for sleep problems. It can cause you to sleep too much or too little.

**Medicines.** Both over-the-counter and prescription medicines can cause sleep problems. Examples of medicines that can interfere with sleep include decongestants (p. 616) and antidepressants (p. 619). If you can't stop taking the medicine, talk to your doctor about the timing of your doses.

**Nicotine.** Smoking can disturb sleep.

**Other medical problems.** Numerous conditions can disturb sleep, including asthma, heartburn, arthritis, menopause, benign prostatic hypertrophy and pain.

**Restless leg syndrome.** If you feel like moving your legs repeatedly before falling asleep, you may suffer from restless leg syndrome. Your legs may even hurt. Several medicines can be used to treat this problem, but it can often be prevented with calf-stretching exercises at bedtime.

**Sleep apnea.** This condition is characterized by brief periods of no breathing that happen several times during sleep. Losing weight, avoiding alcohol and sedatives, and sleeping on your side may help relieve sleep apnea. Discuss other treatments, including surgery, with your doctor.

the road and at work kill or disable thousands of people every year. Yet many accidents can be prevented if proper steps are taken. Learn how to reduce your risk of accidents.

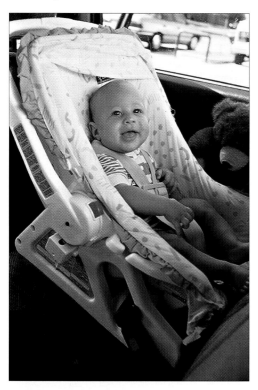

## Car and Vehicle Safety

Put infants and young children in approved car seats. Most states require the use of safety seats in motor vehicles for children under certain ages or weights. Install them properly. Check the directions or call the manufacturer's 800 number (on the back of the seat) for more information. Never use a car seat after it has been in an accident.

Car seats should face the rear of the car until an infant weighs 20 pounds. The middle of the back seat is the safest location for a car seat in your vehicle. Don't put a car seat in the front seat if you have airbags.

Never hold a baby or child on your lap instead of putting him or her in a car seat. It's dangerous.

The most common accidents involving teenagers and adults are car crashes. Always buckle up your seat belt and, if available, shoulder harness. Make sure your passengers wear their seat belts, too. Having other restraint systems in your car, such as air bags, can be lifesaving. Be alert for potential hazards, including other drivers.

Most states hold parents liable for any reckless and damaging accidents caused by their teenagers. Teach your teens proper driving techniques and safety standards.

Never drive after drinking or using drugs. And teach your teens the dangers of driving while under the influence of alcohol. As many as 70% of all highway deaths are related to alcohol consumption.

## Child Safety in Your Home

Once your baby starts crawling, it's time to "childproof" your home. Install stairway gates—and use them— to prevent falls. Put plastic caps on all electrical outlets. Watch out for dangling electrical cords. Children can get serious burns by biting into such cords. Put guards over windows to prevent falls.

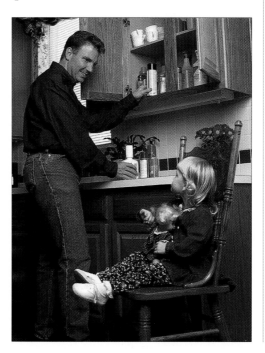

Get rid of the poisonous cleansers under the sink. If you must keep such products in your house, put them up out of your child's reach. If possible, keep them locked in a cabinet.

Keep medicines, both over-the-counter and prescription, out of your child's reach. Vitamins and aspirin are two of the most common medicines that children overdose on. Always use child-resistant caps. Keep medicines in a locked cabinet. Another option: Keep medicines in a tackle box or cosmetic case that locks and then put them up high in a cabinet.

If you keep guns in your home, make sure they're unloaded. Store guns and ammunition separately and keep them both locked up.

Lower your hot water heater to 120° F. Babies and young children can get burned quickly.

Put a fence around an outdoor swimming pool and keep the gate locked. Curious neighborhood children may want to investigate your pool when you're not at home.

## Food Safety

Handling food properly will help reduce your chances of food poisoning. Food poisoning (p. 300) can cause diarrhea, nausea and vomiting, and abdominal pain.

## Preventing Falls

Falling is the most serious preventable health problem for elderly persons. A broken hip from a fall can actually lead to death, a stroke or other serious health problems.

Use nonslip floor mats in the kitchen and bathroom. Get rid of throw rugs that slip or slide. Make sure all areas are well lit. Place

electrical cords so they can't be tripped over. Move other objects that might trip someone. Provide aids for balance and walking, especially in the bathtub.

## Recreation

Any sport or recreational activity, such as swimming, boating, skiing, hunting and bicycling, can be risky if you do it incorrectly or with equipment that's not properly maintained. Make sure you learn the safety requirements and recommendations for each sport and activity, along with the risks.

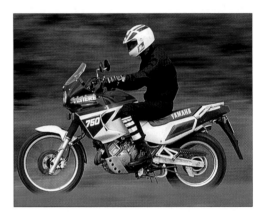

Wear a helmet if you're riding a motorcycle. Make sure you and your children wear helmets while bicycling as well. Helmets can reduce the chances of serious head injuries (p. 50), such as concussions and contusions. Also wear the appropriate protective gear for skateboarding and rollerblading.

## Safety in Your Workplace

The workplace also holds many hazards. Many jobs require the use of noisy tools or power saws or grinders that produce small fragments and dusts that irritate the eyes and respiratory tract. Repeated exposure to industrial chemicals and fumes can damage the skin, eyes or lungs.

---

### Keeping Food Safe

- Wash your hands well before preparing food. Wash them after handling raw meat or poultry.

- Cook food properly. Make sure pork and chicken are thoroughly cooked.

- Place uneaten portions of food in the refrigerator right away.

Know which chemicals, dusts or fumes are common in your workplace and take every precaution to prevent your exposure to them every day you're at work.

Government regulations require employers to provide a safe working environment. This often includes the use of special safety equipment. But this gear is worthless unless you use it correctly and understand the risks of your occupation. Air filters, headgear, safety shoes and protective clothing help prevent injuries.

For example, you can help prevent hearing loss due to job-related noise by wearing ear plugs. Protect your eyes from dusts and other fragments by wearing safety glasses and installing air filters.

People who sit at desks or computer consoles all day also need to heed job-safety suggestions. For example, you can help prevent carpal tunnel syndrome (p. 257) by setting up your work station to avoid positions that contribute to the condition. The best position is the one that bends the wrists the least—up, down or side to side. You may also prevent neck strain and back problems by sitting up straight and keeping your knees a little higher than your hips. Adjust the seat or use a low stool to put your feet on. And don't hold the phone between your head and your shoulder! This is a common position that can lead to neck pain.

Regular exercise, stress-reduction techniques, working in a smoke-free environment and having regular check-ups by your doctor will help to reduce the risks of a sedentary work situation.

## Smoking Cessation

Stopping smoking if you smoke is the single best thing you can do for your health. But this is so much easier said than done! For most people who smoke, smoking is an integral part of their daily lives. Smoking changes your body because the nicotine is addictive. Smoking changes the way you act because it's a *habit*—you have behaviors you're comfortable with that involve lighting and smoking cigarettes.

Many things may trigger the desire for a cigarette—your first cup of coffee in the morning, talking on the phone, driving, feeling tense, socializing. But you won't always crave cigarettes after you quit smoking. The craving will fade over time, and your efforts will pay off in better health!

## Preparing to Quit

Think about when you want to stop smoking. Pick a date that has a special meaning for you, or a date that you think may be as ideal a time as any, given your work and family-life stress. Choose a date two to four weeks away so you can get ready.

Keep a daily diary of when and why you smoke. This may help you understand your habit and form a plan to deal with the times when you'll crave a cigarette. Make a list of reasons you want to quit that are personal to you. Think of things to do instead of lighting a cigarette.

## Quitting

You may feel edgy and irritable right after you quit smoking. You may feel hungrier than usual and have trouble concentrating. You may also have headaches and cough more at first. How you feel depends largely on how addicted to the nicotine you are. You start to feel better after the first few

---

*Reasons to Quit Smoking*

- Bad breath
- Breathing problems
- Cancer risk
- Gum disease risk
- Heart disease risk
- Stained teeth
- Bad smell in clothes, hair, skin
- Cough
- Sore throat
- Faster heartbeat
- Raised blood pressure
- Risk of second-hand smoke to others around you
- Expensive
- Society's negative view of smokers
- Wrinkles

days of not smoking. Most symptoms of nicotine withdrawal go away after a few weeks.

While many people gain a few pounds after they quit smoking, you don't have to gain weight. You can help avoid gaining weight after quitting by watching how much you eat. Keep healthy, low-fat snacks on hand. Start exercising or exercise more. This will help you burn calories and also helps keep you busy so you can't smoke.

If the symptoms of withdrawal are a major problem, talk to your family doctor about whether nicotine gum or nicotine patches would help you. These have worked very well for many people. They help you quit smoking by relieving some of the signs of nicotine addiction while you deal with ending the habit of smoking.

## STD Prevention

The only way to absolutely prevent ever having a sexually transmitted disease (STD, p. 316) is to not have sex (*abstinence*) or to only have sex with one partner who doesn't already have an STD and who isn't having sex with anyone else (a *mutually monogamous* relationship).

If you have more than one sex partner or if you're at all uncertain about whether your sex partner is having sex with anyone else, you may be at risk of catching an STD. The risk increases with the number of sex partners you have. Some people may be offended by a discussion of protective measures for STDs. But many people are at risk,

and it's important to understand which sexual practices can put you and others at risk and how you can reduce that risk.

You can help lower your risk of catching an STD by practicing the following suggestions, known as "safer sex." Keep in mind that these tips aren't guaranteed to protect you and that the only "safe" options are to choose abstinence or to stay in a mutually monogamous relationship.

1. Know your sex partner very well. Tell your partner if you have an STD and ask if he or she has one. Talk about if you've both been tested for an STD, which STDs you've been tested for and if you should be tested again.

2. Look for signs of an STD in your partner. For example, sores around the penis or vagina can indicate an STD. Keep in mind that a person with an STD doesn't always know he or she has an infection.

3. Always use a latex condom when you have sex, including oral and anal sex, if you're at all uncertain about whether your sex partner has an STD or is having sex with anyone else. See page 317 for information on how to use a condom correctly. A condom blocks semen and vaginal secretions and protects the skin. Condoms *reduce* the risk of passing or catching an STD but don't *eliminate* the risk. That's because condoms don't protect all of your skin in the genital area, and sometimes they can break. Condoms shouldn't provide a sense of total security because that might lead to risky sexual activity.

# ATLAS OF THE BODY

## THE BRAIN AND NERVOUS SYSTEM

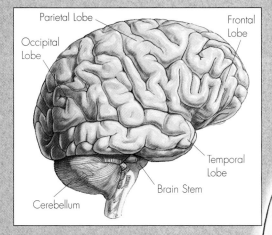

Parietal Lobe
Occipital Lobe
Frontal Lobe
Temporal Lobe
Brain Stem
Cerebellum

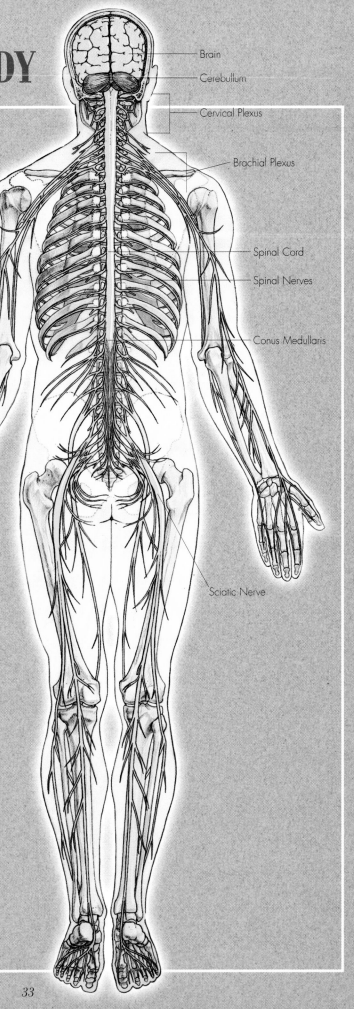

Brain
Cerebullum
Cervical Plexus
Brachial Plexus
Spinal Cord
Spinal Nerves
Conus Medullaris
Sciatic Nerve

The soft, delicate tissues of your brain and central nervous system are found inside your skull and spinal column. The peripheral nerves run from your spine to the rest of your body. Your brain and nervous system are your connection to your environment. This system is responsible for processing all the things that happen around and to you—what you see, hear, smell, taste, feel and think. This system is also responsible for how you respond to your environment because it controls your muscles and other bodily functions. The cortical areas of your brain allow for your "higher" functions, such as sight, speech and thought, as well as movements, personality and memory. The middle of your brain, called the brain stem, deals with the signals from your heart, lungs and digestive tract, and sends signals to regulate these "automatic functions." The back of your brain, the cerebellum, coordinates your motions and your sense of balance.

# THE SENSES

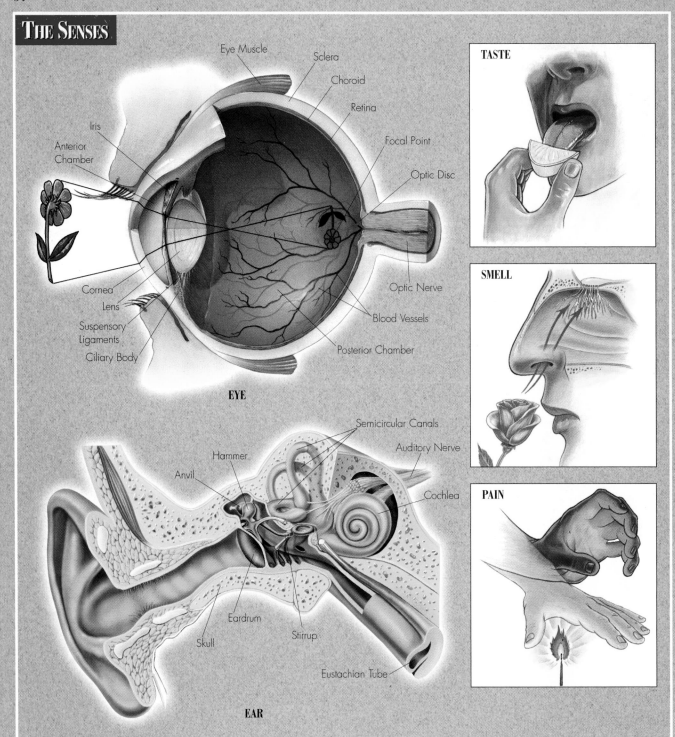

Eye Muscle

Sclera

Choroid

Retina

Iris

Focal Point

Anterior
Chamber

Optic Disc

Cornea

Lens

Suspensory
Ligaments

Ciliary Body

Optic Nerve

Blood Vessels

Posterior Chamber

**EYE**

Semicircular Canals

Hammer

Auditory Nerve

Anvil

Cochlea

Eardrum

Stirrup

Skull

Eustachian Tube

**EAR**

**TASTE**

**SMELL**

**PAIN**

Your brain and nervous system are linked to the outside world through your eyes, ears, mouth, nose and skin. Your eyes take in light, focus images, detect color and shades of light, and transfer images to your brain within fractions of a second. Your ears sense tiny vibrations in the air, translate them into intensity and pitch, and then send the information to your brain for processing. Your mouth, through your taste buds, picks up information about tastes. Taste is closely related to smell, which you pick up through sensors in your nose. Your skin, the largest organ of the body, is an amazing device for protecting your body and also picking up all sorts of information about how something feels to you—soft or hard, hot or cold, rough or smooth. All of these systems send signals to your brain through your nervous system so that you can respond to things around you.

# THE CIRCULATORY SYSTEM

Every part of your body needs oxygen, along with sugar, proteins and other nutrients, to make energy, to grow and to repair itself. Your blood delivers oxygen from your lungs to your body through your circulatory system. Your circulatory system is made up of your heart and your blood vessels. Your heart pumps blood through your lungs and out to your body through your arteries. Your blood returns to your heart and lungs through your veins. While in the lungs, your blood dumps waste products it has picked up as it has traveled through your blood vessels and picks up a fresh supply of oxygen. It then travels back out to your body, repeating the endless cycle.

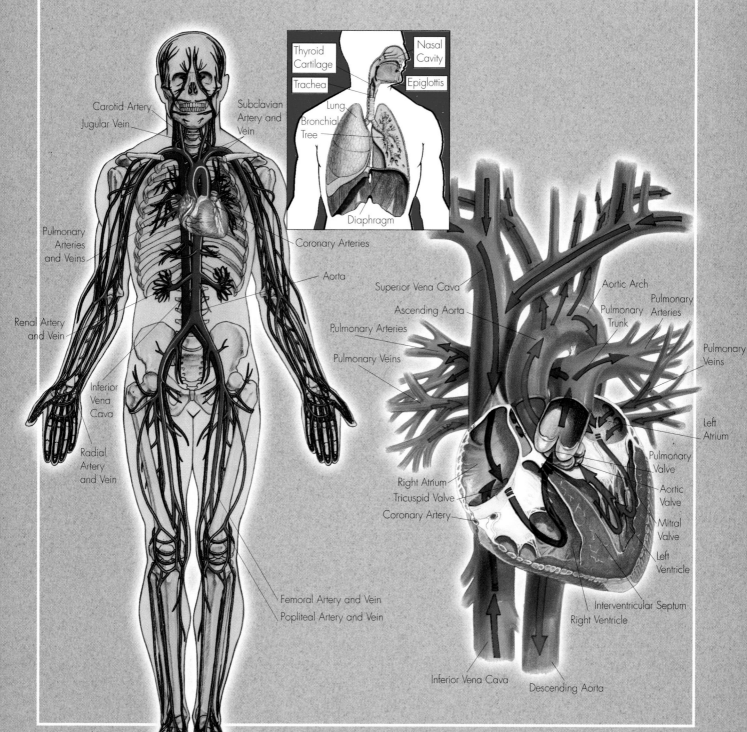

# THE REPRODUCTIVE AND URINARY SYSTEMS

The urinary tract is how your body eliminates fluid waste. Your kidneys filter waste from your blood, and then dump this waste into your bladder through your ureters. When your bladder begins to get full, signals are sent to your brain that you need to urinate to empty your bladder. The urethra is the tube that runs from your bladder to the outside of your body. Without this efficient system of waste removal, the by-products of making energy, or metabolism, would build up and act like a poison, making you very sick.

Sperm are produced in the testicles. The testicles are housed in a sac, called the scrotum, that hangs outside of the body. When a man becomes sexually excited and ejaculates, the sperm travel through the vas deferens and through the urethra in the penis.

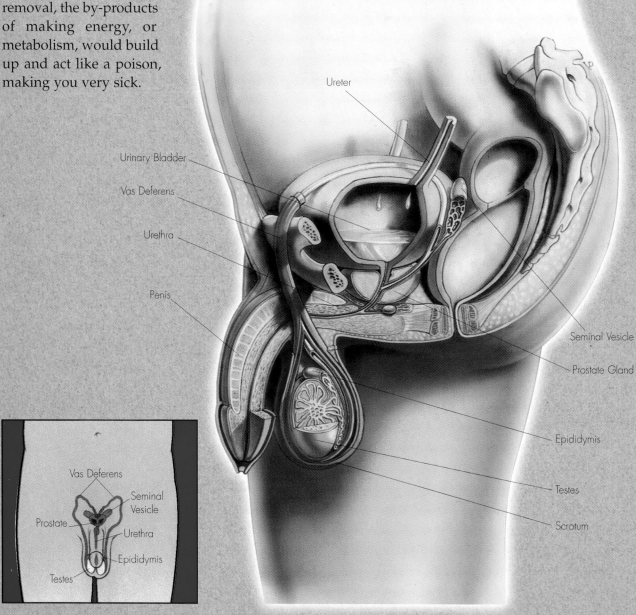

Ureter

Urinary Bladder

Vas Deferens

Urethra

Penis

Seminal Vesicle

Prostate Gland

Epididymis

Testes

Scrotum

Vas Deferens

Seminal Vesicle

Prostate

Urethra

Epididymis

Testes

Women are born with eggs already in their ovaries. The eggs are released by the ovaries when a woman begins to ovulate, usually between ages nine and 16. When a woman ovulates, an egg is released by the ovary, travels through the fallopian tube and into the uterus. If sperm are present in the uterus and one penetrates the surface of the egg, the woman will become pregnant. The fertilized egg will attach to the side of the uterus and begin to grow. If no sperm are present, the egg will pass through the vagina, and the lining of the uterus will be shed. This is called menstruation, or having a "period." It is your body's way of cleansing itself and will usually happen about once a month if you don't become pregnant.

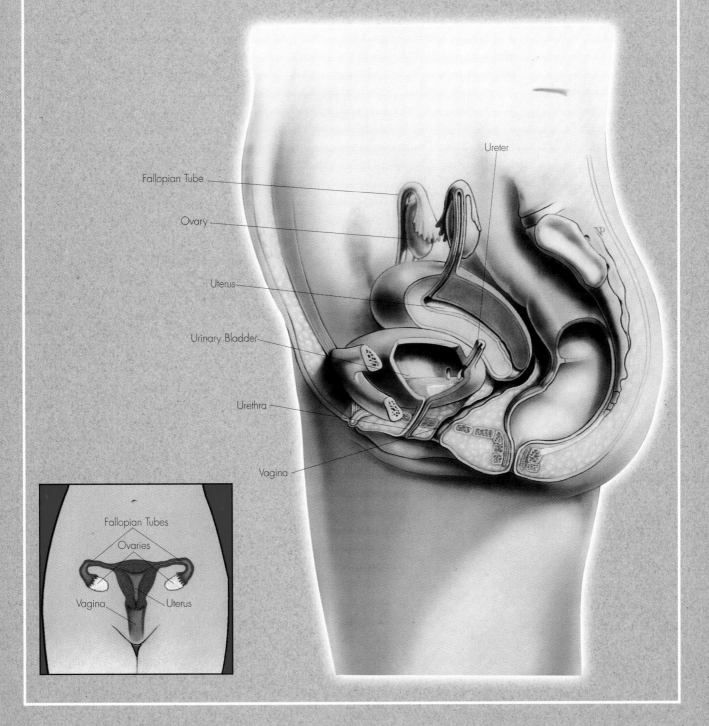

Fallopian Tube

Ovary

Uterus

Urinary Bladder

Urethra

Vagina

Ureter

Fallopian Tubes

Ovaries

Vagina

Uterus

# THE DIGESTIVE SYSTEM

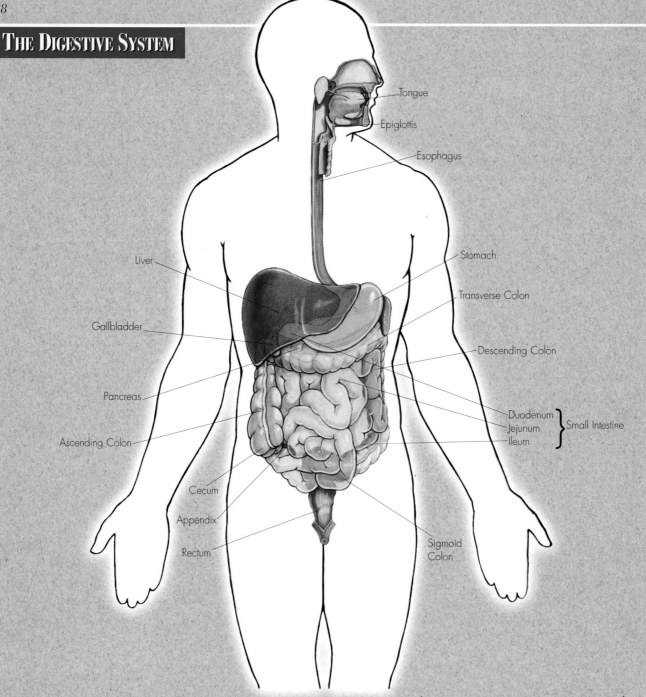

Tongue

Epiglottis

Esophagus

Stomach

Transverse Colon

Descending Colon

Liver

Gallbladder

Pancreas

Ascending Colon

Cecum

Appendix

Rectum

Duodenum
Jejunum
Ileum
} Small Intestine

Sigmoid
Colon

Your digestive system is where what you eat and drink is turned into energy that your body can use to grow and to keep itself healthy. Digestion starts when you chew and swallow. Food moves through your esophagus to your stomach, where strong acids and enzymes mix with the food to begin breaking it down. The food then moves into the small intestine. While in the first part of the small intestine, called the duodenum, many organs help with the digestive process by adding chemicals to the food to further break it down so your body can use the nutrients. The liver adds bile, which is stored in the gallbladder until it's used. The pancreas adds enzymes. Nutrients then move into the lower part of the small intestine, the ileum and the jejunum, where they're absorbed. The remaining water and undigested waste pass into your large intestine. The large intestine is made up of the cecum, appendix, colon, rectum, anal canal and anus. This is where the waste is prepared to pass as a bowel movement through the rectum and anus. The entire digestive tract is between 20 and 25 feet long.

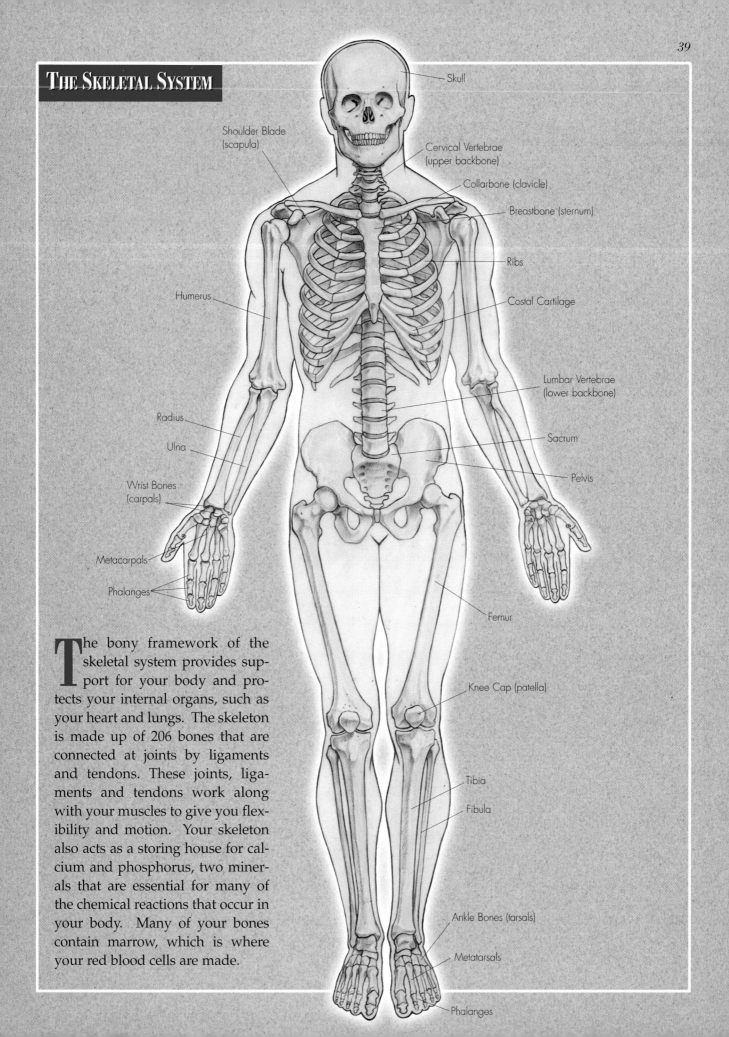

# THE SKELETAL SYSTEM

Skull

Shoulder Blade
(scapula)

Cervical Vertebrae
(upper backbone)

Collarbone (clavicle)

Breastbone (sternum)

Ribs

Humerus

Costal Cartilage

Lumbar Vertebrae
(lower backbone)

Radius

Ulna

Sacrum

Pelvis

Wrist Bones
(carpals)

Metacarpals

Phalanges

Femur

Knee Cap (patella)

Tibia

Fibula

Ankle Bones (tarsals)

Metatarsals

Phalanges

The bony framework of the skeletal system provides support for your body and protects your internal organs, such as your heart and lungs. The skeleton is made up of 206 bones that are connected at joints by ligaments and tendons. These joints, ligaments and tendons work along with your muscles to give you flexibility and motion. Your skeleton also acts as a storing house for calcium and phosphorus, two minerals that are essential for many of the chemical reactions that occur in your body. Many of your bones contain marrow, which is where your red blood cells are made.

# THE MUSCULAR SYSTEM

**M**uscles help give your skeleton the ability to move. They also help you smile or frown, breathe and digest food. Muscles are controlled by the brain and nervous system, which tell them to contract and relax to cause movement. Movement occurs when a shortened muscle pulls on a tendon. The tendon then pulls on the bone, raising or lowering it. Some muscles are voluntary muscles and move only when your nervous system tells them to. Others are involuntary and move without conscious effort, such as the muscles in your digestive tract.

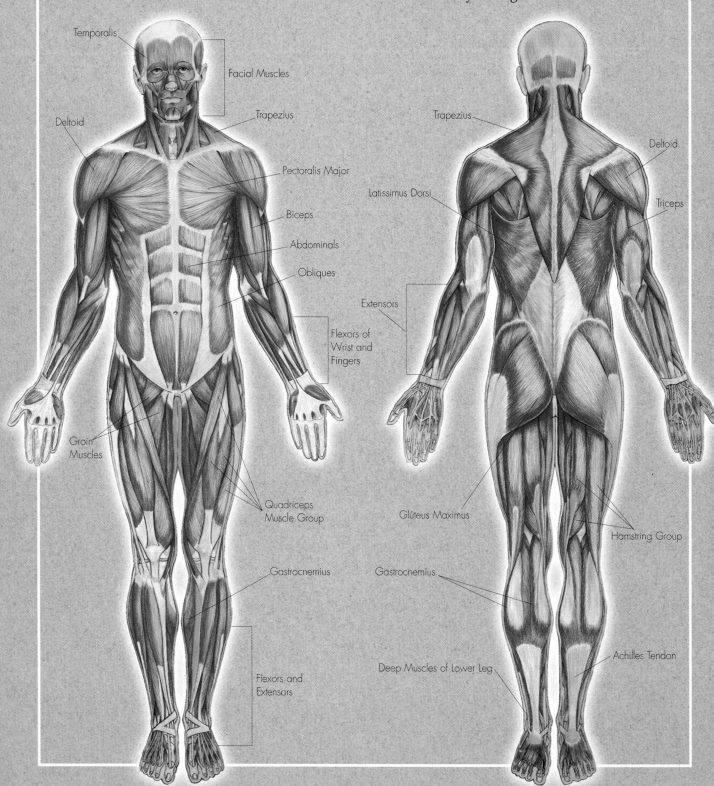

Temporalis

Facial Muscles

Deltoid

Trapezius

Pectoralis Major

Biceps

Abdominals

Obliques

Flexors of Wrist and Fingers

Groin Muscles

Quadriceps Muscle Group

Gastrocnemius

Flexors and Extensors

Trapezius

Deltoid

Latissimus Dorsi

Triceps

Extensors

Glúteus Maximus

Hamstring Group

Gastrocnemius

Deep Muscles of Lower Leg

Achilles Tendon

# PART **2**

# THE BODY

| CHAPTER | | PAGE |
|---|---|---|
| 1 | BRAIN AND NERVOUS SYSTEM | 42 |
| 2 | EYES | 62 |
| 3 | EARS | 76 |
| 4 | NOSE AND SINUSES | 86 |
| 5 | MOUTH | 91 |
| 6 | THROAT | 102 |
| 7 | HEART AND BLOOD VESSELS | 107 |
| 8 | BLOOD | 131 |
| 9 | LUNGS | 141 |
| 10 | URINARY SYSTEM | 158 |
| 11 | GASTROINTESTINAL SYSTEM | 169 |
| 12 | LIVER AND GALLBLADDER | 201 |
| 13 | HORMONES AND GLANDS | 207 |
| 14 | IMMUNE SYSTEM | 220 |
| 15 | BONES, JOINTS AND MUSCLES | 227 |
| 16 | HANDS AND FEET | 255 |
| | PHOTOGRAPHIC GUIDE TO SYMPTOMS | 265 |
| 17 | SKIN AND HAIR | 273 |

# CHAPTER 1 — BRAIN AND NERVOUS SYSTEM

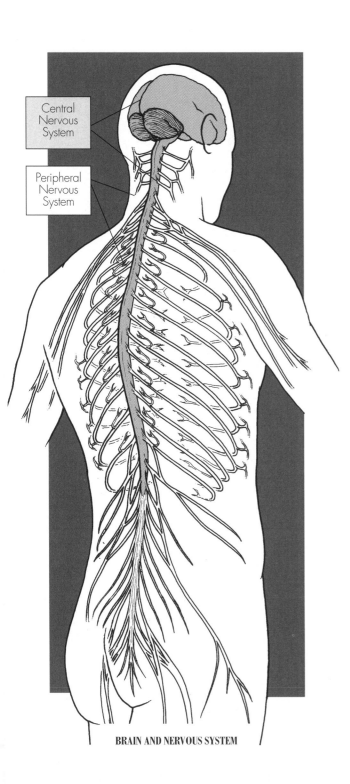

Central
Nervous
System

Peripheral
Nervous
System

**BRAIN AND NERVOUS SYSTEM**

The brain and spinal cord make up the body's *central nervous system.* The nerves that run from the spinal cord throughout the body make up the *peripheral nervous system.* Together, the central and peripheral nervous systems are the body-brain connection.

The brain is a complex organ with many parts that work with the rest of your body to help you see, hear, feel, breathe and function. The brain also gives you your personality and makes you who you are.

The *cerebrum* is the largest part of the brain. It consists of the *cerebral hemispheres,* commonly called the left and right hemispheres. The cerebral hemisphere on the left side of the brain controls the right side of the body, and the hemisphere on the right side of the brain controls the left side of the body. The two hemispheres are connected by the *corpus callosum.* The corpus callosum allows the two hemispheres to communicate with one another.

Each cerebral hemisphere is divided into four lobes: the *frontal lobe* has functions that contribute to personality and emotions, the *parietal lobe* relates to the sense of touch, the *temporal lobe* to hearing, and the *occipital lobe* to vision.

An important part of the frontal lobe is the *motor cortex.* It controls movement. The area that controls speech is near the motor cortex. It's located in the left hemisphere in right-handed people and in the right hemisphere in many left-handed people.

The cerebral hemispheres have an outer layer called the *cerebral cortex.* The cerebral cortex has functions that mostly relate to the coordination of complex nervous activities, such as instincts and perception. The cerebral hemispheres are connected to the spinal cord by the *brain stem.* The *medulla oblongata* is located at the end of the brain stem. Its duties relate to vital

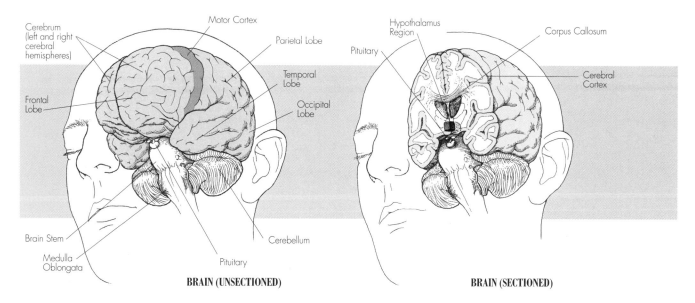

**BRAIN (UNSECTIONED)**                    **BRAIN (SECTIONED)**

functions, such as breathing and the flow of blood.

The *cerebellum* is located under the cerebrum. It's the part of the brain that helps your muscles work together and helps you keep your equilibrium, or balance.

The *hypothalamus* is a small area in the central part of the brain. It's responsible for regulating the temperature of the body, appetite, thirst and sexual behavior, and for controlling the *pituitary gland*. The pituitary gland is the "master gland" of the endocrine system because the hormones it produces control the activity of other glands.

The *cranial nerves* are connected directly to the brain and go mainly to the head and neck. The cranial nerves include nerves responsible for vision, hearing, taste, smell, touch and movement in the head and neck area.

The *spinal nerves* go to all areas of the body below the neck. Their responsibilities include movement and the sense of touch.

The *autonomic nerves* control things that seem to happen "automatically," or at least without conscious thought, such as blood flow, heartbeat, digestion and breathing.

The nerves are made up of nerve cells (*neurons*). The brain and nervous system and the rest of the body communicate through messages that are passed from neuron to neuron.

Neurons consist of a main cell with fibers extending from it. These fibers include *axons*, which usually carry messages away from the main cell, and *dendrites*, which usually carry messages to the main cell.

The neurons pass messages through special impulses that are like electricity.

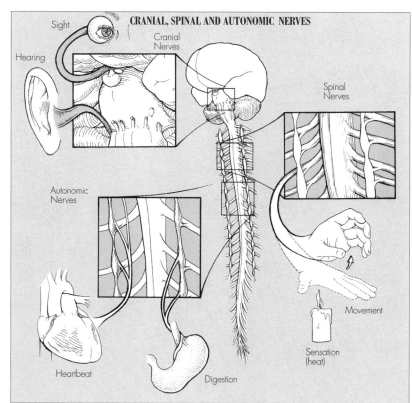

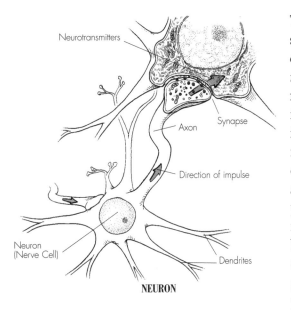

**NEURON**

The impulses are started when chemicals, called *neurotransmitters*, go inside the neurons. Once an impulse is started, it travels from neuron to neuron across connections called *synapses*. This is how your body sends messages to your brain so that you're aware of what's going on around you. It's also how your brain sends instructions to your body so that you can respond to your surroundings.

Of all the tissues in the body, the brain and spinal cord have some of the best protection. The skull provides a solid shield of bone around the brain. The bones of the spine protect the nerves in the spinal cord. Inside these bony covers, the brain and spinal cord are further protected by three layers of membranes, called the *meninges*. The three layers of meninges are the *pia mater, arachnoid* and *dura mater.* The

*cerebrospinal fluid,* or spinal fluid, flows between the pia mater and the arachnoid meninges. The spinal fluid helps cushion the nerves in the brain and spinal cord.

## Amyotrophic Lateral Sclerosis (Lou Gehrig's Disease)

- Weakness
- Problems walking
- Trouble swallowing

*Amyotrophic lateral sclerosis* (ALS), also called Lou Gehrig's disease after the famous baseball player who died from it, slowly kills the nerve cells that tell the muscles to move. This makes it impossible for the brain to communicate with the muscles. When the nerve that stimulates and directs a muscle dies, the muscle becomes weaker and smaller, then *atrophies*, or wastes away. As more nerve cells die, more muscle power is lost and more functions, such as walking, standing, sitting, swallowing and breathing, are damaged.

The cause of ALS is still not understood. It usually affects older adults. No cure is available for ALS, and nothing seems to prevent it. Treatment is aimed at relieving symptoms and improving the general condition of the person.

## Aphasia

- Suddenly not being able to speak, write or understand the meaning of words

Damage to the language areas of the brain can cause you to lose the ability to speak, write or understand the meaning of words. This is called *aphasia*. A stroke (p. 59), bleeding in the brain (p. 45) or a severe head injury can damage the areas that control the understanding of written or spoken language.

**CROSS SECTION OF SPINAL CORD (FROM ABOVE)**

Sometimes a person with aphasia may be able to understand what is said but may be unable to say or write what he or she is thinking. In other cases, a person may not be able to write but be able to speak. Yet in other cases, a person may have trouble finding the correct words to speak. This person may only be able to speak and understand simple words. A person who is totally or almost totally unable to speak, understand or write has *global aphasia.*

### Testing and Treatment

The reason for the aphasia must be determined. If you have aphasia, your doctor will probably do a physical exam, some basic blood tests and a CT scan (p. 632) of the head to check for the cause of aphasia and the extent of the brain damage.

A speech and hearing therapist may be able to help. Some recovery is usual after a stroke or head injury.

## Bell's Palsy

- Drooping of the mouth and eyelid
- Inability to move one side of the face

*Bell's palsy* is a condition in which a nerve in the face becomes inflamed and isn't able to function properly. This can cause one side of the face to become weak and unable to move (*paralysis*), leading to the inability to smile, whistle, keep from drooling and close the eye on that side. The condition usually comes on rapidly, within a few hours, and may be present upon waking in the morning. Some people report pain or tingling on one side of the face within a day or two before the paralysis.

The cause of Bell's palsy isn't known. The condition may be related to a virus that can irritate the nerve and cause it to swell. This may lead to compression of the nerve as it passes through its opening in the bones of the face. The sooner the muscle movement returns, usually in a few weeks, the more likely the paralysis is to have no lasting effects. If the paralysis lasts months, some permanent damage is likely.

### Testing

A few other medical conditions mimic Bell's palsy, so these symptoms should be checked by your doctor. Nerve conduction studies (p. 638) may be ordered to find the source of the problem.

### Treatment

If the facial weakness has no other causes, the "treatment" will probably be a period of patience. If weakness continues, electric muscle stimulation can be used to prevent muscle atrophy and shorten the recovery period. Corticosteroids (p. 622) are sometimes tried. No other treatments are available.

## Bleeding in the Brain

- Confusion
- Headache
- Trouble speaking, seeing, hearing or moving
- Fatigue
- Nausea and vomiting

Bleeding *(hemorrhaging)* in or around the brain can cause severe injury. This type of bleeding may be caused by a weak spot in a blood vessel wall—called a berry aneurysm (p. 108)—that ruptures, a head injury, or untreated high blood pressure (p. 123) and atherosclerosis (p. 111). Bleeding in the brain or into the space around the brain or spinal cord can put pressure on the brain tissues. This pressure can prevent the blood from flowing to the tissues in the brain and the tissues may die from lack of oxygen. People who have high blood pressure or atherosclerosis, or who are on blood-thinning medicine (p. 619), are at greater risk of hemorrhages. Bleeding into or around the brain can occur with stroke, head injury or a ruptured aneurysm. Four areas of the brain can be affected.

**Epidural hemorrhage.** This type of bleeding usually follows a head injury. Blood leaks slowly from a damaged blood vessel into the space between the dura mater and the skull (*epidural space*). Bleeding next to the skull will lead to headache, confusion, increased

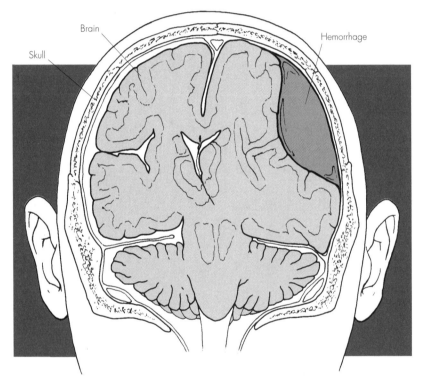

Brain

Skull

Hemorrhage

**BLEEDING IN THE BRAIN**

drowsiness, nausea and vomiting. As with any of these hemorrhages, continued bleeding can lead to coma and death.

**Intracerebral hemorrhage.** Also called *hemorrhagic stroke* or *stroke due to bleeding,* this occurs when blood vessels within the brain tissues rupture or leak, damaging the tissue and causing pressure on surrounding tissues. People who have this type of hemorrhage are usually middle-aged or elderly and have untreated high blood pressure

or atherosclerosis. Symptoms include sudden weakness and confusion or loss of consciousness. The person may also have trouble speaking, seeing or hearing, or moving an arm, a leg or half of the body.

**Subarachnoid hemorrhage.** This occurs when an aneurysm bursts in the *subarachnoid space,* which is between the pia mater and the arachnoid membrane that cover the brain. The bleeding increases spinal fluid pressure, which causes pressure on the brain. Symptoms of subarachnoid hemorrhage include severe headache, dizziness, stiff neck, tiredness, nausea and vomiting. Being bothered by lights is another symptom.

**Subdural hemorrhage.** When blood leaks between the dura mater and the arachnoid layer (*subdural space*), a *subdural hematoma* (a swollen spot that contains blood) forms. A subdural hemorrhage is almost always caused by a head injury. In some cases, the symptoms don't occur until several weeks after the head injury. Symptoms include progressive drowsiness, confusion, headache, weakness or numbness. Some people lose consciousness and may even lapse into a coma (p. 48). Recovery is likely to be faster and more complete if the hematoma is drained through surgery.

### Testing

CT scans (p. 632) will help in the diagnosis. Repeat scans will show whether the bleeding has stopped. The treatment will differ depending on whether the bleeding has stopped or is still going on. X-rays of the skull and possibly a spinal tap (p. 641) may also help find the source of the bleeding in someone who has had a head injury.

### Treatment

Bleeding in the brain is usually treated by lowering blood pressure and using medicines to reduce swelling and prevent further brain damage. Life-support measures may be needed if the bleeding is severe.

Subdural and epidural hemorrhages are usually treated by surgically draining the blood. Sometimes the leaking artery is also repaired. Subarachnoid hemorrhage usually results from a ruptured aneurysm that requires surgery. First, the person's condition must be stable enough for surgery. This may require bed rest in the hospital.

### Prevention

You can help prevent bleeding in the brain by controlling high blood pressure, preventing atherosclerosis, and wearing seat belts when in a car and helmets when riding a motorcycle or bicycle. If any of the symptoms mentioned above occur after a fall or an accident, you should be checked right away by your doctor. This could help prevent further damage and possible permanent disability.

## Brain Abscess

- Headache
- Drowsiness
- Problems with speech, vision or hearing
- Loss of strength or sense of touch
- Fever
- Nausea or vomiting

*Abscesses* are collections of *pus* (a mixture of white blood cells, dead tissue and fluid) surrounded by swollen tissue. They can form anywhere in the body in response to infection with bacteria. If the infection keeps going, pressure from the abscess may build on the surrounding tissues and cause damage. Because the brain is surrounded by the rigid skull, an abscess within the brain can put pressure on the brain. This can result in headache, drowsiness, weakness, trouble talking, seeing and hearing, fever, and nausea and vomiting.

CT scans (p. 632) and MRI scans (p. 637) may be needed to diagnose a brain abscess.

Abscesses in the brain must be drained as quickly as possible to prevent spread of the infection and damage from the pressure. Intravenous antibiotics may also be needed.

## Brain Tumor

- Headaches that are fairly constant and keep getting worse
- Loss of vision or hearing
- Confusion and feeling disoriented
- Changes in personality
- Short-term memory loss
- Nausea or vomiting
- Numbness or weakness of the face, trunk, arm, hand, leg or foot

Tumors of the brain, spinal cord or other parts of the nervous system are rare. Cancerous tumors that occur within the brain tissues are called *primary tumors* of the brain. Cancerous tumors that spread to the brain from other areas of the body are called *secondary,* or *metastatic,* tumors. Tumors in the brain—whether cancerous or non-cancerous, primary or metastatic—are always serious because they may press

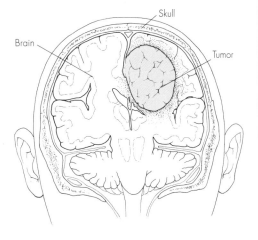

**BRAIN TUMOR**

the soft tissues of the brain against the immovable skull and cause damage.

The first sign of a brain tumor may be loss of some function, such as loss of vision, feeling in the face or strength in the hand. In other cases, the first sign may be headache. The pain may be especially severe when lying down. Persistent vomiting or seizures can also be the first sign of a brain tumor. Personality changes and dementia may also be signs of a brain tumor.

### Testing

Because brain tumors are serious and surgery may be needed, a *neurologist* (a doctor of nerve function), a *neurosurgeon* (a doctor who operates on the brain) or other subspecialist may be called in for diagnosis and treatment. Tests may include a physical exam, CT scan (p. 632) or MRI scan (p. 637). Tests may be done to check for the spread of tumors to other areas of the body.

### Treatment

Surgery to remove the tumor or biopsy of the tumor may be done. Not all brain tumors can be removed by surgery.

Further surgery, radiation therapy (p. 225) or chemotherapy (p. 225) are the usual treatments if the tumor is cancerous. The treatment choices depend on the type of tumor and how fast it is growing. Medicines can also be used to reduce the pressure the tumor is putting on the brain, to relieve the nausea and vomiting, to stop seizures and to relieve pain.

## Coma

- Unconsciousness
- No response to physical stimulus

A *coma* is a state of unconsciousness. Causes of coma include a brain tumor (p. 47) or abscess (p. 47), a contusion (p. 50), epilepsy (p. 56), ketoacidosis meningitis (p. 302), encephalitis (p. 324), a stroke (p. 59) and drug overdoses. Any one of these events can depress the function of the parts of the brain that relate to awareness, and this can lead to coma in some cases. The outlook for a person in a coma depends on the cause of the coma.

A *vegetative state* occurs when the person isn't aware of himself or herself but is still able to breathe. It is similar to a coma but is more serious and is usually permanent. Few people who are in a vegetative state for more than a few months improve, and none have fully recovered. The vegetative state can last for many years before the person dies. *Brain death* refers to a state in which a person has no reflexes and can't breathe without help.

## Compressed Nerve

- Numbness, tingling and weakness in the area supplied by the nerve
- Pain

Repeated movement of your wrist, elbow or ankle while working or playing a sport can lead to swelling in the surrounding tissues. As the tissues swell, they can put pressure on a nerve. The pressure can damage the nerve, slowing or stopping the signals sent through the nerve. This is called *entrapment syndrome*. Different entrapment syndromes can occur, depending on which nerve is affected.

The pain, numbness and tingling of entrapment syndromes can seriously affect the ability to work or enjoy leisure activities. If you have a job that requires the same movements over and over, you're at higher risk for entrapment syndromes. The pain of entrapment syndromes may become worse at night because tissues in the body normally swell during sleep. This puts more pressure on the nerve.

Permanent damage can occur if the pressure on the nerve isn't treated.

**Carpal tunnel syndrome.** This entrapment syndrome affects the *median nerve.* The median nerve runs to your thumb, index and middle fingers through a tunnel in the wrist called the *carpal tunnel.* Pressure on this nerve as it passes through the carpal tunnel can lead to numbness, tingling, and pain in the thumb and index and middle fingers. It can also sometimes lead to weakness of the thumb. Sometimes pain can extend upward from the hand into the forearm. One or both hands may be affected. See page 257 for more information about carpal tunnel syndrome.

**Compartment syndrome.** This occurs when muscles swell slightly during exercise and press on the nerves. This muscle swelling can compress nerves and blood vessels in the forearm or lower leg, causing painful cramps. The cramps usually subside when the muscles are rested. Surgery may be needed to release the pressure for people with chronic swelling. This procedure, called a *fasciotomy,* is particularly common in treating compartment syndrome affecting the front of the lower leg.

**Sciatica.** This is a compression syndrome of the *sciatic nerve,* which runs from the spine to the buttocks and down the back of the leg. Often the cause of compression on the sciatic nerve is a herniated disk (p. 000). For more information about sciatica, see p. 247.

**Tarsal tunnel syndrome.** This occurs when a nerve in the foot is pinched. This can lead to numbness in the toes, or the ball or sole of the foot, along with an aching or burning pain.

**Ulnar nerve entrapment.** This occurs when the ulnar nerve is pinched where it runs through the elbow. The result can be numbness of the ring finger, little finger and thumb.

### Testing

Testing depends on the nerve that's involved. Nerve conduction studies (p. 638) may show where the problem is located. Blood tests may also be used to rule out other problems that could contribute to swelling and irritation of the nerve.

### Treatment

Using the affected area less, either by changing habits or positions or by using a wrist splint or other aids, can give the tissues time to shrink so the nerve can heal. Resting an injury in the early stages isn't always easy if your job requires movement or if you're an athlete, but it's the best way to prevent further or ongoing damage.

Oral anti-inflammatory medicines (p. 615) reduce pain but are often not helpful in reducing the nerve swelling. Corticosteroid injections or surgery are other possible therapies when the entrapment is more severe and doesn't respond to simpler treatment.

---

## Preventing Entrapment Syndromes

- Cut down on alcohol and quit smoking if you smoke.
- Lose weight if you're overweight.
- Get treatment for any disease that may lead to entrapment syndromes, such as diabetes (p. 211) and rheumatoid arthritis (p. 231).

- Take frequent, regular breaks from activities that require repetitive movements.
- Don't sit or stand in the same position all day.
- If you type or do data entry, adjust your chair so that your forearms are level with your keyboard.

Preventing
Head Injuries

- Wear head
  protection when
  you're riding a
  motorcycle or
  bicycle, or doing
  anything in which
  your head could be
  hit or struck, such
  as with a baseball.
- Wear seat belts if
  you're in a car.
- Don't dive into
  water unless it's
  deep enough and
  clear enough that
  you can see there
  is nothing in
  your way.

## Concussions and Contusions

- Brief fainting spells, headache, a
  dazed feeling, amnesia, confusion,
  nausea and vomiting after a blow to
  the head

Many activities can result in a head injury: being tackled in football, falling off a bicycle, slipping on the stairs, even bumping the head while getting into the car. When the brain is bounced inside the bony skull, some of the tissues may become bruised or swollen.

A *concussion* is a jarring injury to the brain. It can be diagnosed when loss of consciousness occurs at the time of a head injury and is followed by mild symptoms that persist for hours to days with no permanent results. A *contusion* means that the brain tissue has been bruised, which can be very serious if the bruising affects a large or critical area of the brain.

Headaches, irritability, bad dreams, trouble sleeping and even some personality changes may follow a head injury. This is called *post-concussion syndrome*. These symptoms go away within weeks to months. More serious head injuries, including contusions, may result in permanent damage to the nerves, emotional problems and personality changes. A serious head injury can cause a coma (p. 48) that lasts for hours, days or weeks. Persistent confusion, speech problems, paralysis, seizures or coma after a head injury suggest that nerve damage, personality changes, and depression and other emotional problems are more likely to follow.

### Testing

Anyone who has lost consciousness, or has numbness, weakness, confusion or drowsiness after a head injury should be seen by a doctor. X-rays, a CT scan (p. 632) or an MRI scan (p. 637) of the head may be needed.

### Treatment

Fortunately, most concussions and contusions don't cause any lasting problems. Treatment can be given to reduce swelling in the brain and minimize long-term damage. Surgery may be needed in about 2% of cases to drain the blood or repair a torn blood vessel.

## Friedreich's Ataxia

- Loss of speech
- Loss of coordination and balance
- Loss of use of the arms and hands

*Friedreich's ataxia* is a rare, inherited neurologic disease. Friedreich's ataxia affects people early in life—from age five to 15. The breakdown of certain nerves leads to increasing problems with speaking, balance and walking, and use of the arms and hands. No treatments or cures are available. If you have Friedreich's ataxia, you may want to get genetic counseling so you can consider the chances of passing it on to your children.

## Guillain-Barré Syndrome

- Muscle weakness, usually
  beginning with the legs and
  moving to the arms

*Guillain-Barré syndrome* is a condition in which the nerves break down, apparently due to an immune reaction following infection, surgery or immunization. It's like the body has an immune reaction to itself—as though the body doesn't recognize its tissues as its own.

Symptoms usually begin five days to three weeks after an infection, surgery or immunization. Weakness may worsen until it leads to complete paralysis.

People who have Guillain-Barré syndrome require hospital care for intravenous fluids so they don't get dehydrated, help with breathing and physical therapy. Special transfusions, called *plasmapheresis*, may be needed. Most people recover completely over a period of months, but about one-third of people still have weakness three years later.

## Headache

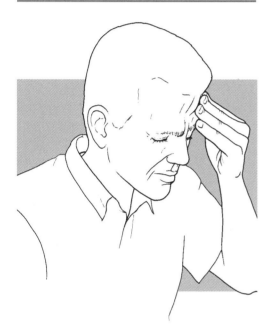

### Cluster Headache

- Sharp, burning, intense pain
- Pain on only one side of the head
- Pain in the eyes or temples
- Watery eyes
- Pupils that shrink
- Drooping of one or both eyelids
- Occurs in groups, or "clusters"

*Cluster headaches* occur in groups— every day for a week or more at a time. The headaches usually start at night. Each headache may last from 15 minutes to three hours. Cluster headaches usually occur once or twice a year. They usually affect older men and often run in families. Once a cluster

period has started, any change in sleep patterns, such as taking a nap, may bring on a headache. Drinking alcohol may also bring on a headache during this period.

### Migraine Headache

- Throbbing or dull aching pain on one or both sides of the head
- Changes in vision, such as blurred vision or blind spots
- Being bothered by light, sounds and smells
- Confusion
- Feeling tired
- Nausea, vomiting, diarrhea

*Migraine headaches* may be caused partly by dilating, or expanding, blood vessels in the brain. In addition to headache pain, migraines may cause nausea and vomiting. Migraines can also cause confusion, lightheadedness and fatigue. Someone with a migraine may be bothered by light, sounds and smells. Migraine headaches aren't usually dangerous.

*Classic migraines* start with an *aura,* or *prodrome.* An aura is a 10- to 15-minute period when the person sees spots or flashing lights, or his or her face becomes numb. The aura usually occurs before the head pain starts. The pain that follows the aura is often sharp and throbbing, and comes on suddenly. Classic migraines account for about 10% of all migraines. The other 90% of migraines don't have a prodrome. These are called *common migraines.* They may start more slowly than classic migraines and last longer. They may interfere more with your daily activities. The pain of both classic and common migraine headaches may occur on only one side of the head.

Migraines seem to run in families. In some people, migraines are triggered by caffeine, foods that are high in

### Foods That May Trigger Migraine Headaches

- Aged cheeses
- Aged, canned, cured or processed meat
- Avocados
- Brewer's yeast
- Caffeine
- Chocolate
- Cultured dairy products
- Lentils
- Luncheon meats, cured meats and other foods containing nitrates
- Monosodium glutamate (MSG)
- Pickled, preserved or marinated foods
- Raisins
- Sauerkraut
- Seasoned salt
- Wine

## Migraine Without Pain

Some people with migraines don't have headaches. Instead, they have symptoms called *migraine equivalents*. These include recurrent numbness, weakness on one side of the body, dizziness, seizure-like spells, nausea and vomiting. These symptoms should be checked by your doctor. If the symptoms are caused by a migraine equivalent, medicine used for classic migraine headaches may help prevent them.

salt, and foods containing nitrates or monosodium glutamate (MSG). See the box at left for a list of foods that may trigger migraine headaches in some people.

### Muscle Tension Headaches
- Dull, squeezing or aching pain around the temples or all over the head
- Tenderness or tightness in the back of the neck and head

These headaches produce dull pain that usually comes on slowly and may last for hours if left untreated. Muscle tension headaches are caused by tense or tight muscles in the scalp, face or neck. Stress, anxiety, tiredness, temporomandibular joint syndrome (p. 252), illness, fever and fatigue from concentrating for long periods are common causes of muscle tension headaches. Whatever the cause, these headaches eventually pass without causing any ongoing problems or disabilities. Most people get them from time to time.

Some headaches may start as a migraine and then become like a muscle tension headache. As the pain begins, the muscles in the scalp tense, and a muscle tension headache then mixes with the migraine.

### Sinus Headaches
- Pain in front part of head
- Pain worse in the morning
- Nasal congestion

Sinus headaches may accompany a viral illness, such as a cold (p. 322) or sinusitis (p. 89). The pain comes from a buildup of pressure in the sinus cavities, which aren't able to drain properly because of the illness or infection.

### Testing
The type of headache is usually apparent by the symptoms. If the symptoms don't make the diagnosis clear, other tests may be needed to make sure the headache isn't caused by something serious, such as bleeding in the brain (p. 45), a head injury (p. 50), meningitis (p. 302), encephalitis (p. 324) or a brain tumor (p. 47). Tests may include blood tests, vision tests and a CT scan (p. 632) of the head in some cases.

### Treatment
The pain of most headaches is relieved by over-the-counter analgesic medicines (p. 614).

The pain of migraine headaches may require prescription medicines (p. 614). These medicines should be taken right when symptoms start to help prevent the pain from getting any worse.

If the pain doesn't ease, a narcotic analgesic (p. 618) may be needed. People who take narcotics can become addicted to the medicine. So narcotics must be used very carefully.

### Prevention
Regular exercise, a nutritious diet and getting enough sleep all help to prevent or reduce stress-related headaches. Maintaining good muscle tone in the neck and back can also help.

Taking breaks to stretch the neck and back during long periods of sitting, and resting the eyes every 30 to 60 minutes when driving, reading or working at a desk or computer can help. Avoid foods that seem to trigger migraine headaches.

Over-the-counter or prescription medicines can be taken to prevent severe, frequent headaches. Over-the-counter medicines include analgesics (p. 614). Prescription medicines include regular headache medicines (p. 615), beta blockers (p. 621) and calcium channel blockers (p. 621).

## Huntington's Chorea

- Mental deterioration
- Personality changes
- Jerky movements

*Huntington's chorea* is inherited and affects both men and women. Symptoms usually begin between age 35 and 50. It can be diagnosed through a CT scan (p. 632) of the brain. While medicines can help suppress the jerky movements, there is no known cure. Special tests can now show if the trait has been inherited. Children of an affected parent have a 50% risk of having Huntington's chorea. If you have a family history of Huntington's chorea, talk to your doctor about genetic testing. You have a risk of passing it on to your children.

## Memory Problems

- Trouble remembering things

Many people become a little forgetful as they get older, but a rapid loss of memory usually indicates a serious problem.

**Amnesia.** This is the loss of the ability to remember. It may be the result of health problems or life events, rather than a disease in itself. It may be a result of damage to the brain from injuries, including head injury (p. 50) or stroke (p. 59), or a result of disease, such as alcohol or chronic drug abuse, or psychologic trauma or stress.

**Dementia.** This is a progressive, permanent decline in all mental ability, including memory. It may also be caused by a head injury, stroke, brain tumor (p. 47) or a degenerative condition of the brain, such as Alzheimer's disease.

*Alzheimer's disease* first causes the person to lose new, or short-term, memories. Many people with early Alzheimer's disease become forgetful—unable to remember where they put their keys or forgetting the way home from a place they don't go often. As Alzheimer's disease progresses, the forgetfulness becomes worse. The person may be confused, lose older memories, become irritable, or have a personality change. The person may not be able to engage in conversation with others. In the later stages of Alzheimer's disease, the person has problems with simple, everyday functions, such as taking a bath or eating, and totally loses interest in any activities. Later, stiffness and trouble moving can occur. Death usually results from an infection or some other problem related to the physical debilitation. The entire process may take from two to 20 years.

Alzheimer's disease rarely begins before the age of 65. It becomes more common after age 65, and affects up to 30% of people after age 85. People who develop Alzheimer's disease before age 65 tend to get worse faster and have more severe symptoms.

For many people with dementia, symptoms will come on slowly and medicines won't help. One way to help the person with dementia is to organize surroundings and apply easy-to-read labels to frequently

*Reducing the Pain of Headaches*

- Lie in a dark, quiet room.
- Put a cold, wet cloth over your forehead.
- Massage your scalp.
- Put pressure on your temples.

*When to See the Doctor*

- You have severe head pain, or the pain is getting worse.
- You have any numbness, weakness, loss of vision or loss of one of your other senses.
- You have a high fever with vomiting.
- You have constant headaches.
- You have several headaches a week.

used items. Eventually, live-in supervision or a move into a nursing home may be needed to allow this person to function safely.

### Testing

A thorough physical exam should be done to find any correctable causes of memory problems. Blood tests, x-rays and a CT scan (p. 632) or MRI scan (p. 637) of the head may help reveal treatable causes of memory problems. Psychological and memory tests can help assess the extent of memory loss.

### Prevention

A healthy diet and adequate rest and exercise can help preserve good health, including mental health. Some memory problems can be prevented. For example, memory problems caused by conditions such as vitamin $B_{12}$ deficiency (p. 134), depression (p. 587) or hypothyroidism (p. 217) can be reversed when the condition is treated.

The memory problems that can occur because of AIDS (p. 325) or because of damage to blood vessels, such as from diabetes (p. 211), high blood pressure (p. 123) or atherosclerosis (p. 111) can't be reversed. But some of these conditions can be prevented. For example, heart disease, diabetes or high blood pressure can be kept under control. If you're at risk for AIDS, following certain precautions (p. 325) can help prevent this infection.

Dementia caused by Alzheimer's disease can't be cured or prevented.

## Motion Sickness

- Nausea and vomiting
- Sweating or salivating
- Dizziness and headache

Some people have motion sickness when they travel by road, air or sea, or when they ride on a carousel or other carnival ride. The constant movement or vibration affects the balance mechanism in the inner ear. The condition is often made worse by fear, anxiety, fumes or a stuffy atmosphere. It may also be worse when the person is moving in relation to what they're looking at.

Motion sickness medicines (p. 625) can help reduce symptoms of motion sickness if taken before travel.

## Multiple Sclerosis

- Episodes of weakness with numbness or tingling in one area of the body, one arm or leg, or one side of the body
- Blurred vision
- Unsteadiness
- Loss of bladder control

The nerves in your body are coated with a fatty, insulating substance called *myelin,* which is like the insulation that covers an electrical wire. Myelin speeds the flow of impulses, or

---

### *Avoiding Motion Sickness*

- Keep your eyes on the distant scene, rather than on nearby objects.
- Don't try to read, because the page is a nearby object.
- Try not to fix your eyes on moving objects.
- Lie down, face up if possible.

- Avoid eating too much or drinking too much alcohol while traveling. Instead, eat simple foods and drink small amounts of fluids often during long travels.
- Open windows for fresh air if possible.

messages, from one end of the nerve to the other. In *multiple sclerosis* (MS), patches of the myelin covering break down, interfering with the messages between the brain and muscles.

Repeated MS attacks damage the nervous system and usually cause the person to be less able to function. Some people have one or two episodes and then have very little or no permanent damage. Others have bad and good periods, while generally losing function in a stair-step fashion with each episode. Still others have a steady downhill course over five to 30 years, with no break in the symptoms.

### Testing

Any weakness, numbness, tingling or loss of function should be checked by your doctor to identify the problem and to decide on the best treatment. The diagnosis of MS is usually made on the basis of medical history and an exam by your doctor or a neurologist. Blood and spinal fluid are usually tested to check for other possible causes of the symptoms. MRI scans (p. 637) and CT scans (p. 632) may be helpful.

### Treatment

Several medicines can reduce the symptoms related to the nerve damage, including muscle spasms. Physical therapy may help strengthen muscles, and various aids can be used to help people with MS get around and stay independent. Because MS can't be cured, the course of the disease depends more on factors such as nutrition, general stress level and other illnesses than on medical therapies.

The long-term outlook for people with MS is unpredictable. Between 25% and 30% of those with MS will have some disability relating to the nerve damage within five years.

# Neuropathy

- Numbness, tingling, pain or weakness

A type of damage to the *peripheral nerves*, which connect the brain and spinal cord with the rest of the body, is called *neuropathy*. Neuropathy reduces the nerves' ability to sense and transfer information. Neuropathy can result from certain industrial chemicals and insecticides, diabetes (p. 211), alcoholism (p. 562), and some vitamin deficiencies, such as $B_{12}$ or folic acid.

When peripheral neuropathy results in loss of feeling, other injuries and damage may result. For example, people with diabetes can develop diabetic neuropathy (p. 212). This puts them at higher risk for such problems as foot infections, in part because they may not feel the pain that normally would be a warning of a foot problem.

### Testing and Treatment

Neuropathy usually happens slowly. Symptoms often come on so gradually that they're ignored for months or even years. Because so many diseases can damage peripheral nerves, a careful search must be made to identify the cause. Blood tests may be helpful to find out if the cause is a nutritional deficiency or a toxin. Nerve conduction studies (p. 638) may be used to show the extent of the damage.

Nerve damage can sometimes be reversed, but not always. Medicines can reduce the pain from the inflamed and injured nerve.

### Prevention

Vitamin deficiencies, diabetes, alcoholism and chemicals used in industry and agriculture are the major causes of neuropathy. All of these causes can be prevented or controlled. Proper nutrition, control of diabetes and avoiding overuse of alcohol can all help prevent peripheral nerve damage.

## Parkinson's Disease

- Shaky hands (*tremor*) and trouble with other motions and balance
- Rigidity
- Loss of memory
- Trouble speaking and moving (late stage)

Symptoms of *Parkinson's disease* stem from a breakdown in a certain area of the brain. Many things are known about Parkinson's disease—such as where the defect in the brain occurs (in the brain stem), the changes that occur (damage to cells) and the problems that result (see signs above)—but *why* it happens is still not known.

Parkinson's disease usually affects older people, but not always. People with severe infections of the brain, or those who take medicine to treat psychosis, and even people who have some types of poisoning (such as carbon monoxide) may have symptoms of Parkinson's disease. Parkinson's disease can also be caused by using the designer drug called MPTP, a synthetic heroin. Most people with the disease, however, get it later in life for no known reason.

The disease starts with a "rest" tremor. For example, the hands may shake when they are at rest, but the tremor vanishes when the person moves. Later, the person's ability to walk may decrease. Instead of taking natural steps with swinging arms, he or she may need to take small, shuffling steps in a hunched-over position. Speaking and writing may become more difficult.

As with any ongoing disease, depression (p. 587) can worsen the symptoms of Parkinson's disease.

Crying spells, loss of appetite, loss of weight and not being able to enjoy favorite activities can be signs of depression.

### Testing

Blood tests and a CT scan (p. 632) or MRI scan (p. 637) of the brain, as well as other special tests, aren't always needed, but may help make the diagnosis of Parkinson's disease if the symptoms and an early exam don't give enough information. Tell your doctor if you're taking any medicines prescribed by a psychiatrist or another doctor.

### Treatment

A number of medicines are available to help reduce the symptoms of Parkinson's disease. Many new medicines are still being tested.

## Seizures

- Stiffening, twitching and jerking of the body
- Falling down
- Staring into space

One of the most misunderstood and frightening sights is a *seizure*, or *convulsion*, as seizures used to be called. Seizures result from problems with the electrical waves of the brain.

**Occasional seizures.** Occasional seizures can be brought on by illness. In babies and young children, fever may cause seizures. Fever-related seizures aren't caused by an underlying brain disorder. Similarly, very low blood sugar in people with diabetes (hypoglycemia, p. 216) may sometimes bring on a seizure.

**Epilepsy.** Epilepsy, on the other hand, is a disorder of the brain that causes recurrent episodes of seizures. Epilepsy seems to stem from nerve cells in the brain that are overly sensitive and release impulses abnormally, resulting in seizures. The exact cause of epilepsy is unknown in most people. In one out of three cases, the cause, such as a brain tumor, brain injury or possibly an infection around the brain or its coverings, can be identified.

*Focal seizures* are caused by an electrical problem in a limited area of the brain. A focal seizure affects the areas of the brain where motion is initiated or regulated. The person almost never loses consciousness and may have no warning of the attack. Symptoms depend on exactly what part of the brain is involved. For example, if the motor cortex is involved (*Jacksonian seizure*), the person may begin to shake or twitch in one small area, such as the fingers. The shaking may spread to the hand, wrist and forearm, and sometimes across the body. Sometimes, a Jacksonian seizure can spread to become a full grand mal seizure that includes loss of consciousness.

*Grand mal seizures* are shaking spells that affect the entire body. People who have epilepsy sometimes can tell when these episodes are coming. Some see lights. Others hear strange noises or think they smell burning rubber. Still others say they sense an *aura,* or a "strange feeling that comes over me." After this warning, they rapidly become unconscious and may fall to the ground. They may become stiff, arch their back and stop breathing. This is called the *tonic phase* of the seizure. Then they may relax and begin to jerk or twitch. This is called the *clonic phase* of the seizure.

Once the clonic phase is over, the person remains in a deep sleep, or *postictal* state, for a few minutes or as long as an hour. Some will awaken confused and combative. A few will urinate during the seizure because the bladder muscle may relax.

Of all the types of seizures, grand mal seizures have the greatest risk of serious injury or even death. The longer the tonic phase, when the person is unable to breathe, the more likely he or she will suffer from brain damage, or inhale saliva or food. The risk of problems becomes more likely the longer the seizures last, the more seizures that come one right after another and the more uncontrollable the episodes are in spite of medicine.

*Petit mal seizures* cause spells of losing consciousness. As its French name suggests, this type of seizure is "smaller" than grand mal seizures. Petit mal seizures occur mainly in childhood. They cause the child to "blank out." The child doesn't fall but for a brief period loses consciousness. The loss of consciousness is so brief that the child's eyes usually don't even close. The child may appear to be "staring" for a short time—from one to 30 seconds. When the seizure ends, no "sleeping" period follows, as with a grand mal seizure. Instead, the child awakens right away but isn't aware of what went on during the seizure.

*Temporal lobe seizures* can cause spells of strange behaviors. Before the seizure, the person may have an aura, or warning symptom, such as sensing the smell of burning rubber. He or she then may curse or laugh in sudden outbursts, or act totally out of character. Involuntary motions can occur, such as tongue moving or chewing motions. Temporal lobe seizures are short, usually lasting only a few seconds to half a minute.

### Testing

A single episode of a seizure related to a fever in a child isn't considered epilepsy. Epilepsy is defined as repeated seizures. Blood tests, a CT scan (p. 632), an MRI scan (p. 637) of the head and an electroencephalogram (p. 634) may be needed to diagnose epilepsy.

### Treatment

Depending on the type of seizures, one or more antiseizure medicines (p. 620) may be prescribed. Antiseizure medicines may reduce the number of seizures or completely stop the episodes. The better the control with medicine, the more activities will be possible and the less likely the seizures will interrupt activities. Doctors usually consider seizures to be under control if none has occurred for six months to a year. If the seizures aren't under control, the person shouldn't drive, operate machinery or perform any activity during which a seizure could endanger the person or others.

Regular blood testing is usually needed to check levels of antiseizure medicine in the blood. This helps ensure that enough medicine is in the person's body to reduce the seizures.

### Prevention

A severe head injury can lead to seizures. So can repeated head injuries, such as in sports. Wearing head protection during any activity that could cause a head injury protects against brain injury during an accident.

Most cases of epilepsy can't be prevented. Proper treatment—taking medicine as prescribed and checking blood levels of medicine—is the best way to reduce or prevent seizures in people with epilepsy.

## Spinal Cord Trauma

- Weakness, numbness, paralysis
- Loss of bladder or bowel control

All feeling and nerve impulses to control the muscles of the body flow through the spinal cord. The spinal cord is surrounded by a flexible canal of bone along with a cushion of fluid,

but severe stresses can still bruise and partly or totally sever the delicate cord. The damaged nerves can no longer send and receive messages. Sensations won't be felt and muscles can't be used in the area served by the damaged nerves. Both sides of the spinal cord are almost always damaged to some extent in a serious injury, although one side may be more affected than the other.

The course of recovery, or *rehabilitation,* following a spinal cord injury is long and difficult. It may take weeks to months. Personality and emotional changes, especially depression, often accompany severe injuries. Group support and individual counseling can help the person recover independence and deal with the psychological impact of the injury.

### Testing

A person who has a spinal cord injury should be transported to the hospital by people who are trained to do so, such as emergency medical technicians or paramedics. X-rays of the spine will be done to determine the extent of damage to the *vertebrae* (the bones surrounding the spinal cord). A CT scan (p. 632), MRI scan (p. 637) or myelogram (p. 638) may be done to check for damage to the cord itself.

### Treatment

The person may need surgery to relieve pressure on the spinal cord. A rehabilitation program will be designed to help the person recover as much function as possible.

## Spinal Cord Tumors

- Back or neck pain
- Tingling, weakness, numbness
- Loss of bowel or bladder control

Primary tumors that start in the spinal cord are very rare. They cause compression of the spinal cord within

---

### Preventing Spinal Cord Injuries

Accidents cause most cases of spinal cord damage. Never dive into a lake or the shallow end of a pool without knowing how deep the water is and what's under the surface. Always wear your seat belt while driving or riding in a car.

the bony spinal canal. X-rays, CT scans (p. 632) or MRI scans (p. 637) can locate the tumor, or mass. Further studies, such as a myelogram (p. 638), may be needed to see the extent of the mass.

An operation can be performed to remove the tumor or relieve the pressure on the spinal cord. Radiation therapy (p. 225) can slow tumor growth and relieve pain and pressure. Rarely, chemotherapy (p. 225) is used, depending on the type of tumor.

## Stroke

- Headache or confusion
- Problems with hearing or sight
- Trouble speaking, writing or understanding
- Sudden weakness
- Numbness or loss of feeling
- Loss of consciousness or coma

A *stroke* is caused by a blood clot or another type of blockage in a blood vessel to the brain. Oxygen in the blood is cut off to the brain and, as a result, the area of the brain supplied by that blood vessel is damaged and may die. Sometimes, when the blood supply is stopped for just a few minutes, the brain tissue is injured but recovers within a few hours or a few days. Other times, when the blood supply is stopped for a longer period, the injury is more severe, and the brain tissue doesn't recover.

Blockages of the blood supply to the brain can be caused by a blood

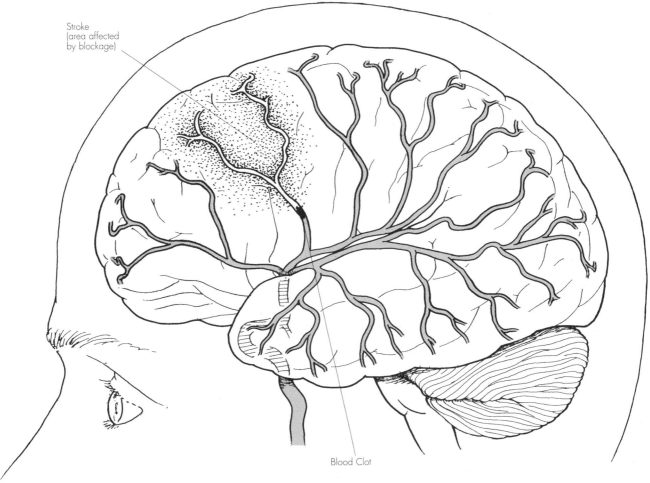

Stroke
(area affected
by blockage)

Blood Clot

**STROKE DUE TO BLOCKAGE**

clot or by a buildup of cholesterol on the walls of a blood vessel (atherosclerosis, p. 111). These blockages can cut off oxygen to the brain and cause a stroke or a *transient ischemic attack* (TIA). A TIA is a ministroke that occurs when oxygen to part of the brain is cut off for a short time. The blockage is usually due to a blood clot or a piece of cholesterol that breaks off from the wall of an artery and becomes stuck in a blood vessel in the brain. Air and fat particles in the bloodstream can also block an artery to the brain.

Symptoms of a blockage can include loss of consciousness, vision, hearing or the ability to speak, or numbness, weakness, paralysis or dizziness. If the symptoms pass within minutes to hours, the attack was probably due to a TIA and the damage won't be permanent. But TIAs are often a warning that a stroke may occur in the future.

Lack of oxygen to the brain causes a part of the brain to die. Anyone who has a sudden and severe headache, stiff neck, drowsiness, fainting, or trouble speaking, seeing or hearing should be seen right away by a doctor. *This is an emergency.*

### Testing

CT scans (p. 632) and MRI scans (p. 637) of the head can show the location and sometimes the extent of the damage to the brain, but they can't show if the brain will recover.

### Treatment

Treatment depends on the cause of the stroke, its severity and the age and health of the person.

Rapid treatment with medicines can dissolve a clot and keep the damage to a minimum. Blood-thinning medicines (p. 619) may prevent repeat episodes in the near future.

Many people who have a stroke are left with problems ranging from permanent weakness or numbness to loss of speech, sight, hearing, or ability to move one or both arms or legs. A few people won't come out of a coma. But most strokes are treatable to a point. Physical therapy, speech therapy and other measures can help people who have had a stroke regain the functions that they lost. Some people recover completely.

### Prevention

High blood pressure (p. 123) is a common cause of strokes and one that can be controlled. High blood sugar in people who have diabetes (p. 211) and high blood cholesterol are risk factors for clots. Early detection and treatment of high blood pressure, high cholesterol and blood sugar levels helps prevent strokes. Unfortunately, many people don't know their blood pressure, cholesterol or blood sugar levels are high.

Smoking contributes to atherosclerosis, which damages the arteries and may lead to clots and stroke. So not starting to smoke or quitting smoking can help prevent strokes.

Atherosclerosis of the carotid artery of the neck, which carries blood to the brain, is a major cause of stroke. *Carotid artery endarterectomy* is a procedure that cleans the plaques, or cholesterol buildup, out of the carotid artery. Carotid artery endarterectomy can be helpful in reducing the risk of stroke in people who have transient ischemic attacks.

---

### *Preventing Strokes*

- Keep your blood pressure under control.
- Keep your blood sugar level under control if you have diabetes.
- Keep your blood cholesterol level within a healthy range.
- Quit smoking or don't start.

## Trigeminal Neuralgia

• Pain, numbness or tingling on one side of the face

*Neuralgia* is pain that results from damage to or irritation of a nerve. Any of the peripheral nerves—in the face and head or the rest of the body—can be involved.

One of the more well-known types of neuralgia is *trigeminal neuralgia.* It involves a nerve in the face, called the *trigeminal nerve.* Trigeminal neuralgia can cause intense, sharp, shooting or burning pain in the face over the eye, on the cheek, on the jaw or in the mouth. The pain is brief—lasting seconds to minutes. It's often brought on by touching a "trigger point" on the face, for example, when washing or shaving. This painful condition usually occurs in people over age 50. The exact cause of trigeminal neuralgia isn't known.

### Testing

A physical exam and medical history often provide enough information to diagnose trigeminal neuralgia. Other tests may be ordered if the diagnosis is in doubt.

### Treatment

Pain-reducing medicine is often the only treatment needed for trigeminal neuralgia. Injecting the nerve with cortisone may also relieve the pain. Rarely, the pain is so severe that other types of injections may be used to numb or destroy the nerve. If the injections don't relieve the pain enough, the nerve can sometimes be destroyed surgically.

Certain antiseizure medicines (p. 620) have shown some benefit in people with trigeminal neuralgia who have severe pain that is not helped with pain-reducing medicines.

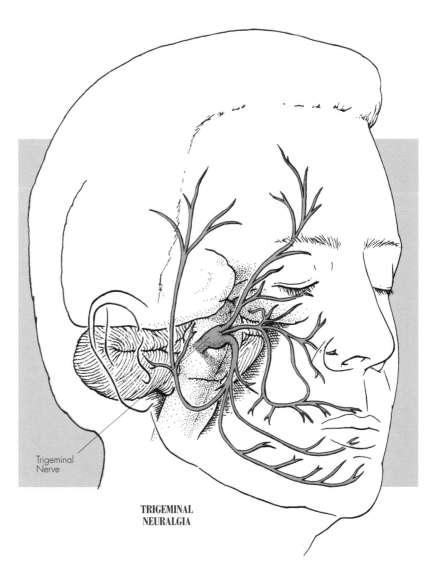

Trigeminal Nerve

**TRIGEMINAL
NEURALGIA**

## Tourette Syndrome

• Moving or jerking without meaning to
• Speaking, shouting or cursing without meaning to

*Tourette syndrome* is an inherited disorder that usually begins during childhood as small tics and grimaces and gets worse. These symptoms may progress to outbursts of grunting or barking and to foul language. The condition is more common in males. Medicines that may be used to help reduce tics in some people who have Tourette syndrome include pimozide (p. 625) and haloperidol (p. 625). Some sedatives (p. 626) can also be used. Tourette syndrome has no cure.

# CHAPTER 2  EYES

The eyes are the body's window to the world. Through a complex process, your eyes send messages to your brain about the shape and size of things around you, about colors, and about lightness and darkness.

The *iris* is the colored part of the eye. The *pupil* is the black circle in the center of the iris. The iris expands and contracts to control the size of the pupil and, thus, how much light enters through the pupil. The *cornea* is the clear coating that covers the iris and pupil. It focuses light through the *lens* to the retina. The lens is a clear disk that lies behind the iris and pupil. It also focuses light on the retina.

The *retina* is a membrane that lines the inside of the back of the eyeball. It's where images of what you see are focused. The retina is made up of nerve cells. Some of the nerve cells are sensitive to colors and light (*cone cells*), and others are sensitive to degrees of light and dark (*rod cells*). The retina has many more rod cells than cone cells. This is why it's easy for you to tell lightness from darkness, but you need

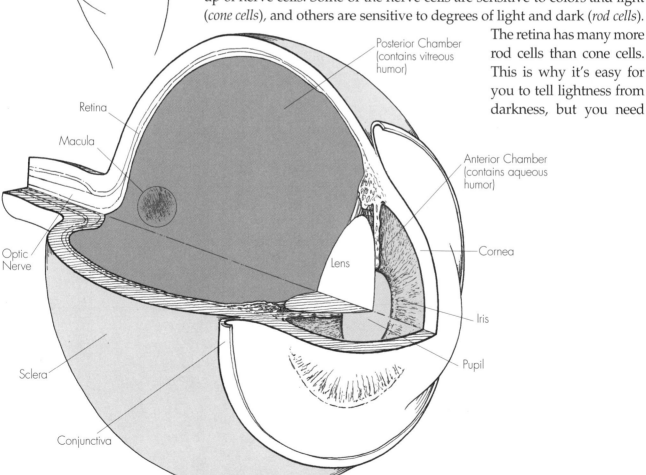

Retina

Macula

Optic Nerve

Sclera

Conjunctiva

Posterior Chamber (contains vitreous humor)

Anterior Chamber (contains aqueous humor)

Cornea

Lens

Iris

Pupil

**ANATOMY OF THE EYE**

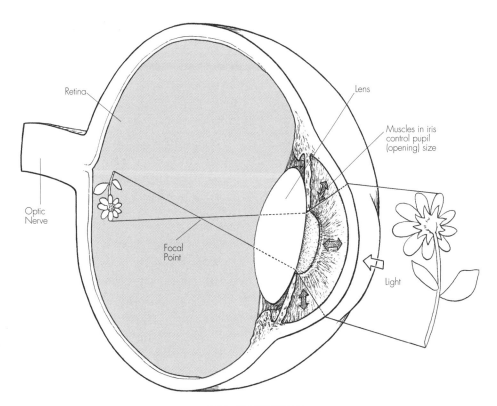

Retina

Lens

Muscles in iris
control pupil
(opening) size

Optic
Nerve

Focal
Point

Light

**FUNCTION OF THE EYE**

more light to see colors. The *macula* is the central part of the retina. It has the highest collection of rod cells and is responsible for detailed vision, or *visual acuity.* The images picked up by the retina are sent to the brain through the *optic nerve.* The images come to the brain upside-down. The brain then interprets these images as they really are, so that you perceive, or "see" them right-side-up.

Other parts of the eye include the *sclera* (the white part of the eye), the *conjunctiva* (the membrane that covers the sclera and the lining of the eyelid), the *vitreous humor* (the jelly-like substance that fills the space in the eyeball called the *posterior chamber*) and the *aqueous humor* (the watery fluid that fills the space between the cornea and the lens, called the *anterior chamber*).

## Black Eye

- Bruising around the eye
- Pain and swelling of or around the eyelids

Even a small injury can cause a bruise in the soft tissues near the eye, called a *black eye.* The black-and-blue markings around the eye are caused by bleeding underneath the skin.

### Testing and Treatment

A black eye alone doesn't necessarily mean that the eyeball is damaged. But if blood is in the eye itself or if vision is changed in any way, the eye should be checked right away by a doctor.

Most black eyes can be treated with ice packs to reduce the swelling. With more serious injuries and when vision is affected, the doctor may order x-rays of the skull, giving special attention to the bones around the eye. These bones are known as the *orbit.* Surgical repair of the orbit or facial bones may be required if they're fractured.

### Prevention

Protect your eyes with goggles, safety glasses or shields designed for your sport or work. Safety shields will help prevent debris from getting in your eyes, and they help prevent black eyes as well.

# Blepharitis

- Redness or swelling and sometimes scaling of the edge of the eyelid

*See photo of blepharitis, page 265.*

People who are prone to eczema or seborrhea (p. 289) often have *blepharitis,* a condition in which the skin at the edge of the eyelid becomes irritated and painful. The eyelid may be red, scaly and swollen. The eyelid may become infected with bacteria, leading to the development of small ulcers and more pain.

### Treatment

Blepharitis is usually easy to treat. Daily self-treatment includes gently scrubbing the scales away with a warm damp washcloth. Antibiotic ointment will probably be prescribed. Eye drops may also be prescribed. Holding a warm damp washcloth over your eye for a few minutes several times each day can help relieve the irritation. Blepharitis may persist or recur, with or without medical treatment.

# Cataracts

- Decreasing vision, usually with aging
- Cloudiness of the lens of the eye

*See photo of cataract, page 265.*

*Cataracts* are a common eye problem. This vision-impairing condition usually, but not always, occurs in older people. Previous injuries to the eye, previous eye infections and diabetes (p. 211) are all potential causes of cataracts. Generally, as people age, the proteins in their lenses begin to *coagulate,* or become sticky. The coagulated proteins cause the normally clear lens

to become cloudy. Vision becomes blurry. Cataracts aren't painful. The changes in vision may occur so slowly that the person doesn't at first notice any difference in vision.

Sometimes babies are born with cataracts *(congenital cataracts).* This can be caused by chromosomal abnormalities or by infections the mother had during her pregnancy.

### Testing

The cataract may be found during a routine physical exam when the doctor checks the eyes. Regular eye exams are especially important for people with diabetes. Causes other than aging should be considered whenever cataracts occur, especially in younger people.

### Treatment

Cataracts can be removed under local or general anesthesia. An artificial lens implant can be put into the eye, or the person can wear eyeglasses or contact lenses to correct the vision problem. Vision testing helps determine if the cloudy lens should be removed. Cataracts generally should be removed as soon as possible in children because they can hinder a child's ability to develop normal vision.

# Color Blindness

- Confusing the colors red and green

Color blindness occurs when there is a problem with the cone cells—the light- and color-sensitive cells—in your eyes. Red and green are usually the colors that are involved. They are seen as the same color. Some people who are color blind only have problems in dim light. Color blindness is much more common in males than in females. It's hereditary. Color blindness usually doesn't cause any serious problems.

## Corneal Ulcer/Infection

- Pain
- White patch on the cornea
- Redness in the sclera
- Blurred vision
- Being bothered by light

An ulcer on the cornea often begins with an injury of the eye or with a condition that causes marked dryness of the eyes. It can also result from poor nutrition, especially vitamin A or protein deficiency. The ulcer may become infected with a bacteria, virus or fungus. Left untreated, this small infection can lead to widespread infection throughout the eye, scarring of the cornea and vision loss.

### Testing

Special stains can be placed in the eye to make the ulcer easier to see and to outline its shape. Seeing the ulcer better is helpful to the doctor in determining what's causing the infection. An exam with a slit lamp (p. 641) may also be needed.

### Treatment

Bacterial infections of the cornea are usually treated with antibiotic drops and ointments, or with oral antibiotics. Viral infections can be treated with antiviral medicine (p. 621), and fungal infections with topical and oral antifungal medicines (p. 615). Serious infections of the cornea or eyeball are treated in a hospital.

### Prevention

Infection from a sore on another part of the body can easily be carried to the eye on unwashed hands. This can happen with the virus that causes cold sores (p. 94). Washing hands carefully after touching an infected area or changing the dressing on an infection will help prevent the spread of infection to the eyes.

## Crossed Eyes

- An eye or eyes that turn in or out
- An eye that wanders

Very young infants sometimes appear to have crossed eyes. This is normal because their eyes aren't yet focusing on specific objects. Very young infants sometimes have an extra fold of skin from the nose to the middle of each eye. This skin fold makes the eyes look crossed even though they are moving and focusing together. As the nose develops, the fold of skin disappears, and the eyes no longer look crossed.

As the infant grows, a consistently crossed eye can become a problem, because the child will begin to use only one eye for vision. This is called *strabismus*. The brain "turns off," or ignores the visual messages of the crossed eye. The eye that quits working is sometimes called a "lazy eye."

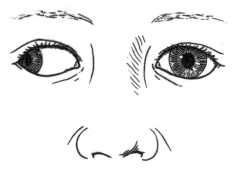

**STRABISMUS**

The muscles that move the eyes are the problem in children with crossed eyes. The problem may be due to differences in the strength or length of these muscles. A child with crossed eyes should have his or her eyes checked as soon as the problem is noticed. The sooner strabismus is diagnosed and treated, the more successful the treatment.

### Testing and Treatment

Special tests can show how the child focuses on various objects. Your doctor may have your child wear a patch over the good eye to make the lazy eye work and the brain begin to communicate with it again. Eye exercises and special glasses may also be used. In some cases, surgery may be needed to lengthen or shorten the eye muscles.

## Double Vision

- Seeing two images when only one is present

Double vision, or *diplopia,* occurs when one eye doesn't focus on the same thing as the other eye. This can sometimes happen to people who have crossed eyes (p. 65). It can also be caused by diseases or disorders that affect the nerves or muscles of the eye. Double vision should always be checked by your doctor.

## Dry Eyes

- Not enough tears in the eyes
- Burning in the eyes
- Mucus in the eyes
- Being bothered by light

Dry eyes can be a condition in itself or can be caused by other disorders and by some medicines. One fairly common cause of dry eyes is Sjögren's syndrome (p. 250), an arthritis-like condition. Dry eyes are more common later in age, and are more common in women, especially after menopause.

The dryness can usually be treated by using artificial tears or eye drops. Using a humidifier in the home to help keep the air moist and avoiding wind to help prevent the tears from evaporating may also help. Sometimes, surgery may be needed to close off the ducts that normally drain the tears away. This surgery can help the eyes stay moist.

## Eyelid Lumps

- A lump, skin tag, flat yellow patch or round reddish bump on the eyelid

Noncancerous lumps on the eyelid are quite common. There are many types, and each type looks different.

**Angiomas.** These are reddish, slightly raised, rounded lesions on the lid, usually present from birth.

*See photo of chalazion, page 266.*

**Chalazions.** These are caused by blockage of a mucous gland under the eye *(meibomian cysts).* They're painless swellings. Chalazions range in size from a BB to a pea. As with most blocked glands, mucus production will usually stop within a few weeks, and the chalazion will shrink within one to two months. Chalazions that don't go away on their own may be removed surgically for cosmetic reasons.

*See photo of papillomas, page 266.*

**Papillomas.** These are very small, soft growths of skin that often occur in bunches. They range from flesh-colored to dark brown. They're a cosmetic nuisance but are otherwise harmless.

**Xanthelasmas.** These are flat, yellowish growths under the skin of the lower lid, often near the nose. They are caused by fatty deposits under the skin, which give them their yellowish tinge. High cholesterol levels in the blood may be the source of these deposits. People who have xanthelasmas should have their cholesterol levels checked. These lesions may be removed for cosmetic reasons.

## Eyelid Weakness

- Drooping of the lower eyelid, often chronic

- Drooping of the upper lid

With aging, the lower eyelid may sag outward (*ectropion*) or it may fall inward toward the eye (*entropion*). Either condition can irritate or dry the sensitive tissues of the cornea, leading to infection in the lid, the conjunctiva and the cornea. With entropion, the eyelashes will also irritate the cornea, causing the constant sensation that something is in your eye.

*Ptosis* is another type of eyelid drooping. It's caused by weakness or dysfunction in the muscle or nerve of the upper lid. Many causes, such as birth injuries, diabetes (p. 211), multiple sclerosis (p. 54) and other muscle diseases, can lead to upper-lid weakness.

### Testing and Treatments

An operation can correct the weakness and prevent the eyelid from sagging. If the upper lid is affected, testing can identify the cause for the ptosis. Surgery may be needed to correct the ptosis.

## Focusing Problems

- Unclear vision of distant or near objects, or both

Many people have problems focusing their eyes. While some of these problems appear during infancy or childhood, most people begin having them when they reach age 40 to 50.

**Astigmatism.** Astigmatism is when the curvature of the cornea is unequal. The cornea normally helps focus the light as it enters the eye. When the curvature isn't equal, the cornea can't focus light evenly on the retina, and objects both near and far are blurry. Glasses or contact lenses with special curvatures can correct astigmatism. These can be hard lenses or special soft lenses. Regular soft contacts don't work as well with astigmatism because they mold to the shape of the cornea.

**Farsightedness.** Also called *hyperopia*, this is when objects in the distance are clearer than objects that are close. This condition occurs when there is too little distance between the lens and the light-sensitive retina at the back of the eyeball. As light comes through the cornea and lens, it's focused on the retina. Farsighted people need an additional lens (in the form of glasses or contact lenses) in front of the eye to focus a sharper image on the retina.

**Nearsightedness.** Also called *myopia*, this is when there is too much distance between the lens and the retina to focus a clear image. Again, glasses or contact lenses can usually correct this problem.

**Presbyopia.** This is when the lenses in the eyes become stiff and less able to change focus—mainly for near vision. Around age 40 to 45, many people suddenly find that they need glasses for reading. Over the next few years, the eyes may need increasing help for close vision, particularly in poor light.

### *Ophthalmologist vs. Optometrist: What's the Difference?*

An *optometrist* is qualified to examine eyes for focusing problems and to prescribe lenses (glasses or contacts) to correct vision problems, as well as eye exercises to help certain other problems. But since an optometrist isn't a doctor, he or she doesn't prescribe medicine or do surgery. An *ophthalmologist* is a doctor who specializes in the health of eyes. An ophthalmologist can prescribe lenses and exercises to help with vision problems and can also prescribe medicine and do surgery.

### Testing

An optometrist or ophthalmologist can test for focusing problems. Vision testing can determine the degree of nearsightedness, farsightedness, astigmatism or presbyopia and help the optometrist or ophthalmologist decide the best way to correct the problem.

### Treatment

Glasses or contact lenses can usually help improve focusing problems. *Radial keratotomy*, surgery to change the curvature of the cornea, has been helpful for some people but not for others. It is worth getting a second opinion from another ophthalmologic surgeon before having this procedure.

## Foreign Substances in the Eye

- Redness and tearing
- Irritation or a feeling that something is still in the eye even after it has been removed
- Pain

*See photo of corneal abrasion, page 265.*

You have probably experienced the discomfort of having a fleck of dirt in your eye. Even tiny particles can be very irritating. If the irritation continues, it's likely that the speck has scratched the cornea. This is called a *corneal abrasion.* The cornea can also be scratched by contact lenses. Chemicals splashed into the eye can cause damage and scarring to the cornea and surrounding area.

### Testing and Treatment

The eye's reaction to foreign substances is excessive tearing, which is your body's attempt to wash the foreign substance out of the eye. Similarly, holding the eye open under a gentle flow of running water may relieve the irritation by washing out the chemical or foreign body. If a caustic chemical has been splashed into the eye, washing it out right away can prevent loss of vision.

If the irritation continues after removal of a particle, or if a chemical has splashed into the eye and washing has not relieved all the irritation, see your doctor promptly.

A scratched cornea may be treated with antibiotic (p. 615) drops to help prevent an infection. A patch is usually applied for one or two days to keep the eye protected.

Sharp objects such as glass or metal may penetrate the eye. Any type of penetrating injury to the eye is an emergency that should be seen right away by an ophthalmologist.

In some cases, x-rays and CT scans (p. 632) of the head may be needed to find an object that has penetrated the eye. Prompt removal of the object and repair of damaged eye structures can prevent loss of vision and infection.

### Prevention

Always wear eye protection when doing anything that could throw debris or splash chemicals into the eye. Welding, mulching and sawing wood are examples of tasks that could easily cause an eye injury. Be particularly careful around power tools.

We don't usually think of a sand pile as a dangerous place. All children like to throw sand, and bits of sand can be hazardous to the eyes. Teach youngsters not to throw objects or dust or to poke at anyone's eyes.

## Glaucoma

- Blurred vision
- Pain and redness in the eye
- Seeing halos around lights

As do other organs in your body, your eyes have their own circulatory system. A watery fluid called the *aqueous humor* normally circulates

### Seeing Spots or "Floaters"

You may sometimes see specks or bits of what appear to be string or hair float slowly across your field of vision. This is normal. These bits of tissue are part of the *vitreous*, the jelly-like substance that fills the eyeball. Sometimes these bits of the vitreous break away and float across your vision. They are harmless and will go away eventually.

from the *ciliary body* behind the iris to fill the *anterior chamber*—the space between the cornea and the lens—and then drains out through a narrow canal called *Schlemm's canal.*

In people who have *glaucoma,* fluid can't drain from the anterior chamber of the eye because the Schlemm's canal is blocked. This causes pressure to build in the anterior chamber and can also cause pressure in the *posterior chamber*—the space inside the eyeball. This, in turn, can put pressure on the retina and optic nerve. The pressure causes the damage by reducing the flow of blood—and the oxygen and nutrients the blood brings with it—to the eye.

Glaucoma may develop slowly over a number of years, resulting in *chronic glaucoma,* which slowly damages vision. Usually, peripheral vision is lost first, meaning that the view gradually shrinks from the outside. Glaucoma may also happen quickly, causing sudden pain, redness and blurred vision. This form is called *acute glaucoma.*

Untreated glaucoma, especially the chronic type, is the most common and preventable cause of blindness in the elderly. Because the early symptoms are so minor and come on so slowly, some vision may be permanently lost before the problem is discovered and treated. The more pressure within the eye, the more damage occurs.

Glaucoma can also occur in newborn babies. This is called *congenital glaucoma.* It usually affects only one eye, causing that eye to enlarge and the cornea to become milky in color and bulge. This condition can lead to blindness if not treated.

### Testing

If you or a family member has signs of acute glaucoma, call your doctor or eye specialist or go to an emergency room right away. The pressure in your eye will need to be measured. One very common method of measuring the pressure uses what is known as the "air-puff" machine.

### Treatment

Acute glaucoma is rare, but it can be very serious. Often the person is admitted to a hospital where special techniques are available to reduce the pressure in the eye quickly. Otherwise vision could be lost completely and permanently. Surgical rerouting of the fluid through a new hole in the iris *(iridectomy)* can be done with local anesthesia. Medicines (p. 624) can also be given to prevent the pressure from building up again.

Chronic glaucoma is treated with oral medicine or medicine in eye-drops to help open the drainage areas around the iris and to reduce the pressure in the eye. If the medicines don't help, an iridectomy can be performed to reroute the fluid.

### Prevention

Regular eye check-ups for changes in vision and for increases in pressure are important. People who are at risk for glaucoma include those over age 65, and those with a family history of glaucoma and farsightedness. If you have a family history of glaucoma and far-sightedness and are 35 or older, see an eye specialist to be checked for this problem. If you have a family history of glaucoma, see your doctor if you have eye pain, redness or blurring of vision. You should also have routine check-ups of your eye pressure, even if you don't have symptoms. Talk to your doctor about how often to have this done.

## Hyphema

- Redness
- Eye pain
- Decreased vision

*Hyphema* results when blood leaks between the lens and the cornea. It's rare but very serious. It's usually caused by a direct blow to the eye.

If you think you or a family member has the symptoms of hyphema after a blow to the eye, call your doctor or go to your local emergency room right away. After a thorough exam and vision testing, the usual treatment for hyphema is bed rest and medicine to reduce the pain and help the person relax. Other medicine to reduce the pressure within the eye is also usually given. The blood can be drained if needed to prevent further scarring or vision loss.

Wearing eye protection during sport and work activities that could cause an injury will help prevent this problem.

## Iritis

* Pain in the eye
* Redness
* Cloudy vision
* Light sensitivity
* Black floating spots

*Iritis* is a painful inflammation of the iris that causes cloudy vision. It's fairly rare. Most cases are thought to be due to autoimmune disorders (p. 223), but some are caused by bacterial infection. Treatment includes medicine given in eye drops, ointments or pills to reduce the inflammation and treat an infection if one is present.

## Night Blindness

* Not being able to see well at night

*Night blindness* can be an inherited visual defect or a symptom of eye disease. It can also be caused by a vitamin A deficiency. Vitamin A is needed to produce *visual purple,* a pigment used by the light-sensitive rods in the retina for seeing in low light. A well-balanced diet, with adequate vitamin A, will help prevent night blindness. Vitamin A is present in liver and in yellow, orange and dark green vegetables.

## Periorbital Cellulitis

* Redness
* Swelling
* Pain
* Fever
* Warmth of the skin around the eye
* Bulging of the eyeball

Infections that occur within the skin, the tear glands, the muscles and the fat around the eye are called *periorbital cellulitis.* This type of infection is rare. It's more common in children than in adults and requires hospitalization for treatment. If left untreated, this type of infection can spread rapidly from the tissues around the eye into the eye socket, and then to the brain and the membranes that cover the brain (meningitis, p. 302). A periorbital infection starts with a scratch or small infection, such as a boil (p. 276), on the skin near the eye or in the sinuses near the eye.

### Testing and Treatment

An exam is important as soon as this type of infection develops. X-rays of the bones in the face and of the sinuses will help confirm the diagnosis. Hospitalization is generally needed for treatment. Because the infection is serious, intravenous antibiotics (p. 618) are given. Medicine to reduce pain (analgesics, p. 614) and fever (p. 616) are also needed. Proper treatment can prevent vision loss or the spread of more serious infection to other areas in the skull.

---

### Light Sensitivity

Light sensitivity *(photophobia)* can be uncomfortable and cause you to squint. Dark glasses will help relieve the problem. Photophobia is common in people with light-colored skin. Iritis can also cause sensitivity to light, as can corneal abrasions. If you suddenly become sensitive to light, see your doctor.

# Pink Eye

- Redness
- Inflammation or swelling of the eyelids
- Mucus-like matter or drainage from the eye
- Itching and watering of the eye

*See photo of conjunctivitis, page 266.*

Infections of the conjunctiva are common, especially in children, because the bacteria or viruses that cause infections are easily carried by the hands to the eyes. Infection of the conjunctiva is called "pink eye." It isn't usually serious and may heal by itself. It's uncomfortable, though, and may spread from one family member or classmate to another. The five common causes of conjunctivitis are allergies, bacteria, chemicals, foreign bodies and viruses.

Conjunctivitis can be serious in some cases. Infection from a virus or bacteria can lead to ulcers of the cornea (p. 65) and, if left untreated, can cause scarring of the cornea, harm vision or even lead to blindness. When the cornea is infected, symptoms are usually much worse and include severe pain and sensitivity to light.

**Allergic conjunctivitis.** This type of conjunctivitis causes redness, itching and tearing. There may be other allergy symptoms, such as sneezing and a runny nose. Staying indoors, particularly when the level of pollen or other allergens is high, may be the main thing you can do to reduce symptoms. Air conditioning also reduces the number of allergens in the air. Over-the-counter antihistamine medicines, such as diphenhydramine (p. 615), can help reduce the itching, redness and discomfort. Prescription medicines, including antihistamine eye drops, may be needed. Allergic conjunctivitis, although very uncomfortable, doesn't usually lead to further complications.

**Bacterial conjunctivitis.** This infection usually causes a more intense redness and inflammation of the eye than viral conjunctivitis. It may cause yellow-green pus.

Bacterial infections are usually treated with antibiotic eye drops or ointment. Cultures of the eye can be used to help identify the bacteria so that the right antibiotic can be prescribed.

**Chemical conjunctivitis.** This type of conjunctivitis can occur if the mucous membranes of the eyes have been exposed to chemicals that the eyes are sensitive to, such as the chlorine in swimming pools. Rinse your eye with water promptly if a chemical gets in it. Ongoing chemical irritation can lead to a bacterial infection that may require antibiotic treatment.

**Foreign-body conjunctivitis.** This may be caused by anything that gets in the eye, such as dust or even a piece of a contact lens. The irritation can lead to tearing, redness and discomfort. The foreign body should be washed out with water. A foreign body that stays in the eye can lead to a bacterial infection. Both foreign bodies and chemicals can damage and scar the cornea if they aren't removed.

**Viral conjunctivitis.** This infection can occur along with a cold, flu or other viral infection. The virus can spread to the mucous membranes of the eyes. If this happens, the cells of the mucous membranes become inflamed and make too much mucus. This is what causes the matter to form in the eye.

If a person has a cold sore and then develops "pink eye," it's very important to have the eyes checked because the herpes virus (p. 325), which causes cold sores (p. 94), can also cause serious eye infections. Severe herpes virus infections of the cornea require treatment with antiviral medicine.

### Testing

Information about how the problem started, other symptoms and previous infections will help your doctor establish the cause of conjunctivitis. An ophthalmologist may use a slit lamp (p. 641) to look closely at the mucous membranes and the cornea.

### Treatment

The cause of the conjunctivitis must be determined before treatment can begin because treatment depends on the cause. Treatment is usually effective within a few days to two weeks, depending on the severity of the infection.

### Prevention

Viral and bacterial conjunctivitis can spread easily. Adults can follow the tips in the box below to help prevent the spread of conjunctivitis. Children can be encouraged to do the same. But because children are less likely to be able to follow these tips, they may need to stay home from school or day care if they have conjunctivitis. Keeping your child at home will help prevent the spread of infection to other children.

People who are allergic to pollen, dust or other substances should try to stay inside when those allergens are in the air. Keeping the windows up while riding in the car will help prevent some allergens from entering the car.

Contact lens wearers are at increased risk of eye infection. Improper lens cleaning and sterilization allow bacteria to infect the lenses. So it's particularly important for contact lens wearers to wash their hands thoroughly and follow instructions on caring for their lenses to avoid infections. If an infection occurs, contact lenses shouldn't be worn. The lenses should be sterilized and stored in a sterile lens solution until the infection has cleared.

## Retinal Artery Blockage

- Sudden loss of vision in one eye

The *retinal artery* is the main blood supply to the retina. If it's blocked for any reason, temporary or permanent blindness can occur if the blockage isn't treated promptly.

### Testing and Treatment

Ophthalmoscopy (p. 639) will probably be needed to examine the eye. Treatment of retinal artery blockage is

---

### *Preventing Conjunctivitis*

- Wash your hands often, especially if you have been around someone with conjunctivitis or another infection anywhere on the body.
- Keep your hands away from your eyes.
- Don't share towels or washcloths.
- Don't rub your eye if you feel something in it.
- Use an eye wash or gentle water spray to wash particles from the eye.

- Antihistamines (p. 615) may help relieve the itching.
- Care for contact lenses according to your eye specialist's instructions.
- Wear eye protection around paint, solvents or irritating chemicals that could splash into your eyes.

an emergency. Medicines or surgery may be used to help prevent permanent vision loss. Retinal artery blockage can be caused by diabetes (p. 211), high blood pressure (p. 123), glaucoma (p. 68) and polycythemia. Good control of blood sugar, blood pressure or pressure in the eye with medicines can reduce the risk of retinal artery blockage.

## Retinal Degeneration

• Gradual loss of vision over the years

Like all tissues of the body, the retina needs oxygen. As the body ages or as certain diseases harden or clog the arteries, the small blood vessels in the eyes no longer feed the tissues enough oxygen. The result is damaged areas of the retina—called *retinal degeneration.* Retinal degeneration can lead to blurred vision or complete vision loss. Many types of retinal degeneration can occur.

**Diabetic retinopathy.** This results from damage to the blood vessels of the retina caused by high blood sugar levels. These blood vessels become harder, and small arteries in the retina can become blocked. New blood vessels form as the body attempts to find a way to compensate for the blockages. The new blood vessels tend to be fragile and bleed into the *vitreous humor* (the jelly-like substance that fills the eyeball), causing problems with vision. Vision may also be impaired by growth of fibrous tissue from the retina into the vitreous humor. The retina may also scar as the body tries to "heal" the affected areas. This scarring of the retina can lead to retinal detachment (p. 74).

Controlling blood sugar levels (p. 212) can slow the damage of diabetic retinopathy. Laser surgery, or photocoagulation, destroys new vessels so that light can still be detected.

**Macular degeneration.** This occurs when the macula (the central part of the retina) begins to lose function. The cause isn't known. It affects the central part of vision. Peripheral vision (around the edges) and color vision usually remain. Macular degeneration is a common cause of vision problems in the elderly. It's more common in white people and it seems to run in families. Early cases can sometimes be helped with laser surgery, but the condition is hard to treat. Smoking may worsen the condition.

**Retinitis pigmentosa.** This is an inherited disorder in which the nerve cells of the retina break down over time. The first symptom is poor night vision. Next, overall vision is affected. Central vision (the part of your vision that sees things the sharpest) is first affected. Then peripheral vision deteriorates. Blindness may eventually occur. No effective treatment to reverse the vision loss is available.

### Testing

If you have any of the symptoms described here, get checked by an eye specialist. An exam of the retina through an ophthalmoscope (p. 639) usually suggests the diagnosis and whether more studies of the retina are needed.

### Prevention

Some of these eye conditions can be prevented by treating the health problems that cause them. Regular tests of blood sugar, blood pressure and pressure in the eyes may help prevent retinal degeneration and allow for early treatment of disorders that may lead to eye problems in the future.

If you have diabetes, see an ophthalmologist on a regular basis and whenever an eye problem develops. Controlling diabetes can help prevent eye problems in people who have diabetes.

## Retinal Detachment

- Bright spots of light or dark webs seen in one eye
- Feeling like a dark "curtain" is being pulled across one eye

*Retinal detachment* begins when a hole forms in the retina. The vitreous humor then begins to leak behind the retina, lifting it away from the back of the eye.

A number of diseases and injuries can cause retinal detachment. An injury that penetrates the eye, diabetic retinopathy (p. 212) or scarring that can occur after cataract surgery (p. 64) can pull on the retina and eventually cause detachment if not treated. Retinal detachment can cause permanent loss of vision.

### Testing

Most family doctors use an ophthalmoscope (p. 639) to look at the retina. But this method doesn't allow your doctor to see the edges of the retina, which is where early signs of detachment appear. If retinal detachment is suspected, your doctor will probably refer you to an ophthalmologist to be examined and treated. A slit lamp (p. 641) is used by ophthalmologists to see the edges of the retina.

### Treatment

Treatment of retinal detachment depends on how much damage has been done and what started it. For example, changes in the retina caused by diabetes may be best treated with *laser photocoagulation,* which involves tacking the retina to the back of the eye with hundreds of tiny burns. The fluid under the retina may have to be surgically drained.

### Prevention

Wearing eye protection during activities that could cause an injury can also prevent retinal detachment. Finding and treating retinal detachment early, before full-blown separation of the retina has occurred, will reduce the risk of vision loss.

## Stye

- Pain, swelling and redness on the edge of the eyelid

*See photo of stye, page 266.*

A stye is an infection of the *hair follicle* of an eyelash. The hair follicle is the small pit that the eyelash grows out of. The eyelid may become swollen and sore. Styes usually come to a head in three to seven days, then burst and heal on their own in most cases. A chalazion (p. 66) can sometimes be mistaken for a stye.

### Treatment

Applying a warm, wet cloth to the tender area may help the stye come to a head and burst. Removing the eyelash from the infected follicle often helps the infection drain. Consult your doctor if the infection comes back. Prescription antibiotic ointment or pills may be needed.

## Subconjunctival Hemorrhage

- A red area or red spots on the white of the eye

*See photo of subconjunctival hemorrhage, page 266.*

Have bloody splotches ever appeared suddenly on the white part of your eye? This is called a *subconjunctival hemorrhage.* It's caused by bleeding *(hemorrhaging)* under the sclera (the *subconjunctival* area). Subconjunctival hemorrhage may result from an eye injury, irritation of the eye or high blood pressure (p. 123). It can appear after sneezing, coughing or vomiting, or for no obvious reason. Sometimes the blood seeps over one side of the eye, right up to the edge of the cornea.

A painless subconjunctival hemorrhage will usually get better on its own within a few days. A painful subconjunctival hemorrhage may be a sign of an infection or a more serious problem and should be checked by a doctor.

## Tumors of the Eye

- Vision problems
- Crossed eyes
- Discoloration in the eyes
- Detached retina

Cancerous tumors of the eye are very rare. The most common of these is *retinoblastoma*, a tumor of the eyeball found in babies and children under the age of five. The child may have some vision problems or have crossed eyes, or the parents may see a discoloration or spot in the eye. There is no pain with this type of tumor. Early laser treatment to destroy the tumor can cure the condition. If laser treatment doesn't work, the eye may have to be removed to prevent the tumor from spreading to other parts of the body. The tendency to develop retinoblastomas appears to run in some families.

Another type of tumor found in the retina is a *malignant melanoma.* Unlike melanoma of the skin, which spreads rapidly, melanoma of the eye is more slow-growing. It occurs in older people. These tumors aren't painful, but they may obstruct vision or cause the retina to become detached. Small tumors can be destroyed with laser surgery. Removal of the affected eye may be recommended to prevent the tumor from spreading.

# CHAPTER 3

# EARS

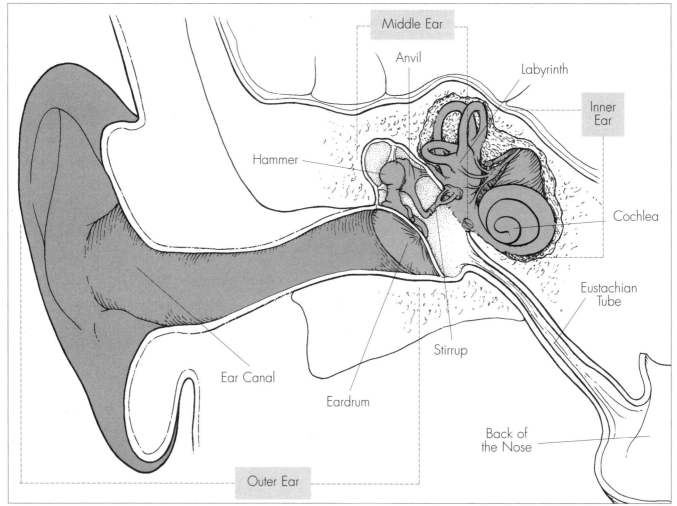

Middle Ear

Anvil

Labyrinth

Inner Ear

Hammer

Cochlea

Ear Canal

Stirrup

Eardrum

Eustachian Tube

Back of the Nose

Outer Ear

**EAR ANATOMY**

The ear works by receiving sound waves and sending messages to the brain. The outer ear includes the ear canal and the part of the ear that can be seen. Sound waves pass through the ear canal and hit the *eardrum*, or *tympanic membrane*. The eardrum is a thin, almost see-through tissue that stretches across the ear canal. Sound waves cause the eardrum to vibrate.

The vibration of the eardrum causes three bones in the *middle ear*, called the *malleus* (hammer), *incus* (anvil) and *stapes* (stirrup), to move. This movement sends the sound waves to the *inner ear,* or *cochlea.* Numerous nerve cells line the cochlea. These are called *sensory nerve cells.* These cells help translate the vibrations into sound messages. The sound messages are then sent to the brain along the *acoustic nerve.*

A part of the inner ear called the *labyrinth* helps you keep your balance. It's located behind the cochlea. It's made up of three canals that are filled with fluid. The canals are lined with tiny hairs that sense the movement of the fluid and send messages to the brain that give information about the position of your head.

The *eustachian tubes* connect the middle ear to the back of the nose. These tubes allow air into the middle ear for proper motion of the eardrum. The tubes drain away middle ear fluids.

## Benign Positional Vertigo

- Severe episodes of dizziness and spinning sensations that last less than 30 seconds
- Twitching of the eyeballs

*Benign positional vertigo* is a condition brought on when the head is held in particular positions, such as when lying on one side or when tilting the head back to look up. The dizziness and spinning sensation are accompanied by twitching of the eyeballs. Benign positional vertigo is caused by tiny deposits of debris in the inner ear that affect how the ear works to detect the position of the head. The best way to control the condition is to avoid the positions that seem to bring it on. Benign positional vertigo usually goes away on its own in a few weeks or months, but it may come back. If it continues for a year or so and is very bothersome, surgery can be done on the inner ear.

## Hearing Loss

- Gradual or sudden loss of hearing
- Some sounds may be heard better than others

Hearing loss can occur at any age and has a number of causes. Some of the most common causes of hearing loss, other than wax buildup in the ear (p. 85), are described below.

**Eustachian tube problems.** Problems can occur if the eustachian tube is compressed or blocked due to an ear infection, allergies or swelling of the *adenoids* (glands near the ear). Any of these things can lead to reduced hearing, at least temporarily. For example, after an ear infection, fluid may remain in the ear and cause eustachian tube blockage and reduced hearing.

Treatment of eustachian tube blockage depends on the cause, but may include the use of decongestants (p. 616) and antihistamines (p. 615). You can also do "eustachian tube exercises" to help air get into the middle ear, which can help resolve the problem. Yawning, chewing, moving your jaw or forceful swallowing can be effective. If you hear or feel a click or pop in your ear, air is getting into the middle ear. The click or pop tells you that you're getting results.

**Noise-induced hearing loss.** This type of hearing loss is caused by exposure to loud noise. It most often affects people younger than 60. It's usually job- or recreation-related—caused by noisy machinery, trucks, jackhammers, airplanes or other loud sounds at work, or by noisy recreational activities, such as shooting a gun, riding a motorcycle or snowmobile, or listening to loud music.

The most damaging sounds are loud, are at high frequencies and last a long time. The loudness of a sound is measured in decibels (dB). Sounds

| Decibels of Sounds | |
| --- | --- |
| Speech at a normal distance | 65-70 dB |
| Lawn mower | 90 dB |
| Chain saw | 100 dB |
| Car horn, rock concert | 115 dB |
| Gun shot, jet engine | 140 dB |

above 85 dB may be dangerous. The frequency, or the range, of sound is measured in Hertz (Hz). High-frequency sounds are also high-pitched and present the greatest risk of damage to hearing.

Hearing loss can be greatly reduced by paying attention to noise levels and by wearing earplugs or ear protectors when you're around loud noise. People have different sensitivities to noise levels. What may be safe for one person might not be for another.

**Otosclerosis.** This is the hardening of the stirrup, which is one of the bones in the middle ear that sends sound vibrations to the inner ear. Otosclerosis begins between the ages of 15 and 35 and may progress to almost total hearing loss. In women, the hearing loss may worsen during pregnancy. Otosclerosis affects about 10% of all Americans and seems to run in families. Surgical removal of part of the stirrup improves hearing for many people, but a few people will eventually have total loss of hearing.

**Presbycusis.** This is a gradual hearing loss that can occur with age. The *sensory nerve cells* within the inner ear normally transmit sound. Over time, they break down and don't transmit sounds—particularly the sounds of normal speech—with the intensity or clarity they once did. A hearing aid may help. Presbycusis affects almost 30% of people over age 65.

**A ruptured eardrum.** This means there's a hole in the eardrum. Any thin object pushed into the ear canal can tear, rip or puncture the eardrum. Fortunately, most of the time a ruptured eardrum heals with little scarring or hearing loss.

The eardrum can also rupture when air pressure builds quickly in the ear, damaging the eardrum before the pressure in the middle ear can equalize with the outside air pressure. This is called *barotrauma,* or pressure-related damage. Pressure-related damage can happen to people in airplanes when the cabin is suddenly depressurized or repressurized. Slapping the ear or being too close to the site of an explosion also can create enough difference in air pressure to burst the eardrum.

A doctor can usually tell by looking at the eardrum if it's ruptured. Antibiotics (p. 615) prevent the damaged area from becoming infected. If the puncture doesn't heal on its own, or isn't expected to heal well, an *otolaryngologist* (a doctor who specializes in diseases of the ears, nose and throat) may apply a temporary plastic patch over the eardrum. If that doesn't help the eardrum heal, an operation called a *tympanoplasty* may be needed to place a tissue graft into the eardrum. Often, only minimal hearing loss results from a damaged eardrum.

Hearing speech is how a child learns to talk. People who are born deaf may have problems learning to speak and understanding the speech of other people. This can lead to

### Deafness

Deafness can be related to a genetic condition, which means it runs in the family. Deafness can also be caused by something that happened during pregnancy. For example, certain infections in the mother can put the baby she is carrying at risk for hearing problems. These infections include German measles (rubella, p. 330), cytomegalovirus, toxoplasmosis (p. 388), influenza (p. 326), syphilis (p. 319) and herpes (p. 325). The baby's hearing also may be at risk if the mother uses drugs, drinks alcohol or is in an accident that damages the placenta.

problems with learning if the deafness isn't diagnosed and dealt with at an early age. Keep in mind that children usually begin forming their first words at one year of age. They usually start forming two-word sentences by two years of age. By age four, normal language is beginning to develop.

### Testing

Besides a general exam of the ear, a number of hearing tests may be needed to determine how much hearing has been lost, what range of sounds can no longer be heard and what the cause of the damage may be. These tests include audiometry (p. 628), tympanometry (p. 643) and tuning fork (p. 643) tests.

### Treatment

Hearing aids can be used to amplify sounds and improve hearing. Most hearing aids use a battery and an amplifier. Many types of hearing aids are available. Some are worn entirely within the ear, some rest behind the ear and others can be placed within eyeglass frames. Others can be worn on the chest. Hearing aids worn on the body are larger and are generally more powerful than hearing aids used in the ears.

A *cochlear implant* can improve hearing for some people. It's an electronic device that is connected to the inner ear through surgery. Cochlear implants are used in people who are completely deaf. They may help the person hear alarms and other loud warning signals.

The cochlear implant will also help the person tell when a word begins and ends, and pick up on the rhythm of speech. It can also help the person hear his or her own speech so he or she can speak clearly enough for hearing people to understand what is being said.

Much can be done to help people who are either born deaf or lose their hearing sometime during their lives. Learning how to lip read (watching people's mouths as they speak) can help people with hearing loss understand those who are speaking to them.

Sign language can be particularly helpful for people who have never been able to hear. The signs, which often involve using both hands and arms, represent objects and activities. Hand signals represent the alphabet so that some words can be spelled out. Classes in sign language are available in larger towns. Your doctor's office staff may be able to help in finding a class.

---

### Preventing Hearing Loss

- Wear ear protection when you're around any loud noise for long periods, such as at work.
- Wear ear protection when you're around explosive noises, such as when you go hunting.
- Never put anything in your ear—even cotton-tipped swabs. Doing so could puncture the eardrum.
- Check any sort of hearing loss with your doctor so that further loss can be prevented, if possible.

---

## Infection of the Ear Canal

- Itching and pain in one or both ears
- Tenderness when ear is tugged
- Draining
- Swelling in the ear canal

Infection of the ear canal, also called *otitis externa* or "swimmer's ear," causes pain or itching in one or both ears. Sometimes fluid may drain from the ear or the ear canal may swell.

Summer is prime time for otitis externa. Moisture may stay in the ear

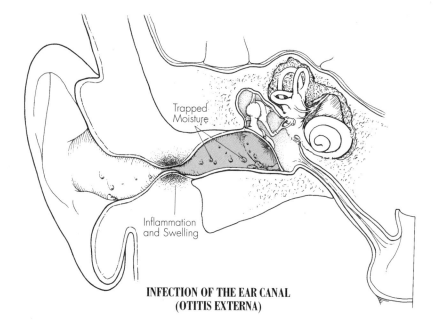

**INFECTION OF THE EAR CANAL
(OTITIS EXTERNA)**

canal after swimming or after a shower or bath. Moisture in the ear, typically combined with repetitive cleaning with cotton-tipped swabs, removes the thin coat of wax that acts as a protective barrier for the ear canal and allows a bacterial infection to gain a foothold. Once the infection begins, the canal may drain or become clogged with a mixture of pus and earwax. The canal becomes red, swollen and tender, and may swell to the point of closing. Cellulitis (p. 276) of the ear canal can develop if otitis externa isn't treated.

### Testing

If your child has recurrent or serious infections, your doctor may swab the ear canal and culture the secretions to find the specific bacteria responsible. Simple and early infections may need no testing before treatment.

### Treatment

Prescription eardrops may be needed to treat the infection and swelling. Analgesic medicines (p. 614) can reduce the discomfort. If the person has a fever, if the nearby lymph nodes are enlarged or if tenderness and swelling have spread beyond the ear

canal, an oral antibiotic (p. 618) may be prescribed to reduce the spread of the infection into the skin of the outer ear and face.

### Prevention

Placing three to five drops of a half-and-half solution of white vinegar and alcohol in each ear after swimming or bathing can help the water evaporate faster and acidify the canal, preventing bacteria from growing. Cotton-tipped swabs should never be used to clean inside the ear.

## Infection of the Middle Ear

- Sharp pain in one or both ears
- Fever
- Temporary hearing loss
- Sense of pressure in ear
- Fussiness in a child

Infection of the middle ear, also called *otitis media,* is most common in children. Two of three children have at least one middle ear infection by their third birthday. Children are more commonly affected than adults because of the small size and horizontal position of their eustachian tubes. These tubes connect the middle ear to the back of the nose and allow air into the middle ear so that the eardrum can vibrate properly. The tubes also drain away middle ear fluids.

The first signs of otitis media may be those of a cold, with sneezing or a runny nose. After a few days, the symptoms may include sharp, stabbing pain in one or both ears, a feeling of pressure inside the ear, fever and some temporary hearing loss. The pain may stop and there may be some drainage of fluid from the ear if the eardrum ruptures (p. 78).

While ear pain and fever are the classic symptoms of an ear infection, middle ear infections are often much more subtle. A child may have little pain with a middle ear infection. He or she may simply become fussy and not want to eat.

Middle ear infections are caused by viruses or bacteria that infect the cells lining the eustachian tube, throat and middle ear. When infected, these cells become swollen and secrete a thick mucus that may clog the eustachian tube and cause fluid and pressure to build behind the eardrum.

Bacterial infections of the ear can lead to complications. For example, pressure can build until the eardrum ruptures. Allergies may put some children at higher risk for recurrent ear infections.

Chronic infections or persistent fluid in the middle ear may temporarily reduce hearing. Hearing loss can interfere with a child's speech development. It's possible that hearing loss caused by ear infections could have the same result.

The bone next to the middle-ear bone, the *mastoid bone,* can become infected. This infection is called *mastoiditis.* Mastoiditis is a serious infection that requires longer antibiotic treatment. It can spread to the *meninges* (the membranes that cover the brain) and brain if not treated.

### Testing

As with infections of the ear canal, most middle ear infections can be diagnosed just by examining the ear with an otoscope (p. 639). A throat culture (p. 642) may also be useful. If the infection is more serious, blood tests, cultures of secretions from the ear (tympanocentesis, p. 643), and x-rays may be necessary to diagnose the extent of the infection.

### Treatment

Analgesic medicines (p. 614) can be used to reduce the discomfort.

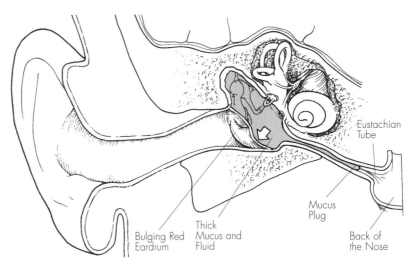

**INFECTION OF THE MIDDLE EAR
(OTITIS MEDIA)**

Antibiotic (p. 615) eardrops may be prescribed to treat a bacterial infection and swelling. Your doctor may prescribe other prescription medicines to help clear the congestion in the middle ear. Long-term antibiotics may be prescribed for infections that keep coming back.

### Prevention

When allergies seem to bring on the infection, ask your doctor about giving the child an antihistamine (p. 615), try to keep him or her in air-conditioned areas, and avoid the pollens, animals or foods that are the culprits.

## Fluid in the Middle Ear

- Muffled sounds
- Bubbling or gurgling noise in ear

Fluid can become trapped behind the eardrum because of a closed eustachian tube. This condition is called *middle ear effusion* or *serous otitis media.*

Fluid behind the eardrum may cause sounds to be muffled and may cause bubbling or gurgling noises in the ear. Fluid in the middle ear usually doesn't cause much pain. Middle ear effusion may follow an ear infection.

### *Preventing Middle Ear Infections*

- Sometimes a low dose of antibiotics every day can help prevent infections from coming back.
- Use allergy medicine if allergies seem to bring on ear infections. Avoid the offending pollens, animals or foods.
- Stay away from smoke to help reduce recurrences.
- If your child drinks from a bottle, try propping him or her up at a 45° angle (not lying flat), and don't let your child take a bottle to bed.

### Testing

Diagnosis of middle ear effusion is usually made by an exam of the eardrum. An otoscope (p. 639) will allow your doctor to see if there are air bubbles or fluid behind the eardrum. The eardrum is usually pulled in (*retracted*) when the eustachian tube is blocked. If a bacterial or viral infection is present, the eardrum may be red and bulge outward. If the infection is serious, blood tests and cultures of secretions from the ear (tympanocentesis, p. 643) may be needed to diagnose the extent of the infection.

### Treatment

Analgesic medicines (p. 614) and cold medicines, such as decongestants (p. 616), are helpful in relieving the symptoms of a cold-virus infection, which is the beginning of many ear infections. If fever, ear pain or drainage from the ear occurs, an exam by the doctor is essential. Your doctor may prescribe antibiotics or other prescription medicines to help clear the clogged middle ear.

A type of operation called *myringotomy* may be needed if fluid pressure builds up behind the eardrum. A myringotomy involves making a small cut in the eardrum. A small *tympanostomy tube* is often inserted into the ear at the same time to allow continuous drainage. A tympanostomy tube will usually fall out of the ear on its own in about six to nine months. Sometimes, a second set of tubes is needed. The child will have to avoid getting water in the ears while the tubes are in place.

## Foreign Objects in the Ear

- Pain, swelling and redness, sometimes with drainage
- Loss of hearing

Adults usually know when something has become lodged in the ear, although the object may not be noticed right away. An insect may enter the ear and become caught in earwax, which may cause the skin within the ear canal to swell, turn red and itch. Sometimes symptoms of infection, such as drainage, redness and pain, may occur. After the object is removed, treatment with antibiotic drops or oral antibiotics may be needed if the ear has become infected.

Small children may push food, toy parts or other objects into their ears. Depending on their age, they may or may not be able to tell an adult if they feel itching or pain. The first signs of the problem may be redness and drainage from the ear. The doctor may be able to identify the object, though the object may be hard to see if a lot of pus or drainage is present. Repeated infections that are only partially responsive to antibiotic drops and don't completely go away may indicate that a foreign body is in the ear. Additional exams by your doctor may reveal the problem.

---

### *Otitis Quick List*

- Middle ear infections may cause fever, pain and irritability, and often follow a cold.
- Ear canal infections cause tenderness when the ear is gently tugged, as well as pain and itching. These infections usually occur after swimming or if you constantly use cotton-tipped swabs in the ear canal.
- Fluid in the middle ear may not cause symptoms, or it may muffle sounds or cause bubbling or gurgling noises.
- Drainage can come from a ruptured eardrum or from an outer ear infection.

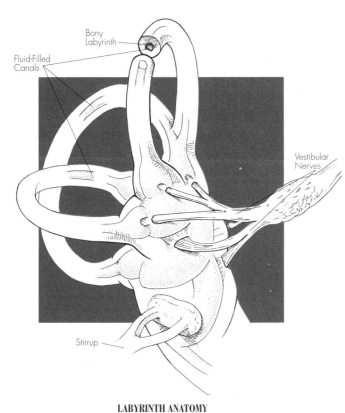

Bony Labyrinth

Fluid-Filled Canals

Vestibular Nerves

Stirrup

**LABYRINTH ANATOMY**

## Labyrinthitis

- Dizziness and a spinning sensation
- Nausea

*Labyrinthitis* is inflammation of the *labyrinth,* a bony structure that is part of the inner ear. The labyrinth consists of three small, fluid-filled canals, called the *semicircular canals,* made up of bone within the inner ear. These canals are lined with tiny hairs that sense the position and motion of the body by monitoring the movement of the fluid. This information is communicated to the brain by the vestibular nerves.

The canals can become infected, usually by a virus. Inflammation from infection disrupts the movement of fluid and how the body's movements are sensed.

Episodes of dizziness or spinning sensations come and go, lasting from seconds to minutes. The infection may take six weeks to resolve. Labyrinthitis caused by a viral infection is uncomfortable, but it is usually not serious and does not lead to long-term problems. Labyrinthitis caused by a bacterial infection (usually one that spreads from a middle ear infection) is uncommon but can lead to deafness or meningitis if not treated with antibiotic medicine.

### Testing

If symptoms of labyrinthitis are severe or don't go away, other problems may need to be ruled out. These problems include a tumor of the brain (p. 47) or of the acoustic nerve, or Meniere's disease (described below). A CT scan (p. 632) or an MRI scan (p. 637), for example, may rule out a serious disorder. Hearing tests and other nerve testing may also be done.

### Treatment

Labyrinthitis caused by a viral infection may be relieved by motion-sickness medicine such as meclizine (p. 625). Antibiotics (p. 615) may be helpful in treating labyrinthitis caused by bacteria. Medicine to reduce nausea also may be prescribed. If symptoms are severe, a sedative (p. 626) may be helpful. Bed rest and limited activity may help reduce recurrent episodes.

## Meniere's Disease

- Ringing in one or both ears
- Feeling of pressure or pain
- Occasional spells of severe dizziness and sensations of spinning, sometimes along with nausea or vomiting
- Hearing loss

*Meniere's disease* is caused by an increase in fluid in the inner ear canals. A feeling of increasing pressure or pain in the ear is sometimes a sign of a coming attack. *Vertigo* (dizziness and a spinning sensation) may cause the person to fall or feel nauseated. In Meniere's disease, unlike other causes of vertigo, symptoms include hearing loss or ringing in one or both ears (*tinnitus*). Episodes of Meniere's disease can occur days to years apart.

### Testing

A wide variety of tests may be used to determine the cause of vertigo. A CT scan (p. 632) or an MRI scan (p. 632) can be used to rule out tumors along the acoustic nerve. Hearing tests can identify hearing loss. Most of the tests done help diagnose Meniere's by excluding other problems. Special tests aren't needed if labyrinthitis (p. 83) or benign positional vertigo (p. 77) are suspected and symptoms resolve after a few weeks.

### Treatment

Most people with Meniere's disease have ringing in the ears, occasional episodes of dizziness and nausea, mild to moderate hearing loss, and anxiety. For early or mild Meniere's disease, oral medicine can help reduce the dizziness, calm the nausea and vomiting, reduce the inner ear fluid and help the person relax. Restricting how much fluid you drink and the amount of salt in your diet may help—this approach prevents episodes for some people and reduces the severity for others.

If Meniere's disease progresses or becomes severe enough to interfere with activities, further treatment may be needed. Two types of surgery have been used. One releases pressure in the inner ear by making a channel through surrounding bone. The other destroys part of the acoustic nerve in the affected ear. The acoustic nerve in the outer ear must be in good working order for this procedure to be helpful. Both procedures carry potentially serious risk because they require surgery within the skull.

Meniere's disease can't be cured. It can lead to permanent deafness in both ears.

## Ringing in the Ear

- Ongoing noise in the ear, usually heard as a ringing sound, but sometimes as a buzzing, roaring, hissing or other constant sound

*Tinnitus* is a constant buzzing or ringing in the ear—much like having an insect constantly buzzing in the ear—that can accompany hearing loss. Many ear disorders, such as serous otitis (p. 82), otitis media (p. 80), Meniere's disease (p. 83) and even wax buildup (p. 85) can bring on tinnitus. Tinnitus can also be a side effect of some medicines. Treating the underlying problem may reduce or stop the annoying noise.

### Testing

The doctor will first examine the ear thoroughly, looking for any visible reason for the ringing. Hearing tests may reveal problems with how the ear is working. CT scans (p. 632) or MRI scans (p. 637) may be used to look for tumors in the brain (p. 47) or the acoustic nerve.

### Treatment

Treatment of ringing in the ears depends on the problem that causes it. For example, removing wax in the canal or fluid behind the drum may stop the ringing. If the noise is caused by Meniere's disease or by something else that can't be cured, a special instrument called a *masking device* may give some relief by "hiding" the sound.

A masking device looks like a hearing aid, but it may be a little larger.

The device is placed in the ear and makes a sound that is the same pitch as the ringing. This sound covers the constant noise and makes it more tolerable. Hearing aids may also improve the situation by amplifying sounds around the pitch of the ring, making the ringing sound more like background noise.

### Prevention

Wearing hearing protection during loud work or recreational activities may help prevent hearing loss and the tinnitus that often accompanies it.

## Tumors of the Inner Ear

- Ringing in the ear
- Dizziness
- Hearing loss

An *acoustic neuroma* is a rare tumor that grows deep within the bony canal that houses the acoustic nerve. The acoustic nerve runs between the ear and the brain and communicates sound messages to the brain.

Early signs of acoustic neuroma include hearing loss and ringing in the affected ear. As it grows, the tumor presses on the nerve, destroying hearing and balance.

Surgery to remove the tumor is difficult. It usually destroys the nerve, resulting in permanent hearing loss in the affected ear.

## Tumors of the Outer Ear

- Growth on the skin of the outer ear

Outer ear tumors of the skin or underlying cartilage are almost as common as skin cancers on the face. Tumors of the outer ear can be cancerous or not. Cancerous skin tumors may begin as nonhealing sores, along with pain, bleeding or hearing loss. The tumor may spread to the skin of the ear canal. Other noncancerous growths, such as warts, can also affect the skin on the outer ear or the ear canal.

## Wax Buildup in the Ear

- Muffled sounds
- Ear pain (sometimes)
- Loss of hearing

The ear secretes a waxy material into the ear canal that collects dirt and debris. This blanket of earwax normally moves gradually outward as you chew food. The earwax is cleaned out of the ears when you wash your ears with a washcloth. In some people, it dries and flakes away by itself. When earwax leaves the ear, it carries dirt and debris with it. Sometimes, the wax builds until it totally clogs the ear canal. Air can't pass through the blocked canal, so sound waves can't pass to the eardrum, and sounds become muffled.

### Treatment

Attempts to remove wax may push it further into the canal and increase the chances of clogging. Your doctor may need to remove earwax buildup. Consult your doctor before using over-the-counter medicine to remove earwax. These products shouldn't be used if the eardrum has a hole in it.

### Prevention

Preventing wax buildup in the ear can be challenging because the canal is hard to clean. Cleaning the ears regularly with an over-the-counter wax-removal product or a mixture of equal parts hydrogen peroxide and water can help prevent wax buildup in people who are prone to it.

The outer portion of the ears can be cleaned with a washcloth or cotton-tipped swab. Do not insert anything into the ear canal. Doing so may force the wax deeper into the canal and damage the eardrum.

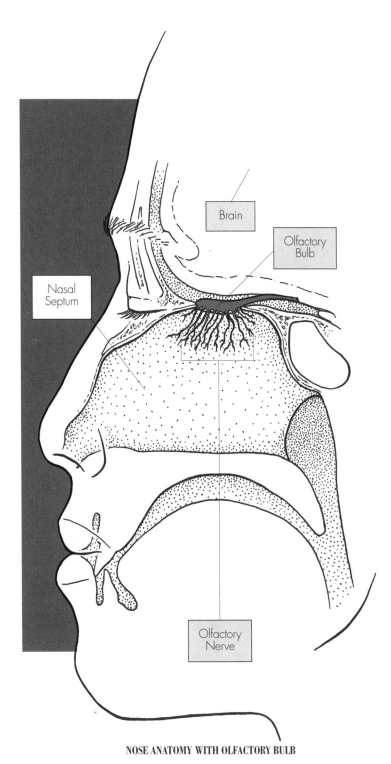

# CHAPTER 4 | NOSE AND SINUSES

The nose is divided in two by the *septum*. The septum is made up of bone and cartilage. The nose has tiny hairs, called *vibrissae*, lining it that clean the air you breathe by catching dust and other substances. The nasal passages are also lined with cells that have tiny hair-like structures, called *cilia*. Other cells in the lining of the nose produce mucus that traps dust and particles in the air you breathe. The air is warmed and moistened as it moves through the nose. This prepares it to go into the lungs.

Your sense of smell comes through the *olfactory nerve*, which projects into the nasal passage in the upper part of the nose. The olfactory nerve picks up the scents from the air you breathe and translates them into nerve impulses, or "messages," that are sent to the

**NOSE ANATOMY WITH OLFACTORY BULB**

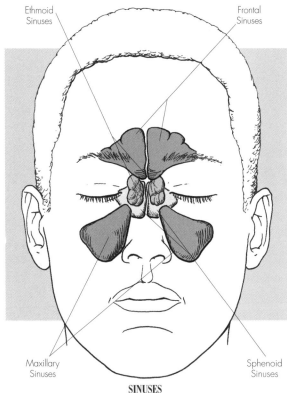

**SINUSES**

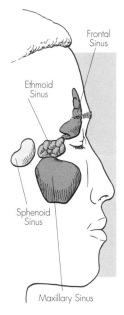

**SIDE VIEW OF SINUSES**

*olfactory bulb* in the brain. The olfactory bulb, which is located at the front of the brain, communicates the scents to your brain. Your sense of smell strongly affects your sense of taste (p. 92).

You have eight sinuses. Two large ones, called the *maxillary sinuses*, are behind your cheeks. Two smaller ones, called the *frontal sinuses*, are in your forehead. The *ethmoid* and *sphenoid* sinuses are beside and behind your nose. Other than making the skull lighter, the function of the sinuses isn't clear.

## Broken Nose

- Nosebleed
- Tenderness or pain
- Swelling
- Bruising

The bones in the nose are broken more than any other bones of the face. Your doctor can usually diagnose a broken nose after hearing you tell what has happened and after an exam and x-ray.

Treatment of a broken nose may involve repositioning the nose and stabilizing by packing it and sometimes splinting it. Splinting is done by taping a v-shaped molded plaster splint to the outside of the nose. This helps hold the bones in position while they heal back together. Packing involves putting gauze or an inflatable latex balloon into the nose. This is usually done either right away, before too much swelling has occurred, or about 10 days later when the swelling has gone down. Ice packs may be used to help the swelling go down.

## Deviated Septum

- Trouble breathing through the nose
- Sinus problems
- Nosebleeds

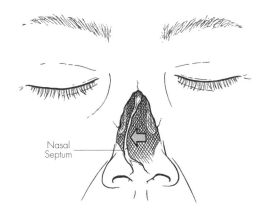

A *deviated septum* occurs when the nasal septum, the wall between the two nostrils, is crooked. This causes one side of the nose to be smaller than the other. Usually this isn't a problem. In some cases, though, the crooked septum can interfere with breathing. It may also cause snoring. People who have a deviated septum may be prone to nosebleeds and sinusitis. Surgery can be performed to straighten the deviated septum if it's causing problems.

## Nasal Polyps

- Stuffy nose that doesn't go away
- Reduced sense of smell

Ongoing allergies (p. 221) can cause *nasal polyps* to form in the passages of the nose. Polyps are like tiny tags of skin. Ask your doctor to check your nose if it's persistently stuffy. You may have nasal polyps. Make sure to tell your doctor if you use over-the-counter decongestant nasal sprays on a daily basis. Continued use of nasal sprays may make symptoms of polyps worse, causing sores and repeated infections.

Once nasal polyps are diagnosed, your doctor may prescribe a special corticosteroid (p. 622) nose spray to help shrink the size of the polyps. Surgical removal of the polyps may be needed if the medicine doesn't help shrink them.

## Nosebleed

- Bleeding from one or both nostrils

The sudden trickle (or gush) of blood from the nose can be very surprising, especially if it isn't caused by an injury. Most nosebleeds stem from dryness of the mucous membranes that line the inside of the nose, from irritation of the nose caused by a viral illness or from picking, blowing or roughly wiping the nose. Diseases of the blood-clotting system or use of aspirin (p. 615) or a blood-thinning medicine (p. 619) can prolong and worsen a simple nosebleed from a cold or minor injury. High blood pressure (p. 123) is a less common cause of recurrent nosebleeds. Blood pressure should be checked at least yearly.

Often, only one side of the nose is affected, and simple pressure stops the bleeding. Holding the nostrils together for five to 10 minutes is usually enough.

### Treatment

A blood count and clotting study may be needed if nosebleeds are severe and recur. These tests may be needed to evaluate the severity of the bleeding and to find out if a disease or another problem is causing the bleeding. For most nosebleeds, the treatment outlined in the box below is enough.

See your doctor if the bleeding is severe and simple measures to stop it don't work. Also see your doctor if the nosebleeds occur often. If your nose is gushing blood, seek immediate treatment at an emergency room.

Treatment may include *cauterization*. Cauterization involves burning the bleeding area to seal the bleeding blood vessel. Sometimes the source of bleeding is so far back in the nose that it can't easily be seen, and the nostril must be packed to stop the bleeding.

### Prevention

You may be able to help prevent nosebleeds caused by viral infections and dry mucous membranes by using a humidifier while sleeping and by using a saline nasal spray. Use the spray as often as needed to relieve dryness—or about four times a day. You can make

---

### *Stopping a Nosebleed*

- Lean forward and pinch both sides of your nose until the flow stops.
- Keep pinching for five to 10 minutes until a clot can form at the site of the nosebleed.
- Don't swallow the blood because it can irritate the stomach, leading to nausea and vomiting.
- Applying ice to the bridge of the nose may reduce the blood flow, allowing it to clot, but this technique is less effective than pinching the nose.
- Using a cotton swab dampened with nasal decongestant (p. 616) to gently rub a slowly bleeding or oozing area just inside the nose may also reduce or stop the blood flow.

the spray yourself by mixing ⅛ teaspoon of salt with one cup of water, or you can buy the spray already mixed. A thin coat of petroleum jelly on the inside of the nose will also keep membranes from drying out. Don't try to remove dry mucous crusts from inside the nostril by picking at them. This is a common cause of nosebleeds.

## Objects in the Nose

- Foul-smelling mucus running from the nose, usually just on one side

Children will sometimes put objects in their noses. This can cause a foul-smelling discharge to come from the nostril. The discharge usually comes from just one side of the nose—the side where the object is lodged.

Call your doctor if a child has placed something in his or her nose that doesn't easily come out on its own with gentle nose blowing. Don't try to remove the object, because this may push it further into the nasal passages.

## Sinusitis

- Runny nose
- Thick nasal drainage
- Pain or pressure in your face, where the sinuses are located
- Tooth pain
- Sore throat
- Cough
- Headache
- Fever

*Sinusitis* can occur if you get a bacterial infection of the mucous membranes that line your nose, sinuses and throat. These mucous membranes are especially prone to viral infections. When the membranes are infected, they swell and become irritated. The infection causes an increase in mucus, which makes a perfect home for bacteria to grow. A bacterial infection of the sinuses may occur after such a viral infection. Sinus pain and pressure can be due to the buildup of mucus in a sinus cavity.

### Testing and Treatment

Your doctor can diagnose most sinus infections based on knowing if you've had a recent cold or the flu, the presence of sinusitis symptoms, and by examining your nose, throat and sinuses. Sinus x-rays are sometimes used to show the extent of the infection and which sinuses are infected.

Treatment of mild sinusitis may begin with decongestants (p. 616) and steam inhalations to clear congestion. If pressure and drainage symptoms don't seem to improve, see your doctor. An antibiotic (p. 615) may also be needed. Serious or recurrent infections may require surgical drainage.

### Prevention

Preventing viral infections and allergies may prevent bacterial infections of the sinus. It's a good idea to wash hands often to prevent colds and other infections. Preventing sinus blockage during a cold, flu or other viral illness may help prevent bacterial sinus infections. Allergies, colds and the flu should be treated with antihistamines (p. 615) or decongestants. These medicines allow sinuses to drain and help reduce the amount of mucus the bacteria can feed on. Staying away from allergens and using air conditioning can help reduce secretions from allergic rhinitis, and so may reduce the risk that sinusitis will develop.

## Vasomotor Rhinitis

- Runny or stuffy nose and sneezing after a change in the air temperature

The mucous membranes that line the nose can be extra sensitive in some people. This can cause reactions to

## Relief for Your Runny Nose and Congestion

*A runny nose can have many causes, including sinusitis and vasomotor rhinitis. It can also be caused by allergies (p. 221) and by a cold virus (p. 322), such as the common cold. No matter what the cause, a runny and stopped-up nose can be annoying. Here are some tips on how to soothe a runny nose and stuffiness, as well as how to care for your nose.*

- Use cold or allergy medicines if they help dry up the mucus in your nose and sinuses.
- Don't use over-the-counter decongestant nasal sprays for more than three days in a row.
- Use soft tissues when you blow your nose, and wipe your nose gently.
- Apply petroleum jelly or another type of ointment to the skin beneath the nose if it seems to help soothe and protect your skin. Talk to your doctor about what to use.
- Drink plenty of fluids. This helps break up the congestion.
- Use a humidifier if it makes you feel more comfortable.

changes in the air temperature. For these people, walking out of hot summer air and into an air-conditioned room, eating cold or hot food, drinking alcohol or being around certain odors, smog or smoke can cause profuse drainage and dripping from the nose. This is called *vasomotor rhinitis*. Many people who experience it have conditions, such as allergies, that make their nasal mucous membranes more sensitive to changes.

Some people overuse nonprescription decongestant nasal sprays (p. 616) to reduce nasal drainage. Overusing nasal sprays can lead to other problems, such as sores and infections. Using nasal sprays for longer than three days could cause your symptoms to be even worse when you quit using them. This is called a *rebound effect*. This can lead to further swelling of the nasal tissues. Special types of nasal sprays can be prescribed to reduce the symptoms of vasomotor rhinitis without risking a rebound effect. These sprays contain corticosteroids (p. 622) or cromolyn sodium (p. 623).

# CHAPTER 5

# MOUTH

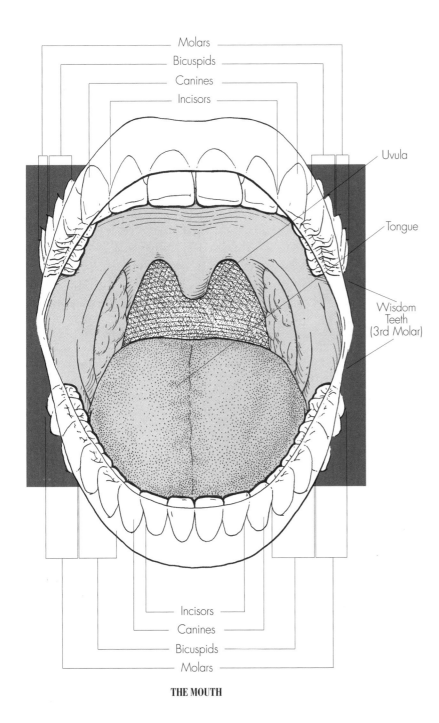

Molars
Bicuspids
Canines
Incisors

Uvula

Tongue

Wisdom
Teeth
(3rd Molar)

Incisors
Canines
Bicuspids
Molars

**THE MOUTH**

Your teeth begin to form even before you're born—as early as during the first three months of pregnancy. They appear in children, or "come in," around six or seven months of age. Most teeth are "in" by age three. These are the *primary* teeth. They're replaced by *permanent* teeth around age five or six. Usually, all of the primary teeth have been replaced by around age 14. The *wisdom* teeth come in later, around age 20. Adults have a total of 32 teeth. Eight of these are along the sides of the mouth (two on each side, top and bottom). They are called *molars*. The wisdom teeth, when they come in, are also molars.

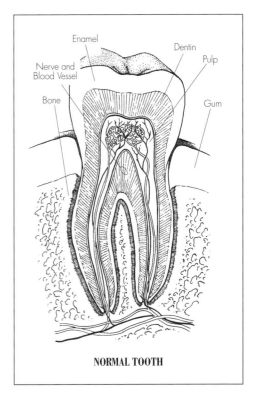

Enamel
Dentin
Pulp
Nerve and
Blood Vessel
Bone
Gum

**NORMAL TOOTH**

And so the total number of molars can be as high as 12. The *bicuspid* teeth are located between the molars and the *canines*, two on top and two on bottom on each side (total eight). The canines number four, one on either side in each jaw. They have the longest, strongest root of all of the teeth. Next to the canines are the *incisors*. They are the four front teeth on top and on bottom. They are the cutting teeth.

The *enamel* is the hard surface that caps the teeth. The supporting part of the teeth is the *dentin*. The *pulp* lies beneath the dentin. It contains the nerves and blood vessels that bring nutrition to the teeth and keep them alive.

*Saliva* is the fluid that moistens the mouth and helps in digestion of food. It's produced by *salivary glands*. The large salivary glands, called *parotid salivary glands,* lie near the back of the cheeks. The small salivary glands located under the tongue are called *sublingual salivary* glands. Saliva is discharged from the salivary glands into the mouth through the *salivary ducts.*

Your salivary glands start discharging saliva when you smell food. Tasting food makes them release more saliva. Saliva contains *mucin,* which helps lubricate the food to prepare it for swallowing and digestion. It also contains a special protein, called *amylase,* that begins to digest the starches in foods while you're chewing.

Your sense of taste comes from your *taste buds* and your sense of smell. Taste buds are sensitive to salty, sweet, sour and bitter flavors. The flavors are picked up by nerves located on the *papillae* (the tiny, "hairy" projections on the taste buds).Taste buds at the back of the tongue pick up bitter flavors, those in the front and side pick up salty flavors. Those in the front also pick up sweet flavors. Those on the sides pick up sour flavors.

The taste of more subtle flavors is triggered by the sense of smell. The *olfactory nerve,* which is located in the upper part of the nose, communicates scents to the *olfactory bulb.* The olfactory bulb communicates taste sensations to the brain. ***See page 86 for an illustration of the olfactory bulb.***

The *uvula* is the tiny sac-like structure that hangs down in the back of your throat. The *palate* is located at the roof of your mouth. It separates your mouth from your nasal passages.

## Bad Breath

- Foul-smelling breath

Bad breath, or *halitosis,* can be caused by a number of things: something that has been eaten or inhaled, decay of food particles in the mouth, gum disease, sinus problems or chronic infection in the respiratory tract. Often people aren't aware of their own bad breath until it's pointed out to them.

## Canker Sores

- A sore in the lining of the mouth

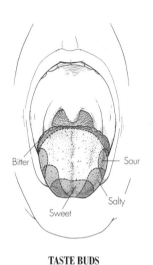

**TASTE BUDS**

### Getting Rid of Bad Breath

- Brush your teeth after you eat.
- Floss your teeth daily to remove bits of food.
- Have any gum problems checked and treated by your dentist.
- If you have a sinus problem or ongoing respiratory infection, have it treated by your doctor.

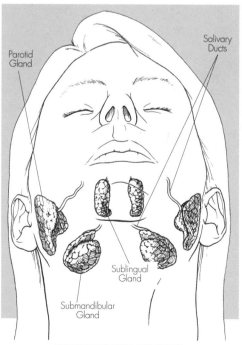

**SALIVARY GLANDS AND DUCTS**

Canker sores, or *aphthous ulcers*, form on the lining of the mouth. The exact cause isn't known. The sore tends to follow irritation of the area and may be related to stress.

Many factors irritate the mouth and lead to sores. These include using alcohol, frequently chewing gum or candy, eating hot foods, or becoming sensitive to mouthwash, candy dyes, toothpaste or other substances. Nutritional deficiencies, such as not enough iron, vitamin $B_{12}$ or folic acid, may increase the risk of canker sores.

Mouth sores are painful but usually harmless. They usually last from 10 days to as long as two weeks.

### Testing and Treatment

Canker sores resolve without treatment, but over-the-counter analgesic medicines (p. 614) and prescription medicines are available to help relieve the pain and discomfort. Dental analgesics (p. 614) are also available to put on the sore. Eating bland foods may help reduce irritation. In severe cases, prescription medicines may include corticosteroid (p. 622) ointments and antibiotics (p. 615).

## Cavities

- No pain in the early stages
- Increasing sensitivity to hot, cold and sweet drinks or foods as decay deepens in the tooth

After eating, food and bacteria wedge in the cracks between the teeth or on the surfaces of the teeth Bacteria grow on the food, causing plaque. Plaque is made of decaying food, thickened mucus and bacteria. The bacteria form acids that can eat away at the tooth enamel and the dentin and cause cavities. Continued decay eats through the dentin to the pulp.

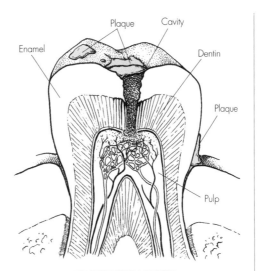

**TOOTH WITH A CAVITY**

Decay of the pulp can cause pain, swelling and infection.

### Testing

Careful inspection of the teeth by a dentist after a thorough cleansing to remove plaque may reveal decay. Dental x-rays (p. 633) are also used to detect early decay between the teeth.

### Treatment

A *filling* is the usual treatment for a cavity. The deeper the decay, the more drilling and cleaning out will need to be done. If decay has destroyed the enamel, dentin and pulp, a root canal may be needed to save the tooth. Severely decayed and neglected teeth may need to be removed.

### Prevention

Brushing, flossing and rinsing the teeth clean plaque off the surfaces and prevent decay. Fluoride hardens enamel and also protects against decay.

Children, even very young children, should brush or have their teeth brushed daily. Children up to about seven years old often need help to do a good job of brushing. Having their teeth *sealed* and treated with fluoride is an excellent yearly habit, starting at age three. Sealing involves brushing a special coating on the teeth to help protect

---

### Home Remedies for Mouth Sores

- Use a numbing sore-throat lozenge or spray.
- Gargle with mild salt water to remove food debris.
- Reduce the pain by taking analgesics (p. 614).

---

### Brushing

Take your time when you brush your teeth. Use a gentle touch. Move the brush in small circles across all of the tooth surfaces. Also gently brush your gums. This stimulates the blood flow in your gums, to keep them healthy.

---

### Preventing Tooth Decay

- Brush with a fluoride toothpaste after eating.
- Floss daily to remove plaque from between teeth.
- Limit snacking between meals unless you brush afterward.
- Use a fluoride rinse to help teeth resist decay.
- Have regular dental checkups.
- Ask your dentist about applying sealants to your teeth.

---

them. Don't let small children or infants sleep with bottles in their mouths. This promotes tooth decay.

Adults should have their teeth checked yearly, so any cavities can be filled and the decay stopped. Toothpastes or rinses, as well as drinking water, that contain fluoride are still useful for adults, but are more important for children. Teeth should be brushed, flossed and rinsed *at least once* daily, but preferably after all meals and snacks. If brushing can only be done once a day, bedtime is the best time to do it. Frequent snacks should be avoided because the bacteria in plaque feed on the sugars and make more acid, which then causes cavities.

## Cold Sores

- A painful, blistering sore that crusts around the mouth or nostrils

*See photo of cold sore, page 266.*

For many people, anticipating an important event—an upcoming prom, job interview or class reunion—seems to bring on a painful, crusted cold sore, or fever blister. Cold sores are caused by the herpes simplex virus (p. 325). Stress and exposure to sun seem to stir up the sleeping virus, bringing about a red, swollen lip.

This virus is contagious. The fluid in the cold sore blister contains the herpes virus. Touching the cold sore can contaminate the fingers and spread the viral infection to other people or other areas of your body. For example, the virus can be spread by unwashed hands to the eye, leading to a corneal infection (p. 65).

### Treatment

Herpes virus infections are hard to treat and can't be cured. They may come back, especially after exposure to sunlight or during times of stress. Topical ointments and oral analgesic medicines (p. 614) can relieve the pain. Applying ice at the first sign of a cold sore helps. Acyclovir (p. 621) may be prescribed for certain people.

### Prevention

Washing hands often and not sharing foods, drinking glasses or eating utensils can help prevent the spread of

---

### Flossing

Flossing is very important to the health of your teeth and gums. Flossing helps disrupt the bacteria that begin to grow between teeth and gums before they can do any harm.

Floss daily by pushing the floss down between two teeth. Move the floss up and down (not back and forth) along the surface of each tooth. Allow it to slide between the tooth surface and the gum. If you have trouble getting the floss out from between your teeth, simply release one end of the floss and pull it through. This will prevent the floss from getting stuck between your teeth.

Don't be alarmed if your gums bleed the first few times you floss. Your gums may need to "toughen up." If they keep bleeding, though, tell your dentist.

viruses. Avoid touching the mouth, nose and eyes with unwashed hands. Wearing a sunscreen lip ointment, eating a nutritious diet, reducing stress and getting enough sleep can help.

## Crowded and Misaligned Teeth

- Underbite
- Excessive overbite, or "buck teeth"
- Crooked teeth

Some people have teeth that fit nicely into their jaw and line up properly. But many people have crowded or crooked teeth or teeth that don't line up properly. This is called *malocclusion*. Many types of malocclusion can occur.

A *crowded bite* is when the teeth are too large for the space allotted to them in the jaw. Some of the teeth may rotate or be crooked or cover other teeth. An *overbite* is when the teeth of the upper jaw are pushed too far in front of the teeth of the lower jaw. An *underbite* is when the lower jaw and teeth are in front of the upper teeth. An *open bite* is when the teeth don't fit together smoothly, resulting in too much space between the upper and lower teeth.

Straight, properly spaced teeth are often the work of an *orthodontist*. An orthodontist is a dentist who corrects the many different types of malocclusion. Correcting malocclusion at an early stage can sometimes prevent the development of other problems, such as temporomandibular joint disorder (p. 252).

### Treatment

Regular dental checkups are the best way to make sure the teeth develop properly and are "straight" or aligned. If problems seem to be developing, your dentist will probably suggest a visit to an orthodontist.

Almost any type of crowding, spacing or alignment problem can be corrected with dental and orthodontic treatments. Braces, once commonly worn only by teenagers to guide permanent teeth into proper position, are now being worn by many adults to correct malocclusion problems.

For some problems, surgery may be needed to remove bone or teeth or to shorten or lengthen the jaw if orthodontic braces will not correct the problem by itself.

## Discolored Teeth

- Stains on the teeth

A host of medical and health-related problems can lead to stained or discolored teeth. Drinking coffee and smoking cigarettes or using other tobacco products can stain the teeth yellow. The death of the pulp can mark or darken the tooth color to tan or gray. So can some medicines. For example, the antibiotic tetracycline (p. 626) can stain a child's teeth yellow, or even brown or violet, if given to a child while the teeth are still developing. It may also stain the child's teeth if the mother took the drug while she was pregnant with the child. Infectious diseases and too much fluoride during childhood, when the teeth are still forming, may result in white or brown spots on the teeth.

### Treatment

Polishing the teeth can remove some stains. *Whiteners* can be used to brighten teeth discolored over time or by food or tobacco stains. Whitening is like a bleaching process that is done gradually or by removing stains with abrasives. *Veneers* can be bonded to the tooth to hide deep stains. A veneer is like a special coating of porcelain or other material that covers the surface of the tooth.

## Infection of the Gums

- Swollen, soft, red gums near teeth
- Gums that bleed easily
- Pulled back, or receding, gum line

**See photos of gingivitis and periodontitis, page 267.**

*Gingivitis* is the term that describes infection and swelling of the gums. It is usually caused by plaque growth near the gum line. The infected gum falls away from the tooth. This allows more space for more plaque—resulting in more infection. The process continues if untreated, until the infection goes into the root of the tooth. Infection around the root of the tooth is called *periodontitis.* The plaque and debris can spread down the root of the tooth and infect both the gums and the bone surrounding the root of the tooth.

*Trench mouth* is a type of gingivitis. It's also called *necrotizing ulcerative gingivitis* or *Vincent's infection.* A sign of trench mouth is heavy bleeding of the gums. Trench mouth is caused by a bacterial infection, but it's rarely contagious.

**Treatment and Prevention**

For most people, proper brushing and, especially, flossing will keep plaque to a minimum and prevent gingivitis. Having your teeth cleaned by a dentist or hygienist regularly is also helpful. In some people, a hardened surface called *calculus,* or *tartar,* develops over the plaque. When your dentist or hygienist cleans the teeth, the plaque and hardened calculus are scraped away. The care of a *periodontist* (a dentist who specializes in diagnosing and treating diseases of the gums and bones around the teeth) may be needed for severe gingivitis. Antibiotic mouthwashes, removal of tartar and, possibly, gum surgery may be required to save the teeth.

## Infection in a Tooth

- Severe pain in the tooth or jaw
- Swelling and redness in the surrounding gums or cheek

Dental abscesses are usually caused by dental decay. An *abscess* is a pocket of pus. Dental abscesses are usually caused by infection of the pulp of a tooth. The infection can spread down into the root of the tooth, then into the jawbone and erode through to the gum, to form a painful *gumboil.* The pain is relieved when the gumboil bursts and discharges pus into the mouth. The infection may also spread to the gums or the cheek, causing a painful, swollen face and swollen neck glands on the same side as the infection.

**Treatment**

Treatment of a dental abscess aims to save the tooth, if possible. The dead tissue and infection will probably need to be drained and removed so the infected area can heal. The dentist will clean, disinfect and fill the cavity and root canal. This process of cleaning and disinfecting the abscess inside a tooth is called a *root canal.* Antibiotics are prescribed to take care of any remaining infection. The pain of a tooth abscess can be reduced with over-the-counter analgesic medicines (p. 614), or your dentist may prescribe a medicine. Warm-water rinses can help "mature" an abscess, or bring it to a head.

**Prevention**

Early detection and treatment of decay can prevent progression to an abscess. Brushing, flossing and rinsing the teeth daily will reduce the likelihood of decay.

## Lichen Planus

- Small, pale bumps forming a white patch of skin inside the mouth
- Sore, dry mouth, sometimes with a "metallic" taste

*See photo of lichen planus, page 266.*

*Lichen planus* is a rash that forms on the inside of the mouth. It looks like white patches. The condition may occur at times of stress and emotional upset, or as a result of poorly fitting dentures.

Learning to reduce and cope with stress may help stop this rash from occurring. Poorly fitting dentures, partial plates or other dental work can be adjusted by a dentist.

No cure has been found for oral lichen planus, but medicine can be prescribed to relieve the pain and swelling.

## Mucocele

- Bluish or clear raised area in the mouth lining

A small bluish knot or lump inside the mouth may develop within a few days after being hit on the lip, for example, with a basketball. The knot is called a *mucocele*. It may continue to grow until it eventually ruptures, releasing a mucus-like substance. Other traumas to the mouth, such as biting the lip, may result in a mucocele. If a mucocele hasn't ruptured by a week to 10 days, check with your dentist or oral surgeon to have it drained, tested or removed.

## Salivary Gland Infection, Swelling or Blockages

- Swollen, warm, red, painful area inside the cheek

Chemicals and proteins in saliva may clump together to form particles. These particles may form into larger particles, or stones. If the stone becomes large enough, it can block part or all of the salivary gland and lead to swelling of the gland after meals. *See page 92 for a picture of the salivary glands and ducts.*

The blockage prevents saliva from discharging. A stone may lead to an infection or recurrent infections of the gland. Salivary glands under the tongue are affected more often than those in the cheek, and older people are affected more often than younger people. This blockage can cause a painful damming up of saliva and result in infection or swelling in the salivary gland, especially if you don't brush and floss your teeth regularly.

Mumps (p. 329) is a viral infection of the salivary glands. If one or both cheeks are swollen, and if you have fever, aches, chills and sore throat, you may have mumps, if you've never had them or a mumps immunization before.

### Testing and Treatment

A swollen, painful salivary gland should be checked by your dentist. Your dentist may use a special x-ray called a sialogram (p. 640) to look for stones or other reasons for the swelling.

Heat, medicine for the pain and antibiotics can reduce the symptoms of a blocked duct and help to cure the infection.

Stones can be surgically removed, often with only local anesthesia, or the entire gland can be removed under general anesthesia if the blockage is extensive.

## Thrush

- Sore mouth or throat
- White patches on the sides of the mouth, throat or tongue

*See photo of thrush, page 266.*

Yeast and bacteria normally live in the mouth and throat in balance with each other. *Thrush* occurs when the yeast *Candida albicans* overgrows. In a person with thrush, white patches may cover part or all of the tongue and inside of the mouth and throat.

Thrush occurs in infants more than in other age groups. The immune systems of infants are less able than the immune systems of older children and adults to fight yeast overgrowth. Children and adults who take antibiotics, those who have immune system problems, such as infection with HIV (p. 325), and people who have diabetes (p. 211) are more likely to have thrush.

### Testing and Treatment

Thrush can usually be diagnosed just by seeing the typical white patches it causes. Infections that keep coming back may make further tests necessary, to find out why treatment isn't working. Blood tests, yeast cultures and, possibly, other tests may be needed.

An antifungal medicine (p. 615) in liquid or tablet form cures the infection in most cases.

## Tongue Abnormalities

- Change in texture of tongue
- Change in color of tongue
- Swelling of tongue

Many changes can occur in the tongue, and the changes can be alarming.

**Geographic tongue.** This is when smooth, red areas form on an otherwise normal tongue. No reason for the change is known. No treatments are available.

**Coated tongue.** This is a change of the tongue that may occur with an illness and fever. A whitish coating is made up of skin cells that have peeled from the tongue and mixed with food and bacteria. The coating often goes away when the illness ends. A condition called thrush (p. 97) has a similar appearance but usually affects the sides of the mouth as well as the tongue.

**Hairy tongue.** This is when abnormally long papillae (the small, hair-like projections on the taste buds that give the tongue its slightly rough texture) become darkly colored as they grow, resembling fuzz or short hairs. Brushing the tongue daily with a toothbrush may return the tongue to its normal look. An oral antibiotic may be the source of the problem, or a fungal infection could be to blame.

**Discolored tongue.** This occurs when the tongue looks dark or black. This is most often caused by bismuth sulfate taken to calm an upset stomach. Yellowish discoloration often results from smoking or chewing tobacco products. Antibacterial mouth rinses and brushing the tongue can restore the color to a more normal appearance. Of course, it's also advisable to quit using tobacco. See p. 31 for tips on quitting.

**Inflammation of the tongue.** Also called *glossitis,* this condition is marked by swelling, redness and tenderness of the tongue, along with an abnormal texture. Sometimes the entire tongue is affected.

Glossitis can be caused by many problems, including infection and burns. Nutritional deficiencies, such as iron-deficiency anemia (p. 133) and other vitamin deficiencies (p. 18), can cause glossitis. Glossitis can also be caused by allergic reactions to medicines. Inflammation and pain on the tongue may be the only sign of this kind of reaction.

These problems may cause the papillae to peel from the tongue. The tongue's surface becomes smoother, redder and more sensitive, just as if the top layer of skin had been peeled from a burn on the hand.

Milder cases of glossitis will probably go away without further treatment. See your doctor if the condition persists or is severe.

A balanced diet or daily vitamin supplement prevents almost all nutritional deficiencies leading to glossitis. Proper care of the teeth and mouth, including daily tooth brushing, can prevent infections that cause glossitis.

## Tooth Loss

- Missing teeth due to an accident, decay or because they never came in

Developing teeth are normally pressed into alignment by neighboring teeth. When a tooth is lost, especially a permanent tooth, neighboring teeth tend to lean into the space, lose their alignment and become crooked.

The uneven bite may affect the jaw joint many years later, leading to arthritis of the jaw and painful muscle

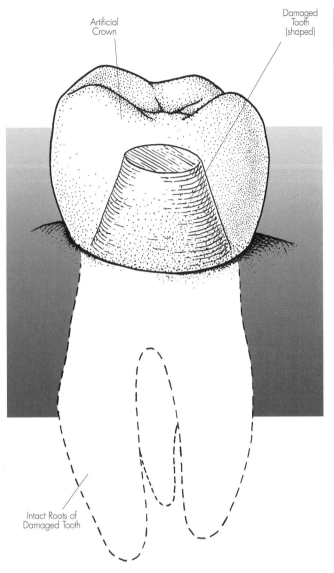

Artificial Crown

Damaged Tooth (shaped)

Intact Roots of Damaged Tooth

**CROWNED TOOTH**

spasms called temporomandibular joint disorder (p. 252).

Teeth may be lost or broken by injury. Teeth can be chipped or fractured, for example, in a fall from a bicycle. A damaged tooth will decay

---

## What to Do if You Lose a Tooth

- Find the tooth (or collect any pieces).
- Wash off the tooth or place it in a warm salt-water solution.
- You may be able to gently replace a full tooth into the socket. If a

gentle bite holds it in place, it can be kept there until you can get to a dentist.
- Always see your dentist about a broken or lost tooth as soon as possible.

more easily, so repair is often required. Neglect and decay are another cause of tooth loss. In a few people, some permanent teeth fail to develop. How the problem of one or more lost teeth can be corrected depends on the location and number of teeth missing.

### Treatment

Many techniques are available to replace or repair damaged or lost teeth. Dentistry aims to conserve as many of the normal teeth as possible.

A *crown* is an artificial top to a tooth that is damaged but has intact roots. The tooth is ground into a shape the crown will fit. The crown is cemented to the top of the tooth.

## Tumors of the Mouth

- Thickening or small lump in the jaw or mouth tissues
- Sores in the mouth

Both noncancerous and cancerous tumors are possible in nearly any part of the body, including the mouth. A biopsy of the tumor can identify the specific kind of tumor and show whether it's cancerous.

Tumors of the mouth or tongue, whether or not they are cancerous, appear to be closely connected to irritation of the surface area. The rubbing of an ill-fitting denture may lead to a thickening, a small lump or a change in the contour of the jaw or the tissues in

### Caring for Dentures

- Clean your dentures daily, removing all food debris.
- Half fill the sink with water and brush your dentures over the water. They will be less likely to break if you drop them.
- If you sleep with your dentures in, brush them before you go to bed.
- If you take your dentures out at night, leave them in a soaking solution, then brush them before you put them back in your mouth in the morning.

A *bridge* is an artificial tooth or group of teeth fixed between two crowns to fill the empty space left by a missing tooth or group of teeth. The two teeth on either side of the missing tooth or teeth are given crowns to anchor the bridge.

*Dentures* are artificial teeth that are embedded into a plastic material that looks like gum tissue. Dentures can fill in a large area of missing teeth, or an entire set of teeth can be created for the upper and lower jaws.

A *root canal* is needed when decay has destroyed the pulp of a tooth. The process involves cleaning out the abscess, and filling and crowning the tooth. A root canal saves the natural tooth.

the mouth. Use of irritating substances, such as tobacco products or alcohol, increases the risk of developing cancer in the mouth.

Noncancerous tumors are almost always painless unless they are bitten or become infected. They usually grow slowly. Cancerous tumors, on the other hand, grow more rapidly, can become tender and often break open into a sore.

Salivary gland tumors are usually not cancerous, although a few can be. They usually grow slowly and occur later in life.

Noncancerous tumors can usually be watched and left untreated. Cancerous tumors will spread and destroy other tissues in the body if not removed promptly.

## Wisdom-Tooth Problems

- Pain, impaction or decay of the wisdom teeth

The last teeth to emerge, usually around age 20, are the very back ones—the third molars, called *wisdom teeth.* Three common problems may arise with wisdom teeth.

*Impaction* occurs when the tooth, as it comes in, becomes trapped by the second molar and can't come in completely. It may stay partly under the gum. Bits of food tend to collect there, causing gum irritation or infection and decay of the tooth.

*Crowding* is when the wisdom tooth grows into place and pushes against the second molar, which in turn may push on the other teeth.

Straight teeth may become crowded or twisted if the wisdom tooth creates enough pressure.

*Gum disease* can occur when a partly emerged wisdom tooth makes an opening in the gum that becomes swollen and tender and forms a pocket that bits of food can get caught in. Infection in this pocket can lead to decay and even loss of the tooth.

### Testing and Treatment

Dentists examine teeth for proper alignment and for emergence of the wisdom teeth. Dental x-rays (p. 633) are used to check for impaction of the wisdom teeth. Unless they push on the second molars, teeth that haven't come out yet are harmless. Removal may be recommended if impaction, decay or gum disease occurs.

# CHAPTER 6 THROAT

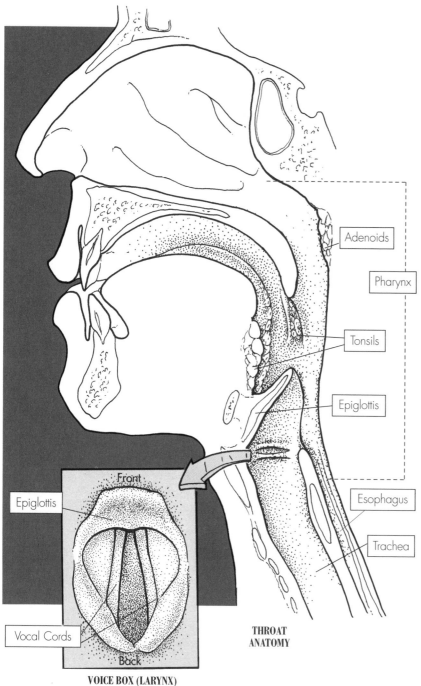

Adenoids

Pharynx

Tonsils

Epiglottis

Esophagus

Trachea

**THROAT ANATOMY**

Front

Epiglottis

Vocal Cords

Back

**VOICE BOX (LARYNX)**

The throat, or *pharynx*, is like a tube with two tunnels running through it. One tunnel, called the windpipe or *trachea*, allows the air you breathe to pass into your lungs. The other tunnel, the *esophagus*, allows food to pass into your stomach. The *epiglottis* acts as a lid for the trachea. It closes when you swallow so that foods and liquids won't get in the trachea and go into your lungs.

The voice box, or *larynx*, is also in the throat. When too much mucus comes up from your lungs or when something tickles your larynx, you cough. Coughing allows your larynx to get rid of whatever is irritating it.

The *vocal cords* stretch across the larynx. When air passes over the vocal cords, they vibrate. This is what allows you to make the sounds you use to form speech. Sometimes, problems with the vocal cords can interfere with speech. Damage to your larynx may affect your ability to speak.

The *tonsils* are located on both sides of the back of the mouth, behind the tongue. Tonsils are part of the body's immune system. They store and organize cells to fight bacteria and viruses that infect the throat. The tonsils usually reach their peak size by six to eight years of age, then begin to shrink. Thus, tonsil problems may diminish as one grows older and the tonsils shrink. Some older children and adults continue to have large tonsils.

The *adenoids* are tissue much like tonsils. Adenoids help fight infection. They're located on either side of the throat. The *uvula* is the tiny sac-like structure that hangs down in the back of your throat.

## Laryngitis

- Hoarseness and loss of voice, sometimes with cold or flu symptoms

*Laryngitis* is an inflammation of the vocal cords, usually caused by an infection of the tender skin (mucous membranes) in that area. With swelling and irritation of the vocal cords, the voice becomes huskier and thicker. Complete loss of the voice is less common. Laryngitis is usually due to a virus if it's caused by infection. It can also occur as a symptom of bronchitis (p. 145), pneumonia (p. 154), influenza (p. 326) and other infections that cause a cough that irritates the vocal cords. Laryngitis can also result if you overuse your voice or if you are around smoke or other irritating fumes.

Persistent hoarseness or loss of voice may indicate a more serious disorder of the larynx and should be checked by your doctor.

Two other conditions involve swelling in the throat or airways. In croup (p. 323), the throat below the vocal cords swells. Croup causes a barking cough and is more bothersome in children than in adults because the airways of children are smaller. Swelling of the epiglottis due to epiglottitis (p. 299) causes fever and inability to swallow, and can lead to dangerous narrowing of the air passage in children.

### Testing and Treatment

Throat cultures (p. 642), blood tests and x-rays may be done to identify the cause of the laryngitis before treatment.

Most cases of viral laryngitis require treatment only for the symptoms and will go away within a few days. Resting the vocal cords, using steam inhalations, taking pain-reducing medicines and drinking warm liquids may help reduce the swelling and inflammation, restoring the voice more quickly.

People who have a fever, a cough and shortness of breath may also have a bacterial infection and will probably require antibiotics to treat the infection and swelling. Their laryngitis may last longer than a week.

## Sore Throat

- Dry, scratchy throat
- Painful, difficult swallowing

Sore throat, or *pharyngitis*, is most often caused by infection with streptococcal (p. 306), or "strep," bacteria, or by such viral infections as the common cold (p. 322) or influenza (p. 326). A sore throat also may be caused by breathing dust or noxious paint fumes, or by smoking.

A sore throat caused by an infection often looks red. Smokers often have chronic redness and inflammation at the back of their throats. Signs of a sore throat in infants may include drooling, refusing to eat or swallow, irritability or fussiness.

Sore throats occur more often in children than in adults because children haven't been exposed to the many different types of viruses and bacteria that cause throat infections. Their immune systems aren't yet able to fight off these infections. Another reason is that hand washing isn't a high priority for most children, and many infections are spread by hand-to-hand contact.

### Testing

Most sore throats caused by viruses begin to improve within a couple of days. Common, over-the-counter medicines help relieve the pain and other symptoms of the infection. If the symptoms last longer than two days or if a rash appears, particularly in a child, see your doctor to check for strep throat. Strep throat is more common in children than adults.

A throat culture (p. 642) or rapid strep test (p. 640) may be used to look for a strep infection. A blood test for mononucleosis (p. 328), which is caused by the Epstein-Barr virus (p. 328), may be done if mononucleosis is suspected as the cause of the sore throat.

### Treatment

Over-the-counter medicines can be used to treat the symptoms of a sore throat caused by a virus, but they don't shorten the time the infection lasts. These infections just have to run their course. Symptoms caused by a cold virus usually go away in seven to 10 days. Symptoms caused by mononucleosis can last for four weeks or more.

Studies suggest that antibiotic treatment for strep throat is most effective if it's started 48 hours to seven days after the symptoms appear and is continued for a full 10 days. Untreated strep can rarely result in rheumatic fever (p. 304). Strep throat can also lead to scarlet fever (p. 305) or kidney problems (glomerulonephritis, p. 161). Fortunately, these complications of strep throat are rare in the United States.

## Thyroglossal Duct Cyst

- Swelling, a red spot or a dimple in the skin under the chin

Long before birth, folds in the neck tissue of the fetus turn into different glands and tissues in the body. Sometimes, a remnant of this tissue persists into childhood and adulthood called a *thyroglossal duct*. The thyroglossal duct can grow, thicken, and become tender and infected. This infection can lead to the formation of a cyst. Thyroglossal duct cysts almost always appear between the jaw and the lower neck. Removal of the cyst is both the recommended treatment and the best means of diagnosis.

## Tonsillitis

- Sore throat
- Pain when swallowing
- Drooling in infants
- Refusing to eat, especially in children
- Fever, aches, chills
- Headache
- Earache
- Swollen neck glands
- Bad breath
- Cough

*Tonsillitis* is an infection of the tonsils that may be caused by a strep infection (p. 306) or a viral infection (p. 320). It's more common in children but can occur in adults. In tonsillitis, the tonsils become swollen. Small

### Home Remedies for Sore Throat

- Rest your voice.
- Take an analgesic medicine (p. 614).
- Drink warm liquids to soothe your throat.
- Suck on throat lozenges or hard candies.
- Use medicated throat sprays.
- Use a vaporizer in the house to keep the air moist.
- Turn down the heat in your bedroom at night. The heater can dry out the air.
- Get a new toothbrush at the end of the infection (to prevent reinfection).

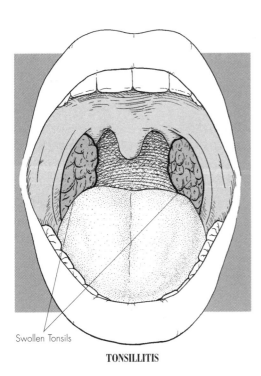

Swollen Tonsils

**TONSILLITIS**

white patches, called *exudates*, may be seen on the tonsils.

Tonsillitis is more common in children because the tonsils are larger and they become infected more easily. Generalized tonsillitis is uncommon in adults, but small pockets of infection in the sides of the tonsils are more common with age.

The infection may spread to the tissues surrounding the tonsil, causing a *peritonsillar abscess* (also known as quinsy). Peritonsillar abscess is seen more often in adolescents and young adults than in children. It's a serious and painful condition that requires prompt medical attention.

You should see your doctor if your symptoms don't get better in two to four days with over-the-counter medicines.

**Testing and Treatment**

Examination will show whether the throat, the tonsils or both are infected. A throat culture (p. 642) will help determine the cause of infection. If the cause is bacterial, antibiotics (p. 615) may help. If the cause is a virus, only the symptoms can be treated. Surgical removal of the tonsils (*tonsillectomy*) and perhaps the adenoids (*adenoidectomy*) may be necessary if tonsillitis keeps coming back or never completely goes away despite treatment.

## Tumors of the Larynx

- Hoarseness that keeps getting worse, sometimes with difficult swallowing
- Pain or lump in the throat

Cancerous tumors can form on the larynx. The earlier the cancer is discovered, the more likely it can be cured. Hoarseness that doesn't go away or keeps getting worse causes most people with this problem to seek help—sometimes after months of waiting for the voice to clear. Smokers and people who drink heavily are at increased risk for cancer of the larynx.

Extensive tumors may require total removal of the larynx, along with radiation therapy (p. 225) to stop the spread of cancer to other areas of the body.

## Vocal Cord Polyps

- Persistent hoarseness and change in the voice quality

A voice change caused by laryngitis usually goes away in a few days. But hoarseness or a voice change that continues without improvement for weeks or months may suggest a different cause. Careful examination of the mucous membrane covering the vocal cords may reveal thickening or small noncancerous growths, called *nodules,* or *polyps.* A cancerous growth may even be present. Vocal cord polyps often result from overusing the voice. Breathing irritating substances, such as dust, fumes or smoke, may also play a part in the development of vocal cord polyps.

*What does a tonsillectomy involve?*

A *tonsillectomy* is the surgical removal of the tonsils. It's usually done as an outpatient surgery. Recovery takes about three weeks, but the patient will feel much better after one week.

### Testing and Treatment

The doctor can usually see growths on the vocal cords by looking into the throat with a mirror or a fiberoptic laryngoscope (p. 637). Removal of polyps is usually a simple surgical procedure that can be done under local anesthesia. The need to rest the voice after removal of vocal cord polyps is probably the most difficult part of the treatment.

### Prevention

Repeated, forceful yelling or frequent, prolonged singing irritate and thicken the mucous membranes of the voice box. The more the voice is over used, the more likely it is that polyps will form. Learning proper techniques of singing and speaking can help prevent this kind of strain. If yelling is a must, use a microphone or megaphone to amplify your voice.

---

## Objects in the Airway

If someone is choking, it's important to know what to do. A person can't live for very long without being able to breathe. See page 601 for tips on how to handle a choking emergency.

# CHAPTER 7

# HEART AND BLOOD VESSELS

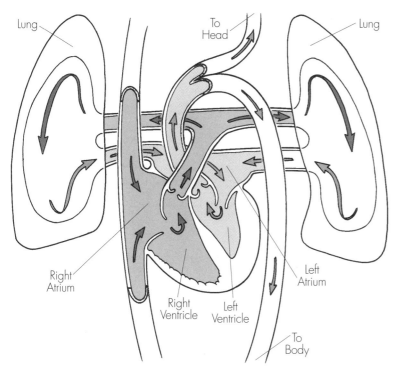

Lung

To Head

Lung

Right Atrium

Right Ventricle

Left Ventricle

Left Atrium

To Body

**CIRCULATORY SYSTEM**

Your *circulatory system* includes your *heart* and *blood vessels*. Your heart is a key part of the circulatory system. It's the muscle that contracts and expands to pump blood through your blood vessels. Your *pulse* is caused by the contractions of your heart—when your heart squeezes blood out. The throbbing this causes in your blood vessels creates your pulse. By counting your pulse beats for 15 seconds and multiplying by four, you can determine your *heart rate*. The "normal" heart rate varies, depending on your age, size and fitness level. See page 5 for more information about heart rates and exercise.

The blood vessels also play an active role in the circulatory system. They *constrict* (narrow), *dilate* (open), and use special valves to help control the amount and pressure of the blood that runs through them to the various tissues and organs of the body.

Blood flows throughout the body in a never-ending cycle. The right and left sides of the heart act as separate but coordinated pumps. When blood leaves the right side of the heart, it travels to the lungs. Here, it picks up oxygen, which you inhale when you breathe. This oxygen-rich blood travels back to the heart. It's then pumped out of the left side of the heart through the *arteries* to the rest of the body. Oxygen, along with sugar, proteins and other nutrients that you get from your diet, provides the energy your body needs to function.

The ends of the arteries turn into *arterioles*, which are tiny arteries. *Capillaries* join the arterioles to the *venules*. The venules turn into veins that carry the blood back from the body to the right side of the heart. The blood carries the carbon dioxide that has built up as a byproduct, or waste, of the body's functioning. When the blood reaches the lungs, it releases this carbon dioxide, which you exhale when you breathe. At the same time, the blood picks up more oxygen and continues its cycle back to the body again.

## Aneurysm

• Usually, no symptoms unless the aneurysm bursts
• Pain at the site of the aneurysm if it bursts or expands rapidly

Damage to a blood vessel wall can weaken the vessel or cause it to balloon out and form an *aneurysm*. This weakness may also be an abnormality present from birth. A similar situation occurs when the layers of a tire tear and the weak area pushes out, forming a noticeable bulge. Increased pressure in an artery with an aneurysm can have serious results, including bleeding, pain and even death.

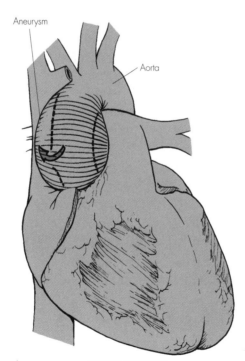

**AORTIC ANEURYSM**

**Aortic aneurysms.** Aortic aneurysms occur in the large artery in the abdomen and chest called the *aorta*. The aorta is a common site of aneurysms because it withstands a tremendous amount of pressure.

Aortic aneurysms can also be caused by damage to the artery wall due to atherosclerosis (p. 111) or syphilis (p. 319), or it can occur after a car wreck or other trauma to the artery. An abdominal aortic aneurysm is when the aneurysm occurs in the part of the aorta that is in the abdomen. The aorta runs from the top of the heart through the chest and abdomen, all the way to the pelvis (about two to two and a half feet long in most adults).

**Berry aneurysms.** These aneurysms occur in an artery of the brain. They are *congenital*, meaning you're born with them. But they rarely cause problems in children, and usually cause no problems for many years into adulthood, sometimes never showing any signs. They may suddenly rupture and cause bleeding in the brain (p. 45). Sometimes, berry aneurysms leak slightly, causing headaches before they rupture.

**Dissecting aneurysms.** Dissecting aneurysms occur when the blood forces its way between the inside wall of the artery and the weakened wall of the aneurysm. This type of aneurysm occurs in the aorta and is often the result of atherosclerosis.

**Ruptured aneurysms.** An aneurysm may rupture when pressure within the artery is so great that the weakness in the wall gives way and blood goes into the tissue around the aneurysm. Persistent or increasing pain in the chest or abdomen, or acute and severe pain in this area, especially in people older than 50, should be checked right away for a possible dissecting or ruptured aneurysm or another serious health problem.

**Ventricular aneurysms.** This aneurysm occurs when an aneurysm forms in the wall of the ventricle of the heart, usually on the left ventricle.

This usually follows a heart attack, but bacterial endocarditis (p. 115) or a trauma, such as a car wreck, can also cause a ventricular aneurysm.

### Testing and Treatment

An arteriogram (p. 628) is the most accurate test for detecting an aneurysm. Standard x-rays will only be helpful if a large aortic aneurysm shadow shows up on a chest or abdominal x-ray. Those in the brain may be diagnosed with an arteriogram, a CT scan (p. 632) or an MRI scan (p. 637). Surgery may be needed if the aneurysm might burst and bleed.

### Prevention

Smoking and a high cholesterol level (p. 14) both contribute to atherosclerosis, which can damage the artery wall and possibly lead to aneurysms. Diabetes (p. 211) and high blood pressure (p. 123) also contribute to artery damage. Stopping smoking and controlling these factors will lead to better health for your heart, your arteries and most other organs. Berry aneurysms can't be prevented.

## Angina

- Discomfort ranging from slight pressure to crushing pain in the chest that may extend to the left shoulder, down the arms or into the throat or the jaw
- Sweating, shortness of breath, nausea, vomiting or faintness or lightheadedness (sometimes)

The heart, like any muscle, requires oxygen to function. And, like any muscle, if it's not getting enough oxygen for its level of activity, it will start to ache. For example, while walking, the muscles in your legs may begin to ache partly because they aren't receiving enough oxygen. When this happens to the heart, it's called *angina*.

Angina is caused by problems in one of the three blood vessels that deliver blood and oxygen to the heart. With age, smoking, a high cholesterol level (p. 14), diabetes (p. 211) and high blood pressure (p. 123), these blood vessels can become stiff, damaged and partly blocked (atherosclerosis, p. 111). This reduces the blood flow to the heart.

Angina often occurs when the workload on the heart is high—with exercise, stress or after eating a heavy meal. With rest, the heart slows down, its workload reduces, and the oxygen it's receiving is enough. The pain may not be as bad or may go away. No permanent damage is done to the heart muscle. But angina can be a sign of a serious heart problem.

Rarely, angina can also be produced by a few other diseases that either increase the demand for oxygen, such as increased thyroid hormone (hyperthyroidism, p. 215), or reduce the amount of oxygen supplied to the heart, such as low blood iron (anemia, p. 133) or atherosclerosis of the valve in the aorta. Also, if the heart enlarges under the strain of high blood pressure, it will need more oxygen to function properly, and angina may occur.

### Testing

Angina shouldn't be ignored. It may be the first sign of heart problems or a coming heart attack. A doctor should be seen right away for testing and treatment if chest pain or pain in the left shoulder or arm occurs.

Blood tests may be done to rule out other possible causes of the pain besides angina. An electrocardiogram (p. 634) may also be done to look for both damage and lack of blood to certain parts of the heart. But even if nothing is found on the electrocardiogram, the pain may still be coming from blocked arteries in the heart.

Next, an exercise stress test (p. 635) may be done. If the pain is serious and the electrocardiogram shows damage, cardiac catheterization (p. 631) may be needed.

### Treatment

Treatment depends on the cause or causes of the angina pain. Mild blockages in the arteries can often be treated with medicines ranging from nitroglycerin (p. 618) or beta-adrenergic blockers (p. 621) to calcium-channel blockers (p. 621). Or a balloon angioplasty (p. 112) may be done. Bypass surgery (p. 112) can also be helpful.

### Prevention

If you have a family history of heart problems, you're at much higher risk for having them yourself. Unfortunately, we can't change our genes. But you can change many other things to reduce your risk for angina (see box above).

## Arterial Embolism

- Often, no symptoms
- Aching in a muscle

An *arterial embolism* is a mass—such as a blood clot, a cholesterol plaque that has broken off the artery wall or an air bubble—that is traveling through the arteries. If this mass, or *embolus,* finds its way to a small artery within a muscle and partly or completely blocks the artery, it can cause no symptoms or possibly a slight ache within the muscle for a few hours. If the arterial embolus finds its way into a coronary artery, which supplies blood to the heart, the heart can be damaged, and a heart attack (p. 115) may result. If the embolus goes into the brain, a stroke (p. 59) may occur.

Heart conditions that can raise the risk of emboli include valve abnormalities, such as mitral regurgitation, and certain arrhythmias, such as atrial fibrillation. Atherosclerosis (p. 111) can also raise the risk of arterial embolism.

### Testing and Treatment

An arteriogram (p. 628) can detect the exact site of a blockage by an embolus. A larger embolus can block the blood supply to an entire limb, such as the leg. Immediate removal of the embolus is essential to avoid death of the tissues in the limb. In the situation where an embolus goes to a limb, Doppler ultrasound (p. 643) and limb blood pressures at various levels can be used to identify the location of reduced blood flow.

In the arteries of people who have severe atherosclerosis, large pieces of plaque may break off and travel to the kidneys or intestines, or into the legs. Clots can also form in the heart and travel to these areas.

In the case of arterial emboli formed of plaque, direct removal may be needed. In the case of blood clots, blood-thinning medicines (p. 619) will usually be needed for a number of months to prevent future clot formation. Other medicines can also be given for comfort.

### Prevention

Smoking, high blood pressure (p. 123), high blood sugar (p. 211) and high blood cholesterol (p. 14) are frequent causes of atherosclerosis. So having regular check-ups to detect and treat these problems can reduce the risk of an arterial embolus.

## Atherosclerosis

- Often, no symptoms, especially early in the process
- Can lead to any number of symptoms and problems, including strokes, transient ischemic attacks, dizziness, angina (p. 109), heart attacks (p. 115), kidney damage, muscle cramps in the legs

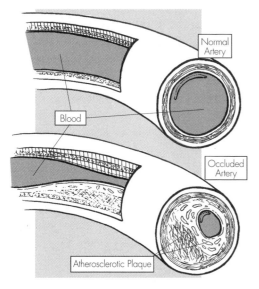

**ATHEROSCLEROSIS: NORMAL VS. OCCLUDED**

*Atherosclerosis*, also called "hardening of the arteries," causes arteries in the body to lose their "bounce," or elasticity. Cholesterol first deposits as small fatty streaks on artery walls. As this material builds up, it forms a thicker deposit, called a *plaque*. Over time, this material hardens, or *calcifies*, and makes the arteries rigid. This makes them less able to dilate and contract, an action that normally helps control the pressure and amount of blood flow. Factors such as high cholesterol (p. 14), high blood pressure (p. 123), diabetes (p. 211) and smoking speed up the "hardening" process.

The lack of elasticity in the arteries can reduce blood flow, especially because the arteries are partly or completely blocked with plaque. The most serious damage occurs not in the artery itself, but in the organ that the artery supplies with blood and oxygen. Blockage of a blood vessel to the brain can cause dizziness, transient ischemic attacks or a stroke (p. 59), and may leave the person paralyzed or unable to talk. Angina or heart attacks can occur when blood flow is reduced through the arteries that supply the heart. Even the toes, fingers or larger parts of the limbs may suffer when atherosclerosis prevents the blood from nourishing those tissues. Atherosclerosis can also affect the way the kidneys clean waste from the blood and so can contribute to kidney failure.

### Testing

Blood tests, a chest x-ray (p. 631) and an electrocardiogram (p. 634) will probably be done. More specialized studies of the arteries may also be needed, such as Doppler ultrasound (p. 643) and arteriography (p. 628).

### Treatment

Treatment options for atherosclerosis have increased over the last 10 years. In many cases, *balloon angioplasty* can be done to open narrow areas of arteries from the inside. This treatment involves passing a deflated balloon through a

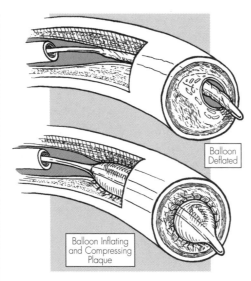

Balloon
Deflated

Balloon Inflating
and Compressing
Plaque

**BALLOON ANGIOPLASTY**

catheter to the point of blockage in the artery and then inflating the balloon to compress the plaque against the artery wall and reopen the artery. It's most commonly used in coronary arteries, which supply blood to the heart.

Other related techniques are being developed to treat atherosclerosis, such as the use of small coiled metal springs, or metal tabs (stents), to keep a vessel open after angioplasty. Lasers can also be used to clear out a blood vessel from the inside.

The techniques of surgical repair of problem areas or removal of plaque from the inside of an artery (*endarterectomy*) have been used for years. Newer laser technologies haven't proved as dramatically helpful as once hoped, but they are still being researched and may be more useful in the future. Endarterectomy is used most commonly in the *carotid arteries,* which travel up the neck and supply blood to the head.

*Bypass surgery* can be done to place grafts of vein and artery so that blood can be diverted around the blockage. It's used mostly in coronary arteries, although large arteries in the legs and arms are sometimes bypassed as well. This type of surgery has become quite safe and common. Bypass surgery with synthetic grafting materials can divert blood around larger areas of blockage.

All of these techniques reduce symptoms but haven't been shown to prolong life. Also, they usually need to be repeated. A bypass, on average, lasts about 10 years.

Medicines can also be used to dilate arteries that are still somewhat elastic or haven't "hardened" completely, to allow blood to pass. A medicine called pentoxifylline (p. 618) can sometimes improve the flow of blood by softening the red blood cells as they slide through very narrow areas of small arteries. Blood-thinning medicines (p. 619) can also be used to prevent clots from forming and causing further damage.

**Prevention**

You can help prevent atherosclerosis by staying active, eating healthy, low-fat foods and avoiding tobacco. See page 2 for more information about what you can do to prevent atherosclerosis and heart disease. If you have diabetes, controlling your blood sugar level can help reduce your risk, as can reducing a high blood cholesterol level and treating high blood pressure.

Women who have gone through menopause (p. 407) tend to have lower levels of high-density-lipoprotein (HDL) cholesterol, which helps protect against heart attacks. If you have gone through menopause, hormone replacement therapy (p. 407) may reduce your

*Wine for the heart?*

Several studies during the past 20 years have shown that drinking one glass of wine a day may reduce your risk of heart disease. Red wine may have a protective effect, while other alcoholic drinks, such as beer or liquor, don't. White wine is less effective.

risk of heart attack by helping to keep your HDL cholesterol level high.

## Cardiomyopathy

- Tiredness
- Shortness of breath
- Dizziness
- Chest pain
- Abnormal heart rhythms
- Swollen ankles

*Cardiomyopathy* is a type of heart disease in which the muscle cells within the heart become damaged, weakening the pumping action of the heart. These faulty cells can arise from a known cause, such as a nutritional deficiency, an inherited disease, poisons or medicine, or for no apparent reason. There are different types of cardiomyopathy.

**Alcoholic cardiomyopathy.** This can occur when someone drinks too much alcohol on a regular basis. The damage to the heart may be caused by the toxic effects of alcohol or by the nutritional deficiencies that are common in people whose calories come only from alcohol. Thirty-year-old alcoholics have been known to die from this disease. Stopping alcohol consumption and rebuilding nutrition are essential for people with alcoholic cardiomyopathy.

**Congestive cardiomyopathy.** Congestive cardiomyopathy is usually a result of damage to the heart caused by heart attacks, high blood pressure or certain kinds of infections. The result is a dilation, or swelling, of the *ventricles*, the pumping chambers of the heart. Congestive cardiomyopathy usually doesn't improve by itself. When possible, treating the condition that is contributing to the cardiomyopathy is essential. Treatment is otherwise similar to that of congestive heart failure (p. 114).

**Hypertrophic cardiomyopathy.** This occurs when the cells toward the center of the heart swell and become less efficient in pumping. As they swell, the wall of the heart thickens and blood is blocked from leaving the heart, forcing the rest of the heart to work harder and swell more. The more the cells swell, the harder they have to work. This condition may lead to heart failure (p. 114) and even death. Early in the disease, some medicines can be tried. In the end stages, a heart transplant may be the only effective treatment. The cause of hypertrophic cardiomyopathy isn't known, but it may be partly related to genetics.

**Toxic cardiomyopathy.** Toxic cardiomyopathy occurs when certain medicines, chemotherapy or industrial toxins cause heart damage, even at "normal" dosages or exposures. Toxic cardiomyopathy may be stopped and, depending on the extent of damage, reversed once the cause is identified.

### Testing and Treatment

The doctor will probably begin by asking questions about work, chemical exposures, medicines, family history and other factors. Blood tests, a chest x-ray and an electrocardiogram (p. 634) are basic tests often used to identify the problem. Further tests may be needed, including an echocardiogram (p. 633). The exams may reveal changes in the heart rhythm, in the sounds and in the location of the main pulse in the chest.

In the case of severe cardiomyopathy, if the condition is not reversible and is deemed bad enough, a heart transplant may be needed.

### Prevention

Limit alcohol from zero to two drinks a day for men and zero to one drink per day for women. If you have trouble controlling how much you drink, ask your doctor for help in quitting. Be aware of chemicals around you at work. Use safety precautions. Learn the effects of the chemicals so any signs or symptoms of exposure will be noticed early. Also, ask your doctor about side effects of any medicines.

## Congestive Heart Failure

- Tiredness
- Cough, wheezing, breathlessness
- Rapid heartbeat
- Sensitivity to cold
- Fluid in the lungs that causes a feeling of suffocation—can't lie down flat comfortably
- Swelling of the legs

One condition that occurs when the heart can't keep up with the body's needs is *congestive heart failure.* This may occur after many years of disease of the heart valves or arteries, atherosclerosis (p. 111), cardiomyopathy (p. 113), pericarditis (p. 125), high blood pressure (p. 123) or rheumatic heart disease. Disease of the liver and kidneys can also lead to an overload on the heart. A past heart attack (p. 115) can also leave a weakened heart that has trouble keeping up with a normal workload.

At first, symptoms may occur only during physical exertion. As the heart failure worsens, symptoms begin to occur even at rest. Pulmonary edema (p. 156) is a very severe form of heart failure.

If the failure involves the ability of the heart to contract and squeeze out blood, symptoms will include weakness and fatigue. If the failure affects the way the heart fills with blood, pulmonary edema may occur. Both types of failure often occur together.

Many other diseases add to heart failure. For example, a sudden increase in blood pressure may put tremendous pressure on the heart, backing up even more fluid into the lungs and causing severe shortness of breath and a cough that produces the pink, foamy sputum. This is classic, full-blown *pulmonary edema.* Liver or kidney disease also can cause excessive fluid to build up in the body, increasing the demands on the heart to pump.

Lack of oxygen in chronic lung disease reduces the efficiency of the heart, while making it harder to pump blood to the lungs. Heart failure may result. Diabetes (p. 211) can damage the blood vessels to the heart, leading to heart attacks (p. 115), a decreased ability to pump, heart failure and pulmonary edema.

For mild congestive heart failure, treatment might include taking a diuretic and propping up the person's head at night. Rest, minimal exercise or activity and limiting salt are also helpful, along with supplemental oxygen for people with more advanced heart problems.

When heart failure becomes very severe, a heart transplant may be an option, but several things must be considered before a transplant will be offered. Transplant operations are only done at larger medical centers, such as university hospitals, which usually participate in a national system of identifying and matching donors with recipients. These hospitals also have programs for the post-surgical support that will be needed after the operation. The risk, cost and shortage of available organs make a transplant a last resort.

### Testing and Treatment

Diagnosis can often be made based on the medical history, a physical exam and laboratory tests. Chest x-rays, echocardiography (p. 633) and cardiac catheterization (p. 631) may also be needed.

If the underlying cause of the congestive heart failure can be treated, that is the preferred approach. Often the cause can't be treated directly, so the symptoms must be treated.

Managing other factors that can be putting more stress on the heart is helpful. These factors include high blood pressure, drinking too much alcohol or eating too much sodium. Treatment also includes rest and sedation. Raising the head of the bed and sitting as much as possible can make breathing easier.

Diuretic medicine (p. 616) can help reduce the amount of fluid in the veins. Digitalis (p. 623) is among the medicines that may be used to help the heart pump better. Vasodilator medicines (p. 626) can also help improve the way the heart works by helping to open the arteries.

### Prevention

Congestive heart failure can be avoided by avoiding the factors that can lead to heart disease. See page 118 for tips on preventing heart disease.

## Endocarditis

- Fatigue
- Fever
- Night sweats
- Weight loss
- Aching joints

*Endocarditis* is an inflammation or swelling of the lining of the heart and the valves of the heart. The most common type of endocarditis is *subacute bacterial endocarditis* (SBE). A heart with defects or abnormal valves may have interior spaces where blood doesn't flow normally. These abnormal valves and defects are the usual locations for this kind of infection.

Fatigue and fever are the most common symptoms. Some people with SBE have small red spots on their skin or under their fingernails. This is a sign that bacteria from the infected heart lining have gone through the bloodstream to the outlying tissues. A new heart murmur is also a common finding, and SBE may lead to an enlarged spleen. SBE may go on for many months before it's diagnosed because the symptoms can be slight and arrive gradually. Eventually, fever, weakness, tiredness or the unusual red spots cause most people to see their doctor.

### Testing and Treatment

Blood tests and cultures can help identify the type and severity of the infection. An echocardiogram (p. 633) will show the bacterial growth on the heart valves. Once the bacteria are identified, intravenous antibiotics are usually given for weeks to get rid of the infection. An abnormal heart valve that has been further damaged by infection may need surgical replacement.

### Prevention

People who have an abnormal heart valve should discuss the risk of endocarditis with their doctor and with anyone who suggests doing dental work or surgery. Bacteria can gain access to the bloodstream in these situations. Antibiotics taken shortly before and after the dental work or surgery can keep bacteria from multiplying and prevent endocarditis.

## Heart Attack

- Sudden, crushing pain under the breastbone, sometimes with sweating, nausea, vomiting
- Pain that extends into or is only found in the jaw or the left shoulder
- Sometimes little or no chest pain, especially in people who have diabetes

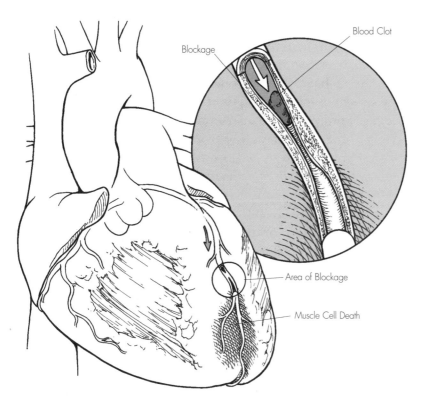

**HEART ATTACK: BLOCKAGE**

A *heart attack*, also called a *myocardial infarction*, occurs when part of the heart muscle dies because it isn't receiving oxygen. This can occur if a *coronary artery*, an artery that supplies blood to the heart, becomes blocked by a clot or embolus, or a spasm occurs inside the coronary artery. Clots are more likely to form where atherosclerosis (p. 111) has narrowed one of the coronary arteries. Similarly, a spasm on top of an existing narrowed area is more likely to cause a problem than a spasm of a normal coronary artery.

When blockages occur in small arteries that supply the heart with blood and oxygen, little or no heart tissue may be damaged. There are often multiple small vessels supplying the same area. But when a larger artery becomes clogged, serious damage can result, including an irregular heartbeat, shock and, sometimes, sudden death. Blockages can interfere with the electrical system that the heart uses to respond to changes in the amount of blood needed throughout the body. For example, if the heart is damaged during a heart attack, it may become hyperactive and begin sending out signals to make the heart beat much too fast. See page 118 for more information about heart rhythm problems.

> ### Emergency Symptoms of a Heart Attack
>
> • A sensation often described as "crushing" chest pressure
> • Sweating
> • Pain extending into the left shoulder, left arm or jaw
> • Nausea and vomiting
> • Shortness of breath
> • Any chest discomfort that doesn't go away
>
> *If you have a combination of these symptoms, don't delay! Treatment received within the first few hours of a heart attack may help reverse the process that's causing the damage to the heart. Call for an ambulance and be transported to the emergency room right away.*

Many people don't know when they've had a heart attack. They blame their pain on indigestion or stress. A few people have heart damage but almost no chest pain or other symptoms—in what is called a "silent" heart attack. Left-shoulder pain or pressure without other symptoms may also be a sign of a heart attack in progress. Any pressure or pain in the chest or into the left upper arm and shoulder should be checked right away by a doctor in the nearest emergency room.

### Testing

When severe chest pain occurs, or when a person faints after having chest pain or pressure, it should be assumed that a heart attack is in progress.

Emergency treatment, including CPR (p. 596), may be needed to restart the heart or to keep its pumping action going. Immediate treatment by emergency personnel may save a life.

If the origin of the chest pain or pressure is in doubt, a number of tests—an electrocardiogram (p. 634), and heart-rate and blood pressure monitoring—will probably be started. Changes in the electrocardiogram may help the doctor decide if any damage has occurred. Heart enzymes in the blood may also suggest that the heart has been damaged.

**Treatment**

Great advances have been made in the treatment of heart attacks. Now, only one out of three people who have a heart attack dies from it. The first six hours are the most critical time after a heart attack. Emergency treatment with rapid transport, CPR and monitoring equipment can be lifesaving. Brain cells die if they don't get oxygen for about five minutes, but the heart may be able to survive for minutes to hours with very low oxygen.

Newer emergency treatments, called thrombolytics, can dissolve blood clots that block an artery. But these clot-dissolving medicines (p. 622) must be given very quickly after a heart attack to preserve the heart muscle. These medicines are given intravenously. Angioplasty (p. 112) is sometimes used.

Someone who has had a heart attack will probably be admitted to an intensive care cardiac treatment unit for careful monitoring and quick treatment of any complications while they rest and heal. Medicines can be given to reduce the work the heart must do and to prevent electrical abnormalities or disturbances. Some of the more common complications include abnormal heart rhythms (p. 118), heart failure (p. 114), inflammation around the heart and an aneurysm in the heart wall (ventricular aneurysm, p. 108).

As recovery progresses, your doctor may recommend gradually increasing activity to prevent working the damaged heart too much. Some doctors ask their patients to take a stress test before leaving the hospital to reveal any other areas of the heart at risk for damage.

> ## Outlook After a Heart Attack
>
> After the initial danger period of six to 12 hours since the heart attack has passed, chances are good—about seven in 10—that the person will live at least another five years. Of course, this depends on the extent to which the other blood vessels to the heart are narrowed and how much the heart has already been damaged. Eating habits, smoking and exercise habits often need to be changed to improve the chances of long-term survival.

What leads to heart attacks? The rate of heart disease rose steadily until the late 1960s, when the public became aware of some of the reasons for heart attacks. Now it's widely known that smoking, lack of exercise, high blood cholesterol (p. 14), high blood pressure (p. 123) and diabetes (p. 211) contribute to heart attacks and deaths from heart disease. As a result, these deaths have declined as more people quit using tobacco, exercise more, reduce the fat they eat, have their cholesterol level checked and treated, watch their blood pressure and control their blood sugar more carefully.

**Prevention**

You can do so much to prevent having a heart attack! The box on the next page lists some things you can do.

> ## Preventing Heart Attacks
>
> - Don't smoke! If you do smoke, see your doctor for help in quitting. See page 31 for more information about how to quit smoking.
> - Have your blood sugar (p. 211), blood cholesterol (p. 14) and blood pressure (p. 123) checked. High levels of all of these are risk factors for heart disease.
> - Decrease the amount of fat you eat and increase the amounts of fruit, fiber and vegetables. For more information about nutrition, see page 13.
> - Try walking briskly for 30 to 60 minutes at a time, three to five times a week. You may prefer other aerobic activities, such as swimming, running, bicycling or rowing. Check with your doctor before you start these activities if you're over 40. For more information about exercise, see page 2.

Talk to your doctor about leading a healthy lifestyle. He or she can help you identify risk factors that you may have for a heart attack and help you find ways to reduce your risk.

## Heart Rhythm Problems

- Fainting, dizziness
- Abnormal heartbeats, skipped heartbeats, fast heartbeats
- A feeling that the heart is "jumping" in the chest
- Shortness of breath

The heart uses an electrical system to respond to changes in the amount of blood flow needed throughout the body. Damage to the heart or another problem can override the normal electrical controls of the heart. For example, when part of the heart quits functioning during a heart attack, that section of the heart may become hyperactive, sending out signals to make the heart beat hundreds of times per minute.

This *fibrillating* heart doesn't rest long enough to fill with blood, so it's constantly moving (almost a shivering motion) but not pumping blood. Other heart rhythm problems, or *arrhythmias*, can be caused by damage to the electrical system itself. Although the heart can pump without the electrical system, it won't be as effective at doing its job.

**Tachycardia.** Tachycardia refers to a condition in which the heart rate is greater than 100 beats per minute. In *paroxysmal tachycardia*, episodes of rapid heartbeat occur for no apparent reason. If tachycardia results from an irritated electrical system in the upper chambers, or atria, it is called *paroxysmal atrial tachycardia*. *Ventricular tachycardia* occurs when the *ventricles* (the lower sections of the heart) are affected. Although a healthy heart may occasionally have an abnormal beat, a diseased heart is more prone to life-threatening episodes of rapid heartbeat. Specific medical problems such as thyroid disease can cause tachycardia.

Atrial tachycardia is usually more uncomfortable than dangerous. Medical tests for causes might find a treatable condition. However, ventricular tachycardia, especially in a person who has heart disease, is serious and needs treatment. The ventricles (not the atria) are the real pumping chambers of the heart. The rapid heart rate of ventricular tachycardia doesn't allow the heart to pump blood efficiently. Ventricular tachycardia can degenerate to ventricular fibrillation (p. 119), which is often fatal.

Usually, medicine can improve the rhythm, but many of these medicines have serious side effects and must be used cautiously. Concern over side effects must be balanced with awareness that these medicines are designed to prevent a condition that is potentially much more serious—that could lead to sudden death.

**Atrial fibrillation.** This occurs when the atria don't beat in harmony with the ventricles but, instead, quiver with rapid, shallow contractions. Sometimes they are said to flutter a slower version of fibrillation. When atrial fibrillation occurs blood can become stagnant within the atria (reservoirs for the ventricles), leading to clots, which may travel out of the heart to clog arteries and perhaps cause a stroke (p. 59).

Atrial fibrillation may occur if the *mitral valves* are damaged (mitral regurgitation, p. 122) or if the atria are damaged, especially in people who smoke a lot and have lung damage. As long as the ventricles keep pumping normally, the heart will only be slightly weakened by this type of fibrillation. If the ventricles are also diseased, the lack of pumping action from the atria may lead to heart failure. If medical treatments have failed in treating atrial fibrillation, *defibrillation* can be used to restore a more normal rhythm. Also called *electric cardioversion*, it involves placing two paddles on the chest that give the heart an electric shock.

**Ventricular fibrillation.** Ventricular fibrillation is the most dangerous type of rhythm disturbance. It can be corrected and treated in the hospital with electric shock or medicines, or both. But if it isn't treated quickly, the person will die. *Cardiac arrest* or *fatal arrhythmia* are other names for this condition.

The usual scenario includes chest pain and shortness of breath during a heart attack. Then the person faints. Damage to the heart results in fibrillation. The extreme drop in blood pressure that occurs with shock can also lead to ventricular fibrillation, by forcing the heart to work harder with less blood return and less oxygen for itself. Eventually, the irritated heart begins to fibrillate.

Cardiac arrest is a life-threatening emergency. Cardiopulmonary resuscitation (CPR, p. 596) will probably be needed until an ambulance arrives. But if no blood is in the circulatory system because of internal or external bleeding, even CPR won't help. Besides giving CPR, emergency medical workers can use electric shock to treat ventricular fibrillation and can administer medicines to stimulate the heart, reduce the irritation of the heart muscle and correct chemical imbalances.

**Atrioventricular block.** Also called heart block, atrioventricular block is a malfunction of the electrical system of the heart resulting from heart damage or blockage of the blood vessels. Symptoms range from none to dizziness and shortness of breath.

Heart block may not be treated unless symptoms occur. Medicine or a *pacemaker* may help. A pacemaker is a tiny device consisting of a wire attached to a battery. The battery can be placed just under the skin, usually in the abdominal area, and the wire attached to the heart muscle itself. The pacemaker helps control the electrical impulses of the heart so that blood pressure is maintained and an adequate number of heartbeats occurs. Without a pacemaker, the prognosis for people with complete heart block is poor.

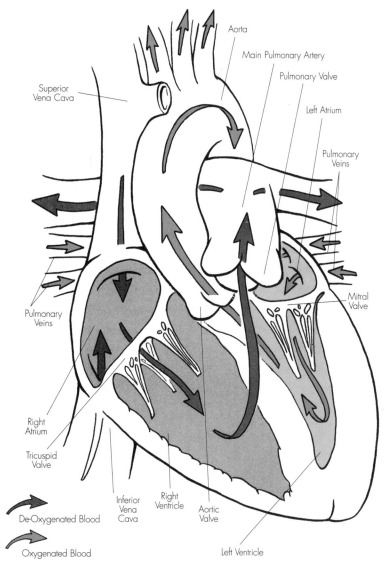

Superior
Vena Cava

Aorta

Main Pulmonary Artery

Pulmonary Valve

Left Atrium

Pulmonary
Veins

Mitral
Valve

Pulmonary
Veins

Right
Atrium

Tricuspid
Valve

Inferior
Vena
Cava

Right
Ventricle

Aortic
Valve

Left Ventricle

De-Oxygenated Blood

Oxygenated Blood

**HEART VALVES SHOWING BLOOD FLOW**

**Premature heartbeats.** Premature heartbeats are fairly common "extra" heartbeats that become apparent on the electrocardiogram (p. 634). Some people feel an *extra* or *skipped* beat when their heart pumps prematurely. Others have no symptoms. Premature beats can occur either in the atria or the ventricles. Certain types of premature ventricular beats can be serious.

Either type can occur in people with healthy hearts, or they may be a sign of heart disease, high blood pressure (p. 123) or heart strain. Premature atrial beats may also show up in

people who use stimulants such as nicotine or caffeine.

**Testing and Treatment**

A careful exam by a doctor can uncover many suspected rhythm problems. But confirmation of the specific type of rhythm problem with an electrocardiogram (p. 634) is important so the proper medicine can be used, if needed. Other tests, including various blood tests, chest x-ray, echocardiogram (p. 633) and even cardiac catheterization (p. 631), may help identify the reason for recurring episodes of abnormal heart rhythm. Treatments are highly specific for each type of rhythm disturbance. Anticoagulants are often used in chronic atrial fibrillation to prevent blood clots. A 24-hour recording of the heart by a Holter monitor (p. 634) may provide information about an arrhythmia and whether or not it's causing symptoms.

**Prevention**

If you prevent heart disease, you may avoid some heart rhythm problems. See the box on page 118 for tips on preventing heart disease. In some cases, avoiding stimulants such as nicotine or caffeine can help prevent premature heartbeats. If arrhythmias continue, medicines and underlying abnormalities that might lead to heart rhythm changes may need to be investigated.

## Heart Valve Problems

- Shortness of breath
- Chest pain

Blood is pushed from the heart to the arteries through one-way valves that keep the blood from flowing "backward." Arterioles (smallest arteries) constrict or dilate to increase or decrease blood pressure. Once pumped by the heart, blood is kept from flowing back into the left ventricle by the *aortic valve* at the base of the aorta, or main artery. The pressure difference maintained by the heart is enough to keep the blood flowing through the arteries and into the tissues. Without this pressure, the blood wouldn't flow into the tissues, oxygen wouldn't be delivered, and the tissues would starve and die.

Veins have valves along their length to keep the low-pressure blood flow always moving in one direction, toward the heart. This keeps blood from falling downward because of gravity. This system of valves maintains the return flow of blood to the heart.

Problems with the heart valves can greatly reduce the heart's ability to function. If its valves are damaged, the heart must work harder to maintain pressure within the system or to maintain sufficient return flow to the heart. Each of the four main heart valves (see p. 120) can become damaged, resulting in a valve that is too loose or too stiff. In some people, this damage occurs because of disease or infection. Other people are born with damaged or deformed heart valves.

Blood flows through the *superior vena cava* and *inferior vena cava* (the large veins that return blood to the heart) and into the right atrium of the heart. Blood passes through the *tricuspid valve* and into the right ventricle. If the tricuspid valve is damaged, it may become so scarred it can't open all the way (*stenotic valve*), or it may be so damaged that blood flows backward because the valve can't close all the way (*incompetent valve*). Severe damage leads to poor blood flow into the right side of the heart and lungs and, eventually, to heart failure.

The next valve in the blood-flow sequence is the *pulmonary valve.* Blood is pushed from the right ventricle

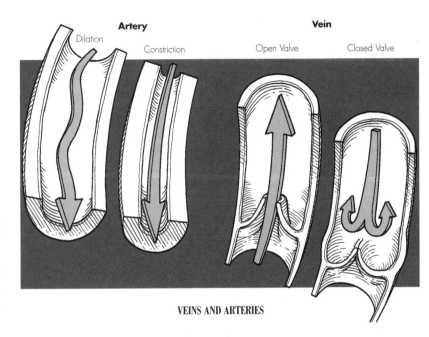

**VEINS AND ARTERIES**

through the pulmonary valve and into the pulmonary artery. If the pulmonary valve is damaged, the right side of the heart must work harder to get adequate blood flow through and into the lungs. See page 351 for information on pulmonic valve stenosis, a condition some children are born with.

Blood is pumped into the lungs by the right side of the heart and returns from the lungs to the heart through the *pulmonary vein* that leads into the left atrium. The blood then passes through the *mitral valve* on its way into the left ventricle.

Scarring of the mitral valve may cause the valve to stiffen. This can force blood to back up in the lungs. A heart attack may also result in mitral valve problems. These problems can cause shortness of breath and congestive heart failure (p. 114). An inept mitral valve makes the heart work much harder, which can lead to heart rhythm problems, such as atrial fibrillation (p. 119) and, eventually, to heart failure.

Some people have a mild deformity called *mitral valve prolapse.* Prolapse means the valve bends backward in response to pressure in the left ventricle.

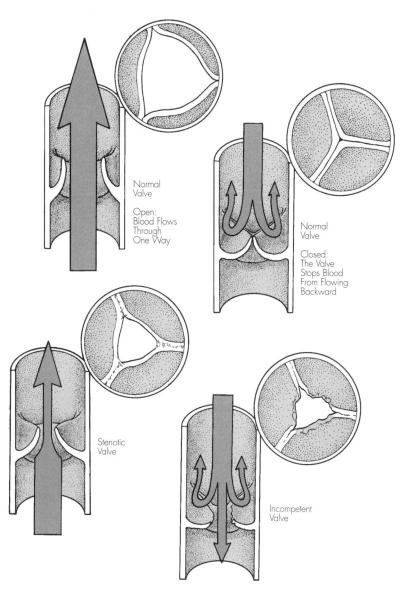

**VALVES: NORMAL, STENOTIC AND INCOMPETENT**

Normal
Valve

Open:
Blood Flows
Through
One Way

Normal
Valve

Closed:
The Valve
Stops Blood
From Flowing
Backward

Stenotic
Valve

Incompetent
Valve

The last valve the blood must go through is the *aortic valve*. Blood is pumped from the left ventricle through the aortic valve and into the aorta. The aortic valve preserves the pressure created by the pumping action of the heart.

Scarring of the aortic valve (*aortic stenosis*) slowly leads to increasing health problems, such as weakness, shortness of breath and angina (p. 109). When the aortic valve can't close, blood may be able to flow back into the ventricle. This can worsen enlargement and thickening of the left ventricle.

The aortic valve can be affected by rheumatic fever. Other causes of problems with this valve include syphilis (p. 319) and birth defects (p. 345).

**Testing and Treatment**

The doctor will listen carefully to the heart, noting any murmurs or abnormal noises, and checking the size of the heart and the clarity of the lungs. A chest x-ray will help the doctor confirm that no lung problems are present. An electrocardiogram (p. 634), echocardiogram (p. 633) and cardiac catheterization (p. 631) may also help in the diagnosis.

Treatment of a heart valve abnormality depends on the severity of the problem. Medicine is used to help the heart work a bit better as a pump with a damaged valve. Surgical treatment or heart valve replacement is sometimes needed if severe disease has affected one or more of the valves.

**Prevention**

Because valves can be damaged by rheumatic fever, it's important to keep simple streptococcal infections from worsening into this serious complication. Medicine can prevent the simple infection from worsening into rheumatic fever.

A person who has an abnormal heart valve should make sure his or her doctor

This deformity can sometimes allow blood to move backward (*regurgitate*) into the left atrium. This condition is quite common, occurring in about 4% of the population. It can cause a rapid heartbeat and minor chest pain.

Some people are born with a severely damaged mitral valve. Most mitral valve damage stems from rheumatic heart disease. This is a complication of untreated strep infections (p. 306) that results in damage to the valves of the heart. If the mitral valve is severely affected, it can be replaced with an artificial valve.

or dentist is aware of the problem before dental work or surgery is done. Sometimes, medicine is given before a procedure to help prevent an infection.

A person who has a damaged heart valve can usually exercise, including aerobic exercises such as walking and golfing. But a doctor should be consulted before playing basketball or racquetball, or using free weights for strength training.

## High Blood Pressure

- Usually no apparent symptoms
- Can increase your risk of atherosclerosis (p. 111), an enlarged heart, heart attacks (p. 115), strokes (p. 59), kidney failure and vision problems

Pressure within the circulatory system provides the force that moves blood from the heart, through the arteries and back through the veins. The heart, acting as a pump, generates this pressure. But the blood vessels, by dilating and contracting, control the pressure and amount of the flow. When this pressure is higher than normal, it's called *high blood pressure,* or *hypertension.*

Blood pressure is written as two numbers separated by a slash—like 120/80. The first number is the *systolic blood pressure,* which is the peak blood pressure when the heart is squeezing blood out. The second number is the *diastolic blood pressure,* which is the pressure when the heart is filling with blood, or relaxing between beats. A blood pressure below 130/85 is considered normal. A blood pressure above 130/85 is high. There are three kinds of hypertension.

**Essential hypertension.** Essential hypertension, also called *primary hypertension,* accounts for more than 90% of persons with high blood pressure. The exact cause remains unknown. Lack of exercise, a diet that's high in sodium, being overweight and drinking too much alcohol are factors that can elevate blood pressure. Stress may also have an impact on blood pressure. It may not necessarily be the amount of stress someone is under but, rather, how their body reacts to stress.

Essential hypertension occurs more commonly and is often more severe in blacks and often runs in families. It's more common in older people, occurring in 75% of people over 75 years of age. And it's more common in men, at least until women reach menopause, at which point it becomes equally common between the genders.

In the early stages, mild essential hypertension can be treated by reducing sodium intake, exercising and losing weight (if needed). Medicine to help the kidneys get rid of extra fluid, called diuretics (p. 616), can also lower blood pressure. Taking diuretics doesn't eliminate the need to cut back on sodium in the diet. While diuretics are still useful, they're no longer the usual first-choice medicine to treat high blood pressure. Many other types of medicine can also help treat high blood pressure. They are called antihypertensive medicines (p. 619).

**Secondary hypertension.** This is a type of hypertension caused by other disorders. Causes include various disorders of the hormones, such as too much adrenal hormone, thyroid hormone or aldosterone. Secondary hypertension occurs in some people taking oral forms of female hormones such as birth control pills (p. 550). Kidney disease causing fluid buildup in the blood vessels and fluid retention associated with pregnancy can also lead to secondary hypertension. Treating these medical conditions can reduce blood pressure. Blood-pressure elevation during pregnancy, also called toxemia (p. 395), must be treated aggressively to prevent complications in the baby and the mother.

**Malignant hypertension.** This is an uncontrolled, extreme rise in blood pressure to very high levels that puts the person at immediate risk of a stroke (p. 59) or heart failure (p. 114). It is an emergency. This type of hypertension occurs in about 5% of people with either essential or secondary hypertension. It's important that this type of hypertension be treated right away with antihypertensive medicines to prevent stroke or heart failure.

### Testing

For all their ill effects, blood pressure problems may be among the easiest to diagnose and treat. A simple and painless test with a blood-pressure cuff (p. 629) gives an accurate reading of the blood pressure.

Ambulatory blood pressure monitoring (p. 629) allows the blood pressure to be followed while the person goes on with normal daily activities.

A physical exam, including blood and urine tests and an electrocardiogram (p. 634), might help determine the extent of damage caused by the abnormal blood pressure. These tests can also be used as a baseline—which means they can be used to compare with future tests to find out if damage is occurring.

### Prevention

Persistently elevated blood pressure may shorten your life, while treatment of high blood pressure can prolong life. Treatment also reduces disease complications along the way. Blood pressure should be checked every one to two years or more often, especially if blood pressure problems run in your family.

## Low Blood Pressure

* No symptoms unless the low blood pressure is associated with poor blood flow
* Dizziness, lightheadedness, fainting

Low blood pressure, or *hypotension,* is a blood pressure below 90/50. See page 123 for information about what these numbers mean.

In *orthostatic hypotension,* the blood pressure drops suddenly when a person sits up or stands. Many people

### *Reducing High Blood Pressure*

* Don't use tobacco. Nicotine products make your body release *adrenaline.* Adrenaline causes your blood vessels to constrict and your heart to beat faster, which raises your blood pressure. See page 31 for tips on quitting nicotine use.
* Lose weight if you need to. Every 10 pounds of excess weight that you lose reduces your diastolic blood pressure number by two to three points. See page 26 for tips on losing weight.
* Exercise regularly. This can help you lose weight and also seems to lower high blood pressure by itself. See p. 2 for information about how to be more active.
* Limit the amount of sodium you eat to less than 2,300 mg (p. 17) a day.
* Limit the amount of alcohol you drink to no more than two drinks a day.
* Eat enough potassium, calcium and magnesium. These minerals may help lower blood pressure. See page 20 for information about foods containing these minerals.
* Eat less fat and cholesterol to help reduce your risk of atherosclerosis. Atherosclerosis can worsen high blood pressure by stiffening the blood vessels and making them less able to control blood pressure. See page 20 for information about a low-fat diet.
* Try relaxation techniques or biofeedback. Stress may affect blood pressure. See page 571 for more information about stress.

experience this kind of hypotension now and then. If it happens often, it may be caused by medicines, neurologic disorders, a hormone deficiency or heart problems.

Low blood pressure itself usually isn't treated because symptoms rarely occur. But if the low blood pressure is caused by another problem, the underlying condition may require treatment.

## Pericarditis

- Chest pain that extends into the left shoulder and increases with a deep breath, movement or when lying down
- Shortness of breath
- Low-grade fever

*Pericarditis* is an inflammation of the sac around the heart, called the *pericardium*. People who have had pericarditis sometimes describe the chest pain as "almost unbearable." A deep breath or cough brings on a stabbing sensation. They try to move to find a comfortable position, only to experience an increase in their pain. And if they do find a comfortable position, it's usually sitting up and leaning forward so it's often impossible to sleep. Viral infections are the most common cause of pericarditis.

The smooth inner surface of the pericardium becomes roughened, almost like sandpaper. Each beat of the heart produces a sickening rubbing sensation against the heart wall. Fluid can gather in the sac and put pressure on the heart. This condition is called *pericardial effusion*. The more fluid that pools in the sac, the more pressure is produced and the harder it is for the heart to pump blood. Heart failure can result if the fluid isn't removed.

Much less common causes of pericarditis include bacterial, fungal and viral infections, and other diseases, such as rheumatoid arthritis (p. 231) and systemic lupus erythematosus (p. 252). Pericarditis can also occur when the heart is damaged in a heart attack or a car wreck. Most often, pericarditis leaves no permanent damage to the heart or the pericardium.

### Testing

The chest x-ray (p. 631) will show an enlarged heart shadow if fluid is accumulating, because the fluid around the heart will make its shadow appear abnormally large. The electrocardiogram (p. 634) will also show changes characteristic of pericarditis. An echocardiogram (p. 633) is the best tool for determining whether fluid is accumulating around the heart and if it's restricting the heart's function.

### Treatment

Because of the pain and discomfort, and the sometimes rapid deterioration of people with pericarditis, most people with this condition are hospitalized and watched. Treatment may start with a medicine that reduces inflammation, such as indomethacin (p. 615). Steroids are used when the inflammation is more serious, along with pain-relieving medicine for comfort. Insertion of a needle to drain fluid or surgery to open the pericardial sac may be needed.

If another disease, such as tuberculosis (p. 307), is causing the inflammation, that problem must also be treated in addition to the pericarditis.

## Raynaud's Phenomenon or Disease

- One or more fingers change color, often appearing bluish, then return to normal

- The skin of the hand, foot, arm or leg appears mottled and bluish

*Raynaud's phenomenon* affects the circulation. It makes the fingers and toes extra sensitive to cold temperatures and vibrations. In response to these stimuli, the arteries in the fingers and toes contract, reducing the flow of blood to the area. The fingers or toes turn a white or even a bluish color. Although no pain develops, a tingling and sometimes numb sensation can be felt. After warming or gently rubbing the fingers or toes, the arteries relax and the color returns to normal.

Nerve damage is quick to occur in the absence of oxygen. In very severe Raynaud's phenomenon, the arteries may become so tight and stay contracted so long that the tissue in the fingers or toes dies, leading to infection and gangrene.

This condition has been linked to arthritis-like disorders, such as systemic lupus erythematosus (p. 252). Inflammation of the connective tissues or the joints leads to irritation, inflammation and contraction of the arteries for no apparent reason. If symptoms last for at least two years and no cause is found, the condition is referred to as *Raynaud's disease*. Women are affected more often than men.

*Acrocyanosis* is a condition similar to Raynaud's phenomenon, but it affects larger areas, such as the hands and feet. Sometimes it is called *Raynaud's sign*. The skin takes on a mottled, bluish appearance that is intensified in cold temperatures. No tissue damage or pain comes from this kind of arterial spasm.

### Testing and Treatment

Your doctor will rely on your description of the problem. A sure sign of Raynaud's phenomenon is that some fingers turn white or bluish while others remain their normal color. Your doctor will probably perform tests to see if another condition is responsible for the symptoms.

Usually warming the hands alleviates the problem. For more severe and recurrent episodes, treatment includes medicine that widens blood vessels or surgery. For Raynaud's phenomenon, treating the underlying disease may cure the symptoms.

### Prevention

To prevent attacks of Raynaud's phenomenon, dress warmly, even in moderate temperatures; wear gloves while shopping for cold or frozen foods. Try to avoid cold temperatures and jobs or hobbies in which vibrations can affect your hands. Because smoking can intensify Raynaud's disease, it's a good idea to quit. In addition, certain medicines may provoke attacks because they can cause blood vessels to contract. These include diet pills and decongestants containing phenylpropanolamine (p. 616), and birth control pills.

## Temporal Arteritis

- Flu-like symptoms, followed by an ache in one or both temples

### What to Avoid if You Have Raynaud's Phenomenon

- Smoking
- Cold temperatures
- Phenylpropanolamine (a common ingredient of decongestants and diet aids)
- Diet pills
- Birth control pills
- Heavy vibrations

- Tenderness over the sides of the head
- Vision loss or changes

*Temporal arteritis* occurs when the arteries in the temples, usually in people more than 50 years old, become inflamed, causing throbbing headaches, pain in the forehead and tenderness over the arteries. Not only are the headaches painful, but inflamed arteries may thicken and the blood flow through them may be restricted. This can affect vision if the inflammation isn't treated. An estimated 50% of people with untreated temporal arteritis will have vision problems, and a few will go blind. Women above age 55 are most likely to have this condition.

### Testing and Treatment

A history of dull, throbbing headaches, tenderness in the temple, changes in vision and blood tests that show the presence of inflammation may lead the doctor to order a biopsy of the temporal artery. Arteriography (p. 628) may also be done if the chronic inflammation of the arteries is more widespread than just the temples or if the cause for certain symptoms is unknown.

A number of corticosteroid medicines (p. 622) can be used. They're usually given orally. After an initial high dose of the medicine, the dose is usually lowered to prevent side effects that may occur when high doses of corticosteroid medicines are used over long periods. The medicine must be taken for long periods and tapered off, because stopping the medicine too quickly can result in uncomfortable symptoms.

### Prevention

The vision problems caused by temporal arteritis can't be corrected, but

they can be prevented if the arteritis is caught early. Early recognition of temporal arteritis as the source of headaches and associated symptoms can prevent vision loss or further damage to the eyes.

## Varicose Veins

- Bluish, soft, sometimes tender lumps just under the surface of the skin

Under normal conditions, the actions of your leg muscles during movement propel blood through the veins and back toward the heart. Varicose veins develop when the wall of a vein is weak and the valves in the vein are damaged or

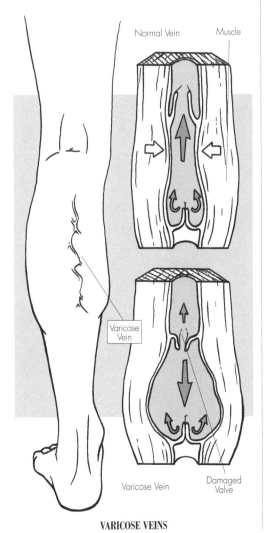

**VARICOSE VEINS**

aren't working properly. Gravity can then cause the blood to pool in the vein. Varicose veins can appear in the smaller, superficial veins near the surface of the skin. This type of varicose vein causes blue veins, sometimes even lumps, to show through the skin. Varicose veins can also occur in the deep, hidden veins of the leg. Varicose veins raise the risk of venous thrombosis (p. 129).

Varicose veins are most common in the legs. The longer a person stands without moving, the more blood pools in the veins. As more blood pools in the veins, the veins stretch, causing the overlying skin to bulge. Also, the weakness of one valve puts more pressure on other valves that are working, because the working valves must support a heavier amount of blood.

In rare cases, varicose veins can become a more serious problem. Pooled stagnant blood has a tendency to clot. This clotted blood can temporarily, or permanently, block the vein. If clotting occurs, or if the deep veins of the leg become varicosed, overall circulation in the leg may become poor. This may lead to swollen ankles and dry, scaly skin, itchy skin or darkening of the skin. This condition is called *venous stasis.* The result is tissue that can be injured easily. The leg may become infected. Small scrapes and bumps may not heal easily and may become open sores or ulcers. These are called *venous stasis ulcers.*

Very tiny veins of the legs can also dilate. These are called *spider-burst varicose veins,* because of the spider-web pattern they form. They are *not* related to real varicose veins. They don't hurt or lead to any other problems, but some people are bothered by the way they look.

**Testing**

The tendency to have varicose veins seems to run in families. If varicose veins are common in your family or if you believe you have early signs of varicose veins, have them checked by your doctor.

Tests aren't usually needed. The diagnosis can usually be made just by examining the legs. Venograms (p. 644) may be needed if deep-vein thrombosis (p. 129) is a suspected source for the swelling of the smaller veins. Doppler ultrasound (p. 643) may also be used if more information about the blood flow is needed.

**Treatment**

Raising the legs when sitting may help reduce the pain, swelling and complications of varicose veins. Custom-fitted support stockings can also help.

Venous stasis ulcers may require prescription medicines, medicated wraps or physical therapy.

### Preventing Varicose Veins

- Take breaks from standing and raise your feet when you can.
- Wear well-fitted support stockings to reduce your long-term risk of getting varicose veins.
- Avoid wearing tight knee-high socks, garters, girdles and pantyhose.
- Avoid sitting with your legs crossed.
- Take short walks during your workday, walk in place while you work or even wriggle your toes frequently. This allows the action of the muscles to pump the blood in your legs and helps prevent blood from pooling in the veins.

Sometimes other diseases, such as diabetes (p. 211) or heart failure (p. 114), add to the problem. Treatment may include frequent or almost constant elevation of the legs, along with elastic wraps, and antibiotic pills or creams for the skin. Severe ulcers, especially in people who have diabetes or heart failure, may take months to heal, even with the best possible care.

## Venous Thrombosis

- Swelling, redness and tenderness along a vein
- A wide variety of symptoms, depending on which vessel is blocked

*Venous thrombosis* occurs when the blood forms clots (also called *thrombi* or *emboli*) within the veins. This is especially likely in the veins where blood moves more slowly. For example, the downward pull of gravity on the blood within the leg slows the blood flow from the leg back to the heart. Lying still for many days, as might occur during an illness, also allows small, stagnant areas to form within the veins, increasing the risk of clots. Even sitting for several hours of travel, as in a car or airplane, can lead to venous thrombosis. Some medicines and diseases may also increase the risk.

Have you ever hit your arm or leg and later developed a hard, tender knot or cord that was slow to go away? Did the site of an injection or intravenous line turn red and tender, then swell or develop into a clot along a vein? These are common symptoms of venous thrombosis in smaller veins near the surface of the skin. This is called *superficial phlebitis* or *superficial thrombophlebitis*. Venous thrombosis in the smaller veins can

impair blood flow. Over time, this can starve the tissues for oxygen and nutrients. In chronic, untreated conditions, the tissues become more susceptible to injury and infection.

A clot within the larger veins of the leg, the *deep veins,* is called *deep-vein thrombosis.* This is a serious condition that requires immediate attention. A blood clot in a deep vein can pass through the heart and into a lung. A large clot that lodges in the pulmonary artery may block the blood supply to the lungs and cause serious lung damage or even death This is called a pulmonary embolism (p. 157).

### Testing

Your doctor can often diagnose thrombosis of the small veins just by examining the affected area and by hearing how the symptoms started. Possible deep-vein thrombosis may require further testing. Swelling, tenderness and redness in a leg, especially in people at risk or with a history of clots in the deep veins, should be checked right away by a doctor. Venography (p. 644) and Doppler ultrasound (p. 644) may be used to identify reduced blood flow and a probable clot.

### Treatment

If the problem involves the veins close to the skin, it may heal by itself. Medicines, especially anti-inflammatory medicines (p. 615), can help reduce both the inflammation and the pain. Keeping the affected area elevated may help, as may short periods of using a heating pad on a low setting. Wearing special elastic stockings may help maintain better blood flow if a leg is involved. Special elastic wraps can also be helpful on a leg or an arm.

Because deep-vein thrombosis can cause a clot to lodge in the lung, immediate treatment (usually in the hospital) is important. Intravenous blood thinning medicines (p. 619) will probably be given until the swelling and redness improve. Clot-dissolving medicine (p. 622) can be given through a catheter.

A pulmonary embolus may cause chest pain and severe shortness of breath or cause relatively few symptoms. Pulmonary embolism is an emergency that requires attention in the emergency room. In life-threatening situations, a pulmonary arteriogram (p. 628) may be done to evaluate the need for surgical removal of the clot or treatment with thrombolytic medicine.

After the clot has been treated, oral anticoagulants will probably be needed to ensure that new clots don't form. A mesh can be surgically placed in the *inferior vena cava* (the vein that returns blood to the heart) to prevent future clots from traveling to the lungs.

**Prevention**

Some things that can lead to venous thrombosis can be avoided. These things include smoking, taking estrogen, going long periods without activity and being overweight. If you've had clots in your legs, keep taking anticoagulants according to your doctor's instructions. When traveling, try to get out of your car (or your seat on an airplane) and move around every two hours. This may prevent a clot from forming in your leg. Special stockings that help maintain good blood flow in the legs may also prevent problems.

Let your doctor know about any swelling in your legs. Discovering and treating deep-vein thrombosis before it moves to the lungs can save your life.

# CHAPTER 8 — BLOOD

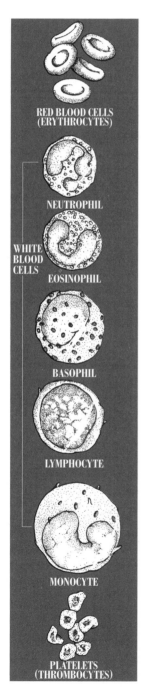

**RED BLOOD CELLS (ERYTHROCYTES)**

**WHITE BLOOD CELLS**
NEUTROPHIL
EOSINOPHIL
BASOPHIL
LYMPHOCYTE
MONOCYTE

**PLATELETS (THROMBOCYTES)**

Blood is the life-sustaining liquid that provides your body with oxygen and nutrients. Blood carries nutrients, obtained from food, to tissues. Blood also carries medicines, alcohol, nicotine and other tobacco products that are absorbed into the blood through the lungs. Blood maintains body temperature and fluid balance, and carries hormones produced by endocrine glands (p. 207) to the rest of the body.

Blood is made up of red and white blood cells, platelets and plasma. The red blood cells, platelets and most of the white blood cells are made inside the bones, in the *bone marrow*.

Red blood cells, or *erythrocytes,* contain *hemoglobin*. Hemoglobin is the red pigment, or coloring, within the blood cells. Hemoglobin carries oxygen that's absorbed as the blood cells move through the lungs and into the body. Red blood cells also help rid the body of carbon dioxide.

White blood cells, or *leukocytes,* are an important part of the immune system. They protect the body from infection and help remove dead cells so repair of tissues can take place. White blood cells include *lymphocytes, monocytes, basophils, eosinophils* and *neutrophils.* See page 296 for more information on how your body fights infection.

Blood also contains platelets, or *thrombocytes.* Platelets play an important role in helping blood clot so bleeding slows down. *Plasma,* the liquid part of the blood not including the cells and platelets, contains nutrients, proteins, fats and salts. Both platelets and plasma contain components called *clotting factors* that are involved in making your blood clot to stop bleeding. A blood clot starts when platelets collect at the site of injury where blood vessels have been damaged. After a natural chain reaction, a substance called *fibrin* is produced. Fibrin surrounds the platelets and the components of the chain reaction to hold them in place and form a clot. Problems with clotting factors cause bleeding disorders, such as hemophilia (p. 136). Serum is the clear or amber-colored liquid that's left after the blood clots. It separates from blood during the clotting process. It has no cells, platelets or clotting factors.

**Blood types.** Blood is classified into different types. Two main classification systems are the *ABO classification system* and the *Rh system.* Blood can be A, B, AB or O. It can also be either Rh positive or Rh negative. Your blood type is inherited.

The ABO classification system is based on the presence of either A or B *antibodies* in the serum of the blood and A or B *antigens* on the surface of the red blood cells. Antigens are protein-like substances that occur naturally in the body or enter the body from the outside (such as an infection by a virus or bacteria). The body often makes antibodies to destroy foreign antigens. This is how the body fights infections. But when antibodies act against the body's own antigens, it causes what's called an autoimmune reaction. Auto-immune disorders (p. 223) can be very serious illnesses.

People with *type A* blood have the A antigen on the surface of their red blood cells and the B antibody in their serum. People with *type B* blood have the B antigen on the red blood cell surface and the A antibody in their serum.

People with *type AB* blood have both antigens on the surface of their red blood cells but neither antibody in their serum. These people can receive blood of any type—because their blood doesn't contain any antibodies to A or B antigens.

People with *type O* blood have neither the A or B antigen on the red blood cells and both types of antibody in their serum. That's why they can only receive type O blood—because their blood contains both antibodies and will attack any blood cells that have A or B antigen.

People who have *Rh positive* blood have the Rh factor antigen on the red blood cells. People who have Rh negative blood don't. This difference between the two groups can cause problems if an *Rh negative* woman is pregnant with an Rh positive baby. This situation is called Rh factor incompatibility (p. 345).

**Donating blood.** Donating blood is important because blood can save lives. Donating is easy and very safe. You aren't at risk of catching AIDS or any other disease by giving blood. A new sterile syringe and needle are required and used every time someone donates blood.

When you give blood, you'll probably be asked some questions and a small sample of blood will be taken to check your hemoglobin level. You'll probably also have your temperature, pulse and blood pressure taken. About one pint of blood can be given at a time. The average adult man who weighs about 155 pounds has about seven quarts of blood flowing through his veins. Blood can be donated every two months.

You can donate blood if you're older than 17 and weigh 110 pounds or more. You shouldn't donate blood if you have hepatitis, heart disease, cancer, severe

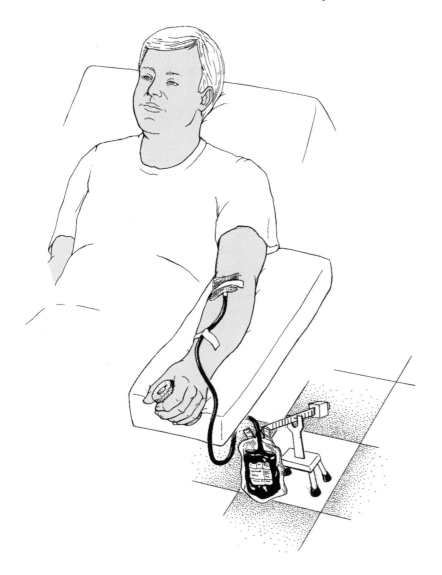

**PERSON GIVING BLOOD**

asthma (p. 142), a bleeding disorder (p. 135), seizures or AIDS (p. 325), or if you're at risk for HIV infection (p. 325). Other health problems also take you off the donor list, at least until they're resolved. These include anemia (below), malaria (p. 312), exposure to malaria or hepatitis, pregnancy, major surgery, high blood pressure (p. 123) and low blood pressure that's causing symptoms (p. 124).

**Blood transfusions.** Blood transfusions can be given to help replace blood lost, for example, in an accident or during surgery. Transfusions can also be used when certain types of anemia cause a lack of hemoglobin in the blood. Transfusions may include all the blood components, called *whole-blood* transfusions, or just certain parts of the blood, such as the red cells or platelets.

Sometimes people give their own blood in advance to use when they plan to have surgery. This is called an *autologous* transfusion. Using your own blood is safest because it eliminates the risk of an allergic reaction or infection. You can begin donating blood several weeks before a planned surgery. Your blood is stored until your surgery.

## Anemia

- Light-headedness
- Headaches
- Chest pain
- Pale skin
- Weakness, tiredness and breathlessness with activity

*Anemia* can occur when the hemoglobin level is low. Hemoglobin carries oxygen to the body's tissues, so a low hemoglobin level can cause symptoms like those listed above. If you feel tired, you may suspect you have anemia and wonder if you should take iron supplements. But

tiredness is only one symptom of anemia, and not all types of anemia are caused by a lack of iron in the blood.

**Anemia of chronic disease.** Anemia often occurs in people with chronic diseases, probably because the body doesn't produce as many red blood cells when a disease or infection is present. Kidney disease is a very common cause of anemia. Rheumatoid arthritis (p. 231) and chronic infections such as tuberculosis (p. 307), hepatitis or AIDS (p. 325) are diseases in which anemia often occurs. Treatment of the disease may improve the anemia.

**Hemolytic anemias.** These anemias occur when the blood cells are destroyed faster than they're replaced. This situation can lead to a shortage of oxygen-carrying cells— and to symptoms of anemia. There are a number of causes for hemolytic anemias. The action of artificial heart valves, for example, can destroy red blood cells when the blood flows through the valve. Toxins or poisons can damage red cells and cause them to break open. Antibodies in a mismatched blood transfusion can destroy red cells.

Hemolytic anemias also can be caused by medicines, which should be stopped as soon as they're identified as the cause. Some people with hemolytic anemia need a *splenectomy* (removal of the spleen) to reduce the severity of the anemia.

**Iron-deficiency anemia.** Iron-deficiency anemia can result from a low intake of iron or poor absorption of iron from food. Blood loss, such as that caused by colon cancer (p. 175) or a bleeding ulcer (p. 197), can also lead to iron-deficiency anemia. Even heavy menstrual periods can cause iron-deficiency anemia. This type of

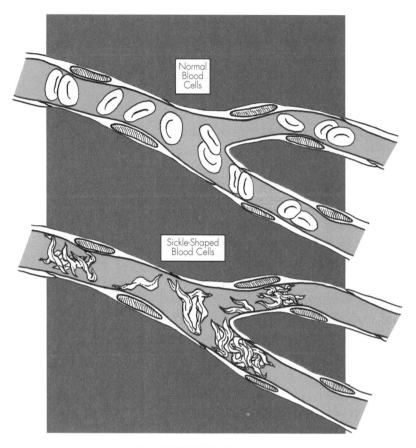

**BLOOD CELLS: NORMAL VS. SICKLE**

and antibiotics if the episode was brought on by an infection.

Sickle-cell anemia is inherited from both parents. Each parent must pass a sickle cell gene to the child for the child to have sickle cell anemia. If only one parent passes a gene, the child will have the *sickle-cell trait.* This means he or she has inherited only one faulty hemoglobin gene and is able to make enough hemoglobin to prevent most symptoms. A trait carrier can pass the defective sickle gene to his or her children.

Sickle-cell anemia is usually discovered during childhood. It occurs almost exclusively in black families. About 1% to 3% of blacks carry the sickle-cell trait, and one in 400 have sickle-cell disease.

**Thalassemia.** This is another type of inherited hemoglobin defect that leads to anemia. It's found mainly in people from Mediterranean countries, such as Italy and Greece, the Middle East and parts of India and Pakistan. It's a type of hemolytic anemia. The hemoglobin cells are destroyed in the bone marrow because they're seen by the body's defenses as abnormal or foreign.

There are two types of thalassemia. People who have only one thalassemia gene have a condition called *thalassemia minor.* They may have chronic anemia, but generally they have few symptoms. People who have two genes have *thalassemia major,* the full-blown disease. Thalassemia major is a severe disease that can affect many organs, such as the liver, spleen and heart. Thalassemia major is usually treated with blood transfusions, but people with the disease have a shortened life expectancy.

**Vitamin-deficiency anemias.** These anemias can occur in people who don't get enough vitamin $B_{12}$ or folic acid. These vitamins help the body form red blood cells and hemoglobin. A common

anemia can be corrected with an improved diet, iron pills or injections of iron. The cause of the abnormal blood loss has to be identified and treated to prevent continued problems.

**Sickle-cell anemia.** This is a hereditary disease that results in an abnormally shaped hemoglobin cell. The cells are shaped like a sickle. These "sickled" cells are fragile. They stick together and break. Sickled blood cells clog small arteries in the bones, spleen, liver, lungs and other tissues. The result is episodes of terrible pain, especially in the chest, abdomen and joints. These painful episodes are unpredictable but may be triggered by infection and by hot or cold weather.

Sickle-cell anemia has no cure, and treatment can only reduce the severity of the anemia. Painful episodes are usually treated in the hospital with strong pain medicines, fluids, oxygen reason for this type of anemia is poor nutrition from chronic alcoholism.

*Pernicious anemia* occurs when a person's digestive tract can't absorb vitamin $B_{12}$ from food. Pernicious anemia is usually diagnosed in people over 50 years old or in people who are strict vegetarians and eat *no* animal products.

Vitamin deficiencies can be corrected with oral or injectable forms of vitamins.

### Should I take a vitamin and iron supplement?

If you eat a balanced diet with fresh fruits, vegetables, lean meats, milk, whole grains and beans, you probably won't need vitamin or iron supplements. People whose diets include large amounts of fast foods and junk foods may benefit from vitamin supplements. A healthy diet is still the best choice.

Overdoses of iron supplements can lead to toxic levels of iron in the liver, along with stomach irritation and constipation. Iron supplements should only be used if you can't get enough iron in your diet. If you're thinking about taking an iron supplement, talk to your doctor first.

### Testing

After anemia is diagnosed, the cause of the anemia must be found through blood tests. It's important to find out which type of anemia is present before treatment is started. For example, taking supplements to treat one kind of anemia can hide the damage other types of anemia can cause. The number, size and shape of the blood cells and a family history of anemia can help your doctor identify the exact cause for your low blood count or low hemoglobin level. Then the right treatment can be started.

### Prevention

The only types of anemia that can be prevented are iron-deficiency and vitamin-deficiency anemias that are caused by inadequate amounts of iron, vitamin $B_{12}$ or folic acid in the diet. Make sure your diet contains adequate sources of iron and B vitamins. Sources include meats, dairy products and dark-green, leafy vegetables.

## Bleeding Disorders

- Nosebleeds or bleeding gums
- Bruising easily
- Bleeding from cuts or scrapes that doesn't stop easily
- Small red dots under the skin resembling a rash

When the skin is damaged, the blood vessels contract, reducing the blood loss. Then platelets gather at the open, bleeding site and begin to form a plug, or *clot*. Clotting factors in the blood, a component called *fibrinogen* and the cells caught in the clot act together with platelets to firm up the plug. White blood cells also come to the area to fight off any foreign substances or invading bacteria.

Clotting disorders result because of low levels of platelets, poorly functioning platelets and low levels of clotting factors or fibrinogen. These problems can occur for many reasons, including inherited disorders, infections, medicines, toxins and vitamin deficiencies. These are the different types of clotting disorders:

**Disseminated intravascular coagulation (DIC).** DIC can occur as a result of the trauma of surgery, a major accident or an infection. In subacute DIC, the blood may clot (*coagulate*) very easily, sometimes causing blood clots that block arteries and veins. In acute DIC, the clotting factors become depleted and the blood isn't able to form clots. Healing incisions or cuts start bleeding again, sometimes profusely.

DIC can be life-threatening, and transfusions of whole blood or blood components may be needed to stop further bleeding. The underlying cause of DIC must be treated. If clotting is out of control, anticoagulant medicines (p. 619) may be needed.

**Factor deficiencies.** These are inherited traits. They include factor VIII deficiency (*hemophilia A*), von Willebrand's disease, factor IX deficiency (*hemophilia B*) and factor XII deficiency. Levels of clotting factors decline because the person's body doesn't make these factors or makes very small amounts of them. Bruising easily, bleeding into the joints, nosebleeds and blood in the urine or stool are the most common symptoms of a factor deficiency.

Transfusion of the missing factor or factors is essential after a bleeding episode has begun. A new medicine called desmopressin (p. 623) is being used in people with hemophilia A to stimulate production of clotting factor VIII. The increased level of factor VIII slows or stops the bleeding.

**Thrombocytopenia.** Thrombocytopenia occurs when the platelet count falls to very low levels. Bruises or small red spots that look like a rash may be signs of thrombocytopenia. Viral infections, radiation therapy, a large number of medicines and some forms of arthritis (p. 229) and autoimmune disorders (p. 223) can cause thrombocytopenia. Treatment involves treating the underlying cause, such as a viral infection. Some cases have no known cause.

**Vitamin deficiencies.** Serious vitamin deficiencies can cause bleeding problems. Bleeding gums and easy bruising occur when there's a severe lack of vitamin C, called *scurvy*.

Vitamin C deficiency can lead to damage and weakness of the blood vessel walls, which in turn leads to bleeding.

Vitamin K deficiency can lead to clotting problems because this vitamin is needed for the production of many of the clotting factors. Because the clotting factors are produced in the liver, damage to this organ may result in bleeding problems. Alcoholic liver damage can affect intestinal absorption of vitamin K. If this problem occurs, injected vitamin K may be used to stimulate clotting.

### Testing

The source of a bleeding problem can usually be found through blood tests that check blood cell counts, platelet counts and clotting factors. The blood can also be examined to find deficiencies in specific clotting factors or problems with the way the platelets function.

### Prevention

You can prevent bleeding disorders caused by scurvy by making sure you include enough vitamin C in your diet. You can also prevent clotting factor problems from vitamin K deficiency by making sure you include vitamin K in your diet as well. See page 19 for more information about these vitamins. The clotting problems from alcoholic liver damage can be prevented by limiting the amount of alcohol you drink.

## Bone Marrow Problems

- Bleeding easily
- Weakness
- Infections
- Bone pain

The *bone marrow* inside the bones produces all the red blood cells, platelets and most of the white blood cells. These cells are needed to transport oxygen and nutrients, to stop

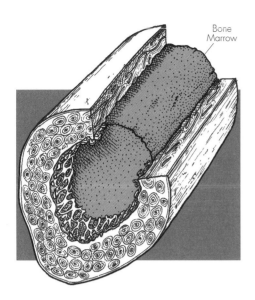

Bone
Marrow

**BONE CROSS SECTION (LENGTHWISE)
SHOWING MARROW**

bleeding by forming clots and to fight infections. When the bone marrow is diseased, it doesn't produce enough of these cells, or it doesn't produce healthy cells. Treatment depends on the cause of the bone marrow problem.

**Agranulocytosis.** This disorder occurs when no *granulocytes,* a type of white blood cell, are being produced by the bone marrow. Medicines, infections or cancer of the bone marrow (leukemia, p. 138) may cause this problem. Agranulocytosis can also lead to infections because of the reduced number of white blood cells to fight infection.

**Aplastic anemia.** Aplastic anemia occurs when the bone marrow completely stops making all types of blood cells, including red and white cells and platelets. Infections, easy bleeding and weakness may be the first symptoms. Medicines, toxins and infections have been known to cause this serious problem, but many cases have no known cause.

**Multiple myeloma.** This is cancer in a certain type of white blood cell called *plasma cells,* which are produced in the bone marrow. Plasma cells normally produce *antibodies*— the proteins created by the body to destroy bacteria, viruses and other invading agents. In someone with multiple myeloma, normal plasma cells change into cancer cells. The bone marrow is pushed out of the way, and red cells, other white cells and platelets can't be produced. Instead, an excessive amount of an abnormal antibody protein is produced. This excess antibody protein can be measured in the blood, and also in the urine in some cases. This measurement helps doctors diagnose the disease. Early symptoms of multiple myeloma include bone pain, infections, weakness or easy bruising.

**Polycythemia.** Polycythemia occurs when too many red blood cells are produced. This can happen as the result of a disorder called *polycythemia vera* that stimulates the bone marrow to produce too many red blood cells. Or polycythemia may occur as a result of heart or lung disease or smoking. The heart disease or lung disease causes low oxygen levels in the blood, which stimulates the bone marrow to overproduce red cells. The blood becomes very thick, and the person's complexion appears reddish. The person may feel weak or dizzy, have a constant dull headache and be at risk for both bleeding and blood clots. The more severe symptoms generally occur in people with polycythemia vera. Polycythemia can also produce intense itching of the skin, especially when part of the body is warm or hot, such as after a hot bath.

### Testing

Tests can be done on a blood sample or on a sample of the marrow taken directly from the bone (p. 630). Samples of bone marrow can reveal problems that don't show up in a blood test or urine test. They also can supply other helpful information to your doctor.

## Bruising

- Blue, purple or brown markings on the skin

*Bruising* occurs when blood vessels break and bleed into the surrounding tissue under the surface of the skin. Usually this happens after the area has been hit. A black eye (p. 63) is one example of this type of injury.

Bruises usually aren't serious. Most small ones go away on their own in seven to 10 days. For more severe bruises, ice packs (p. 243) can be applied in the first 24 to 48 hours to help reduce swelling. Ice packs can also help slow bleeding and lessen bruising. You should raise the bruised area above heart level, if possible, to help reduce swelling.

If you begin to bruise much more easily than you usually do, see your doctor. This may be a sign of a blood disorder. Another serious situation is bruising of a deep muscle. This can occur after a crushing injury, such as in the case of a thigh or calf injury. These deep bruises can lead to a blood clot, so talk to your doctor right away.

## Leukemia

- Bruising easily
- Fatigue
- Weight loss
- Weakness
- Enlarged lymph nodes (sometimes)
- Infections

*Leukemia* occurs when the white blood cells, both granulocytes and lymphocytes, become cancerous. The cancerous blood cells can quickly spread throughout the bloodstream to many different areas of the body, invading and destroying organs and tissues. Some types of leukemia are more aggressive and severe than others. The outlook varies with the age of the person.

**Acute lymphocytic leukemia.** This form of leukemia occurs when lymphocytes become cancerous. The cancerous cells can be found in both the bone marrow and the lymph nodes. Acute lymphocytic leukemia is the most common type of leukemia in children. Bone pain, bruising easily, infections and fever are common symptoms. Bone-marrow samples will reveal large quantities of cancerous cells. Chemotherapy (p. 225) cures the disease in more than seven out of 10 adults and nine out of 10 children.

**Acute myelogenous leukemia.** This leukemia stems from cancer of the granulocytes. While this form of leukemia can be rapidly fatal, chemotherapy can bring about a long-term remission in about half of the people with the disease. Death can occur within one to two weeks from the start of symptoms if the illness isn't treated or if it doesn't respond to treatment. Early symptoms of acute myelogenous leukemia include bruising, rashes and infections in the mouth and throat.

Chemotherapy is used to try to stop the cancer cells from spreading to organs and tissues. Transfusions and bone-marrow transplants are used to replace the cancer cells with healthy cells.

**Chronic lymphocytic leukemia.** This form of leukemia is marked by fatigue, swollen lymph nodes, infections and weight loss. It usually occurs in elderly people, and it progresses slowly. Some people won't require treatment. Others may need chemotherapy or corticosteroids (p. 622). Removal of the spleen can reduce some complications and can stop or slow the disease.

**Chronic myelogenous leukemia.** This type of leukemia is more aggressive than chronic lymphocytic leukemia because the cancer cells multiply

## Bone Marrow Transplants

A bone marrow transplant is an option for people with leukemia and can be an option for cancers that can spread, such as breast cancer. It's done in people who have severe disease with the hope of improving their life expectancy.

The first step is finding a compatible bone marrow donor. Possible donors can come from family members or from the National Bone Marrow Registry. To find out if a donor is compatible, possible donors must have a test for *human lymphocyte antigens* (HLA test). The HLA test examines proteins, or HLAs, found on the white blood cells and other cells in the body. The HLAs of the donor and the recipient must match for a bone marrow transplant to be considered.

The procedure involves first destroying the recipient's diseased bone marrow. This is done with radiation and medicines. Bone marrow is taken from the donor's hip bone. The bone marrow can either be used the same day or frozen and stored until the recipient is ready for the procedure. The donor's bone marrow is injected into the recipient's veins. The bone marrow flows through the bloodstream to fill the bone marrow space and make new cells.

To avoid the risk of infection or complications, the bone marrow recipient must stay in the hospital for four to six weeks, and may receive intravenous antibiotics (p. 618). Complications can include infection, a severe reaction called *graft-versus-host disease* or pneumonia.

rapidly. Chemotherapy is usually needed, and bone-marrow transplants may offer the best chance of a complete cure.

## Lymphoma

- Persistent cough
- Fever
- Fatigue
- Night sweats
- Weight loss
- Painless swelling of the lymph nodes at the base of the neck, armpit or groin

*Lymphoma* is cancer of the lymph nodes. Many types of lymphoma can be treated, but finding and treating it early are the keys to curing the disease.

Although lymphoma can occur anywhere in the body, swelling of a lymph node in the neck is often the first sign. Because the middle portion of the chest, called the *mediastinum*, has many lymph nodes, it's also a common site of swelling. There may be few apparent symptoms until the tumor is quite large. Then, pressure on the bronchial tubes may lead to a chronic cough. Weight loss, night sweats and fatigue may be the first signs of lymphoma.

**Hodgkin's lymphoma.** This type of lymphoma often starts in the chest with a persistent cough or chest pain. The lymph nodes at the base of the neck or armpits may become swollen. Fever, weight loss, night sweats and fatigue are other common symptoms. Most cases occur in people in their late teens to early forties, but the disease can occur earlier or later in life. Cure rates are good: greater than 90% for people whose disease is detected in the earlier stages and greater than 50% for those whose disease is discovered later.

**Non-Hodgkin's lymphoma.** This type of lymphoma often results in enlarged lymph nodes in the neck, armpit and groin. It may cause symptoms of unexplained sweating, fevers, tiredness, loss of appetite and weight loss. Non-Hodgkin's lymphoma tends to occur in people over 40 years old. The cure rate for non-Hodgkin's lymphoma is lower overall than that for Hodgkin's lymphoma, but it depends on the particular type.

## Testing and Treatment

Don't panic if you find an enlarged lymph node. Most nodes are enlarged because of a nearby infection. For example, colds and sore throats often lead to enlarged lymph nodes in the neck. When the infection goes away, the nodes shrink back to normal size within a few weeks.

If you notice a rapidly growing lymph node that isn't near a site of infection, see your doctor. If a tumor is suspected, a biopsy, or removal of one of the enlarged lymph nodes, may be needed. The biopsy will show if it's lymphoma and identify the specific type of lymphoma. Blood tests and chest x-rays (p. 631) may also be needed. If cancer is diagnosed, other tests will be needed to determine the best treatment.

Chemotherapy (p. 225) destroys cancer cells but also affects healthy tissue. Radiation therapy (p. 225) can be focused to selectively destroy cancer cells. Both chemotherapy and radiation therapy may be used to treat lymphoma. Surgery isn't used for treating most people with lymphoma. It's sometimes used to explore the abdomen to determine the severity of the disease or to decrease the size of a tumor when the lymphoma involves the stomach. A bone-marrow transplant can be used in very severe cases, when the lymphoma has spread throughout the body.

# CHAPTER 9   LUNGS

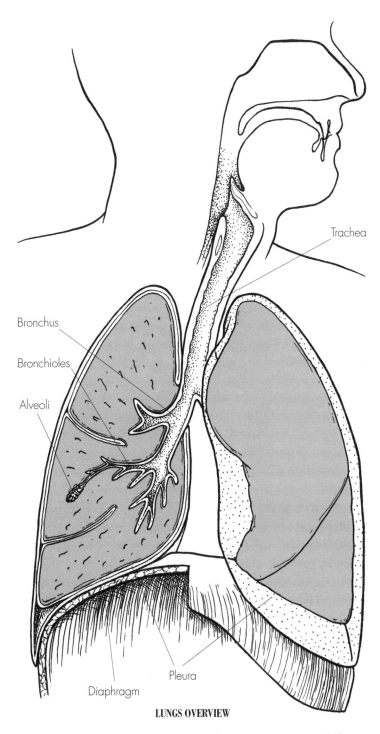

Trachea

Bronchus

Bronchioles

Alveoli

Pleura

Diaphragm

**LUNGS OVERVIEW**

The air you breathe goes into your *lungs*. Two important functions take place in your lungs: oxygen is picked up by the blood, and carbon dioxide, a waste, is removed from the blood and exhaled. Your lungs are made up of several *lobes,* roundish compartments or areas of your lungs that are smooth and shiny.

Air inhaled through the nose and mouth goes through a series of tubes. It flows through the windpipe, or *trachea,* in the throat, through the main air passages in the lungs called *bronchial tubes,* through smaller air passages called *bronchi,* through the even smaller air tubes called *bronchioles,* and then to the tiny air sacs in the lungs called the *alveoli.* Alveoli have very thin walls through which gases, such as oxygen and carbon dioxide, can pass.

The alveoli are surrounded by tiny blood vessels called *capillaries.* Veins carry the blood to the capillaries in the lungs. The blood carries carbon dioxide and other wastes of normal body functions. When it reaches the capillaries, the blood releases the waste into the alveoli. This waste is discharged from your body when you exhale. While the blood is in the capillaries, it also absorbs the oxygen that you have inhaled into the alveoli. The oxygen in the blood travels throughout your body to nourish your tissues.

Exhaling and inhaling are things you do without even thinking. Your body keeps track of the levels of carbon dioxide and oxygen in your blood. Nerve cells in the tissues send signals to the brain if the level of carbon dioxide gets too high or the level of oxygen gets too low. This causes you automatically to breathe faster and deeper.

The main muscles responsible for breathing are the *diaphragm* and the muscles that control the ribs. The diaphragm stretches across your mid-section underneath your lungs. When you inhale, your lungs expand, your diaphragm moves down and your ribs move out to make room for the air in your lungs. When you exhale, the opposite occurs.

Your lungs are surrounded by the *pleura,* a slick, two-layered membrane that holds a fluid between its layers to help the movement of your lungs in your chest.

## Asthma

- Wheezing
- Coughing
- Shortness of breath
- Tightness in the chest

*Asthma* is a disease that affects the bronchial tubes, or airways, of the lungs. The airways of people with asthma are extra sensitive to substances that they're allergic to, called *allergens,* and to other irritating things in the air, called *irritants,* or to emotional stress. These things can cause the bronchial tubes to swell, or become inflamed, leading to an asthma attack.

An asthma attack can occur when someone with asthma is exposed to an allergen, an irritant or emotional stress. Some people are prone to asthma attacks when they eat certain foods or when they take certain medicines.

Whatever the triggering factor, the swelling in the airways causes mucus to form inside the air tubes and causes the muscles around the tubes to contract. This makes the airways smaller, making it harder for air to pass through quickly. The mucus can also reduce the air flow, causing wheezing and breathing problems.

Over the past few years, a radical change has occurred in the understanding of asthma. Until recently, most doctors considered the shrinking, or *constriction,* of the bronchial tubes as the major problem in asthma, so treatment was aimed at relieving the constriction. Some of these treatments produced unpleasant side effects.

Doctors knew irritants and allergens played a role in asthma, but for a long time they didn't know how these agents affected the muscles in the airways. It's now known that airway inflammation is the primary factor in asthma, and since more is known about asthma, better treatments are available and symptoms can be better controlled.

### Testing

Your symptoms will help your doctor diagnose asthma. Asthma is suspected if you have spells or attacks of wheezing and shortness of breath or coughing for no known reason. Pulmonary function tests (p. 640) may show problems that indicate airway constriction. A dose of asthma medicine may be given during the test to see if the constriction can be reversed.

### Treatment

Asthma medicines fall into two main categories: those that relieve airway constriction (bronchodilators, p. 621) and those that reduce the swelling, or inflammation, such as corticosteroids (p. 622), cromolyn (p. 623) and nedocromil (p. 622). All of these medicines can be inhaled or given by pill, and most can be given through the vein if a serious attack occurs.

**Bronchodilators.** Bronchodilators relax the muscles of the bronchial tubes, increasing the size of the tubes and restoring normal air flow. Bronchodilators come in an inhaled form for very rapid relief of an asthma attack. But it's important that you follow directions

---

## Things That Can Trigger an Asthma Attack

- Air pollution
- Dust
- Emotional stress
- Exercise
- Fumes
- Infections of the respiratory tract, such as viral infections
- Molds
- Perfume or cologne
- Pollen
- Sinus infections
- Smoke
- Foods that you're allergic to
- Medicines that you're allergic to
- Spray-on deodorants
- Sulfite, a preservative used in red wine, beer, salad bars, dehydrated soups and other foods
- Temperature changes

for their use. Overuse can cause serious side effects and sometimes even death. When bronchodilators are used frequently for relief, it may mean that airway swelling hasn't been treated as much as needed. Bronchodilators may mask symptoms of swelling. This is why it's dangerous to self-treat what could be asthma. See your doctor if you have symptoms. Bronchodilators also can be given more regularly in pill or liquid form to treat or prevent attacks.

**Anti-inflammatory medicines.** When used regularly, an anti-inflammatory medicine can also be effective. Anti-inflammatory medicines help reduce the swelling in the airways. Often, anti-inflammatory medicines are taken every day to prevent attacks. They take hours, even days, to begin working, and usually don't work well unless taken regularly. Anti-inflammatory medicines include corticosteroids, such as prednisone (p. 620), cromolyn and nedocromil. Inhaled steroids have fewer side effects than oral forms.

Many people with asthma use more than one kind of asthma medicine because one medicine can

> ## *Using an Inhaler*
>
> - To make sure your inhaler has medicine in it, place the canister (not the mouthpiece) in water. If it floats sideways, it's empty. If it tips up, it's partly full. If it sinks, it's full.
> - Shake the canister.
> - Assemble the canister and mouthpiece.
> - Remove the cap and hold the inhaler upright.
> - Tilt your head back and breathe out.
> - Put the inhaler 1 to 1½ inches away from your mouth. If you're using a *spacer*, put the end of it in your mouth and seal your lips around it. A spacer is a tube that you attach to your inhaler. It makes the inhaler easier to use and more efficient.
> - Press down on the inhaler to release the medicine. At the same time, breathe in slowly for three to five seconds. If you use dry powder capsules, close your mouth tightly around the mouthpiece of the inhaler and inhale rapidly.
> - Hold your breath for 10 seconds so the medicine can get deep into your lungs.
> - Repeat as many times as your doctor suggests. Wait one minute between puffs to let each puff get deeper into your lungs.

often enhance the way another medicine works.

With newer and safer medicines to open the airways, an important older medicine, theophylline (p. 626), is used less often. Theophylline has helped a number of people through the years

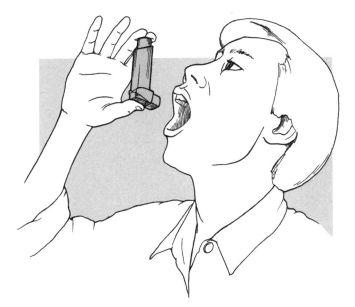

**USING AN INHALER WITHOUT A SPACER**

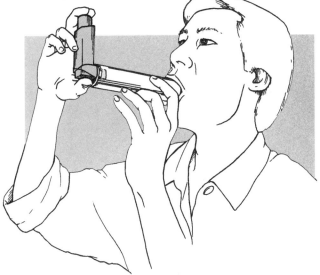

**USING AN INHALER WITH A SPACER**

but can have unwanted side effects, such as heart problems and confusion. When theophylline is prescribed, blood levels of the medicine must be checked on a regular basis to ensure that it's not harming you.

If an asthma attack is severe, emergency treatment in the hospital may be needed. Emergency treatment includes an injection or inhalation of a bronchodilator and administration of injected or inhaled steroids. Intravenous fluids, close observation and oxygen may help ensure a safe and speedy recovery from a serious attack.

### Prevention

Allergies, infections and tobacco smoke are common triggers of asthma attacks. Try to avoid these triggers as much as possible.

People with allergies may benefit from antihistamines (p. 615) in addition to avoiding the causes of their allergies. Allergy shots (p. 619) are also available for some allergies.

If allergies cause serious asthma attacks that come on rapidly, it may be important to always carry an injectable form of a bronchodilator in case a serious attack occurs. The injectable bronchodilator contains adrenaline and is commonly called a *bee sting kit*. Quick access to this medicine can be lifesaving.

A *peak flow* meter is an important part of controlling asthma. It's a simple hand-held device that measures how fast the air can go out of your lungs. To use a peak flow meter,

take a deep breath and blow as hard as possible into the mouthpiece. Look at the number the meter records. Do this three times and write down the best result. This is your "peak flow."

Measure your peak flow twice a day for two weeks when your treatment starts. Use these numbers to create your *peak flow chart*. The chart will only work for you if you measure your peak flow regularly. It will allow you to find your personal best peak flow value. After you know your best peak flow value, your doctor can prescribe an asthma medicine that meets your needs.

Measuring your peak flow regularly will also help you know when early symptoms of asthma are occurring—before they become severe. Medicine can be taken right away to help prevent an attack.

If your peak flow is in the *green zone*, or 80% to 100% of your personal best, you are probably fine and need no additional medicine. If your peak flow is in the *yellow zone*, or 50% to 80% of your personal best, you may need to call your doctor and ask about additional medicine. If your peak flow is in the *red zone*, or less than 50% of your personal best, this is an emergency. Use a bronchodilator and call your doctor right away.

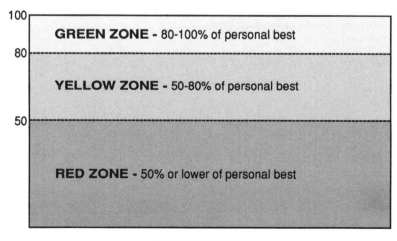

**PEAK FLOW ZONES**

> ## Asthma Can Be Life-Threatening!
>
> If you or a family member has asthma, make plans ahead of time for handling a serious attack. Talk with your doctor about keeping an injectable bronchodilator in the house in case it is needed. Have all emergency phone numbers posted in case you need to call. Purchase a peak flow meter, know what your normal reading is and know at what level you need to go to the hospital.

## Bronchitis

- A cough that produces mucus
- Chest tightness
- Shortness of breath

*Bronchitis* is a swelling, or inflammation, of the large airways. In response to irritation from the swelling, thick mucus is secreted into the air tubes. This causes an urge to cough. If enough mucus collects, the smaller air passages become clogged, restricting air movement and causing shortness of breath.

*Acute bronchitis* occurs when a viral or bacterial infection invades the respiratory tract. Less often, fungal infections cause acute bronchitis.

*Chronic bronchitis* is usually the result of exposure to irritants rather than an infection. It may occur in people who smoke and those who have been exposed to fumes, dust, chemicals or other irritants for many years. Chronic bronchitis usually causes a chronic cough that produces yellow, gray or brown mucus. This chronic irritation, along with infection, slowly damages the lungs. Many years of this irritation will lead to shortness of breath and trouble with even simple physical tasks. People with chronic bronchitis often have emphysema (p. 147), too. This combination of chronic bronchitis and emphysema is called *chronic obstructive pulmonary disease.*

### Testing

Diagnosis of acute bronchitis can usually be made based on the symptoms. These include a cough that produces mucus, shortness of breath or wheezing. Fever isn't usually present.

A chest x-ray (p. 631) and pulmonary function tests (p. 640) can help your doctor diagnose chronic bronchitis. The chest x-ray may show infection within the lung tissues near the bronchial tubes. Low-grade pneumonia (p. 154) and an infection of the lung tissue may have similar symptoms, but an x-ray will show shadows in the lung from pneumonia that won't be present in bronchitis. In people with chronic bronchitis, the chest x-ray often shows signs of emphysema.

The mucus may be tested for bacteria if an infection is severe, if it doesn't respond to the usual treatment or if another type of infection, such as tuberculosis (p. 307), is suspected.

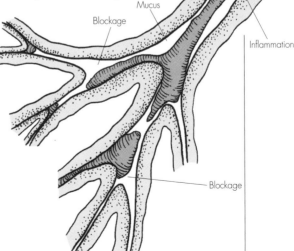
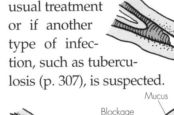

**BRONCHITIS**

### Treatment

Many cases of mild acute bronchitis caused by viruses go away on their own within a few days or a week. Most cases of acute bronchitis caused by bacteria will also disappear within four to eight weeks. However, bacterial infections may occasionally become pneumonia if not diagnosed and treated with antibiotics (p. 615). Your doctor may recommend treatment with an antibiotic to help stop the infection and prevent it from getting worse.

Over-the-counter analgesic medicines (p. 614) and cold medicines may comfort and soothe the irritated mucous membranes within the nose, throat and lungs when you have bronchitis. If wheezing is present, a bronchodilator (p. 621) may be helpful.

### Prevention

Preventing acute bronchitis is difficult because it's often caused by highly contagious viruses. To keep from catching such infections, wash your hands often and don't share foods and eating or drinking utensils.

To reduce your chances of developing chronic bronchitis, stay away from smoke and other noxious fumes. These fumes make the bronchial tubes more susceptible to infection. Also, don't smoke.

## Collapsed Lung

### Atelectasis

- Persistent dry cough
- Shortness of breath
- Low fever (sometimes)

Following surgery or after a rib fracture, many people take small, shallow breaths to prevent pain. Without the pressure from normal breathing, small areas of the lung or even entire lobes can collapse—a condition known as *atelectasis*, or collapsed lung. Anything that completely blocks a large or small airway, such as a tumor or foreign body, will also lead to atelectasis in the area of lung that's blocked.

Atelectasis may cause a cough, sometimes severe, and a low fever. Changes in the lung will show up on a chest x-ray (p. 631), which will confirm the diagnosis of atelectasis.

Deep breathing re-expands the collapsed areas if nothing is pushing on the lung or on a nearby bronchial tube. Coughing, blowing up balloons or using a breathing device called an *incentive spirometer* forces the person to increase the air pressure in the lungs and re-expand the collapsed section. If a tumor is the cause of atelectasis, it must be removed.

Deep-breathing exercises should be done as soon as possible after a rib fracture or surgery to prevent a collapsed lung.

### Pneumothorax

- Sudden shortness of breath
- Pain on one side of the chest

*Pneumothorax* occurs when air gets into the space between the rib cage and the outer surface of the lung, causing the lung to collapse. This may happen if a small area in the lung lining bursts or leaks air around the lung.

Usually the chest wall and the wet, slippery surface of the lung stick together. When air gets in this space, the lung can't expand fully. Breathing becomes very hard. The person usually has no cough or fever, just trouble catching his or her breath.

Diagnosis can often be based on the symptoms—sudden mild to severe shortness of breath—along with sounds in the lungs that are different from one side of the chest to the other. A chest x-ray will reveal the problem

---

### Home Remedies for Bronchitis

- Drink plenty of fluids. This will help break up the mucus that's clogging your airways.
- Use a humidifier to add moisture to the air. Cool-mist humidifiers may be the most helpful.
- Take over-the-counter medicines to suppress a dry cough or loosen a moist cough. Talk to your doctor about which ones to use.
- Avoid smoke and fumes.

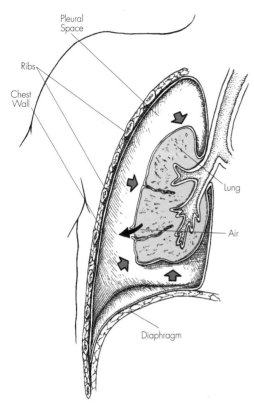

**PNEUMOTHORAX**

and show the amount of air that has leaked into the space between the rib cage and the lung.

Small leaks will probably only need to be watched. No treatment is usually needed because the leaks tend to go away on their own. For larger leaks, in which 25% or more of the lung volume is lost, a small plastic tube is inserted into the space between the rib cage and the lung to remove the air. The tube is left in the space for a few days to make sure the leak doesn't recur. When the leak has healed itself, the tube is removed.

## Emphysema

- Blue tinge to mouth and fingernail beds
- Use of shoulder muscles and exaggerated chest movements to breathe
- Chronic shortness of breath that worsens gradually over time
- Weight loss

*Emphysema* causes overinflation in the lungs. The lungs become damaged from chronic irritation, such as from smoke. As a result, the small air sacs, called *alveoli*, begin to break down and form larger and larger air sacs. The thin membranes that surround these air sacs are destroyed. It's in the membranes that oxygen from the air diffuses into the blood. Their destruction reduces the amount of oxygen that can get into the bloodstream. Membrane destruction also tends to collapse the breathing tubes when you exhale, making it harder to get air out of the lungs in preparation for the next breath. As the supply of oxygen decreases, the shortness of breath gets worse. Emphysema can also lead to weight loss and a bluish color around the mouth and on the fingernail beds.

Cigarette smoking for many years is the cause of most cases of emphysema. The typical person with emphysema has had many bronchial infections, a few episodes of pneumonia (p. 154) and a gradual increase in shortness of breath after many years of smoking. Besides smoking, occupational exposure to dusts, fumes or chemicals can also lead to emphysema. In some cases the chronic lung damage is caused by a genetic deficiency in an enzyme called *alpha$_1$-antitrypsin*, which normally protects the lungs.

The outlook for people with emphysema depends on their age, occupation, smoking history, number and severity of infections and the severity of asthma (p. 142), if present. The more severe the damage from any one or more of these factors, the faster emphysema progresses, eventually leading to death unless the damage is stopped.

### Testing

Your doctor will probably be able to diagnose emphysema after taking a medical history and doing an initial exam. The doctor will ask about smoking, frequent bronchial infections and occupational exposures.

An arterial blood gas test (p. 628) can measure how much oxygen and carbon dioxide are in the blood to find out how well the lungs are working. A chest x-ray (p. 631) may show signs of emphysema.

### Treatment

Several treatments can help lungs that are already damaged work the best they can. Many people with emphysema need *oxygen therapy*—oxygen given from a canister to relieve oxygen shortage. Oxygen therapy may be needed either during activities, during sleep or all the time. Depending on the severity and type of problems you have, your doctor may prescribe bronchodilators (p. 621), which open the airways, antibiotics (p. 615) to treat an infection if you have one, and anti-inflammatory medicines, such as corticosteroids (p. 622), to slow the progress of the disease.

When medicines no longer work, a heart-lung transplant can be done, although this option is used only rarely. A relatively new surgery involves removing a portion of the lung so the overinflation doesn't hamper breathing as much.

### Prevention

Smoking is the major risk factor for emphysema. Even if emphysema has started, you should stop smoking to keep the emphysema from getting worse. See page 31 for tips on quitting the smoking habit.

If you work around fumes, dusts or chemicals, or have frequent lung infections, protect your lungs. Wear a mask or other types of protection while you work and treat infections aggressively to keep them under control.

If you have family members who don't smoke but have emphysema, ask your doctor about getting tested for alpha$_1$-antitrypsin deficiency. Talk to your doctor about ways to preserve as much lung power as possible.

## Hyperventilation

- Shortness of breath
- Weakness
- Tightness in the throat
- Chest pressure
- Numbness of the hands, feet or the area around the mouth
- Anxiety

If you start breathing too hard because you feel like you're out of breath, you may be suffering from *hyperventilation*. The body functions best when there's a careful balance of oxygen and carbon dioxide in the blood. If panic or anxiety causes you to breathe faster, you lose too much carbon dioxide. This tends to make you even more anxious, so you breathe even faster. Eventually, you can pass out unless you slow down your breathing.

Numbness of the hands, feet and the area around the mouth can result from the low carbon dioxide level in the blood.

Some people hyperventilate when they're nervous, scared or during a panic attack. Other people hyperventilate when they run or exercise too hard, and still others hyperventilate when they have stomach cramps. Other health problems, such as asthma (p. 142), can also cause hyperventilation.

### Testing

Only one test specifically diagnoses hyperventilation—the arterial blood gas test (p. 628). It may show a low carbon dioxide level. Other changes in the blood may be present as well, helping to confirm hyperventilation as the cause of the symptoms.

Because shortness of breath and chest pressure can have many serious causes, the problems should be checked by your doctor. Intense chest pain can be caused by a heart attack (p. 115), blood clots that clog the lungs (pulmonary embolism, p. 157) or a separation of the layers in the main artery, the *aorta*, that takes blood away from the heart (aortic dissection). Pulmonary function tests (p. 640) and other tests may be needed for people who have severe shortness of breath and chest pain.

### Treatment

You can relieve the symptoms of hyperventilation by breathing into a paper (never plastic) bag held loosely over your nose and mouth. This forces you to breathe in more carbon dioxide, which will help put the carbon dioxide levels in the blood back into balance.

Practicing relaxation techniques (p. 572) may also help if anxiety is the cause of hyperventilation. These techniques usually involve lying down, relaxing, closing your eyes and concentrating on breathing slowly. This may be enough to stop the episode within 10 minutes or so. During recovery from hyperventilation, you may have a mild weak feeling and sometimes a headache.

### Prevention

If you begin to feel weak, short of breath or numb in your hands, feet or around your mouth, stop what you're doing right away. Relax and concentrate on taking slow, shallow breaths. If a panic attack or asthma is causing hyperventilation, treatment of those problems will help prevent hyperventilation.

## Interstitial Lung Disease

- Coughing that may bring up mucus
- Gradual shortness of breath
- Tiredness
- Weight loss
- Chest pain (rarely)

The membranes within the lung tissue, called *interstitial lung tissue* because it is located within the lung, are very thin so that oxygen breathed into the lungs can be released to the blood and carbon dioxide in the blood can be traded back to the air in the lungs. Thickening of these membranes reduces the ability of oxygen to get into the blood. The membrane thickening is called *interstitial lung disease*. The reason for this thickening varies, but the effect may be inflammation within the lung tissues.

**Goodpasture's syndrome.** This interstitial lung disease usually affects young men. A cough is the main symptom. Sometimes the cough produces blood, because of bleeding in the lungs. The bleeding may stem from antibodies that turn against the body itself (autoimmune disorders, p. 223). Goodpasture's syndrome is a serious, sometimes life-threatening, disease that also affects the kidneys.

**Idiopathic pulmonary fibrosis.** Another form of interstitial lung disease, this condition usually affects people in middle to older age groups. *Fibrosis*, or scarring, of the lung tissue follows the breakdown of the interstitial membranes. The cause is unknown. The disease usually keeps getting worse, often resulting in death within five years of the diagnosis.

**Pulmonary alveolar proteinosis.** This is a rare lung disease. It causes a thick, jelly-like material to form in the small air sacs, the *alveoli*, of the lungs. The cause isn't known. It usually affects men between the ages of 20 and 50.

---

### How do I know I'm hyperventilating?

- You felt anxious or nervous before the breathing symptoms started.
- You feel just like you did during an episode of hyperventilation you had before.
- You feel as if you are out of breath.
- You feel numb in your hands and around your mouth when you're short of breath.

*It's always wise to be checked by a doctor if you're not sure what's causing your symptoms. Relaxing, lying down, closing your eyes and breathing into a brown paper bag often work when practiced with patience.*

**Sarcoidosis.** Sarcoidosis is a disease that affects tissues throughout the body. It almost always involves the formation of small, round bumps in the tissue and thickening of the air sacs. The condition often affects other areas of the body, such as the skin, lymph nodes, heart and nerves. The cause is unknown. Fever and tiredness accompany shortness of breath. Fortunately, most people recover and never have another episode. But a small number of people have gradual lung failure or other organ failure and eventually die.

### Testing

With interstitial lung disease, a physical exam may reveal no changes in breath sounds or any other signs that would suggest the disease. A chest x-ray (p. 631) may show changes that suggest interstitial lung disease, or it may reveal few changes.

A sample of lung tissue may be tested to confirm the diagnosis. Pulmonary function tests (p. 640) and other tests may also be used to help your doctor form a treatment plan.

### Treatment

Corticosteroids (p. 622), by mouth or by injection, are the mainstay of therapy for most interstitial lung diseases. Inhaled steroids have little effect but may be used to keep the air tubes from shrinking, or constricting. Bronchodilators (p. 621) can also be used.

Treatment of Goodpasture's syndrome that involves the kidneys may also require dialysis (p. 164) to cleanse the blood of wastes that have built up. Lung transplants are sometimes used in people who have severe idiopathic pulmonary fibrosis. Treatment for pulmonary alveolar proteinosis includes *bronchial lavage.* In bronchial lavage, a bronchoscope (p. 630) is used to push a special fluid through the lungs to rinse the mucus away and open the airways.

In cases of sarcoidosis that don't improve with corticosteroids, certain chemotherapy (p. 225) medicines may be used.

## Lung Abscess

- Coughing up mucus that may be foul-smelling and blood-streaked
- Rough breathing (*rales*)
- Dull chest pain
- Sweating and fever
- Loss of appetite

An *abscess,* or collection of pus, can form in the lung when bacteria have been inhaled. The bacteria may come from an infection in the nose, sinuses, throat or teeth. Bacteria may be inhaled into the lungs, or *aspirated,* if you breathe in mucus from your mouth, airways or throat, or contents of your stomach that carry bacteria. This may occur after drinking too much alcohol or taking a sedative, or during a seizure or anesthesia.

Sometimes a lung abscess breaks open and the area fills with fluid and air. This area needs to be drained so that the abscess can heal. When an abscess breaks open, more mucus and pus will be coughed up.

### Testing and Treatment

A lung abscess may be diagnosed based on the symptoms. Chest x-rays (p. 631) will show signs of an abscess and will probably be repeated to follow the progress of the treatment. The mucus may be tested to find out which type of bacteria, if any, is present. Antibiotics will probably be prescribed to treat the infection.

### Prevention

You can help reduce your chances of developing a lung abscess. Good dental care will reduce the number of bacteria that could be inhaled into the lungs. If you have a seizure disorder, follow instructions to keep it under control. Don't go overboard on alcohol or medicines that act as depressants, such as sleeping pills.

## Lung Cancer

- Cough with bloody mucus
- Shortness of breath
- Chest discomfort
- Loss of appetite and weight loss

Lung cancer is one of the most common and preventable cancers in the United States. It's common because of one factor—smoking. Of the thousands of men and women who die each year of lung cancer, more than 85% have gotten the disease from smoking. Living around someone who smokes and constantly breathing in the tars and other cancer-causing substances in second-hand smoke can also lead to cancer. Smokers 50 or older have the greatest risk of cancer.

*Radon* is another known risk factor for lung cancer. Radon is a gas produced by the breakdown of uranium within the soil in some parts of the country. When uranium is in the soil, it can get into buildings, including homes. *Asbestos* exposure is also a risk factor for lung cancer.

Four types of tumors arise directly from the lung tissues.

**Adenocarcinoma.** This type of tumor arises from the mucous membrane cells lining the smaller air tubes and air sacs. Because these tumors occur in the outer edges of the lungs, they don't block any main airways. Because they don't produce symptoms like coughing, they're often quite large when they're diagnosed. This cancer spreads through the bloodstream to organs and tissues outside the lungs.

**Large-cell carcinoma.** This cancer is found most often in the edges of the lungs. It spreads through the bloodstream to other organs and tissues outside the lungs. Like adenocarcinoma, this type of cancer is also usually large before it's discovered.

**Small-cell carcinoma.** Small-cell carcinoma is also called *oat-cell carcinoma* because the cancer cell is shaped like an oat grain when viewed through a microscope. It's one of the faster-growing and faster-spreading lung cancers. Small-cell carcinoma is usually found in the central portions of the lungs. The tumors cause symptoms when they push against or block a large bronchial tube, leading to infection or partial collapse of the lung.

**Squamous-cell carcinoma.** This tumor arises in the cells lining the larger airways. The cancer cells can sometimes be seen in samples of lung secretions. This type of cancer may be found earlier than other cancers, but it's still hard to treat.

Because all blood passes through the lungs to be recharged with oxygen, cancer from other areas in the body spreads to the lungs. This is called metastatic cancer, because it has *metastasized*, or spread, from another part of the body. These tumors most commonly start in the colon, breast, testicle, bone, thyroid or prostate.

### Testing

Lung cancer can be found in many ways. Some people have no symptoms, and the tumor is found during a chest x-ray (p. 631) done for another reason. Other people seek treatment for a chronic cough. When the cough doesn't go away after treatment, a chest x-ray may reveal the cancer.

Some people with lung cancer first see their doctors because they have noticed worsening shortness of breath, weakness and weight loss. They may also see their doctor because of an infection or other lung disorder.

A CT scan (p. 632) can be used to further identify the tumor or assess its spread to other areas of the lungs. Samples of mucus taken from the air tubes may show cancer cells when the mucus is looked at under a microscope. A bronchoscope (p. 630) may also be used to assess the tumor.

### Treatment

Treatment of lung cancer depends on the type of tumor. All cancer treatments, including surgery, radiation therapy (p. 225) and chemotherapy (p. 225), may be used to treat lung cancer.

But chemotherapy doesn't make many of these tumors get smaller. And both surgery and radiation therapy may damage the lungs. This damage to the lungs further decreases the ability to breathe, which may already be limited by years of smoking.

The outlook for people with lung cancer is poor, unless it's caught at a very early stage. With most cases, there's very little chance of survival past five years.

### Prevention

You can help prevent lung cancer. Don't start smoking and quit if you already smoke. Avoid second-hand smoke. Buildings can be checked for radon using an inexpensive testing kit. Changes in the venting can help lower the radon level. Most newer buildings are free of asbestos but be aware that it can be present in older buildings. Asbestos can be in the shingles, tiles and insulation. Before doing any renovation on an older building, get an expert opinion about the presence of asbestos.

## Occupational Lung Diseases

- Cough and wheezing
- Gradually increasing shortness of breath
- Tiredness
- Chest pain (rarely)

Many jobs involve the risk of lung disease. Firefighters, for instance, may damage their lungs by breathing hot, smoke-filled air and fumes. The lungs of farmers can become infected and irritated by exposure to fungal molds, dusts from hay and fumes from moist silage. Coal miners damage their lungs by breathing in the same coal dust that blackens their faces, hands and clothing. Any dust, fume, chemical vapor, solvent, smoke, mold or gas can damage the lungs if enough is breathed in. If you smoke and also have a job that exposes you to these damaging substances, the damage to your lungs will be even greater, and symptoms will appear sooner.

**Anthracosis.** Also called "black lung," *anthracosis* is produced by repeatedly breathing in coal dust.

**Asbestosis.** Asbestosis is caused by breathing in asbestos fibers. Asbestos has been used in the past in fireproofing materials, pipe insulation and other building products. Breathing in asbestos fibers causes lung inflammation, or *asbestosis*, and years later may lead to cancer of the lining of the lung, called *mesothelioma*.

### Why should I stop smoking after so many years?

Even if you have been smoking for 20 years or more, giving up your habit *now* has health benefits. The risk for cancer goes down, and risks for heart disease and stroke return to normal within two to five years after quitting. The longer you smoke, the more permanent damage you do, but some of that damage can be reversed if you stop. See page 31 for helpful tips on how to quit smoking.

**Byssinosis.** This is the name given to lung damage caused by breathing the dust from cotton, hemp or jute—a fiber used mostly in burlap and twine.

**Farmer's lung.** This is a fungal infection. Mold enters the lungs when the farmer breathes the moist air around drying hay. Fever, chills, shortness of breath and cough are possible symptoms. Antifungal medicine (p. 615) is used to treat this infection.

**Occupational asthma.** Occupational asthma occurs in people who work around wood dust, soldering flux or synthetic dyes. It can usually be prevented by wearing a breathing mask, working in a well-ventilated area or avoiding the materials that provoke an asthma attack.

**Silicosis.** *Silicosis* occurs mostly in people who work in mines or who do stone cutting or quarrying and breathe silicon particles into their lungs. These tiny quartz crystals can cause severe damage to the lungs.

**Silo-filler's lung.** This lung disease occurs when the nitrous oxide fumes produced by decaying silage burn the lining of the small airways and the deeper tissues of the lungs, reducing the ability to breathe.

### Testing and Treatment

A history of chronic exposure to dusts and fumes in the workplace should raise suspicions about the cause of lung problems. Your doctor will probably do some tests, which may include a chest x-ray (p. 631), pulmonary function testing (p. 640) and an exam of mucus samples from the lungs.

Once the damage is done to the lung tissue, it can't be reversed. But ending the constant exposure to dusts, molds or fumes will prevent further damage. The lungs may heal enough to produce a small increase in lung function.

Medicines can sometimes be used to maximize the ability to breathe. Bronchodilators (p. 621), corticosteroids (p. 622) and oxygen can help make breathing more comfortable.

### Prevention

Preventing these diseases is by far the most effective method of limiting their impact. If you work with chemicals, be sure to use the protective equipment and practices prescribed by the Material Safety Data Sheets (MSDS). Employers are required by the Occupational Safety and Health Administration (OSHA) regulations to have an MSDS for every chemical a worker is exposed to. The employer is required to follow all of the precautions outlined on the MSDS. It's also important to avoid smoking.

When working with wood dust, insulation, solvents, paints or other chemicals at home, be sure to wear a protective mask and make sure the work area is well ventilated, so fumes or dusts aren't inhaled. Avoid being around chemicals or solvents that have caused severe reactions in the past. Don't mix chemicals or solvents.

## Pleurisy

- Chest pain with deep breathing, coughing or sneezing
- Cold or flu symptoms (sometimes)

*Pleurisy* is an inflammation of the double membrane, called the *pleura,* that surrounds the lung and holds the fluid that allows the lungs to expand in the chest with little friction. Pleurisy, which is sometimes referred to as *pleuritis,* can make every breath painful.

The cause is usually a viral infection that irritates the smooth, slippery surface of the lung. Occasionally more

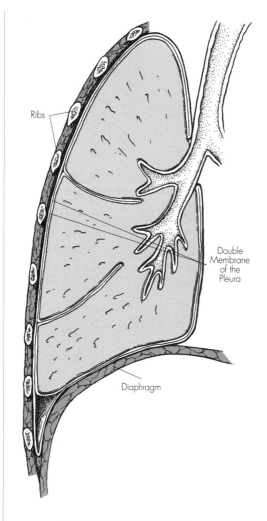

Ribs

Double
Membrane
of the
Pleura

Diaphragm

**CHEST CAVITY INCLUDING PLEURA**

serious problems, such as pneumonia (p. 154), a lung abscess (p. 150), tuberculosis (p. 307) or a blood clot in the lung (pulmonary embolism, p. 157) can lead to pleurisy.

### Testing and Treatment

No specific test can prove the presence of pleurisy. A chest x-ray (p. 631) will often show nothing wrong, but it may show changes in the lung near the site of the pain. A blood test, an electrocardiogram (p. 634), a CT scan (p. 632), pulmonary function tests (p. 640) and tests for blood clots will probably be normal.

In mild cases, treatment may be the most helpful test—if the symptoms respond to the treatment, the problem was probably pleurisy.

Oral medicines alone, such as indomethacin (p. 622), aspirin (p. 615) or ibuprofen (p. 617), are usually the only treatment needed. Oral cortisone (p. 623) can also be used. All of these medicines can reduce the swelling of the pleura. In severe cases of pleurisy, hospitalization may be needed so intravenous medicines can be used to reduce the swelling.

## Pneumonia

- Cough
- Fever
- Shortness of breath or wheezing
- Rapid breathing in infants and toddlers
- Aches
- Chills
- Fatigue

The air spaces within the lungs must stay open and clear from fluid so oxygen and carbon dioxide can be exchanged. When the air tubes are irritated and infected, mucus forms on their walls, causing bronchitis (p. 145). When the air spaces at the ends of the air passages, the *alveoli*, fill with infected fluid, the result is *pneumonia*.

---

### Home Treatment for Mild Pleurisy

- Take aspirin or ibuprofen (adults only).
- Apply a heating pad to the aching area.
- Wrap an elastic bandage around your chest. The support may provide some comfort.
- Change position. The pain may go away if you move.
  *Talk with your doctor if the pain is severe. Never assume that pleurisy is the cause of chest pain.*

Chapter 9 Lungs 155

Different types of infections can lead to pneumonia. Some types of pneumonia are deadly, especially in older people and people whose immune systems are damaged. Other types of pneumonia are so mild they may not require medical attention.

Pneumonia may develop in young children if bronchitis or other airway infections are untreated. A few children with pneumonia become ill with fever, aches, chills, nausea and vomiting but no cough or shortness of breath. Typically, children have a cold or flu that worsens over three to seven days, until the child is very ill with pneumonia.

**Atypical pneumonia.** This type of pneumonia is usually caused by a type of bacteria called mycoplasma. This bacteria acts like a virus. Mycoplasma infection usually produces mild fever, cough (often at night), tiredness and sometimes headache over three to five days. The fever rarely exceeds 101°F. Young adults are the age group most often affected. The old name for this type of pneumonia was "walking" pneumonia.

**Bacterial pneumonia.** Bacterial pneumonia is generally the most dangerous type of pneumonia. It's commonly caused by pneumococcal (p. 303) and *Haemophilus* (p. 301) bacteria. Bacterial pneumonia comes on quickly, giving the person shaking chills, nausea, vomiting, extreme tiredness, shortness of breath and a cough that produces thick, dark or even blood-tinged mucus. The temperature may rapidly rise to 104°F. Bacterial pneumonia can be fatal in weak elderly people and people who have serious health problems, such as congestive heart failure (p. 114), cancer or emphysema (p. 147).

**Pneumocystis pneumonia.** This type of pneumonia often affects people who have extremely damaged immune

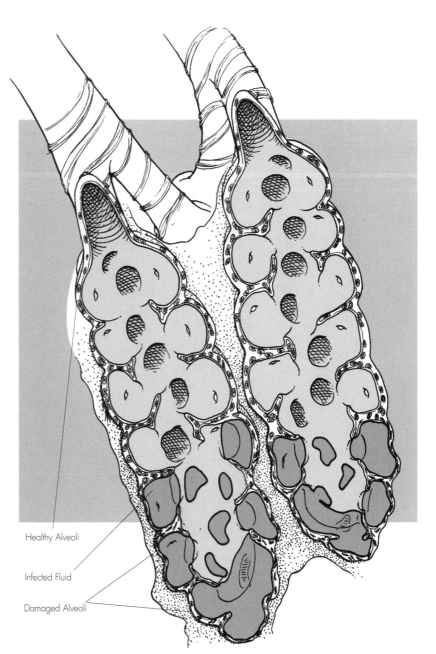

Healthy Alveoli

Infected Fluid

Damaged Alveoli

**PNEUMONIA: ALVEOLI FILLED WITH FLUID**

systems, such as people who have AIDS (p. 325). This type of pneumonia is caused by the small organisms called *Pneumocystis carinii*. The fever may be very high and come on very quickly. More often the fever is low and comes on slowly. Shortness of breath can become severe.

**Viral pneumonia.** Viral pneumonia is commonly caused by influenza (p. 326), respiratory syncytial virus and cytomegalovirus. Viruses cause three-fourths of the cases of pneumonia. This type of pneumonia usually begins with cough, fever and fatigue that increase gradually over a few days to weeks. The fever usually stays around 101°F, only rarely going to 103°F and above.

While bacterial pneumonia is usually more dangerous, even viral pneumonia can be fatal, especially in the elderly. Depending on the type of virus and the general health of the person, viral pneumonia can be a very mild illness or a life-threatening disease.

### Testing and Treatment

The type of pneumonia can sometimes be identified by symptoms alone. The pattern seen on a chest x-ray (p. 631) is often helpful. For example, a bacterial infection may cause a high fever, and the chest x-ray may show a whited-out area in part of a lung.

Treatment of pneumonia depends on the type of pneumonia and its severity. Analgesic medicines (p. 614) and fever-reducing medicines (p. 616) may help relieve discomfort. If oral antibiotics are prescribed, be sure to take all of them.

A person with bacterial pneumonia, including atypical pneumonia, may require hospitalization, along with intravenous antibiotics to target the specific type of bacteria that is the suspected cause of the pneumonia.

Antibiotics can't destroy viruses, which are the cause of viral pneumonia. However, many people with viral pneumonia need hospitalization for supportive and potentially life-saving care, including intravenous fluids, oxygen and therapy to help remove mucus from the lungs.

### Prevention

Because influenza can lead to pneumonia, a yearly influenza vaccination can protect you, especially if you're elderly, a health-care worker or susceptible to complications of the flu. A medicine called amantadine (p. 621) is used to treat influenza type A. A vaccine for the bacterial pneumonia caused by the pneumococcal organism is also available. One dose of this vaccine protects you from bacterial pneumonia for life. This vaccine is especially important for the elderly, who are at highest risk of pneumonia complications or death.

Limit your exposure to air pollutants, particularly tobacco smoke, which increases the risk of pneumonia.

## Pulmonary Edema

- Severe shortness of breath, especially when lying flat
- Coughing up pink, foamy mucus
- Swelling in the ankles and legs
- Anxiety, restlessness or sweating

*Pulmonary edema* is a life-threatening excess of fluid in the lungs. It can result from uncontrolled congestive heart failure (p. 114). The heart is still beating and pumping blood, but it's not keeping up with the body's needs. Fluid gathers in the lungs, causing severe shortness of breath. Pulmonary edema is a severe form of congestive heart failure that needs immediate treatment.

### Testing

Steadily increasing tiredness often leads people who have pulmonary edema to see their doctor. After a physical exam, the doctor may decide to do further testing. A chest x-ray (p. 631) may be used to look for fluid in the lungs, or an electrocardiogram (p. 634) to assess damage to the heart, and blood tests to find other diseases that can lead to congestive heart failure. A blood sample may be taken to check the blood oxygen level (arterial blood gases, p. 628). Special monitoring is important because heart or blood pressure problems or breathing difficulties may be signs of a life-threatening illness.

### Treatment

Several medicines can be used to help reduce fluid in the lungs. Medicines that reduce blood pressure may help reduce the work of the heart, and medicines that stimulate the heart may help it pump more effectively. A diuretic (p. 616) is often given to help the kidneys rid the body of excess fluid.

### Prevention

Many lifestyle habits and behaviors lead to heart attacks (p. 115), which can then lead to congestive heart failure and pulmonary edema. Examples of these habits include smoking, lack of exercise and a high-fat diet. A healthy lifestyle reaps great rewards in later life by preventing disease. Treatment of high blood pressure also helps prevent heart failure.

## Pulmonary Embolism

- Chest pain
- Severe shortness of breath
- Sometimes, no apparent symptoms

A *pulmonary embolism* is caused when a blood clot lodges in the pulmonary artery and blocks the blood supply to the lungs. For example, a pulmonary embolism can occur if a blood clot in the deep veins (deep vein thrombosis, p. 129) of the legs breaks loose and travels to the lungs. Pulmonary embolism can cause serious lung damage or even death. About one out of four persons who have a pulmonary embolism will die from the blockage. Report any swelling, redness or problems of the lower leg to your doctor. These symptoms could mean that

deep vein thrombosis is present. The clot could move from your leg to your lungs.

### Testing and Treatment

Pulmonary embolism is a serious problem that requires attention in an emergency room. Doppler ultrasound (p. 634) may be used to identify reduced blood flow and find a clot. In life-threatening situations, a pulmonary arteriogram (p. 628) helps evaluate the need for surgical removal of a clot or treatment with a clot-dissolving medicine (p. 622). Blood-thinning medicines (p. 619) will probably be given by vein.

After the clot has been treated, oral anticoagulants will probably be needed to ensure that new clots don't form. Surgery can be performed to place a mesh in the *inferior vena cava* (the vein that returns blood to the heart) to prevent future clots from traveling into the lungs.

> ### Emergency Symptoms of Pulmonary Edema
>
> - Sudden onset of severe shortness of breath
> - A cough that produces pink, frothy or foamy mucus
> - An increase of fluid in the feet, ankles and legs, over a few days
> - Anxiety, restlessness or sweating
>
> *If you have these symptoms, call an ambulance and go to the nearest emergency room for treatment right away.*

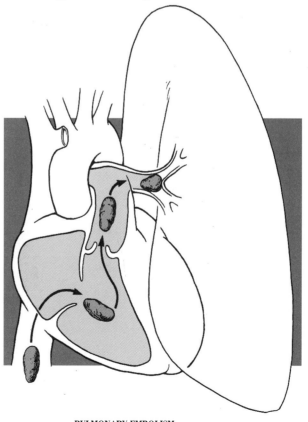

**PULMONARY EMBOLISM**

# CHAPTER 10 URINARY SYSTEM

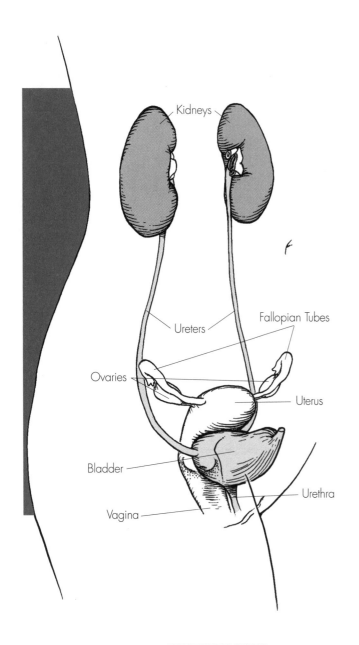

Kidneys

Ureters

Fallopian Tubes

Ovaries

Uterus

Bladder

Urethra

Vagina

**FEMALE RENAL SYSTEM**

After your body breaks food down into energy and uses the protein to build and repair tissues, it produces a waste material called *urea*. As blood flows through your body to deliver oxygen and nutrients, it also picks up urea and other wastes, such as extra sodium and potassium. These wastes must be removed from the blood. If they aren't, they build up in the body and eventually damage the organs.

The waste travels through the bloodstream to the *kidneys*, where it's filtered from the blood. All blood passes through the kidneys. The waste is removed from the blood and concentrated into urine by millions of tiny filtering units in the kidneys, called *glomeruli*. The urine is kept in channels within the kidneys.

Tubes, called *ureters*, carry the urine from the kidneys to the *bladder*. The bladder is like a storage tank that holds the urine until you urinate. When the bladder is full, *stretch receptors* in its walls send messages to your brain that it's time to urinate.

When you urinate, the urine travels through the *urethra*, the final tube of the urinary tract, and leaves your body.

The *urinary system* is closely related to the reproductive systems in both men and women. The organs of both systems lie close to one another, and problems with one system can often affect the other. The reproductive systems are discussed in the Special Groups section, beginning on page 333.

## Cancer of the Urinary Tract

- Blood in the urine
- Pain when urinating
- Difficulty urinating
- Recurrent urinary tract infections
- Weight loss, nausea and vomiting, fever

In adults, a cancerous form of kidney tumor is called *renal cell cancer.* Cells from this tumor can invade nearby tissues, as well as spread to the lungs or bone through the bloodstream. They can also spread to the lymph nodes.

In children, the name for cancer in the kidney is Wilms' tumor. Symptoms include weight loss in a child less than five years of age, a painless tumor in the abdomen, pale skin and high blood pressure. Cancer that spreads from a Wilms' tumor is more aggressive and more destructive than its adult counterpart. This type of cancer is very rare.

Tumors can also occur in the bladder and ureters. The lining of the bladder or the ureters can become cancerous when it becomes irritated by toxins inhaled through smoking or by exposure to certain industrial chemicals.

Blood in the urine can be the first symptom of cancer of the kidneys, ureters and bladder. Pain in the abdomen can occur if the flow of urine is blocked by a tumor in one of the ureters. Pain can also occur if the tumor presses on the tissues.

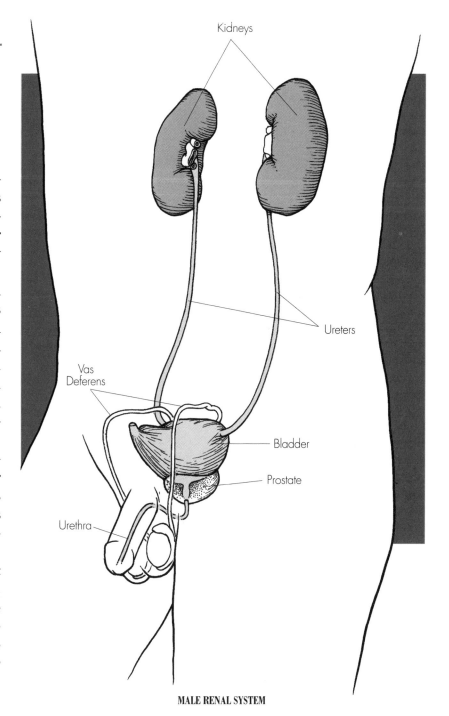

**MALE RENAL SYSTEM**

### Testing

If you have any of the symptoms just described, your doctor will probably begin by checking your urine for blood and signs of infection. Blood tests may also be needed. An IVP (p. 636) will show any changes in the shape of the kidneys or any abnormalities such as a kidney stone within the bladder or ureters. A CT scan (p. 632), ultrasound (p. 643), MRI scan (p. 637) or nuclear scans (p. 639) may be used to detect the full extent of the disease, such as the spread of the tumor.

### Treatment

A cancerous tumor must be removed surgically to prevent it from spreading and destroying other organs within the abdomen. If cancer is found, the affected kidney will have to be removed. The remaining kidney will increase its filtering power to make up for the missing kidney.

If a cancerous tumor is in the bladder, a procedure called *fulguration* can be used to destroy the tumor if it's small. In this procedure, an instrument is used to burn away the bladder tumor. To remove a large bladder tumor, abdominal surgery may be needed, and the entire bladder may have to be removed. In this case, urine will be directed to a bag worn on the outside of the body but attached to an opening in the abdominal wall. This is called an *ostomy*.

For a cancerous tumor of the kidney or bladder, chemotherapy (p. 225) and radiation therapy (p. 225) may be used along with surgery to reduce the risk of the tumor spreading.

Regular follow-up exams are recommended for at least five years after cancer of the urinary tract has been diagnosed. The outlook depends type of tumor and how far it ha gressed when it was diagnosed.

### Prevention

Studies show that smoking, as well as working around certain chemicals and solvents, such as aniline dyes, may increase your risk of bladder cancer. Because of the risk of cancer, don't start smoking. If you already smoke, ask your doctor for help quitting (p. 31). Talk to your employer about safety issues. The Occupational Safety and Health Administration (OSHA) requires that workplaces using potentially hazardous materials keep a list of these chemicals, the risks associated with them and ways to reduce the risks.

## Cysts of the Kidney

- Often no symptoms
- Back pain or blood in the urine as the cyst enlarges

Cysts of the kidney usually don't cause symptoms. They're often found during tests for another problem. Most cysts of the kidney are single, fluid-filled sacs attached to the kidney wall. They may grow quite large, leading to back pain or blood in the urine. These cysts are almost never cancerous, but it's good to have further tests to make sure.

### Testing and Treatment

Many cysts of the kidney are found during an ultrasound (p. 643), a CT scan (p. 632) or an IVP (p. 636) done to evaluate another problem.

If a cyst is found, your doctor may remove some of its fluid through a needle to check for cancer cells. This is called a needle biopsy (p. 636). Large cysts may be drained to take pressure off the affected kidney. This will allow the kidney to function better. Repeated checkups with ultrasound may be needed.

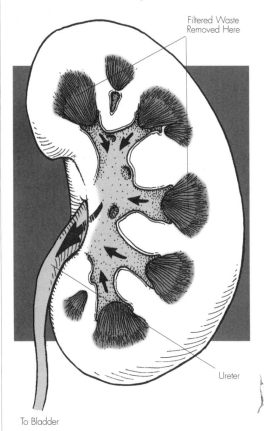

Filtered Waste Removed Here

Ureter

To Bladder

**NORMAL KIDNEY**

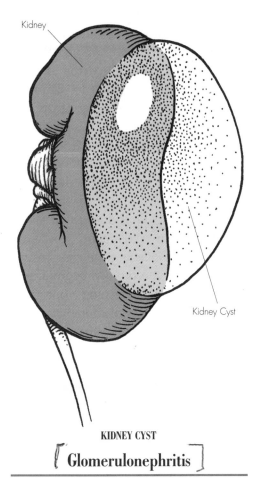

Kidney

Kidney Cyst

**KIDNEY CYST**

## Glomerulonephritis

- Dark, tea-colored or bloody urine
- Lower back or flank pain
- Achiness throughout body
- Fatigue and lethargy
- Low fever
- Swelling of hands, feet and face (late symptom)
- Shortness of breath (late symptom)

When the filtering units in the kidneys, called the glomeruli, are damaged, the resulting condition is called *glomerulonephritis*. The kidneys don't function properly when the glomeruli are damaged. Waste and extra fluids build up in the body, and blood and protein leak into the urine, making it look dark or bloody. Glomerulonephritis leads to kidney failure, which causes swelling, or *edema*, and high blood pressure.

A common cause of damage to the glomeruli is an autoimmune response to an infection caused by a virus or bacteria. Your body normally begins making antibodies to fight the infection. Antibodies and the virus or bacteria clump together and get stuck in the glomeruli. White blood cells are sent by the body to break up these clumps. But the white blood cells can damage the delicate membranes of the glomeruli.

*Acute glomerulonephritis* is short-term. It may last from a few days to a few weeks. It usually doesn't cause any permanent damage to the kidneys. On the other hand, *chronic glomerulonephritis* is more ongoing. It may be present for years with no symptoms. Chronic glomerulonephritis can lead to complete kidney failure (p. 163).

Rarely, a streptococcal bacteria (p. 306), such as those that cause strep throat (p. 306) or impetigo, may lead to *post-streptococcal glomerulonephritis*. This disorder occurs in children and young adults ages three to 21. Post-streptococcal glomerulonephritis begins about two weeks after the initial streptococcal infection. This condition has become more and more uncommon over the past 20 years because of effective treatment of streptococcal infection.

### Testing

If you have symptoms of glomerulonephritis, your doctor will probably test your urine for blood and protein. An ultrasound (p. 643) of the kidneys, ureters and bladder may be done to see if there are other reasons for the blood and protein in the urine. Special urine and blood tests may help identify the cause of the glomerulonephritis. Sometimes, a small sample of kidney tissue is taken by needle biopsy (p. 636) for examination and further testing.

### Treatment

Mild cases of glomerulonephritis don't require treatment, only close monitoring by your doctor. He or she may tell you to rest, limit your intake of fluids and salt, and reduce the amount of protein in your diet. More severe and chronic forms of glomerulonephritis may be treated with corticosteroids (p. 622) and other medicines to stop further damage of the glomeruli. Diuretics (p. 616) may help rid your body of extra water and reduce swelling.

### Prevention

Always finish the full course of antibiotics for an infection, such as strep throat, to prevent the risk of glomerulonephritis.

## Infections of the Urinary Tract

### Cystitis
- Burning sensation when you urinate
- Feeling like you need to urinate often
- Foul-smelling urine
- Low abdominal pain and low back pain
- Blood in the urine (often can only be seen with a microscope)

This term, *cystitis*, means the bladder is inflamed or swollen. It's usually brought on by an infection. That's why the condition is commonly called a *bladder infection* or *urinary tract infection* (UTI). Cystitis can also be caused by a tumor in the bladder or an allergy or unusual ulcers on the bladder walls.

Bladder infections are more common in women, whose *urethras* (the tube that carries urine outside the body) are much shorter than men's. In women, bacteria can move up the urethra and into the bladder more easily. Women sometimes have a bout of cystitis after having sexual intercourse for the first time. This used to be called "honeymoon cystitis." Some women get cystitis just about every time they have sexual intercourse.

In men, bladder infections are rare. They can be caused by other problems in the urinary tract, such as an enlarged prostate that may block the flow of urine. This causes urine to sit in the bladder, where bacteria can grow and lead to an infection.

Your doctor may want a sample of your urine to look for infection and to identify which type of bacteria is causing the infection. When a sample of urine is needed, your doctor will ask for a "clean-catch midstream" specimen. This requires cleaning the area around your urethra thoroughly, beginning to urinate and then catching your urine midstream in a special container.

The sample of your urine can then be checked under a microscope. The sample can also be cultured (p. 633) to identify the type of bacteria causing the infection.

Blood tests can confirm the presence of a serious infection. Sometimes an ultrasound (p. 643) of the kidneys may be done to check for tumors or blockages.

Oral antibiotics (p. 618) are all that's needed to treat bladder infections in otherwise healthy young people. The symptoms improve in 48 to 72 hours. Phenazopyridine (p. 618) is a medicine that can be used to numb the urethra so urination won't be so painful. Drinking plenty of fluids may seem to cause discomfort at first, but the increase in fluids causes more frequent urination and helps your body get rid of the infection. Your doctor may also prescribe aspirin (p. 615) or acetaminophen (p. 614) for pain and fever. It's important to take all the antibiotics you're given and to have your urine recultured when you finish your prescription. The length of treatment for a bladder infection depends on the bacteria involved, the exact site of the infection and other factors. Be sure to follow the directions your doctor gives you about taking your antibiotics.

> ## How to Reduce Your Risk of a Bladder Infection
>
> - Drink lots of fluids. Cranberry juice and blueberry juice may be particularly helpful. These juices contain a chemical that may prevent bacteria from sticking to the bladder cells.
> - Urinate often—at least every three to four hours.
> - Urinate before and after having sex.
> - For women: wipe from front to back after a bowel movement.
> - For women: use enough lubrication during sex. Try putting a small amount of vaginal lubricant (p. 617) around the opening of your vagina before having sex if you're a little dry. Be sure to use a water-soluble lubricant. Petroleum products can make condoms or diaphragms ineffective as birth control.
> - For women: don't use a diaphragm for birth control if you get bladder infections often. The diaphragm may push against the urethra and make it harder for you to empty your bladder completely. The urine that stays in the bladder is more likely to collect bacteria and cause an infection. Ask your doctor about other birth control choices.
> - Have your sexual partner get treated with antibiotics too if you have recurrent bladder infections.

## Pyelonephritis

- Sudden onset of shaking chills and fever of more than 102°F
- Constant ache in the side
- Burning sensation when you urinate
- Urinating often
- Fatigue
- Nausea and vomiting

Bacteria in the bladder can spread up into the ureters and kidneys and cause *pyelonephritis*, or a kidney infection. This is more likely to happen if one of the valves that normally keeps urine from flowing into the ureters from the bladder is abnormal. A stone in the kidney may also lead to a kidney infection. Infections can spread to the kidneys from other parts of the body.

People with a tumor of the kidney or bladder, men who have an enlarged prostate that partially blocks the urinary tract and women who are pregnant are at increased risk for infections of the kidneys.

Acute infections of the kidneys usually cause severe illness: high fever, aches, chills, nausea, vomiting and intense back pain, along with the other urinary tract symptoms. Repeated infections can lead to damaged kidneys, reduced kidney function and, eventually, kidney failure (p. 163).

Infection can be confirmed by bacteria in the urine. Treatment consists of fluids and antibiotics (p. 615) and can often be done without hospitalization. If the infection is severe, hospitalization may be needed for intravenous antibiotics and fluids.

### Kidney Failure

 Urinating in small amounts
- Swelling of the body
- Nausea and vomiting
- Fatigue
- Confusion, convulsions and coma (late symptoms)

The kidneys are needed for the body to function normally. When the kidneys fail, toxic wastes build up in the blood. Even the levels of blood salts, especially sodium and potassium, can't be properly regulated by the body when the kidneys stop working. When these wastes aren't cleansed from the body, a fluid and chemical imbalance occurs. This imbalance can cause fluid retention, swelling, irregular heartbeat, heart failure and death.

**Acute kidney failure.** This is usually a temporary condition related to an infection, kidney inflammation, ingestion of poison, serious injury, massive blood loss, burns or medicine. A sudden drop in blood pressure, dehydration, a blocked blood vessel to a kidney and other factors may damage the kidneys. With time and treatment of the underlying problem, the kidneys begin to work normally, and the fluid and chemical balance of the body are restored.

**Chronic kidney failure.** Chronic kidney damage can be caused by diabetes (p. 211), poorly controlled high blood pressure (p. 123), glomerulonephritis (p. 161), congenital kidney problems, recurrent kidney infections, a kidney stone (p. 165) or an enlarged prostate that blocks urine flow. Other diseases, such as systemic lupus erythematosus (p. 252), can also lead to chronic kidney failure. The function of the kidney is lost slowly over many months or years. Many people don't notice any symptoms until much of the damage has been done. Damage from chronic kidney failure is usually not reversible.

**End-stage kidney failure.** The fluid and chemical imbalance in the body will eventually become serious if severe kidney damage can't be reversed. When this occurs, kidney dialysis or kidney transplant is required.

### Testing

Kidney failure is diagnosed by blood and urine tests. These tests show the abnormalities that result when wastes aren't removed from the body. Special blood tests, an ultrasound (p. 643) or CT scan (p. 632) of the kidneys and, possibly, a biopsy of the kidneys may be needed. These tests help identify the cause of the kidney failure.

### Treatment

The first step in treating kidney damage is to treat any diseases that are causing it. Better control of diabetes and high blood pressure will reduce damage to the blood vessels and glomeruli within the kidneys. Treatment of high blood pressure in people with diabetes is especially important to protect the kidneys.

Intravenous fluids and transfusions can improve acute kidney failure associated with severe blood loss. Some medicines can reduce the inflammation of chronic glomerulonephritis, lessening the chance of irreversible kidney damage. Surgery may be needed to correct a blocked blood vessel to the kidney. If an enlarged prostate or kidney stone is blocking urine flow, surgery may be required to remove the obstruction, which will usually restore kidney function.

*Dialysis* may be required two to three times weekly if the kidney damage is irreversible. Dialysis eliminates wastes in the blood after the kidneys can't do it anymore. Two forms of dialysis are available. *Hemodialysis* uses a machine to cleanse the blood of waste. The blood is removed through a tube connected to an arm or leg artery. The blood passes through the dialysis machine and is "cleansed." *Peritoneal dialysis* requires insertion of a plastic catheter into the abdomen so that fluid flows into the space around the intestines. Waste then drains into this fluid and is removed from the body.

For some people, a kidney transplant may be an option to replace the kidneys that have failed. Kidney transplants are the most common of the transplant surgeries and also the most successful. The healthy kidney may be donated by a close blood relative or by an unrelated organ donor. The chances of kidney rejection are reduced if the organ comes from a blood relative. With any transplant, immunosuppressants (p. 624) must be taken for the rest of the recipient's life. Immunosuppressants keep the body from rejecting the new organ.

Not everyone is a candidate for a kidney transplant. Factors that are considered include the person's age, general and chronic health conditions, reasons for past kidney failure and availability of a donated organ that is a close match.

### Prevention

The most common causes of kidney failure are diseases that can be treated, such as diabetes and high blood pressure. See your doctor for regular exams and screenings for these and other treatable health problems. You can reduce the impact of these diseases on your health by carefully following treatment recommendations.

## Kidney Stones

- Severe pain in lower back and groin
- Nausea and vomiting
- Blood in the urine (often can only be seen with microscope)
- Recurrent infections
- Sometimes no symptoms if stone remains in kidney

When the kidneys filter out unneeded fluid and wastes, a number of chemical reactions take place in the kidneys. The chemicals and salts form small crystals that are passed harmlessly from the kidneys through the bladder and urethra. Sometimes, though, these crystals may form larger

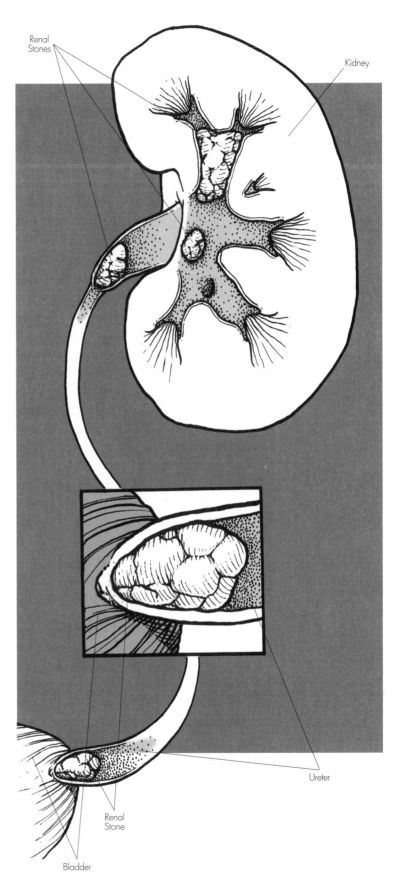

**KIDNEY (RENAL) STONES**

structures—solid stones that may not easily pass through the urinary tract.

The amount of pain and irritation a kidney stone causes depends on how big it is. Small stones—less than $1/25$ inch in diameter—usually pass with little or no discomfort. Larger stones—$1/5$ inch or larger in diameter—may be too large to enter the ureter. They tend to stay in the kidney. Stones between $1/25$ inch and $1/5$ inch may start to pass out of the kidney but become wedged in the ureter. This can cause spasms of excruciating pain and bleeding into the urine. Stones that remain in the kidney often cause no symptoms. Larger ones may cause bleeding and recurrent infections.

Many people say the pain caused by kidney stones is the most excruciating pain they've ever had. The pain begins in the small of the back, near the lower rib cage. It's a ripping, stabbing or burning sensation that moves toward the front of the body and the groin. The pain starts when the stone enters the ureter and stops when the stone is passed from the ureter into the bladder. The pain may begin again if the stone passes from the bladder through the urethra.

### Testing and Treatment

Your doctor may examine your urine under a microscope to check for signs of bleeding or infection. Kidney stones are most easily located with an IVP (p. 636) or ultrasound (p. 643) of the kidneys, ureters and bladder.

Taking medicine for pain and drinking lots of fluids may be the only treatment needed to help you pass a small stone. But many people experience such severe pain that hospitalization, injections to relieve pain and intravenous fluids are needed.

Stones caught in the ureter may be snared through a device called a cystoscope. The cystoscope goes into the bladder and grabs the stone with a tiny basket. The stone then comes out with the cytoscope. This procedure is performed under anesthesia in an operating room.

An ultrasonic "stone blaster," called a lithotriptor, is sometimes used to break up large stones in the kidney. This shock-wave technique breaks up the stone until it becomes a powder, which easily passes through the urethra and out of the bladder.

Some stones caught within the kidney itself may be too large to break apart and may require surgical removal.

In rare cases, kidney stones can lead to significant urine blockage, infection and kidney damage, requiring surgical removal of the affected kidney.

### Prevention

Drink lots of fluids. Water is best. The more water your kidneys handle, the less likely the various chemicals and salts will form into crystals or stones. Drink at least eight glasses a day or, better yet, add eight glasses of water to the fluid you currently drink.

If you have had a certain type of kidney stone, such as a calcium, cystine or uric acid stone, or if someone else in your family has had one, your doctor may suggest changes in your diet to help prevent such stones from forming. For example, avoiding too much oxalic acid, which may contribute to some stones, may be helpful. Oxalic acid appears in rhubarb, spinach, cocoa, nuts, pepper and tea.

## Nephrotic Syndrome

• Extreme swelling of the feet, legs, hands, face and abdomen

Nephrotic syndrome is a condition in which the kidneys are leaking large amounts of protein from the blood-stream into the urine because the glomeruli, the filtering units of the kidneys, are damaged. The loss of protein in the blood triggers a series of reactions that lead to fluid retention, or edema. The feet, legs, hands, face and abdomen may swell.

Numerous conditions and illnesses can lead to nephrotic syndrome. Causes include diabetes (p. 211); infections, such as endocarditis, hepatitis B (p. 205) and AIDS (p. 325); drugs or toxins, such as gold, mercury, heroin and antivenoms; cancers, such as Hodgkin's disease and leukemia (p. 138), and other diseases, such as systemic lupus erythematosus (p. 252) and rheumatoid arthritis (p. 231). Sometimes, the cause of nephrotic syndrome isn't known.

Nephrotic syndrome can affect people of all ages. Some types are more common in children.

### Testing

The gradual or sudden onset of swelling may signal nephrotic syndrome. Your doctor will probably test the urine and blood for protein. A sample of blood may also be tested to measure kidney function. Special blood tests for possible causes of the nephrotic syndrome may also be needed. In rare cases, a kidney biopsy may be required.

### Treatment

Limit the amount of salt you eat and get enough protein in your diet. Salt can lead to fluid retention, which is already a major problem in people with nephrotic syndrome. Some types of nephrotic syndrome can be treated with corticosteroids (p. 622). Diuretics (p. 616) may be helpful. In severe or prolonged cases, immunosuppressants (p. 624) may be needed.

Children with nephrotic syndrome often respond quickly to treatment and improve in a few weeks to months. Adults may take longer to respond to treatment. Medicines and a modified diet may be needed for several months or years. Adults often develop chronic kidney failure (p. 163) as a result of nephrotic syndrome.

### ⟨ Urinary Incontinence ⟩

• Not being able to hold your urine

The tissues near the bladder and the muscular rings (*sphincters*) that keep the bladder closed may weaken and stretch with age or as a result of injury, such as that caused by childbirth. When this happens, physical stress such as coughing, laughing or even bending to lift a book may put pressure on the weakened sphincter and cause urine to spill. This is called *stress urinary incontinence*.

In some cases, the sphincter may not close properly because the bladder opening is too inflamed, from an infection in the bladder, urethra,

---

## Bladder Retraining

• Urinate at regular intervals, beginning with every 30 minutes and gradually increasing the interval to every three to four hours.

• When you have the urge to urinate between intervals, practice tightening your muscles to keep from urinating.

• After the urge passes, wait five minutes and then urinate. Gradually increase the wait from five minutes to 10 minutes, then to longer periods.

• Bladder retraining may take three weeks to three months before the effects are noticeable.

prostate or vagina. Some injuries to the brain or nerves, such as a stroke (p. 59), spinal cord trauma (p. 58) or damage to the nerves around the bladder, can also result in urinary incontinence.

### Testing

Urine and stool tests, blood tests and possibly x-rays will help determine the cause of urine leakage. In some cases, special tests of the bladder's strength and capacity are needed. If nerve damage is suspected, nerve conduction studies (p. 638) may be done.

### Treatment

If inflammation or irritation of the bladder, urethra, prostate or vagina is the source of incontinence, it can be treated with antibiotics (p. 615). In women who have gone through menopause, estrogen (p. 623) in the form of pills or a vaginal cream may decrease vaginal and urethral dryness and irritation, which can lead to infection. These medicines can also improve the strength of the tissues around the urethra.

Other treatments can be tried when the cause of incontinence isn't infection or inflammation. Bladder retraining helps some people establish control by simply using the toilet regularly and frequently. Kegel's exercises (see box at right) can also strengthen

---

### Kegel's Exercises

Kegel's exercises can give women better bladder control by strengthening the *pubococcygeus muscle,* which is in the pubic area. To do the exercise, locate this muscle by sitting on the toilet with your knees as far apart as possible. Begin to urinate and then squeeze to stop the flow. The muscle you feel is the one that needs to be strengthened.

Practice squeezing that muscle on a daily basis. Squeeze the muscle for a count of three and then relax. Begin with 10 and work up to 30 squeezes at a time. Do 10 to 30 squeezes five times a day. Practice regularly for a few months before looking for results. The end result should be a stronger, more toned pelvic muscle that can cut off or hold urine.

Maintain the muscle tone with 10 to 30 squeezes two to three times a day.

---

the pelvic muscles in women who have stress urinary incontinence.

Surgery to tighten muscles around the bladder's internal opening may also help women, especially those with pelvic muscles that are stretched from pregnancy and delivery. Various incontinence aids, such as pads, allow you to remain active. No one should "just live" with incontinence. Many recent innovations and treatments are available.

# CHAPTER 11

# GASTROINTESTINAL SYSTEM

Your digestive, or *gastrointestinal*, system turns what you eat and drink into the energy your body needs to grow and keep working. Digestion begins in your *mouth*. You chew food into small pieces that can be digested more easily. An enzyme in the saliva helps break down carbohydrates.

Food moves from your mouth through your *esophagus* and then to your stomach. The esophagus is a muscular tube that uses wave-like motions to move the food to your stomach.

When food arrives in your stomach, it mixes with strong acids and enzymes. The strong muscles of the stomach churn the mixture of food, acids and enzymes. This mixture is called *chyme*.

Your stomach periodically releases chyme into the first section of the *small intestine*, called the *duodenum*. The small intestine is the place where most digestion occurs. Substances from the *pancreas*, *gallbladder* and *liver* are secreted to help change carbohydrates, fats and proteins into particles that are small enough to be absorbed. After chyme passes from the duodenum, it moves to the last two parts of your small intestine, the *ileum* and *jejunum*, where nutrients are absorbed into the bloodstream. These nutrients provide the energy your body needs.

The pancreas is located behind the stomach. It secretes enzymes into the

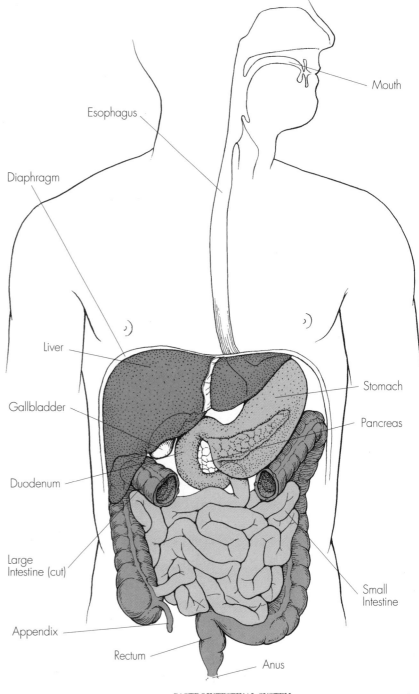

Mouth

Esophagus

Diaphragm

Liver

Gallbladder

Duodenum

Large Intestine (cut)

Appendix

Rectum

Anus

Stomach

Pancreas

Small Intestine

**GASTROINTESTINAL SYSTEM**

duodenum to help digest fats and proteins. The liver, the largest gland in the body, plays a part in digestion by producing *bile*, which breaks fats into small globules, or tiny drops. Bile is sent to the gallbladder and then the gallbladder secretes bile into the duodenum. The liver also helps the body process glucose, proteins, vitamins and fats. See page 201 for more information about the liver and gallbladder.

After nutrients are absorbed in the small intestine, water and undigested waste, such as fiber, pass into the *large intestine*. The mixture of water and waste is called *feces*. The large intestine is made up of the *cecum, appendix, colon, rectum, anal canal* and *anus*. The walls of the colon, which is the largest section of the large intestine, absorb water until the feces is solid enough to pass as a bowel movement. Movement in the large intestine causes the feces to pass through the intestine to the rectum. The rectum holds the feces until the urge to have a bowel movement is felt. The bowel movement then passes into the anal canal and out the anus.

## Anal Abscess

- Rectal pain
- Fever
- Discomfort with bowel movements, sometimes with a pus-like drainage
- Pain, redness and swelling of the skin near the anus
- Pain, blood or mucus with a bowel movement
- Fever (sometimes)

An *abscess* is a small pocket of pus surrounded by irritated, swollen tissue. A skin abscess near the rectum is called a *perirectal abscess*. An abscess in the rectum is called an *anorectal abscess*. The anal canal is lined with anal glands, which are in small, recessed folds. If a bacterial infection begins in one of these folds, it can quickly become an abscess. Fever, pain and sometimes pus in the rectal area with each bowel movement are signs of an anal abscess. Left untreated, such an infection can spread in the rectal area and even into the blood, causing severe illness.

**Testing**

If you have symptoms of an anal abscess, your doctor will probably perform a digital rectal exam (p. 633). Then your doctor may use either a proctoscope (p. 640) or a sigmoidoscope (p. 640) to look into your rectum and colon. If a deep rectal abscess is suspected, your doctor may refer you to a surgeon.

**Treatment**

Warm *sitz baths*, which involve soaking your anal area in a solution of warm salt water or warm soapy water, may reduce the swelling of perirectal abscesses and make the area more comfortable.

An anorectal abscess is almost always treated with surgical incision and drainage of the abscess. This is usually done in the hospital under general anesthesia. Antibiotics and fluids are given intravenously until the infection gets better. Analgesic medicines (p. 614) may also be given.

**Prevention**

Careful hygiene, gentle daily cleansing of the anal area and early treatment of any infections can help keep an abscess from turning into a more serious problem.

## Anal Fissures

- Pain with a bowel movement
- Bleeding or itching around the anus

An *anal fissure* is a "split" in the skin of the anal opening. It's sort of like

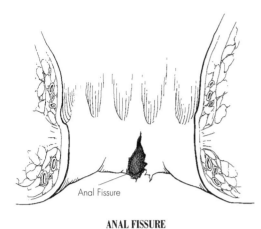

Anal Fissure

**ANAL FISSURE**

a split lip. The lips and the anus are made of the same type of skin. As would happen with a split lip, a split in the anal skin causes tenderness and bleeding. An anal fissure forms when a bowel movement is too hard or the muscles that close the anus are too tight. When a bowel movement passes through the anus, a crack occurs in the delicate anal skin. This may cause pain and itching in the anal area.

### Treatment

If you think you have an anal fissure, talk to your doctor to make sure your pain or rectal bleeding comes from a fissure and not from another condition, such as hemorrhoids (p. 189) or a serious rectal infection. Softening your bowel movements by getting plenty of fluids and fiber in your diet (p. 16) is usually all that's needed to heal the fissure. Warm sitz baths may reduce the symptoms and help the fissure heal. Fissures may come back. Fissures that don't heal even after using fiber supplements and sitz baths may, rarely, require surgery.

## Anal Itching

- Annoying itch in the anal area

Anal itching has several common causes. Possible causes are described below:

**Hygiene problems.** Not wiping enough after a bowel movement may allow feces to remain on the skin and lead to irritation. Too much wiping and cleansing of the anal area can also dry or irritate the skin. Wipe your anal area completely but gently. When you bathe or shower, don't scrub the anal area too hard and don't use a rough washcloth. Use a mild soap.

**Infestations.** A pinworm infestation can cause anal itching at night, when the adult worm comes to the surface of the skin to lay eggs. Treatment consists of taking an oral medicine to kill the worms. A steroid cream, such as hydrocortisone cream (p. 616), may relieve itching. See page 315 for more information on pinworm infestation.

**Skin conditions.** Fungal infections, psoriasis, eczema or contact dermatitis may cause itching anywhere on the body, including the skin around the anus. Antifungal medicines (p. 615) can help relieve the symptoms and kill the infection. Hydrocortisone cream can help relieve the itching.

**Other problems.** Hemorrhoids (p. 189) or loose muscles around the anus can result in fluid leakage from the anal canal, which irritates and chaps the skin. The skin irritation usually causes itching and pain in the rectal area. Treatment of the problem usually relieves the itching.

## Appendicitis

- Pain and tenderness in the abdomen that keeps getting worse and often moves to the lower right side of the abdomen
- Low fever of about 99°F to 101°F
- Loss of appetite
- Nausea and vomiting

The appendix is located on the right side of the abdomen. It's a finger-like tube that branches from the large

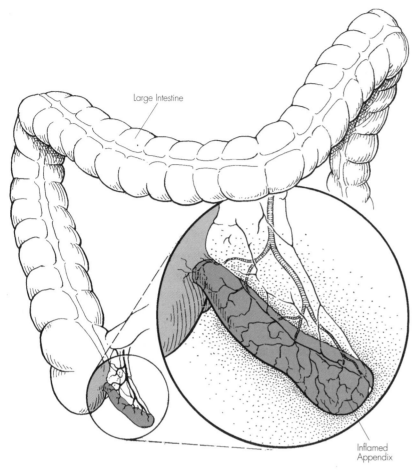

Large Intestine

Inflamed
Appendix

**APPENDICITIS**

intestine. In adults, it's about three and a half inches long. Its function is unknown, but when it becomes inflamed, a condition called *appendicitis* is the result.

Appendicitis can be the result of a blocked opening to the appendix, an infection, a parasite in the appendix lining or a condition in which the sides of the appendix stick to one another, closing it off. The appendix becomes inflamed when one of these conditions is present. Appendicitis occurs most often in teenagers and young adults, especially males.

For most people, the pain of appendicitis comes on quickly and gets worse over the first 24 to 48 hours. The pain usually starts as a constant, mild pain in the middle abdomen. As the pain worsens, it often moves to the

lower right side of the abdomen, near the hip bone. Loss of appetite, a slight fever, and nausea and vomiting are also common.

If appendicitis isn't treated, the appendix can burst, spilling its contents into the area around the appendix and spreading infection to the entire abdomen. This is a serious condition. A temperature higher than 101°F, along with the other symptoms of appendicitis, may indicate that the wall of the appendix has burst. If you suspect this has happened, go to an emergency room right away.

Sometimes symptoms of appendicitis develop more gradually. In some people, the appendix is in a slightly different location. If it's in a different location, the pain may not be in the usual area. When the usual symptoms aren't present, appendicitis is more difficult to diagnose.

### Testing

If your abdominal pain keeps getting worse or is severe, see your doctor or go to the emergency room right away. While you're waiting to see the doctor, bend your knees in a squatting position or bring your bent knees to your chest to help relieve the pain.

Your doctor will listen to your description of the pain and then examine your abdomen. He or she will press down on your abdomen to check for a rigid area and may listen to the sounds of your bowels with a stethoscope. A lack of normal bowel movement sounds is a sign of appendicitis. A high white blood cell count, which is a sign of infection, and urine tests can help determine if appendicitis is the cause of symptoms or if another problem is present.

### Treatment

The inflamed appendix must be surgically removed to prevent rupture and further infection. This operation is called an *appendectomy.* If leaking or rupture has occurred, the area will be cleaned during surgery, any damaged tissue will be removed and at least one surgical tube will be left in your abdomen to drain the infection. You'll be given intravenous antibiotics for several days. Within a few days the infection subsides, and the tube is removed.

If the appendix hasn't ruptured, the surgeon may do the appendectomy through a laparoscope (p. 637). This type of appendectomy requires a very small incision and usually shortens your recovery time.

## Bowel Blockage

- Vomiting (small-intestine obstruction)
- Severe, cramping pain in the abdomen
- Swollen belly (large-intestine obstruction)
- Lack of bowel movements
- Diarrhea (partial obstruction)

The small and large intestines, sometimes called the bowel, can become kinked, twisted or blocked as a result of several conditions. When this happens, your intestines can't move fecal material. Your intestine moves it through the digestive tract as far as the blocked area. The fecal bulk builds up at the blockage, causing increased pressure in the area.

As the growing bulk stretches the intestine, the blockage is sometimes partially relieved and some of the bulk gets through. This is called a *partial obstruction.* When a *complete obstruction* occurs, nothing moves through the area.

Symptoms of bowel blockage vary and depend on the location of the blockage—in the small intestine or the large intestine. Abdominal pain and vomiting are usually more severe if the obstruction is in the small intestine. The abdomen may swell if the blockage is in the large intestine. The longer the blockage exists, the worse the symptoms become. As more fecal material builds up, the vomited substance may begin to look like feces.

Intestinal blockage is most commonly a result of a tumor. But it can occur as a result of a hernia (p. 190), when a part of the intestine is twisted and pushed through a small hole in the abdominal wall. Other causes of blockage include a build-up of scar tissue that may be the result of previous surgery or intestinal damage. A build-up of solid waste within the bowel, called *fecal impaction,* or inflammation caused by a bowel infection can also be causes of blockage. In infants and young children, a blocked intestine may occur when part of the intestine slides back into another section, like a telescope sliding inward. This condition is called *intussusception.*

### Testing

After your doctor examines you, he or she may also want to do an x-ray of your abdomen to see the obstruction. The x-ray may show the cause of the blockage. A barium enema (p. 628) may also be needed. Blood tests, including a white blood cell count, may help your doctor find the cause.

### Treatment

Because a blocked intestine is serious, you'll probably stay in the hospital until the problem is taken care of, and the reason for the obstruction is identified. Intravenous fluids will be given to relieve dehydration from vomiting or not being able to drink. Sometimes, surgery is required to identify the cause of small or large intestinal obstruction.

In cases of bowel impaction, a suppository, enemas or oral medicine to soften the feces may allow you to pass the blockage on your own. In some cases of partial obstruction, a tube may be used to remove material from the bowel. Intussusception is frequently relieved by the barium enema used to diagnose it.

Often surgery is needed, especially to treat complete blockage of the bowel. The surgeon opens the abdomen to find and free the blockage. A twisted colon (*volvulus*) or a loop in the small bowel can be fixed surgically. Antibiotics (p. 615) may be given to fight infection if the bowel contents may have leaked into the abdomen.

## Carcinoid Tumors

- Flushed face
- Wheezing and shortness of breath
- Diarrhea and cramping

A *carcinoid* is a rare tumor that can develop from specialized cells, called *argentaffin cells*, in the stomach and intestinal walls. The tumor is cancerous but grows very slowly, enlarging and spreading over 10 years or more. The tumor secretes a hormone, called *serotonin*. This hormone is what causes most of the symptoms. The tumor rarely blocks the intestine.

### Testing

Your urine may be tested for evidence of serotonin if you have recurrent severe diarrhea with cramping and facial flushing. X-rays or a CT scan (p. 632) may be done if a tumor is suspected, or your doctor may recommend surgical exploration to look inside your abdomen. This exploration can sometimes be done with a laparoscope (p. 637), which requires only a small incision and allows direct visual examination of the intestine. A small sample of the tumor may be obtained at the time of surgery and sent to the laboratory for testing. The sample helps your doctor make the diagnosis.

### Treatment

Your doctor can prescribe medicines, such as cyproheptadine and phenoxybenzamine, to reduce the facial flushing, diarrhea and wheezing. The medicines are usually given before surgery is done to remove the tumor. When the entire tumor can't be removed, chemotherapy (p. 225) may limit its spread to other organs. Radiation therapy (p. 225) isn't effective.

## Colon Polyps

- No apparent symptoms
- Bleeding from an irritated polyp

Colon *polyps* are smooth, finger-like growths that form in the large intestine, or colon. When the colon becomes irritated, it produces extra lining to protect itself from further damage, and polyps form in this lining. Polyps may become irritated when waste moves through the bowel and pulls on them.

Polyps are believed to occur most often as a result of a low-fiber, high-fat diet, although the reasons they develop aren't completely understood.

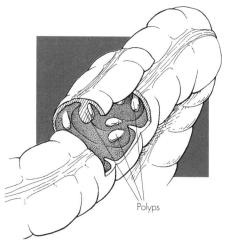

**COLON POLYPS**

A high-fiber diet causes waste to move more quickly through the colon. This quick movement limits the amount of time the bowel lining is exposed to waste toxins. Over the years, the faster passage of the waste causes less irritation of the bowel lining. Years and years of eating a low-fat diet may also limit the irritation, because this kind of diet requires a smaller amount of acidic secretions for digestion. On the other hand, eating a low-fiber, high-fat diet for years may cause irritation of the bowel lining, because waste doesn't move quickly through the intestine and because more acid is secreted to digest the fatty foods.

Less often, the tendency to develop polyps is inherited. The most common of these conditions is *familial polyposis*, but it affects only one in about 8,000 people.

Some polyps have a tendency to become cancerous, especially if they are left untreated for a long time and grow larger than an inch in diameter. The most common precancerous polyps are called *adenomatous polyps*. These polyps are like glands because they secrete hormones. People who have a family history of colon polyps tend to have precancerous polyps. If you have such a family history, have your colon checked regularly. Any polyps should be removed because they may become cancerous.

### Testing

Polyps may be found during any type of colon exam. Your doctor may suggest that a screening sigmoidoscopy (p. 640) be done to view your rectum and sigmoid colon. A screening sigmoidoscopy is recommended for people over age 50. If you have a family history of polyps or colon cancer, or if you've had a polyp removed before, your doctor may want to perform a screening exam periodically. A colonoscopy (p. 632) may also be done. Colonoscopy allows doctors to look at the entire colon. A piece of tissue from the polyp may be taken during these procedures so that it can be tested for cancer.

### Treatment

Small polyps may be removed during a sigmoidoscopy or colonoscopy. They may also be removed during a procedure called a *polypectomy.* However, a large, cancerous-looking polyp may not be removed this way. Instead, surgery may be done to remove the part of the colon that contains the polyp. Before this type of surgery, your doctor may order a CT scan (p. 632) or other tests to see exactly where the growth is located and if it has spread to any other area of the colon.

### Prevention

Eat a diet rich in fresh fruits, vegetables and grains. Reduce your intake of high-fat foods. See page 13 for more information about nutrition.

## Colorectal Cancer

- Abdominal pain
- Changes in your bowel habits, such as diarrhea or constipation
- Blood in bowel movements
- Thin bowel movements
- Weight loss
- Fatigue

Cancers of the colon and rectum are grouped together and called colorectal cancer. The reasons colorectal cancer develops aren't completely understood. Diet may be a factor. People who eat low-fiber, high-fat diets have an increased risk of getting these cancers and colon polyps, which sometimes lead to colorectal cancer. Both colon polyps and colorectal cancer can run in families.

In colorectal cancer, abnormal cells develop into cancerous tumors that invade normal tissues of the colon or rectum. The cancer can grow through the intestines and into other tissues or spread to other parts of the body, such as the lymph system or liver.

The most common symptoms of colorectal cancer are abnormal bowel movements, such as constipation or diarrhea, very dark or bright red blood in the bowel movement or abdominal pain. People who have colorectal cancer, especially rectal cancer, may feel that the bowel is never quite empty. If a tumor is blocking the bowel, the bowel movement may become narrow. Weight loss, loss of appetite, fever, anemia and fatigue may occur.

### Testing

Early detection of colorectal cancer—before symptoms occur—may improve the outcome. Early detection is usually done with a digital rectal exam (p. 633), tests for blood in the stool (fecal occult blood testing, p. 635) and sigmoidoscopy (p. 640) or colonoscopy (p. 632). If you have any risk factors for colorectal cancer, such as a family history of colorectal cancer or polyps or a history of colon polyps in yourself, see your doctor for an exam of your colon. If you're over 50, your doctor may want to perform an exam of your colon even if you don't have a history of polyps or colorectal cancer in your family or yourself.

Other tests may include a barium enema (p. 628). This test may help detect a tumor in the large intestine. Once cancer has been found, a CT scan (p. 632) and other scans can check for spread to other organs and to bone. Blood tests may also be done to identify any spread of the cancer beyond the colon.

Measurement of substances produced by tumors, called *tumor markers*, may prove to be useful in the future. A test for the blood level of a tumor marker called *carcinoembryonic antigen* (CEA) can help monitor the progress of people being treated for colorectal cancer. But it can't detect the disease until symptoms appear and, in some people with known colorectal cancer, the CEA level isn't abnormally high. In addition, the CEA level may be high because of reasons not related to cancer. For example, smokers and people with inflammatory bowel conditions or noncancerous growths in the colon may have a high CEA level in the blood. For these reasons, CEA test results often are unreliable.

Following the diagnosis of colorectal cancer, other tests will be needed to determine how advanced the cancer is and how best to treat it. The amount of spread—or lack of spread—and the aggressiveness of a colon cancer are used to determine the stage of the cancer and the best treatment for it.

### Treatment

When possible, a colorectal tumor is surgically removed to help prevent the spread of cancer. Many different techniques are used to remove tumors while keeping as much normal bowel function as possible. But sometimes, a large section of the colon or the entire rectum must be removed. This procedure is called a *partial colectomy*. If the rectal part of the colon is removed, the end of the colon is moved to an opening in the skin on your abdomen. This procedure is a *partial colostomy*. The new opening is called a *stoma*. The opening is connected to a bag that collects the waste and is emptied periodically. The stoma may be permanent or temporary until healing has occurred.

Colorectal cancer can be cured about half of the time. The cure rate depends largely on how deeply the cancer has spread into the colon wall and whether it has spread to other sites. Spread of the tumor can be treated with chemotherapy and sometimes radiation therapy.

**Prevention**

Eat a diet high in fiber and low in fat. This means eating plenty of fresh fruits and vegetables, along with fiber-rich cereals and grains, and eating fatty foods in moderation. See page 13 for more information on nutrition.

## Constipation

- Cramping pain with the desire to have a bowel movement
- Hard, painful, dry bowel movements

Many different factors—including a low-fiber diet and stress—can affect the consistency of bowel movements. You can remedy occasional bouts of constipation by making a simple change in your diet, by drinking extra liquids or by taking bulk-forming laxatives (p. 617). Constipation can also be caused by medical conditions, such as low thyroid hormone levels, blocked or twisted bowel, diverticulitis or colorectal cancer.

**Testing and Treatment**

**Infants and children.** Infants often have one or more bowel movements a day, but sometimes they skip a day or two. Hard, pellet-like stools may be caused by lack of fluids, too much iron in the formula or a rectal problem. A rectal exam by your doctor will rule out any problem in the rectum. X-rays of the colon are rarely required to determine the cause of constipation in children.

Add extra fluid to your infant's formula or consult your doctor about decreasing the formula's iron content. If your child is old enough to drink juice and eat solid food, increase the amount of fruits, vegetables, fruit juices and water in your child's diet.

Constipation should respond to these simple measures. If it doesn't, see your doctor. Don't use suppositories or enemas without talking with your doctor first.

**Adolescents and adults.** A change in diet or in the amount of fluid you drink may interrupt your normal cycle of bowel movements. Many people have a bowel movement every two or three days. Others have two to three each day. A few people have only one bowel movement a week. No matter what your schedule is, as long as you don't have abdominal pain, consider it normal.

> ### Serious Causes of Constipation
>
> - Blocked or twisted bowel (p. 173)
> - Colorectal cancer (p. 175)
> - Diverticulitis (p. 183)

> ### Home Remedies for Constipation
>
> - Drink extra liquids.
> - Eat a diet high in fiber, such as fresh fruits and vegetables.
> - Use fiber supplements, such as psyllium powder (p. 617).
> - Use an occasional laxative to ease discomfort.
> - Get more exercise, such as walking.

You can often loosen constipated bowels by adding fiber to your diet—eating high-fiber cereals, fresh fruits and vegetables—and by drinking more water or juice. You can also get your bowels moving with exercise, such as walking, running or an aerobic workout. Avoid using harsh laxatives, such as mineral oil or castor oil, unless your doctor recommends them. Excessive laxative use can lead to dependency. It's okay to use bulk-forming laxatives, which work naturally to add bulk and water to your bowel movements so they pass through your intestines easier.

## Crohn's Disease

- Crampy abdominal pain, often in the lower abdomen on the right side
- Diarrhea, sometimes mixed with blood
- Weight loss
- Fever

*Crohn's disease* is part of a group of disorders known as inflammatory bowel diseases (IBD). As this name implies, their common feature is long-lasting inflammation, or swelling, in the small or large intestine. The other common inflammatory bowel disease is ulcerative colitis (p. 198).

Crohn's disease affects the lower part of the small intestine, or the *ileum,* and also affects the colon. It causes swelling of the deep layers of the lining of the intestine. The cause of Crohn's disease is unknown.

The disease usually begins in young adults, causing a low-grade fever along with diarrhea and crampy abdominal pain, often in the lower right side of the abdomen. In some cases, the swelling occurs in other parts of the gastrointestinal system, from the mouth to the anus, as well as the intestine. Continued swelling in the intestine can cause the bowel wall to thicken with scar tissue, which can result in bowel blockage (p. 173).

Other problems can occur in people who have Crohn's disease. For example, some people have arthritis-like joint swelling and pain, skin, eye, liver, kidney or gallbladder problems. Children with the disease may have stunted growth. In addition, channels, called *fistulas,* sometimes form in the intestine, connecting the bowel wall with tissue or structures around it. For example, the fistulas may connect with other sections of the intestine, the bladder, the vagina or the skin. The rectum and anus are particularly prone to fistula formation with the skin, vagina and bladder, because they are so close to the rectum and anus. Seven of 10 people with Crohn's disease need surgery to correct fistulas or obstructions.

Crohn's disease lasts for a lifetime, though periods may occur when symptoms subside.

### Testing

Crohn's disease is easily confused with ulcerative colitis because the symptoms are so similar. If you have the symptoms of an inflammatory bowel disease, diagnosis begins with routine blood tests that include checking for low red blood cell count or high white blood cell count. Your doctor will probably do a colonoscopy (p. 632) to look

---

### *Symptoms of a Serious Bowel Problem*

- Bleeding from the rectum or with a bowel movement
- Abdominal pain, with severe cramping
- Change in bowel movements (ongoing diarrhea or constipation), with severe cramping
- High fever, along with other symptoms
- Prolonged nausea and vomiting
- Weight loss, along with other symptoms

*Any of the symptoms listed above could mean a serious health problem. See your doctor if you have a history of any of these symptoms and don't know the cause.*

at your rectum and colon and obtain a sample of the tissue for testing. The tests will confirm the diagnosis of Crohn's disease. A barium enema (p. 628) or small bowel x-ray can also be used to look for signs of Crohn's disease.

### Treatment

Controlling the inflammation with prescription medicines is the primary aim of treatment. These medicines include special drugs to treat bowel inflammation, such as sulfasalazine (p. 626) or mesalamine (p. 624). Corticosteroids (p. 622), such as cortisone (p. 623), given by mouth or by enema, may be needed for severe inflammation. For severely ill people, hospitalization to receive intravenous fluids and nutrition, intravenous corticosteroids and antibiotics may be needed.

Surgery to remove scar tissue or fistulas and even partial or complete removal of the colon may be needed when medicine or other treatments fail. But surgery isn't a cure. Even when diseased parts of the bowel are removed, inflammation usually returns to nearby areas of the intestine.

Some people with severe disease decide to have the colon completely removed, a procedure called a colectomy.

Although Crohn's disease requires long-term medical care, it's possible to live a productive life despite its symptoms. Most people are able to have full-time jobs, and women who have the disease are usually able to have children.

## Dehydration

* "Doughy" skin that tents up when you pinch it
* Crying without producing tears in a child
* Dry mouth
* Thirst (babies may show thirst by crying, being irritable and being eager to drink when something is offered)
* Decreased urination in adults and fewer wet diapers in infants
* Urine that's darker than usual
* Lethargy

Your body's fluids are made up of a complex array of chemicals, including water, calcium, sodium and potassium. Body fluids must be mixed at the right levels for your body to function properly. This balance can be upset during an illness that causes vomiting or diarrhea. *Dehydration* can occur when you're not able to take in enough fluids to keep up with the amount of fluids you're losing. Fever may contribute to dehydration.

Dehydration can be a serious problem. It can lead to seizures, coma and death if fluids aren't replenished so the chemical balance can be regained. Because children don't have as much of a reserve of fluids as adults, children are more prone than adults to dehydration as a result of diarrhea and vomiting. They should be watched carefully for signs of dehydration if they are vomiting or have diarrhea.

### Testing

Your doctor will probably be able to tell if you're becoming dehydrated just by listening to your symptoms, especially if you've been ill with diarrhea or vomiting, and by examining you. Tests aren't often needed, but blood and urine tests can confirm dehydration. In adults, blood pressure changes are sometimes helpful.

### Treatment

If you notice signs of dehydration in your baby, take him or her to a doctor right away. Dehydration can happen very fast in babies.

Infants older than three months can be given an oral rehydration solution (ORS) during periods of illness to ensure they get the right balance of salt and sugar along with fluids. ORS is a special drink that contains the right mix of salt, sugar, potassium and other chemicals to help replace body fluids.

There are many ORS brands available in stores. Some come as powders that you mix with water and others are already mixed with water. See page 180 for information about ORS brands.

Whether or not you should keep feeding your infant while providing ORS will depend in part on whether your baby has diarrhea alone or with vomiting. If your baby is also vomiting, you may need to start giving ORS gradually, giving just an eye dropper or spoonful every minute or so until the baby can keep it down.

If vomiting continues, you may need to wait 30 to 60 minutes before trying to give the ORS again. After the vomiting stops, you can increase the amount of ORS you give at a time, and you can lengthen the time between feedings to once every three to four hours. Keep giving ORS until your child's bowel movements become normal and the vomiting stops.

If you breast feed, keep nursing your baby and also give ORS. If you've been using formula, you may want to stop the formula and use just the ORS for 12 to 24 hours, and then switch back to formula. If your child is eating solid foods, try giving ORS for 12 to 24 hours and then start giving solid food again. If diarrhea or vomiting persists, call your doctor.

Home remedies, such as apple juice, chicken broth, cola or tea, shouldn't be given to children under two years of age. These drinks don't contain the right mix of sugar, salt and other chemicals. Soft drinks with caffeine shouldn't be given because caffeine is a diuretic and may only worsen dehydration. Even plain water can be harmful because it may dilute the levels of salt or sugar in the blood. Home remedies may be fine to use in older children and adults. Talk to your doctor.

**Prevention**

Dehydration can be prevented in most babies by starting ORS soon after he or she becomes ill with diarrhea and vomiting, or even before symptoms begin if you suspect dehydration may occur. Older children and adults can prevent dehydration by drinking plenty of fluids during an illness. See page 181 for more information on diarrhea and page 199 for more information about vomiting.

---

### Preventing Dehydration in Adults

- Don't force yourself to drink large amounts of liquids if you're vomiting.
- Sip liquids slowly. Very cold or hot liquids may aggravate cramps.
- You may need to use ORS if your vomiting or diarrhea is frequent and goes on for more than a couple of days.
- Antinausea and antidiarrheal medicines may be helpful. (Note: Antidiarrheal medicines can prolong the problem in young children and are not recommended for short-term symptoms.)

*See your doctor right away if you think you're becoming dehydrated! Dry mouth, infrequent urination, fatigue and lethargy are warning signs.*

## Diarrhea

- Cramping before a bowel movement
- Loose or watery bowel movements

Loose or watery bowel movements have many different causes. Most episodes of diarrhea are due to viral infections in the bowel lining. The infection causes water to be secreted into the bowel and results in runny bowel movements. After the bowel has "flushed" itself a few times, the infection is usually relieved.

Sometimes a virus infects the bacteria that normally live in the large bowel. These bacteria may make up 50% or more of the bulk of bowel movements. When this kind of infection occurs, the bowel movements may remain loose or watery for weeks, until the bacteria that normally live in the intestine can replace themselves. Eating yogurt with active lactobacillus cultures helps replace these bacteria and can help slow or stop this type of diarrhea within days.

A bacterial infection can cause severe irritation of the bowel lining, which can lead to cramps, nausea, vomiting and diarrhea. Such an infection can be spread by food that's improperly cooked, improperly refrigerated or improperly prepared by infected food handlers. There are many types of food poisoning (p. 300).

*Traveler's diarrhea* is a type of diarrhea caused by bacteria. It's called "traveler's" diarrhea because this illness develops in people traveling in a different country. The culprit is often a different strain of the bacteria in the food or water than normally live in the large intestine. Intestinal irritation that leads to cramping and diarrhea, seldom with fever, is the usual symptom. To prevent traveler's diarrhea, your doctor can prescribe simple medicines, including oral antibiotics (p. 615) or bismuth sulfate, that you can take regularly during your trip.

Nonbacterial causes of diarrhea include *giardiasis,* a parasitic infection that causes mild but prolonged diarrhea, gas, bloating and abdominal discomfort. Giardiasis is easily treated with antibiotics and usually has no complications. The illness can be contracted through eating contaminated food or drinking contaminated water. Giardiasis can be a problem in day-care centers when an infant or child has the infection and spreads it to other children and caretakers.

*Amoebic dysentery*, another parasitic cause of diarrhea, is contracted from exposure to infected food or water in areas of poor sanitation. In addition to intestinal infection, it may cause pockets of infection, or abscesses, to form in the liver. Cramping and bloody diarrhea are common symptoms.

Diarrhea has other causes besides infection or infestation. Nervousness and fear can cause the bowels to empty with a flurry of cramps and diarrhea. Undigested food can irritate the intestine and cause diarrhea. Increased hormone activity can lead to rapid emptying of the bowels. Diarrhea is also a symptom of irritable bowel syndrome (p. 193), which can cause severe cramping with alternating diarrhea and constipation. In addition, diarrhea can result from hyperthyroidism (p. 215) or reactions to medicines, such as antibiotics (p. 615).

### Testing and Treatment

**Infants and children.** Many newborns and small infants have soft bowel movements each time they nurse or take a bottle. This is normal and shouldn't be considered diarrhea. If a child younger than three months has large amounts of watery diarrhea,

### Serious Causes of Diarrhea

- Cholera (p. 298)
- Crohn's disease (p. 178)
- Diverticulitis (p. 183)
- Food poisoning (p. 300)
- Ulcerative colitis (p. 198)

### The BRAT Diet

Bananas
Rice cereal
Apple juice or
    apple sauce
Toast

*Use the BRAT diet when you start your baby on foods again after an illness with diarrhea or vomiting. Be sure to include plenty of clear fluids.*

take him or her to see your doctor. The risk of dehydration, especially in babies, is high.

Some changes in diet may help slow or stop diarrhea. If your baby is younger than three months of age, consult your doctor before changing his or her diet. In infants older than three months, try giving oral rehydration solutions (ORS, p. 180) to prevent dehydration.

With older babies and young children, stop giving milk and dairy products until the child takes other foods well and the diarrhea has stopped for 24 to 48 hours or longer. Dairy products shouldn't be given because diarrhea causes a temporary inability of the intestine to digest the sugar in milk, called lactose. Because of this, dairy products may make diarrhea worse. You may also need to use lactose-free formula for a few weeks if you feel your infant is bothered by the usual formula. Other foods to avoid include those with a lot of sugar or fat, such as ice cream, pudding and fried foods. You may try the BRAT diet (bananas, rice cereal, applesauce, toast) plus liquids to provide some solid food without causing the diarrhea to come back.

Over-the-counter medicines, such as bismuth sulfate, are usually safe and helpful in children older than two years. But treatment with these medicines may prolong an intestinal infection. Some antidiarrheal medicines have ingredients that could produce a toxic reaction in babies and young children. Carefully follow the directions on the package or contact your doctor if you have any questions.

If possible, the best therapy for diarrhea is to replace lost fluids. When needed, intravenous fluids can be given to replace fluid losses from severe diarrhea. Intravenous therapy is seldom needed if ORS is given promptly.

**Adolescents and adults.** Many cases of diarrhea related to stress, food or minor illness don't need treatment unless the cramping is uncomfortable or the diarrhea persists. Over-the-counter medicines for diarrhea usually work for mild viral gastroenteritis or other common causes of diarrhea. Your doctor can recommend or prescribe medicines that reduce cramps and nausea. Drinking only clear liquids may be necessary for people with persistent diarrhea or cramping after meals. As mentioned earlier, yogurt with active cultures can replace the essential colon bacteria that some illnesses destroy.

Prolonged diarrhea, diarrhea accompanied by other severe symptoms, or bowel movements mixed with blood or mucus can be serious. See your doctor as soon as possible.

If a bacterial cause is suspected, your doctor may order an exam and culture of the stool. The consistency of the stool, the presence of blood or mucus, and the presence of Giardia, amoebas, cysts or eggs of other bowel parasites will help your doctor make the diagnosis and prescribe the right treatment.

Most cases of bacterial diarrhea subside within a few hours or days without antibiotics. Prolonged cases should be evaluated by your doctor so any needed antibiotics can be prescribed. People with a severe case of diarrhea, including dehydration and fever, may require hospitalization for treatment with intravenous antibiotics and fluids.

### Prevention

If you travel to foreign countries, you may want to take along medicine to prevent traveler's diarrhea. Wash and peel fresh fruits and vegetables. Drink boiled water or bottled water that's unopened in countries where the water supply is unreliable. When camping, don't drink water that hasn't been boiled, filtered or treated with chlorine to remove or destroy bacteria. Always cook eggs and poultry completely, and wash your hands after handling raw meat or poultry.

Your doctor can prescribe an antibiotic you take once daily to prevent traveler's diarrhea. Bismuth sulfate, taken four times a day, has been shown to prevent traveler's diarrhea but, unfortunately, it can't cure the problem once it has started. Some medicines used to treat diarrhea can cause bacterial diarrhea to become worse. If your symptoms don't improve after taking over-the-counter medicines for a few days, contact a doctor as soon as possible.

## Diverticulosis and Diverticulitis

- No symptoms (diverticulosis)
- Minor abdominal pain or tenderness, muscle spasms
- Severe abdominal pain and cramps, fever and bleeding during bowel movements (diverticulitis)

As you age, the walls of your large intestine get weaker. Sometimes the weak areas develop into little pouches in the intestinal wall, called diverticula. This very common condition is called *diverticulosis.* Most people with diverticula never have symptoms or problems. If there are symptoms, they are usually limited to minor pain, tenderness or muscle spasms in the area near the diverticula.

But the diverticula can become infected and swollen. This more serious condition is called *diverticulitis.* Diverticulitis occurs in only about 20% of all people with diverticulosis, and it

becomes serious in just a few of those cases. Rarely, an infected diverticulum forms an abscess, which causes swelling, fever, blood with bowel movements and even a blockage of the intestine. Rarely, inflamed diverticula rupture, spilling fecal material into the abdomen and causing peritonitis (p. 195).

### Testing

Many people with diverticulosis never know they have the condition. It's usually detected on an x-ray or during a sigmoidoscopy (p. 640) or colonoscopy (p. 632) performed for another, unrelated reason.

If you develop severe abdominal pain, blood with bowel movements or any other persistent bowel problem, consult your doctor for further diagnosis. Blood tests and x-rays of the intestine will help your doctor make a diagnosis. He or she can use

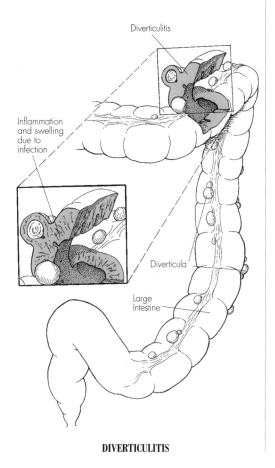

Diverticulitis

Inflammation and swelling due to infection

Diverticula

Large Intestine

**DIVERTICULITIS**

a colonoscope or sigmoidoscope (p. 640) to search the large intestine for signs of infection or diverticula. A barium enema (p. 628) can outline diverticula, in addition to revealing other bowel problems.

### Treatment

Most diverticula don't become infected, so usually no treatment is needed. Your doctor may recommend that you eat a high-fiber diet and avoid excessive use of laxatives and enemas. If pain and diverticulitis occur, your doctor may prescribe oral antibiotics (p. 618), along with analgesic medicine (p. 614) or anticramping medicine (p. 620). People with more serious bouts of diverticulitis may require hospitalization for treatment with intravenous fluids and antibiotics. Suction of the stomach and intestinal contents, done with a nasogastric tube, may be needed if blockage occurs. Surgery may be needed if a diverticulum ruptures or peritonitis is suspected. Rarely, surgical removal of the weakened bowel area may be required if bouts recur.

### Prevention

People who include fiber in their diet seem to have fewer weak intestinal areas than people who eat a low-fiber diet. In fact, a diet filled with fiber-rich foods may also decrease your risk for colorectal cancer (p. 175). Fiber may cause bloating or other abdominal discomfort if you aren't used to it, so start with small amounts and gradually increase the fiber until your bowel movements are bulky and soft. High-fiber diets should always include three to five glasses of water or other liquids each day.

## Esophageal Cancer

- Problems with swallowing
- Coughing
- Hoarseness
- Throat pain
- Vomiting (sometimes bloody material)
- Heartburn
- Pain in the chest
- Weight loss

Esophageal cancer is uncommon in the United States, accounting for less than 1% of all cancers. Unfortunately, almost all tumors of the esophagus are cancerous, and esophageal cancer is usually fatal. Esophageal tumors often spread into lymph nodes, the windpipe and other structures of the chest before symptoms start.

People who drink alcohol or smoke heavily are at highest risk of esophageal cancer. The primary symptom is a gradually increasing difficulty with swallowing, especially with solid foods. Sometimes bloody material that smells like rotten food is vomited. These symptoms, along with constant indigestion or heartburn, contribute to difficulty with eating and weight loss.

### Testing

Anyone who has trouble swallowing or who vomits blood should see a doctor right away. A barium swallow (p. 629), the test most likely to show

---

### Preventing Esophageal Cancer

Smoking and excessive drinking are risk factors for esophageal cancer. These two habits also have other health consequences. Stop smoking and stop excessive use of alcohol. See page 31 for tips to quit smoking. If you need help to kick the alcohol or nicotine habit, talk with your doctor. He or she can refer you to a support group or treatment program in your area and provide medical therapy.

an esophageal cancer, may be needed. The doctor also may use an endoscope (p. 634), inserted into the mouth and down the esophagus, to see the tumor and obtain a sample. If a test of the sample confirms cancer, a CT scan (p. 632) may be done to show how much the tumor has spread.

### Treatment

Radiation therapy (p. 225), alone or combined with surgical removal of the tumor, is the main treatment. Surgical opening, or *dilation*, of the esophagus to ease swallowing can help relieve some of the swallowing problems.

## Esophageal Varices

- Vomiting bright red blood in someone who has cirrhosis of the liver

*Esophageal varices* result from liver damage caused by cirrhosis (p. 201) that prevents blood from passing through a scarred liver. This blockage causes pressure to build up in the veins near the abdomen, including those at the bottom of the esophagus. The veins may swell like a hemorrhoid and bleed when food passes by. The bleeding from these swollen esophageal veins, called *varices*, can be severe and lead to death.

### Testing and Treatment

Bleeding in the esophagus is often life-threatening. The source of the bleeding must be found, and the bleeding must be stopped. Most people with severe bleeding require intravenous fluids and blood transfusions. An endoscope (p. 634) can be used to see whether the bleeding comes from the esophagus or the stomach. If bleeding esophageal veins are the problem, a balloon-like tube can be expanded within the esophagus to put pressure on the bleeding veins until the blood clots

in the area and the bleeding stops. These enlarged veins can also be hardened, or *sclerosed*, by injecting them with a substance that causes scars on the veins and makes them stop bleeding. Surgery to stop the bleeding may save the person's life if the source of the bleeding can be found in time.

### Prevention

Excessive use of alcohol can lead to cirrhosis of the liver and esophageal varices. Talk to your doctor if you need help to stop drinking.

## Gas

- Belching
- Abdominal bloating and discomfort
- Flatulence

Most people produce a pint to a half-gallon of gas each day. Gas produced by the body must be released either from the mouth (belching) or the rectum (passing gas, or *flatulence*). Abdominal bloating and discomfort may occur when gas builds up in the digestive tract.

There are many causes of intestinal gas. One common cause is swallowed air, which contains oxygen, carbon dioxide and nitrogen. Air enters the digestive tract each time you swallow. The amount of air you swallow may be increased if you smoke, chew gum, eat too fast, have poorly fitting dentures or have blocked nasal passages that make you breathe through your mouth. Carbonated beverages, which contain carbon dioxide, may also increase intestinal gas.

Certain foods, such as beans, cabbage, Brussels sprouts, cauliflower and high-fiber grains, can cause excessive gas production. Part of the reason for this is that the body lacks the enzymes needed to completely digest these foods. When the undigested portion enters the colon, the bacteria that normally live in the colon ferment the food, a process that produces hydrogen and methane gas, as well as carbon dioxide and oxygen. Over time, most people adjust to a diet that's higher in fiber and find gas becomes less of a problem.

Some people lack an adequate supply of *lactase*, an enzyme needed to digest *lactose*, a milk sugar. This makes them lactose-intolerant (p. 194). The undigested part of the milk ferments and causes gas. Eating fatty foods doesn't produce more gas, but fat delays stomach emptying, allowing gas to build up.

Conditions that may cause excessive gas build-up include hiatal hernia (p. 191), gallbladder problems and anxiety.

Although most of the gases in the intestine don't cause any odor, gases that do smell bad, such as hydrogen sulfide, are produced in small amounts as a result of food decay in the colon.

### Preventing Gas

- Eat fewer fatty foods.
- Avoid overeating gas-producing foods, such as beans and cabbage.
- Limit the number of carbonated beverages you drink.
- Exercise to help stimulate digestion and the passage of gas. Taking a walk after dinner may help decrease the amount of time gas is allowed to accumulate in your digestive tract.
- Limit the amount of time you chew gum.
- If you wear dentures, check with your dentist to make sure your dentures fit properly.
- Take supplementary digestive enzymes, such as lactase, to help digest food completely.

If you have irritable bowel syndrome (p. 193), you don't produce excessive gas, but you may have abdominal discomfort in response to normal amounts of intestinal gas.

### Testing

Bloating usually isn't a sign of a serious problem, but it can be a symptom of bowel blockage (p. 173). If your doctor suspects blockage, he or she may perform an x-ray of your abdomen, or a lighted-scope exam, such as a colonoscopy (p. 632), of your lower intestine.

If lactose intolerance is suspected, your doctor may order a blood test to check levels of the enzyme lactase. A breath test, which detects the hydrogen produced by bacteria during fermentation, may also be done to check for lactose intolerance. You may be asked to consume fewer dairy products for a period of time to see if this reduces the amount of gas.

### Treatment

Antigas medicines (p. 614) and supplementary digestive enzymes, such as lactase, are some of the over-the-counter medicines that may help relieve excessive gas.

If the gas is related to anxiety, relaxation therapy (p. 572) or counseling may break the cycle of swallowing air and passing gas. Reducing the fat in your diet will allow more rapid emptying of the stomach and reduce belching.

## Gastroenteritis

- Vomiting
- Nausea
- Cramping
- Diarrhea
- Fever

Commonly known as the "stomach flu," *gastroenteritis* is an infection that's usually caused by bacteria or viruses. It causes inflammation of the stomach and intestines, which leads to abdominal cramps, diarrhea and, in some cases, nausea, vomiting and fever.

Most cases of gastroenteritis are mild and go away without treatment, so seeing your doctor may not be necessary. Most bouts last from two to five days.

See your doctor if you run a high fever, if the diarrhea contains blood or mucus, if you suspect dehydration, if the pain in the abdomen becomes severe or if the illness continues longer than a few days. Signs of dehydration include dry mouth, decreased urination and lethargy. Children are more prone to dehydration as a result of diarrhea and vomiting, so they should be watched carefully for these symptoms. See page 179 for more information on dehydration and how to prevent and treat it.

### Testing

Because gastroenteritis is usually mild, lasts only two to five days and goes away without complications, most people don't need to see a doctor. Infants, young children, the elderly or those with chronic diseases, such as diabetes (p. 211), may need their doctor's advice for control of symptoms and prevention of dehydration.

### Treatment

Treatment depends on the source of the infection and its severity. Most people find that if they stop eating and drink plenty of clear liquids, their diarrhea and vomiting will slow and the cramping will ease. Rest, fever-reducing medicine (p. 616) and anticramping medicine (p. 620) also help.

Gastroenteritis can be much more serious in children than adults. Children may require an oral rehydration solution (ORS) to prevent dehydration.

See page 180 for more information on ORS.

As the illness leaves, you can gradually add simple, plain foods to your diet, such as gelatin, broth and cooked cereal, or use the BRAT diet (p. 182)—bananas, rice, applesauce and toast. Avoid milk products and fruit juices, which can prolong diarrhea.

Rarely, dehydration may require treatment with intravenous fluids. Any illness with severe abdominal pain should be checked right away by your doctor to make sure the appendix (p. 169) or another part of the digestive tract isn't seriously infected, swollen or injured.

### Prevention

Most viral illnesses are spread by hand-to-hand, hand-to-mouth or hand-to-rectum contact. An important step toward preventing these illnesses is to wash your hands before preparing food, especially after visiting a sick friend, using the toilet or changing diapers.

## Heartburn

- A burning pain in the chest or upper abdomen
- Belching an acidic fluid
- Pain when you swallow

If you've ever eaten spicy food or overindulged in a big meal, you've probably had the burning sensation in your chest or stomach called *heartburn.* Heartburn is often caused by acid and food coming back up from the stomach into the esophagus, usually because the stomach is overloaded or irritated. This is called *reflux.* If this happens often, the acid in the food can cause the esophagus to become irritated. This is called *reflux esophagiti*s, which can cause heartburn and pain while swallowing. Lying down after a meal or eating within one or two hours of bedtime may bring on or increase heartburn. Other causes of heartburn include gastritis (p. 197) and ulcers (p. 193).

At times the pain can become intense, especially if you have a weakness in your diaphragm called a hiatal hernia (p. 191). A hiatal hernia allows part of the stomach to push up into the chest, aggravating heartburn. This pain, along with the burning and irritation of heartburn, can produce great discomfort, even causing some people to think they're having a heart attack. Heart attacks can cause a similar pain in the chest. Overweight people have more problems with the reflux of stomach contents into the esophagus and are more likely to develop a hiatal hernia.

Most of the time, heartburn is caused by eating too much, by smoking or by drinking too many caffeinated beverages, such as coffee, tea, colas or hot chocolate. Acidic juices, such as orange juice, may also cause discomfort.

**Testing**

After listening to your symptoms, your doctor may simply begin treatment or may order an upper gastrointestinal series, a set of x-rays to look at your esophagus, stomach and duodenum. An endoscope (p. 634) can be used to look directly into the esophagus and stomach to see the linings of these two organs.

Special tests can be performed on the esophagus to detect increased spasm or laxity as a possible source of the reflux that causes the pain. To make sure no other cause of pain exists and to rule out heart attack, an electrocardiogram (p. 634) or chest x-ray (p. 631) may sometimes be done.

**Treatment**

Antacid (p. 614) liquid or tablets relieve most symptoms of heartburn. Famotidine (p. 626) and cimetidine (p. 626) may also be helpful. If the pain becomes chronic or gets worse, seek the advice of your doctor. If needed, your doctor can prescribe other medicines to reduce stomach acid secretion.

Bland diets haven't been shown to prevent heartburn. But avoid any foods that seem to aggravate your symptoms. Alcohol and tobacco can worsen heartburn and should be avoided. Consider eating smaller meals four to six times a day instead of two or three larger meals. Don't eat within two or three hours of your bedtime.

Surgery may be needed if a hiatal hernia becomes large and symptoms

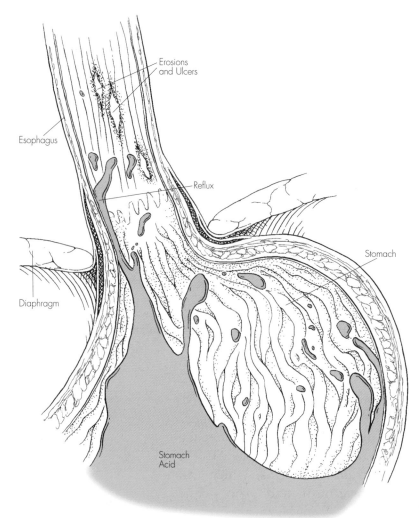

**ESOPHAGITIS**

### Preventing Heartburn

- Reduce the size of your meals.
- Lose weight.
- Don't drink alcohol or caffeine-containing beverages.
- Don't smoke.
- Limit your intake of coffee.
- Avoid citrus fruits, tomato products, chocolate, mints or peppermints, fatty foods, onions and spicy foods.
- Avoid aspirin (p. 615), ibuprofen (p. 617) and naproxen (p. 617), all of which can be irritating to the stomach.
- Try taking two tablespoons of liquid antacid with each meal and at bedtime.
- Loosen your belt and wear loose-fitting waistbands.
- Ask your doctor whether any medicines you're taking can make heartburn worse.
- Don't lie down or go to bed until at least two to three hours after you eat.
- Raise the head of your bed so stomach contents are less likely to go back into the esophagus.

are severe. In most cases, heartburn gets better by avoiding alcohol and tobacco, using over-the-counter medicines and making some minor changes in diet.

## Hemorrhoids

- Soft, tender, swollen veins in the rectum that may bleed during a bowel movement
- Itching in the rectal area
- Burning in the rectal area

When you stand, sit, lift heavy objects, strain to have a bowel movement or exercise, you put pressure on the veins in and around your rectum. Just as varicose veins (p. 127) in your legs bulge when you stand because the force of gravity fills them with blood, the veins of hemorrhoids bulge when pressure builds in the rectum. The

more pressure, the more likely you are to have hemorrhoids.

Hemorrhoids are more common in people who have constipation or diarrhea, pregnant women, people who are overweight and people who stand for long periods of time or lift heavy objects.

*External hemorrhoids* are hemorrhoids that involve the veins outside of your anus. External hemorrhoids can be itchy and painful. When a vein on the inside of the anal canal bulges, an *internal hemorrhoid* may form. There is little or no pain with internal hemorrhoids, but bleeding often occurs with a bowel movement. The hemorrhoid may stretch down and bulge outside your anus. This is a *prolapsed hemorrhoid*. Prolapsed hemorrhoids can be itchy or painful. A very tender, hard knot on the outside of the rectum may be a *thrombosed*, or clotted, hemorrhoid. Thrombosed hemorrhoids may bleed and cause pain, especially with a bowel movement.

### Testing

Your doctor can usually diagnose the problem by examining your anal area. An internal hemorrhoid can be seen with an anoscope (p. 628), a short, rigid, lighted scope. If the source of the bleeding isn't hemorrhoids, your

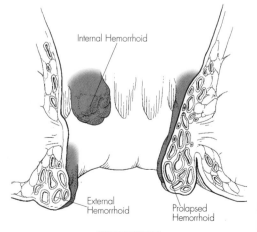

**HEMORRHOIDS**

doctor will probably order several other tests, such as a sigmoidoscopy (p. 640) or barium enema (p. 628), to find the source.

### Treatment

Because hemorrhoids are often a result of constipation, treating constipation is a good start. See page 177 for ways to prevent and treat constipation. Over-the-counter preparations to soothe the irritation and reduce the swelling may be useful, although many haven't been proven to work. Talk to your doctor about which hemorrhoid preparation to try.

Warm baths help relieve distress and itching in the anal area. Clean your anus after each bowel movement by patting it with moist toilet paper or moistened pads, such as baby wipes. Don't rub hard, because this may irritate the skin.

Ice packs may help relieve swelling, and analgesic medicines (p. 614) may help relieve the pain. Witch hazel or a numbing ointment may help soothe itching and pain, as may a cream that contains hydrocortisone (p. 616). Stay off your feet for a day if you're having a lot of pain.

Surgical treatments for internal hemorrhoids include *rubber-band ligation*. In this procedure, tight rubber bands are fastened around the hemorrhoid. The hemorrhoid falls off within days to weeks. More extensive, recurrent bouts may require surgical removal of the hemorrhoids. Thrombosed hemorrhoids can be opened by your doctor and the clot removed if it's done within the first day or two of symptoms.

### Prevention

Drink lots of water and eat plenty of fiber (p. 16), especially water-soluble fiber, such as oat bran. Try not to strain when you have a bowel movement. Straining increases the pressure in that area and increases your risk of developing hemorrhoids. Avoid becoming constipated. Constipation can contribute to hemorrhoids by causing you to strain during a bowel movement, which increases the pressure on anal veins.

## Hernias

A *hernia* occurs when an organ, such as the intestine, protrudes through the muscular wall that surrounds it. There are many different kinds of hernias. Those related to the gastrointestinal system include the abdominal wall hernia, hiatal hernia and inguinal hernia.

### Abdominal Wall Hernia
* Bulge in the middle of abdomen
* Intestinal blockage

An *abdominal wall hernia* results when the large muscles in the abdomen split or when there's a weak area in the muscle because of an old surgical scar. The intestine bulges through the muscle and can be seen under the skin. The bulge is usually most apparent when you lie flat on your back and raise your head. Abdominal wall hernias can occasionally be dangerous because the intestines may be pinched and not be able to function properly. This can lead to intestinal blockage or serious infections.

Abdominal wall hernias are usually diagnosed by physical exam. Abdominal wall hernias that aren't likely to pinch part of the intestine or another organ may be left alone. Other abdominal wall hernias require surgery. Emergency surgery to put the intestine back in its proper place and strengthen the weakened area may be needed if part of the intestine is pinched.

## Hiatal Hernia

* Fullness or pain in the upper abdomen and chest after large meals, especially when lying down

A *hiatal hernia* is a protrusion of a portion of the stomach through the diaphragm. The *diaphragm* is a muscle that separates the chest cavity from the abdominal cavity. It aids breathing by moving up and down to help bring air into and out of the lungs. The stomach lies beneath the diaphragm. The esophagus passes through an opening in the diaphragm to join the stomach. If the opening in the diaphragm becomes stretched, part of the stomach can slide upward through the hole in the diaphragm.

Hiatal hernias are usually brought on by increased pressure within the abdominal cavity, which can occur because of coughing, vomiting, straining when having a bowel movement or exerting yourself in intense physical activity. Hiatal hernia is especially common among overweight older people and pregnant women.

If you have a hiatal hernia, you may notice an increased back-up (*reflux*) of acidic fluid into the esophagus after you eat a large or spicy meal. This is heartburn (p. 187) and it can be severe. Symptoms are worse if you eat a meal and then lie down before it has left the stomach.

Your doctor may be able to diagnose a hiatal hernia based on your symptoms: increased heartburn after large meals eaten an hour or so before you go to bed. An upper gastrointestinal series (p. 629) will usually reveal the problem. Other tests, such as x-rays, electrocardiogram (p. 634) or an endoscopy (p. 634), might also be needed to exclude other problems.

Treatment for a hiatal hernia includes learning about the problem

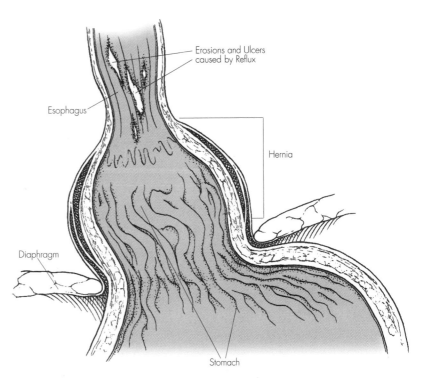

Esophagus — Erosions and Ulcers caused by Reflux

Hernia

Diaphragm

Stomach

**HIATAL HERNIA**

and its posture-related solutions. For example, sleeping on a wedge or a few pillows arranged in a wedge lets gravity keep food in your stomach. This helps reduce the symptoms of a hiatal hernia. Eating smaller meals, especially late at night, reduces reflux. Over-the-counter antacids (p. 614) and prescription medicines can reduce the acid in your stomach and the irritation caused by the acid in the esophagus. Avoiding smoking and alcoholic beverages reduces irritation in the esophagus and stomach. Surgical correction of a hiatal hernia is recommended only for people who have severe pain after trying all other medical and posture-related treatments.

## Inguinal Hernia

* Bulge in the groin, especially after straining, heavy lifting or coughing
* Pain in the area of the scrotum in men

Inguinal hernias are common. An *inguinal hernia* occurs when a loop of

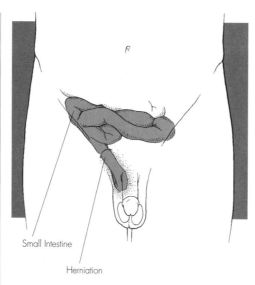

Small Intestine

Herniation

**INGUINAL HERNIA**

intestine protrudes into the *inguinal canal*, a tubelike passage through the deeper layers of the lower abdominal wall. In males, the inguinal canal leads to the scrotal sac. If an inguinal hernia is present, the intestine may fill the scrotal sac.

Part of the intestine can push through the inguinal canal and cause a bulge in the groin. Rarely, the intestine becomes trapped and causes a complete bowel blockage (p. 173). If this occurs, there may be abdominal cramps, bloating and inability to pass a bowel movement. In men, pain in the

scrotum can occur if the intestine slips into the scrotal sac.

If you go to your doctor because of a bulge in the groin, especially when lying down or straining, or because of pain in the groin, a physical exam will often reveal the problem.

Treatment for inguinal hernia involves surgery to repair the weakness in the muscle and to prevent the intestines from becoming trapped.

## Ileus

- Pain in the abdomen
- Abdominal bloating
- Nausea and vomiting
- Constipation

*Ileus* is obstruction of the intestines. If the normal, coordinated movement of food through the intestines is interrupted, the food stops moving through the intestine and becomes stagnant. Gas builds up, and the intestines swell. This can happen as a result of bacterial or viral infections. Ileus associated with gastroenteritis usually clears up within 24 to 36 hours. Other causes of ileus include any type of serious infection, particularly pneumonia, certain medicines and abdominal surgery. If ileus

### Hiccups

Hiccups are the result of spasms of the diaphragm. Rapid closing of the vocal cords cause the characteristic "hiccup" sound. The diaphragm is the muscle that divides the chest cavity and the abdominal cavity, and aids breathing by moving up and down to bring air into and out of the lungs. Common causes of hiccups include indigestion and eating too fast.

Hiccups may be annoying, but they don't usually cause problems. An attack of hiccups typically lasts for a few minutes at most, but occasionally hiccups may last longer or occur often.

Hiccups usually go away without any special treatment. You can try one of the fabled remedies for hiccups, such as holding your breath, breathing into a paper bag or swallowing a teaspoon of sugar. In rare cases when hiccups don't stop after a long period of time, your doctor may prescribe a sedating medicine.

lasts for more than a few days and is untreated, the bowel can sometimes become so swollen or stretched that it may rupture or leak, causing peritonitis (p. 195), a serious infection of the lining of the abdominal cavity. Peritonitis can lead to shock or death if it's not treated promptly.

**Testing and Treatment**

Increasing abdominal pain with nausea and bloating suggests ileus. X-rays will show enlarged loops of intestine filled with gas and fluid. Hospitalization for placement of a nasogastric tube to remove the gas and fluids in the stomach and intestines will relieve the pressure and prevent a rupture. Intravenous fluids are given, and antibiotics may be prescribed to treat an infection. Ileus usually stops when the cause is treated.

## Irritable Bowel Syndrome

- Abdominal cramping, often after eating
- Abdominal bloating
- Constipation
- Diarrhea
- Sometimes alternating constipation and diarrhea

Just about everyone has an occasional bout of abdominal pain and a change in bowel movements. But some people are bothered by regular episodes of cramping, abdominal pain, intestinal spasms, and alternating constipation and soft stools or diarrhea. This condition is called *irritable bowel syndrome* (IBS), or *spastic colon*.

The cause of IBS is unknown. Unlike inflammatory bowel diseases, such as Crohn's disease (p. 178) and ulcerative colitis (p. 198), in which the walls of the large intestine are inflamed with white blood cells, no specific intestinal changes have been found in IBS except extra mucus-gland

secretions. IBS affects more women than men and often first appears in late adolescence or early adulthood. Some researchers believe the disorder is related to anxiety and increased nerve input to the intestine.

**Testing**

Most people with IBS have a history of alternating diarrhea with constipation and abdominal cramping—all in an irregular pattern. After hearing these symptoms, your doctor may suspect IBS and try some simple treatments to see if your symptoms get better.

If you have excessive mucus or blood in your stool or if your symptoms don't follow the typical pattern, your doctor may order tests of the blood and stool to rule out other disorders. Stool cultures and stool exams might reveal an infection or another gastrointestinal problem. Abdominal x-rays with a barium enema (p. 628) or a barium swallow (p. 629) may be done.

**Treatment**

When the diagnosis of IBS has been made by ruling out more serious problems, your doctor will probably suggest some diet changes. Fiber

---

*Home Remedies for Irritable Bowel*

- Exercise regularly to reduce stress.
- Limit the fat, caffeine and alcohol in your diet.
- Slowly add psyllium powder or oat bran to your diet.
- Try reducing the dairy products in your diet.
- Use an over-the-counter pain medicine, relaxation therapy and heat applied to your abdomen when you have a bout of cramps and pain.

(p. 16), especially water-soluble fiber, such as oat bran or psyllium powder, may be helpful. But too much fiber may aggravate the problem or cause other symptoms. Medicines are available to help reduce the spasms of the large intestine and ease emotional distress. Because many of these medicines can have unwanted side effects, they may be prescribed only if you're having severe problems. IBS doesn't have complications or lead to more serious problems, such as cancer. Treatment is aimed at reducing stress and relieving the symptoms.

### Prevention

Eat a high-fiber diet to lessen the symptoms of IBS. Reduce stress and get enough sleep and exercise to help ease the symptoms. Limit the amount of caffeine in your diet to help reduce cramping and discomfort. Avoid any foods that bring on symptoms.

## Malabsorption

*Malabsorption* is the inability of the intestines to absorb certain nutrients or completely digest food. A host of medical conditions can lead to malabsorption.

### Bacterial Imbalance
* Crampy abdominal pain
* Gas
* Diarrhea
* Weight loss

An overgrowth of one type of bacteria in the intestine can cause diarrhea, bloating and weight loss. Too few bacteria in the intestine allows overgrowth of yeast and fungi. This problem can be identified by doing a stool culture to find out if the balance has been thrown off in the intestine. Bacterial imbalance is rare and usually occurs after bowel surgery, with other intestinal problems or after antibiotic

treatment. This condition will usually correct itself. Occasionally, another antibiotic will be needed to correct the problem.

### Celiac Disease
* Short height
* Infertility
* Anemia

Also called *gluten enteropathy* or *non-tropical sprue, celiac disease* is an inability to digest *gluten,* a protein found in some grains, including wheat. The lining of the intestine becomes irritated from undigested gluten, which leads to malabsorption of other nutrients. The cure is to stop eating barley, oats, rye and wheat—permanently. Celiac disease runs in families.

### Lactose Intolerance
* Diarrhea
* Bloating

People with lactose intolerance can't digest lactose, the sugar in milk and milk products. These people don't produce enough of the enzyme *lactase,* which helps digest lactose. The amount of lactase produced may decrease as a person ages. Thus, lactose intolerance is very common in adults. The reason for reduced production of lactase isn't clear. Asian and Mediterranean people are also likely to be lactase-deficient.

A list of the types of foods that upset you may be the most helpful information you can give your doctor to help sort out the cause of your symptoms. If you have bloating and gas after eating milk products, try switching to yogurt or other dairy products that contain lactase, or take lactase enzyme (p. 617) supplements.

### Pernicious Anemia
* Weight loss
* Constipation mixed with diarrhea

- Abdominal pain
- Burning of the tongue
- Tingling or numbness of feet and sometimes hands

*Pernicious anemia* is caused by vitamin $B_{12}$ deficiency due to poor absorption of the vitamin from the digestive tract. The $B_{12}$ deficiency leads to anemia, because $B_{12}$ is needed to produce red blood cells, the cells that carry oxygen to the body. The reason the intestine stops absorbing vitamin $B_{12}$ is unknown. Oral $B_{12}$ supplements don't help because the $B_{12}$ won't be absorbed in the intestine. Injections of vitamin $B_{12}$ are needed.

## Post-Surgical Malabsorption
- Bloating
- Diarrhea
- Cramping

After part of the intestine is removed or after gallbladder removal, some people don't absorb nutrients as they did before. This can lead to bloating, diarrhea and cramping pains. These symptoms can be treated with nutritional supplements that are easier to digest than unprocessed foods.

## Whipple's Disease
- Anemia
- Darkening of the skin
- Arthritis
- Weight loss
- Diarrhea

This rare bacterial infection of the intestines leads to severe malabsorption. Treatment with antibiotics (p. 615) over many months or years may suppress the infection and allow normal absorption to resume. A barium enema (p. 628) may be needed to help identify the reason for your symptoms. A sample of the small intestine is needed to confirm that Whipple's disease is the problem.

## Peritonitis

- Severe abdominal pain that's either just in one spot or more widespread
- Fever
- Vomiting

*Peritonitis* is an inflammation of the *peritoneum*, the lining of the *peritoneal cavity*. The peritoneal cavity houses your abdominal organs. The peritoneum is a membrane that encloses each abdominal organ and the inner surface of the entire wall of the abdomen. Peritonitis can be caused by an infection of the peritoneum, by problems with the organs it surrounds—such as a hole in part of the gastrointestinal tract—or by an infection in another part of the body that contaminates the blood and leads to an infection of the peritoneum. Examples of problems that can lead to peritonitis include appendicitis (p. 171), an ulcer (p. 193) that produces a hole in the stomach lining and pelvic inflammatory disease (p. 417). Peritonitis can become serious, even leading to shock and death, if not treated.

### Testing and Treatment

If peritonitis is suspected, x-rays of the abdomen will probably be done, as well as a laparotomy to find the cause of the infection.

Treatment depends on the cause of the peritonitis. Surgery may be needed in some cases, such as appendicitis. Intravenous antibiotics (p. 618) are usually needed to help fight the infection.

## Proctitis

- Blood, mucus or pus in the stool
- Feeling a constant need to have a bowel movement
- Severe rectal pain
- Fever

*Proctitis* is an inflammation of the mucous membrane inside the rectum and anus. Possible causes include Crohn's disease (p. 178), ulcerative colitis (p. 198), sexually transmitted disease (STDs, p. 316), injury from other diseases, radiation treatment for cancer or damage to the area during anal intercourse. Proctitis can be very painful. It can cause bleeding and mucus secretions with each bowel movement.

### Testing

Some causes of proctitis, such as radiation therapy, will probably be apparent based on your history. If you've been exposed to STDs, such as gonorrhea (p. 318) or herpes (p. 325), usually through anal intercourse, your doctor will do rectal cultures. Proctitis can be the first sign of Crohn's disease and ulcerative colitis. To rule out other diseases, a barium enema (p. 628) and sigmoidoscopy (p. 640) or colonoscopy (p. 632) may be needed.

### Treatment

Treatment for proctitis depends on its cause. Most bacterial infections respond to oral antibiotics (p. 618). Herpes infections may or may not respond to acyclovir (p. 621). Proctitis after radiation therapy is treated with soothing local ointments and heals with time. Crohn's disease or ulcerative colitis must be treated to improve associated proctitis.

### Prevention

Only infectious proctitis or proctitis due to injury is preventable. Safer sexual practices (p. 32), especially the use of condoms for anal intercourse, will prevent most cases of infectious proctitis.

## Stomach Cancer

- Feeling full after a small meal
- Nausea
- Vomiting, sometimes bloody
- Loss of appetite
- Abdominal pain
- Black, tarry bowel movements
- Weight loss
- Anemia

Cancer of the stomach is believed to be related to a high intake of certain foods, such as barbecued meats, smoked or pickled fish, nitrate-preserved foods and alcohol. Vitamin A and magnesium deficiencies may also increase the risk of stomach cancer. It's more common in people with blood type A and in certain families.

Pain with eating or pain relieved by eating is a common symptom of ulcers (p. 193), but it also may be the first symptom of stomach cancer. Weight loss is often noted in people with stomach cancer. Vomiting with blood is a sign of stomach cancer and should be checked by your doctor right away to make sure cancer isn't the cause. Feeling full after only a small meal and loss of appetite can also be symptoms of stomach cancer.

### Testing

A barium swallow (p. 629) can usually identify an ulcer or tumor in the stomach. In early stomach cancer, the x-ray findings are similar to those of a stomach ulcer, so endoscopy (p. 634) and biopsy may be needed. A CT scan (p. 632) or ultrasound (p. 643) may be done to check for spread of the cancer to the liver.

### Treatment

Stomach cancer is surgically removed. Chemotherapy (p. 225) may be needed to kill any small pockets of cancer cells left behind. If the entire cancer can't be removed because it's too large, chemotherapy can slow its progress and relieve symptoms. Radiation therapy (p. 225) is of little help by itself but may add to the benefits of chemotherapy.

## Ulcers

- Pain in the stomach area about 1½ to 3 hours after eating
- Relief of pain with eating

The membrane that lines the stomach and duodenum is extremely resistant to the acid that the stomach secretes to digest food. But sometimes, the amount of acid becomes too great and irritates these membranes. Ulcers are most common in the duodenum rather than in the stomach.

While ulcers used to be blamed on stress and alcohol use, infection with *Helicobacter pylori* (a type of bacteria) is now known to contribute to many ulcers.

An ulcer begins with mild inflammation, or *gastritis*. This may lead to more serious roughening of the lining and then breakdown or ulceration. This process takes weeks to months. The healing of an ulcer with medicines also takes weeks to months, as the stomach lining rebuilds.

Symptoms of ulcers vary. Some people have pain in the stomach when they eat. Others have pain that's relieved by eating. Most people have pain a few hours after eating. Some have nausea. Others have vomiting, too. Weight loss and anemia can also occur. Smoking, caffeine, stress, anti-inflammatory medicines (p. 615) and alcohol can cause stomach irritation and hasten ulcer disease.

Rarely, an ulcer destroys an artery in the stomach, causing what is known as a bleeding ulcer. Bloody vomiting may be a symptom. This is an emergency. Go to an emergency room right away if this happens.

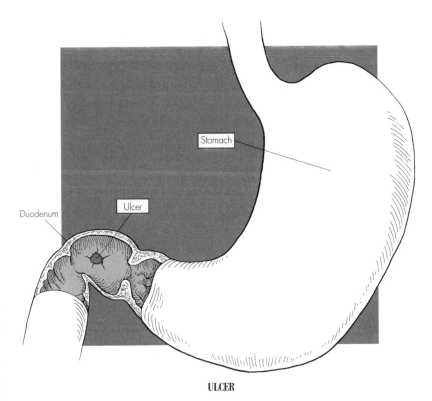

**ULCER**

### Testing and Treatment

Your history of pain in the area of your stomach, along with tenderness in your upper abdomen, will suggest the possibility of an ulcer to your doctor. Your doctor may decide to treat you with anti-ulcer medicine and antibiotics, without further tests, to see if the symptoms are relieved.

If additional tests are required, your doctor may perform an exam of the stomach through an endoscope. This usually answers most questions about what's causing your pain. A red blood cell count can help check for anemia, which can be caused by blood loss from an ulcer. A barium swallow (p. 629) may miss a small ulcer but can provide other information about the movement of material through the stomach. If the source of the pain is still in doubt, further x-rays or ultrasound (p. 643) of the abdomen may be needed. If you have vomited blood, angiography (p. 628) can identify the bleeding site in case surgery is needed to stop the bleeding.

For many people, self-treating gastritis with over-the-counter antacids (p. 614) is enough to keep the discomfort under control. Stronger medicines are available by prescription to reduce the acid secreted by the stomach, allowing the irritation to heal. Antibiotics may be used to treat *Helicobacter pylori* infection. A stomach ulcer that doesn't heal should be tested to make sure it isn't cancer.

### Prevention

Smoking, drinking alcohol, excessive stress and use of coffee or other caffeinated beverages may contribute to gastritis and ulcers. Avoid these things to help prevent the problem. Stress reduction includes adequate sleep, regular exercise and communicating clearly to prevent misunderstandings. The most important step you can take to avoid stomach ulcers and many other health problems is to stop smoking.

## Ulcerative Colitis

- Crampy abdominal pain
- Loss of appetite
- Diarrhea mixed with blood and mucus
- Anemia from rectal bleeding
- Fatigue
- Weight loss
- Involvement of other parts of the body, leading to skin and eye problems, arthritis-like joint pain, liver problems

*Ulcerative colitis* is a serious, chronic colon disease, one of a group of disorders known as inflammatory bowel diseases. In ulcerative colitis, the intestine becomes so inflamed that the lining *ulcerates*, or forms small, open sores. The characteristic symptom is bloody diarrhea, although a few cases start with abdominal pain without diarrhea. Other symptoms may result if these small sores, or ulcers, destroy the wall of the intestine and puncture other tissue. This leads to high fever, nausea, vomiting and peritonitis (p. 195). In this case, the abdominal pain is intense.

The cause of ulcerative colitis is unknown. The disease results in small abscesses or areas of infection within the lining of the large intestine. This characteristic sets ulcerative colitis apart from Crohn's disease (p. 178), another type of inflammatory bowel disease. Small abscesses and areas of infection aren't part of Crohn's disease. Ulcerative colitis increases the risk of colon cancer more than Crohn's disease does, so ulcerative colitis may be treated more aggressively.

Ignoring the disease's symptoms for a long time may lead to fever and blood poisoning from a "toxic *megacolon*," a massive enlarged colon that leaks toxic substances into the bloodstream. Complications of ulcerative colitis include inflammatory skin and eye problems, arthritis-like joint pain and malfunction of other organs, such as the liver. This may be caused by an overaggressive response of the immune system to the disease (autoimmune disorder, p. 223).

Unlike Crohn's disease, which can skip some areas of the intestine, ulcerative colitis always involves the rectum and part of the colon from the rectum toward the small intestine.

### Testing

Your doctor may suspect an inflammatory bowel disease based on your symptoms. Tests must be done to determine which one. A sigmoidoscopy (p. 640) may help your doctor see the characteristic ulcer pattern of ulcerative colitis. In addition, barium enema (p. 628) or other tests can help determine the extent of the disease.

**Treatment**

Sometimes, avoiding spicy foods and milk or other dairy products can help decrease irritation of the intestinal ulcers. Your doctor may prescribe sulfasalazine (p. 626) and anti-inflammatory medicines (p. 615). For people who can't tolerate those medicines, corticosteroids (p. 622), such as prednisone (p. 620) and hydrocortisone (p. 616), may be prescribed.

For severely ill people, hospitalization to receive intravenous fluids, steroids, nutrition support and antibiotics (p. 615) may become necessary. The risk of colon cancer in people who have ulcerative colitis may be 32 times that of people without ulcerative colitis. Because the risk of colon cancer is so high for people who have ulcerative colitis, surgical removal of the colon, called a colectomy, may be recommended.

When the colon is removed, an ileostomy is needed. An *ileostomy* involves creating a small opening, called a *stoma*, in the waistline area of the abdomen. The ileum, or the last part of the small intestine, is attached to the stoma. The stoma is connected to a bag that collects the waste and is emptied periodically.

## Vomiting

- Nausea
- Loss of appetite

Few symptoms of disease are disliked as much as nausea and vomiting. Nausea results from inflammation of the stomach wall, along with stoppage of digestion. The secretions, food or fluid go slowly through the stomach or may not move at all.

The body's reaction is to expel the stomach contents.

Many conditions can cause nausea and vomiting. Gastroenteritis (p. 186) is the most common cause. Infections of the respiratory or urinary tract can bring on nausea and, occasionally, vomiting. Head injuries, infections or bleeding around the brain can lead to vomiting by irritating the part of the brain that sends signals of nausea.

Vomiting can be an important warning sign in meningitis (p. 302), encephalitis (p. 324), appendicitis (p. 171) and bowel blockage (p. 173). Other possible causes of nausea and vomiting include certain medicines, swallowed mucous secretions or blood from the nose, and bleeding and irritation from an ulcer (p. 193), diverticulitis (p. 183) or other abdominal infections.

In infants, "spitting up" may be confused with vomiting. Spitting up formula or breast milk doesn't mean the baby has an infection or is allergic to the milk. Spitting up may act as an overflow mechanism when the baby has had enough milk. Air in the stomach from inadequate burping can also cause spitting up. As the baby grows, spitting up happens less often and eventually stops completely.

If vomiting in an infant or young child is accompanied by diarrhea, fever or cold symptoms, or if the vomiting is excessive or projectile (projected a few feet from the baby's mouth), your doctor should see the child.

**Treatment**

When a child or adult has an illness that causes vomiting, food and drink shouldn't be taken until the vomiting wanes. To avoid dehydration, it's best to start with small amounts of liquid, which may stay

*Serious Causes of Nausea and Vomiting*

- Appendicitis (p. 171)
- Head injury (p. 50) or bleeding in the brain (p. 45)
- Meningitis (p. 302)
- Encephalitis (p. 324)
- Blockage of the bowel (p. 173)

down when larger quantities won't. See page 180 for tips on preventing and treating dehydration.

Infants under three months of age who show any signs of an illness, including vomiting for six or more hours, should always be checked by your doctor. Older children with nausea and vomiting can usually be treated at home and watched carefully.

If you're nauseated but haven't vomited for an hour or two, begin drinking small amounts of clear liquids and eating gelatin or frozen flavored ice (such as Popsicles). Make sure you drink and eat very slowly. Some people sip warm, flat soda pop to combat nausea. Infants should be given an oral rehydration solution (p. 180) to ensure that they get the right balance of salts and sugar along with fluids.

Once the nausea ends, you can start eating bland foods such as crackers or dry toast. Follow the BRAT diet (p. 182)—bananas, rice cereal, apple juice and toast—for a day or two. A normal diet can slowly be resumed. Wait to add milk and dairy products until the nausea is completely gone.

Some time-honored home remedies, such as cola syrup or burnt toast, haven't been proved helpful, but seem to make some people feel better. They aren't likely to be harmful to adults.

## Call Your Doctor If:

- Nausea is accompanied by a headache or stiff neck, and even normal light hurts the eyes.
- Nausea is accompanied by a high fever.
- Your child is vomiting and has a dry mouth or cries without producing tears or, if the child is an infant, has few wet diapers.
- The vomiting is excessive or violent.
- The vomit contains blood.
- There is severe abdominal pain and diarrhea.
- Vomiting with fever or diarrhea lasts longer than 24 hours in children under six years of age, or when older children have vomiting, fever and diarrhea longer than 48 hours.
- Excessive sluggishness, drowsiness or weakness develops.

# CHAPTER 12 LIVER AND GALLBLADDER

The *liver* is the body's largest internal organ. In adults, the liver weighs about three to five pounds. It's located in the upper right part of the abdomen, under the diaphragm. The liver is divided into two main sections, called lobes—a large right lobe and a smaller left lobe. The liver needs a rich blood supply to carry out many functions. This organ is often referred to as the "chemical factory" of the body, because it performs more than 500 different functions. These functions include:

- *Detoxifying*, or cleansing, substances from the body, such as alcohol and drugs.
- *Metabolizing*, or breaking down, carbohydrates, proteins and fats.
- *Converting* digested food into energy.
- *Storing* such substances as iron and vitamins A, $B_{12}$ and D.
- *Producing* bile, which breaks down and aids digestion of fats.

The *gallbladder* is a pear-shaped pouch three to four inches long that's located under the liver. It stores bile—about four tablespoons of it. It then releases the bile into the *duodenum*, or the part of the small intestine that's near the stomach.

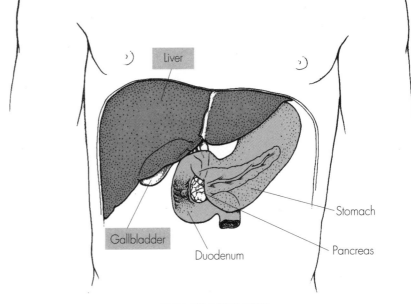

**LIVER AND GALLBLADDER**

## Cirrhosis

- No symptoms in the early stages
- Loss of appetite, nausea and vomiting
- Fatigue
- Swelling of the abdomen, arms and legs
- Weight loss
- Muscle wasting
- Jaundice
- Easy bruising
- Itching

Many cells in the body can repair themselves if they're damaged. But

*201*

when the liver cells are damaged and can't repair themselves, they die and are replaced by scar tissue and fat. The resulting condition is called *cirrhosis.* This condition reduces the body's ability to use calories and nutrients, causing weight loss and fatigue.

When the liver is scarred, blood can't flow easily through it. This results in a condition called *portal hypertension.* To compensate, other blood vessels open to allow blood to return to the heart from the intestines, without having to pass through the liver. When these blood vessels are in the esophagus, they're called *esophageal varices.* These vessels have thin walls and rupture easily. When esophageal varices tear or rupture, the resulting bleeding can be profuse and fatal.

In people with cirrhosis, the liver is unable to cleanse the body of poisons and wastes. When these products build up, they can cause symptoms such as confusion, agitation, tremors and coma. Cirrhosis also causes fluid to build up in the abdomen (*ascites*).

The liver also regulates the male hormone testosterone. Cirrhosis can decrease levels of testosterone, causing impotence, reduced muscle mass and shrinking of the testicles.

**Alcoholic cirrhosis.** This is the most common form of cirrhosis. It's caused by drinking too much alcohol. Alcoholic cirrhosis may be advanced by the time it's discovered, because it may not cause any symptoms at first. Each person has a different threshold for liver damage caused by alcohol. Women are more susceptible to liver damage than men. In the early stages of liver damage, avoiding alcohol may improve liver function.

**Biliary cirrhosis.** This type of cirrhosis can occur in two ways. In the *primary* form, the small ducts in the liver become inflamed. What causes the inflammation isn't known. It may be related to autoimmune disorder (p. 223). In the *secondary* form, the bile ducts are blocked by gallstones, scars or tumors. Bile can't leave the liver, leading to inflammation.

Both types of cirrhosis can cause permanent liver damage and, eventually, liver failure. Removal of gallstones can improve the liver function. Few other treatments exist. For people with advanced cirrhosis, a liver transplant may be the only hope for survival.

**Postnecrotic and postviral cirrhosis.** These forms of cirrhosis are the result of serious liver injury. The injury sometimes is a result of viral hepatitis. Postnecrotic cirrhosis may be caused by inherited disorders, such as alpha$_1$-antitrypsin deficiency (p. 147), galactosemia, glycogenoses, or rare metabolic disorders, such as Wilson's disease (storage of too much copper, p. 663) or hemochromatosis (storage of too much iron, p. 653). In some people, certain medicines, such as methotrexate (p. 625) and arsenic (p. 621), may damage the liver.

### Testing

If no symptoms are present, cirrhosis is often first suspected when blood tests show that the liver isn't functioning properly. When symptoms are present, they're probably similar to those caused by other chronic diseases. To pinpoint the problem, your doctor will ask about your symptoms, your exposure to toxins, your use of alcohol and any medical conditions you or your family have.

Further testing will be needed to reveal the type and extent of liver damage. These tests may include an ultrasound (p. 643) or a CT scan (p. 632). Special tests can identify the cause of the cirrhosis. The diagnosis of cirrhosis may be confirmed with a liver biopsy.

### Treatment

Once you have cirrhosis, it can't be reversed. But the symptoms can be treated. To reduce ascites, your doctor may prescribe a salt-restricted diet and a mild diuretic, such as spironolactone (p. 623). Antinausea medicines (p. 620) can improve appetite and reduce nausea. The antihistamine diphenhydramine (p. 615) may relieve the itching caused by jaundice (p. 205). Blood transfusions, fresh-frozen plasma and vitamin K help stop bleeding from esophageal varices and replace lost blood. A liver transplant may be the only hope for people who have severe cirrhosis.

### Prevention

You can prevent alcoholic cirrhosis by not drinking alcohol excessively. If you think you drink too much, ask your doctor or an alcohol-treatment center for help.

You may also prevent cirrhosis by avoiding infection with hepatitis. Hepatitis B is a type of viral infection that's spread through contact with infected blood or sexual intercourse with an infected partner. Using safer sex practices (p. 32) can reduce your risk for hepatitis B. Children should be immunized (p. 11) against hepatitis B.

If you have a metabolic disease such as Wilson's disease or hemochromatosis, removal of the excess copper or iron from your blood can prevent or slow cirrhosis.

## Gallbladder Cancer

- Constant and increasing pain in the right upper side of the abdomen
- Indigestion
- Jaundice
- Recent weight loss

Cancer of the gallbladder is rare. It's four times more common in women than in men. It generally strikes the elderly, especially those who have had gallstones.

Ultrasound (p. 643) or a CT scan (p. 632) may show the tumor. Sometimes, the cancer is discovered during surgery for other reasons.

The most common treatment is removal of the cancerous gallbladder. Unfortunately, many tumors are discovered too late and can't be completely removed.

## Gallstones

- No symptoms if stones remain in the gallbladder
- Sharp pain in the upper right side of the abdomen, and sometimes in the back
- Nausea and vomiting
- Low-grade fever
- Jaundice
- Symptoms sometimes brought on by eating rich or fatty foods

Gallstones are formed when the chemicals dissolved in the gallbladder build up. When the stones are small, they may be squeezed out of the gallbladder and through the common bile duct into the intestines. Larger stones can become stuck in the duct, causing pain and a backup of bile in the

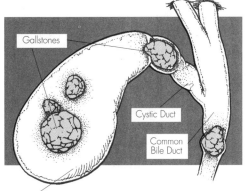

**GALLBLADDER WITH STONES**

gallbladder. When this happens, the stones must be removed.

When a stone is pushed from the gallbladder into the bile duct, it can cause extreme pain in the upper right abdomen. This pain is called *biliary colic*. Biliary colic comes and goes in waves and may spread to the right shoulder or back. If the duct remains blocked, the gallbladder can become inflamed (*cholecystitis*) and infected.

The pain of cholecystitis is usually severe and associated with decreased appetite, nausea, vomiting and a low-grade fever. Taking deep breaths may make the pain worse.

### Testing

If you suspect you have gallbladder disease, see your doctor. Pain after eating fatty or fried foods, and tenderness in the right upper part of the abdomen suggest a gallbladder problem. Your doctor may order x-rays or an ultrasound (p. 643). The ultrasound can identify stones in the gallbladder and the common bile duct. Blood tests reveal infection, the extent of gallbladder inflammation or abnormal liver function.

### Treatment

Gallstones are often discovered during a routine chest x-ray or other x-ray. You and your doctor will have to decide whether or not to remove the gallstones. Reasons for removal include a history of diabetes (p. 211), a history of recurrent biliary colic or the presence of a large stone. Some people choose to live with their gallstones until they have symptoms.

When surgery isn't possible, medicines can be used to dissolve gallstones. The medicines take one to two years to dissolve the gallstones completely. Surgical removal of the gallbladder is generally preferred to prevent gallstones from recurring.

Surgical removal of the gallbladder, an operation called *cholecystectomy*, is done through a large incision in the abdomen. Another method uses a laparoscope, called a *laparoscopic cholecystectomy*. It requires a number of smaller incisions and has a shorter recovery period.

### Prevention

Eating patterns can increase your risk of gallbladder problems. For example, prolonged fasting or a very low-calorie diet increases the risk of gallbladder disease. High-calorie or high-fat diets may make stone formation more likely. So it's safest to eat moderately and lose weight moderately. See page 13 for more information about nutrition.

## Hepatitis

- Headache
- Nausea
- Abdominal pain
- Tea-colored urine
- Grayish bowel movements
- Jaundice
- Weakness and fatigue

*Hepatitis* can be caused by viruses that attack the cells of the liver, causing jaundice (p. 205), fever, nausea, vomiting and abdominal pain. The viruses can be spread through contaminated food or water, shared intravenous needles, sexual intercourse and contact with infected blood. The most common viruses that cause hepatitis are known as hepatitis A, hepatitis B and hepatitis C.

**Hepatitis A.** This type is also known as "infectious hepatitis." It's usually spread by contaminated food or water and is common in countries with poor sanitation. It can also be spread by infected food handlers who don't wash their hands before touching food. Occasional outbreaks occur from eating shellfish taken from sewage-filled water. The hepatitis A virus causes a flu-like illness that's sometimes followed by jaundice, dark urine and clay-colored bowel movements.

**Hepatitis B.** This type is also called "serum hepatitis" because it's spread through blood and other body fluids. It's often passed through sexual contact and sharing intravenous needles. In some cases it causes no symptoms, but it usually results in an illness that may be more severe than hepatitis A. Hepatitis B may lead to long-term liver disease.

**Hepatitis C.** This type of hepatitis used to be called non-A, non-B hepatitis. Type C hepatitis may cause short-or long-term illness. It can be transmitted through contact with infected blood and by sharing intravenous needles. It can also be spread by sexual contact.

*Acute viral hepatitis* is an acute, or short-term, illness that can be caused by any of the hepatitis viruses. The symptoms may resemble those of the flu. In some people, the symptoms are more severe, and jaundice, dark-colored urine and clay-colored bowel movements develop.

*Chronic viral hepatitis* can occur as the body tries to clear the liver of the hepatitis virus. The immune reaction of the body can damage the liver. This can result in *chronic active hepatitis* or *chronic persistent hepatitis*. With chronic active hepatitis, the disease progresses steadily toward cirrhosis (p. 201) and liver failure if treatment is unsuccessful. Symptoms resemble an irregular pattern of acute hepatitis. In contrast, chronic persistent hepatitis progresses slowly and the person usually remains free of symptoms.

**Reactive hepatitis.** Symptoms of hepatitis caused by toxins are similar to those caused by viral hepatitis. Removing the toxin and avoiding alcohol or drugs are essential to stop further damage to the liver.

### Testing

Blood tests can determine which type of hepatitis is present. Other tests are used to make sure the liver recovers. A liver biopsy can show how severe the damage is and help your doctor decide what medicines to use.

### Treatment

No antibiotic will destroy the hepatitis virus and return the liver to normal. Medicines can relieve the persistent nausea, occasional vomiting and abdominal pain of hepatitis. Corticosteroids (p. 622) may be prescribed for the inflammation if the hepatitis becomes chronic. Hospitalization may be required for severe acute illness. Removal of the poisonous substance in toxic hepatitis is essential to prevent continued liver damage.

### Prevention

Immunizations are available for hepatitis A and hepatitis B. People who are exposed to family members with

---

## Jaundice

Sometimes the skin turns yellowish. This is known as *jaundice*. Jaundice shouldn't be ignored because it may mean there's a problem with the liver. Jaundice is especially noticeable in the whites of the eyes and the palms of the hands. The urine may also be dark brown. The skin can become intensely itchy. The yellow color is caused by a build-up of *bilirubin*, a pigment generated by the breakdown of old red blood cells in the liver. If the liver is injured or swollen, or if the bile duct becomes clogged or compressed by a tumor, the bilirubin level in the blood rises because the liver can't get rid of the bilirubin.

hepatitis A and health care workers who are exposed to hepatitis B should consider immunization (p. 11). Children should be immunized against hepatitis B in the first year of life (p. 11).

If you're sexually active, practicing safer sex (p. 32) can help reduce your risk of infection. If you know your partner is infected, abstain from sex. Intravenous drug users are at risk when they share needles. Be wary of any needles that may be reused, such as those for ear piercing, tattooing or acupuncture. If you choose to have your ears pierced or get a tattoo, make sure the person uses new and sterile needles.

## Liver Abscess

- Fever
- Nausea and vomiting
- Fatigue
- Weight loss
- Pain in the upper right side of the abdomen
- Jaundice

An infection in the liver can cause an *abscess*, or pocket of pus, to form. Such an infection may have spread to the liver from the intestines due to diverticulitis (p. 183) or appendicitis (p. 171), from inflamed bile ducts or from infection elsewhere in the body. An abscess can also be due to an infection caused by parasites or to an injury to the liver. In the United States, liver abscesses are very uncommon.

An ultrasound (p. 643) or CT scan (p. 632) will confirm the liver abscess. Then a needle is inserted into the liver to draw a fluid sample to identify the cause of the infection. A tube may be inserted into the abscess to allow it to drain.

Antibiotics or antiparasitic medicines are given. Weeks of intravenous antibiotic therapy may be needed.

## Liver Cancer

- Nausea and vomiting
- Pain in the abdomen or where cancer has spread
- Weight loss
- Jaundice

The most common types of cancer found in the liver are *metastatic* tumors that have spread from other sites in the body. Most liver cancers occur in people with cirrhosis (p. 201), so their major symptoms are those of cirrhosis.

### Testing and Treatment

An ultrasound (p. 643) or a CT scan (p. 632) can show any abnormal areas of the liver. Blood tests can suggest the presence of liver cancer. A liver biopsy can identify the type of tumor.

Treatment of liver cancer is usually difficult because the cancer is often discovered late in the course of another disease, such as cirrhosis. Newer screening tests can aid early detection and removal of the cancer. Liver cancer may be treated with chemotherapy (p. 225) or rarely, surgery. A catheter is sometimes used to put medicine directly in the liver.

### Prevention

If your job exposes you to chemicals, find out as much as you can about their toxicity and how to protect yourself. Avoid excessive alcohol intake. If you have a drinking problem, get treatment to help prevent cancer associated with alcoholic cirrhosis. Unsafe sex and sharing intravenous needles puts you at high risk of contracting hepatitis B, another risk factor for liver cancer. If you're sexually active, practicing safer sex (p. 32) can help prevent hepatitis B. And don't share needles to inject illegal drugs. Make sure infants complete the hepatitis B vaccine series (p. 12).

# CHAPTER 13 HORMONES AND GLANDS

Hormones are chemicals made by glands and organs in your body. They regulate many of your body's activities, including your temperature, growth, cell repair and immunity to disease. Hormones also play an important role in metabolism. Metabolism is the rate at which your body uses and stores energy.

There are two main types of glands. The *endocrine glands* release hormones directly into the bloodstream. The hormones then travel in the blood to the part of the body where they're needed. Endocrine glands include the adrenal glands, thyroid gland, pituitary gland, testes (p. 429) and ovaries (p. 416). *Exocrine glands* release chemicals through a tube or duct. The pancreas, salivary glands (p. 92), sweat glands, mammary glands (p. 480), mucous glands and sebaceous glands are exocrine glands. The pancreas, for example, releases enzymes through the common bile duct and into the small intestine, where they help digest food.

**Adrenal glands.** The adrenal glands look like a cap on the top of each kidney. The adrenal glands have two sections—the outer cortex and the central medulla. The outer cortex produces two types of steroid hormones: the *mineralocorticoids* and

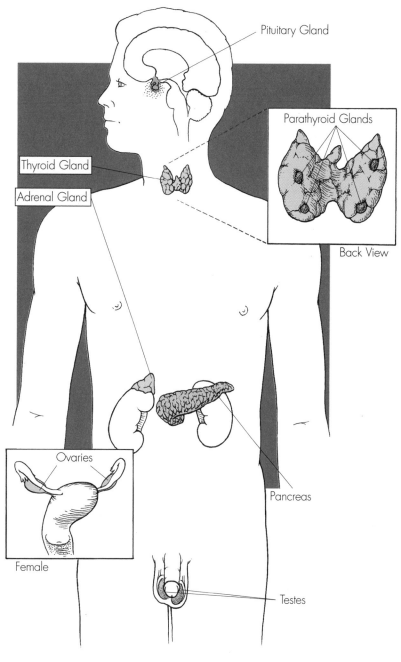

Pituitary Gland

Parathyroid Glands

Thyroid Gland

Adrenal Gland

Back View

Ovaries

Female

Pancreas

Testes

**HORMONES AND GLANDS**

the *glucocorticoids.* The mineralocorticoids help regulate the body's salt, water and blood pressure levels. Glucocorticoids regulate metabolism and the body's response to stress. In addition to these two types of steroids, the outer cortex produces at least 50 other steroids, including small amounts of the male hormone *androgen* and the female hormone *estrogen.*

The central medulla of the adrenal gland is important in the production of *epinephrine,* or adrenaline, which prepares the body to deal with a crisis—the "fight or flight" response. Most people have felt the adrenal rush when they're surprised or frightened.

Overproduction or underproduction of any of the adrenal hormones can produce disease. Dysfunction of the adrenal glands can lead to Addison's disease (p. 209) and aldosteronism (p. 210). But malfunction of the adrenal glands is uncommon.

**Pancreas.** The *pancreas* is located behind the stomach and small intestine. It produces enzymes needed to digest food. It also releases *insulin,* the hormone that allows your cells to use *glucose,* or blood sugar. The pancreas can be damaged if the abdomen is punched or struck during a car accident. Dysfunction of the pancreas can cause diabetes (p. 211).

**Parathyroid.** The *parathyroid* glands are located on either side of the thyroid in the neck. Most people have several small parathyroid glands. They produce *parathyroid hormone,* which has a direct effect on the level of calcium in the blood. Calcium is important in muscle movement, especially functions of the heart muscle. It's also very important for your bones. Too much parathyroid hormone can lead to hyperparathyroidism (p. 214). Too little can lead to hypoparathyroidism (p. 216).

**Pituitary.** Although the pituitary gland is small, it's important. The pituitary is attached to the hypothalamus in the bottom of the brain. Combined with the hypothalamus, the pituitary directs the body's hormone operations. The pituitary and hypothalamus control metabolism by regulating the thyroid, control growth by regulating the production of growth hormones and control breast-milk production by regulating the hormone *prolactin.* The pituitary and hypothalamus also provide instructions and information to the adrenal glands, ovaries and testes. Most problems with the pituitary gland are caused by a tumor or decreased blood flow to the pituitary gland. Dysfunction of the pituitary gland can lead to acromegaly (below) and Cushing's syndrome (p. 210).

**Thyroid.** The thyroid gland produces two thyroid hormones that regulate your *metabolic rate*—the amount of energy your body burns. This butterfly-shaped gland is located near the base of the front of the neck. It can become inflamed in a number of diseases, leading to an increase or decrease in the amount of thyroid hormones produced. Malfunctions of the thyroid can result in hyperthyroidism (p. 215) or hypothyroidism (p. 217).

## Acromegaly

- Coarsening of the facial features
- Abnormal thickening or enlargement of the bones, especially the skull, jaw, hands and feet
- Increased hat size, ring size or shoe size

When the pituitary gland produces too much growth hormone for years in an adult, a condition called *acromegaly* results. If the pituitary gland overproduces in adult years, the main overgrowth of bones occurs in smaller bones, such as those in the jaw, hands and feet. If the pituitary gland goes into overdrive in children or teenagers, whose bones are still able to grow lengthwise, *giantism* occurs, and the child may reach a height of seven or eight feet. Most cases of acromegaly are caused by a pituitary tumor.

## Testing

Blood tests can measure the level of growth hormone. A glucose tolerance test (p. 636) may also be done. Glucose usually suppresses the release of growth hormone. In acromegaly, the growth hormone level doesn't go down after a large glucose ingestion. If acromegaly is suspected, x-rays can show the thickening of the bones in the skull and the hands. CT scans (p. 632) or MRI scans (p. 637) may be used to look for a tumor on the pituitary gland.

## Treatment

Bromocriptine is the medicine used to treat acromegaly caused by a pituitary tumor. It reduces the production of growth hormone. If medicine isn't successful or causes too many side effects, radiation and surgery may be used to stop the overproduction of growth hormone. Sometimes, all three—bromocriptine, radiation and surgery—are used to control the disease.

### WARNING: Don't Stop Taking Steroid Medicines on Your Own

If you've been taking oral steroids for more than two weeks, don't stop your medicine without talking to the doctor who prescribed the medicine. You could go into an *adrenal crisis*, which may lead to shock and death.

## Addison's Disease

- Nausea and vomiting
- Abdominal pain
- Tiredness
- Weakness
- Weight loss
- Darker color to the skin, especially on skin folds, scars, knees, elbows and knuckles, and in the mouth.

*Addison's disease* is rare. It's caused by low production of the steroid hormones in the adrenal glands. The adrenal glands may stop making enough of the hormones if the body mistakes the adrenal glands for foreign tissue and destroys them. The reason for this type of response, called an autoimmune disorder (p. 223), is unknown. Symptoms of Addison's disease may appear slowly over months or years.

In about 25% of people with the disease, infection, injury, surgery or stress causes an adrenal crisis. This condition is life-threatening. Extreme weakness, severe pain in the abdomen, lower back or legs, dehydration, confusion or even coma are symptoms of an adrenal crisis. If an adrenal crisis isn't treated quickly, the kidneys stop working and death occurs from dehydration (p. 179) and shock (p. 597).

## Testing

Your doctor will probably test the levels of sodium and potassium in your blood. The sodium level is low and the potassium level is high in people with Addison's disease. Blood tests will also be done to check the levels of steroid hormones, such as cortisol, produced by your adrenal glands. Low levels of steroid hormones in your blood and urine can indicate adrenal failure or Addison's disease.

## Treatment

In an adrenal crisis, hospitalization and rapid hormone replacement are needed. Long-term oral replacement of the adrenal steroids is possible, but you'll have to take these hormones daily for the rest of your life. Talk with your doctor about increasing the dose when you're under stress or have an injury, infection or surgery.

## Aldosteronism

- Fluid retention
- Excessive urination and thirst
- Muscle weakness

*Aldosteronism* results when your adrenal glands produce too much of the hormone *aldosterone,* which regulates fluids and salt in the body. Overproduction of aldosterone may be caused by a tumor of the adrenal gland. This condition is called *Conn's syndrome.* Or, aldosteronism may be the result of another condition, such as heart failure (p. 114), cirrhosis (p. 201) or pregnancy.

### Testing and Treatment

If you have high blood pressure (p. 123) and low potassium levels but aren't taking diuretics (p. 616), your doctor may want to do blood and urine tests to check your hormone levels.

If a tumor is responsible, it may be removed with surgery. Medicine may help control problems associated with overactive adrenal glands.

## Cushing's Syndrome

- A rounded face
- Extra facial and body hair
- Obesity
- Fat deposits on body, especially between shoulder blades, often called "buffalo hump"
- Stretch marks on skin
- Bruising easily
- Weakened muscles
- Menstrual disorders
- Rapidly changing emotions

*Cushing's syndrome* can occur when the pituitary gland makes too much of a hormone called ACTH. The oversupply of ACTH stimulates the adrenal glands to produce cortisol and other steroid hormones. High levels of these hormones cause symptoms such as weight gain, a rounded or "moon" face, extra hair on the face and body (called *hirsutism*) and other symptoms. Cushing's syndrome can be the result of a tumor on the pituitary gland. Identical symptoms can occur as a result of a tumor on the adrenal gland in people who take steroids—including people who take them for body building—or in people who have a cancer that makes an ACTH-like substance that acts like a pituitary hormone.

### Testing

Blood and urine tests can measure the levels of cortisol in the body. Your doctor may want to measure your cortisol levels over the course of several hours to see how the levels change throughout the day.

Dexamethasone (p. 622), a synthetic corticosteroid, may be given to you by injection or orally to see if it lowers the cortisol level. X-rays and CT scans (p. 632) may be used to look for tumors on the pituitary or adrenal glands.

### Treatment

If Cushing's syndrome is caused by a pituitary tumor, the tumor is removed surgically. Surgery can be combined with radiation therapy (p. 225). In some cases, radiation kills the tumor without the need for surgery. Cushing's syndrome caused by adrenal tumors is also treated by removing the tumor.

Cushing's syndrome caused by steroid use is treated by gradually decreasing the dosage. Steroids should only be taken under the careful supervision of your doctor and should never be stopped suddenly.

## Diabetes

- Thirst
- Frequent urination
- Fruity smell on the breath
- Weight loss, even with increased eating
- Weakness, fatigue
- Loss of consciousness or marked confusion
- Changes in vision
- Numbness in hands or feet
- Recurrent infections

*Insulin* is a hormone released by the pancreas. Insulin makes it possible for cells all over the body to absorb *glucose*, or blood sugar. Glucose is the primary energy source for the cells and the body. To understand how insulin works, think of a key and a door. Insulin is like the key. It's needed to unlock the "door" of the cell and allow sugar, or glucose, to pass into the cell. Without insulin, the cell would just about starve. People who have diabetes have a problem with their insulin. They either don't make enough insulin or their bodies don't use the insulin properly.

When insulin isn't available, sugar can't be absorbed into the cell. So sugar gathers in the bloodstream. This is called high blood sugar, or *hyperglycemia.* The high blood sugar leads to most of the symptoms of diabetes. It causes excessive urination as the body tries to get rid of the extra sugar.

If hyperglycemia is severe, it can lead to dehydration (*ketoacidosis*), coma and death. Ketoacidosis is the result when glucose can't be used as energy by the body. The cells then try to use fat and protein for energy. This leads to a build-up of wastes (called *ketones*) in the blood and urine, which in turn leads to high acid levels in the blood. If ketoacidosis isn't treated quickly with fluids, insulin (p. 624)

and potassium, the person may die. The sudden onset of ketoacidosis often follows illness, such as a viral or bacterial infection.

Symptoms of diabetes may come on slowly, with weight loss, weakness and fatigue, or can appear rapidly, with thirst and increased urination that's usually associated with a viral infection. There are two types of diabetes.

**Type I diabetes.** This type of diabetes is often called *juvenile-onset diabetes mellitus* or *insulin-dependent diabetes mellitus,* because it typically begins when the person is young and requires insulin to control the disease. The pancreas produces little or no insulin, which is what the body uses to keep the blood sugar level under control. The inability of the pancreas to produce enough insulin is believed to be caused by the combination of an inherited defect, certain types of viral infections and an autoimmune disorder (p. 223).

Type I diabetes is usually discovered in children or teenagers. The onset is usually abrupt. The child or teenager rapidly develops a very high blood sugar level, and in a period of one to three days begins having symptoms of tiredness, a fruity smell to the breath, confusion and may even fall into a coma. In older people with type I diabetes, the symptoms develop more slowly.

**Type II diabetes.** Also called *adult-onset diabetes mellitus* or *non-insulin-dependent diabetes,* this type of diabetes comes on slowly. Blood sugar may be mildly elevated for months to years before the problem is discovered. Symptoms aren't always obvious. They include changes in vision, numbness in the hands or feet, weight loss, weakness or fatigue, and recurrent infections.

People who have type II diabetes have a normal or near-normal level of insulin in the blood. The problem is that the body is resistant to insulin. Greater amounts of insulin are needed to keep the blood sugar under control. People who have type II diabetes may receive insulin injections to help control the blood sugar, but they don't need insulin to survive the way people with type I diabetes do.

Type II diabetes may be discovered when a routine blood test is done. Like type I diabetes, it tends to run in families.

### Testing

A simple blood test can show the level of blood sugar. Adult-onset or type II diabetes is often identified during routine blood tests done for other reasons. Very high levels of blood sugar may be enough to diagnose diabetes. If the blood sugar level is only slightly high, a glucose tolerance test (p. 636) can be

performed. Before the test you will be asked not to eat for 12 hours. First, the blood sugar level is measured. Then a sugar "load" is given, usually in the form of a super-sweet drink. Blood samples are then taken every 30 minutes for three hours to see how high the blood sugar levels rise in response to the sugary drink. Specific levels of blood sugar at one, two and three hours after the drink tell your doctor if you have diabetes.

### Treatment

Control of the blood sugar level requires a different treatment plan for each person with diabetes. It generally requires a combination of diet, exercise, oral medicine and insulin. The doses of oral medicine and insulin depend on the severity of the diabetes. Your doctor will work with you to plan the treatment that's just right for you. You can help prevent or reduce

## Complications of Diabetes

*Diabetes can be a dangerous and even deadly disease. One reason is that a number of serious complications can occur, especially when blood sugar levels aren't well controlled. Persistent high blood sugar levels damage the arteries, which can lead to damage in various organs.*

**Brain.** Damaged arteries decrease the blood flow to the brain, which can lead to stroke (p. 59).

**Heart.** People with diabetes are at much greater risk of atherosclerosis (p. 111) and heart disease. This can lead to a heart attack (p. 115).

**Kidneys.** If the small blood vessels in the kidneys become damaged, the kidneys can no longer filter waste as effectively and may eventually fail. Dialysis (p. 164) may be needed.

**Eyes.** If the small blood vessels within the retina are damaged, blindness can result. This is called diabetic retinopathy.

**Nerves.** Damage to the blood vessels in the legs can cause an insufficient supply of blood to the nerves of the legs. This is called diabetic neuropathy. Numbness, tingling or a burning feeling in the feet and legs can result.

**Peripheral vascular disease.** This disease occurs when blood vessels are damaged and not enough blood flows to the legs. People with peripheral vascular disease have a much greater risk for infections and sores that won't heal. Gangrene (p. 300) can result. Sometimes the gangrene is so severe that the affected part of the body must be amputated.

## Home Glucose Monitoring

*Home glucose monitoring* is a test you can do at home to measure your blood sugar level. Home monitoring allows you to change insulin doses, food intake and exercise to fit each day's activities. Careful control of blood sugar can reduce the risk of complications. Home glucose monitoring is important for people with type I diabetes and may also be useful for people with type II diabetes.

One way to check your blood sugar level with a home glucose monitoring test is to prick your finger to get a drop of blood. The needle is in a spring-loaded device, which makes the process simple and less painful. The device pricks your finger when you press it against your skin. You then place a drop of blood onto a test strip. The strip changes colors. You insert the strip into a blood sugar meter or compare the color of the strip with a color chart. This will tell you your blood sugar level.

In addition to checking your glucose level, your doctor may also want to check your blood for *hemoglobin $A_{1c}$*. This test is done in your doctor's office and shows how well your blood sugar has been controlled during the previous six to eight weeks. It can help you and your doctor decide which changes you may need to make in your treatment plan so that it can be as effective as possible in controlling your blood sugar level.

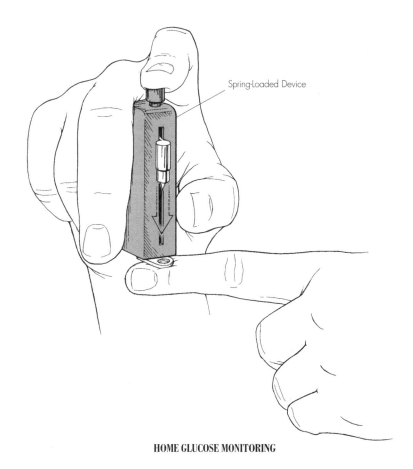

Spring-Loaded Device

**HOME GLUCOSE MONITORING**

keep your blood sugar level more constant by keeping your body weight within a healthy range. Eat the right amount of calories, limit the amount of fat and simple sugars in your diet, and exercise regularly. When planning meals, focus on complex carbohydrates instead of sugar and fats. See page 13 for more information about nutrition.

Exercise is important to help burn calories and keep your body fit, regardless of whether you have type I or type II diabetes. Proper diet and exercise can go a long way to bring down blood sugar levels and help prevent the complications of diabetes.

People with type I diabetes require injections of insulin. Most people require more than one injection of insulin each day. Instead of insulin injections, some people use a device called an "insulin pump." The pump constantly delivers a small

many of the complications of diabetes by keeping your blood sugar level as close to the normal range as possible—from 80 to 120 milligrams per deciliter.

Diet is a very important part of treating both type I and type II diabetes. The main thing to remember about your diet is to eat a variety of healthy foods and avoid junk foods and foods high in sugar. You can help dose of insulin under the skin and provides a larger amount of insulin at mealtimes, just as the body does under normal circumstances. Insulin pumps are surgically placed under the skin of the abdomen.

Transplanting insulin-producing *islet* cells into the pancreas is a successful treatment for diabetes in some people, making other treatments unnecessary. Islet cell transplantation is reserved for people who have type I diabetes.

Sometimes, type II diabetes can be controlled through a combination of diet and exercise alone. In other cases, medicine that stimulates insulin production is also needed. When oral medicine and diet fail to control blood sugar in people with type II diabetes, insulin may be given instead of, or in addition to, the oral medicine.

Learning about diabetes is important for all people with the disease. The more you know about how it works and what you can do to help yourself, the better chance you'll have to prevent complications. Diabetes education classes can help you learn about diet, exercise and the daily adjustment of insulin doses.

### Prevention

Currently, diabetes can't be prevented. But it's possible that maintaining a proper weight, along with regular exercise and a healthy diet, can delay the disease in people who have inherited the tendency to develop diabetes.

## Hyperparathyroidism

- Kidney stones
- Fatigue
- Increased urination and thirst
- Indigestion

*Hyperparathyroidism* results when one or more of the parathyroid glands make too much parathyroid hormone. Parathyroid hormone is important for your body's use of calcium. Too much parathyroid hormone causes a too-high level of calcium and a too-low level of phosphorus in the blood. Too much calcium can cause kidney stones. Hyperparathyroidism is most often caused by an *adenoma* (tumor) on one of the parathyroid glands.

### Testing

Half of people with hyperparathyroidism have no symptoms. The condition is often found when a routine blood test is done. Blood tests

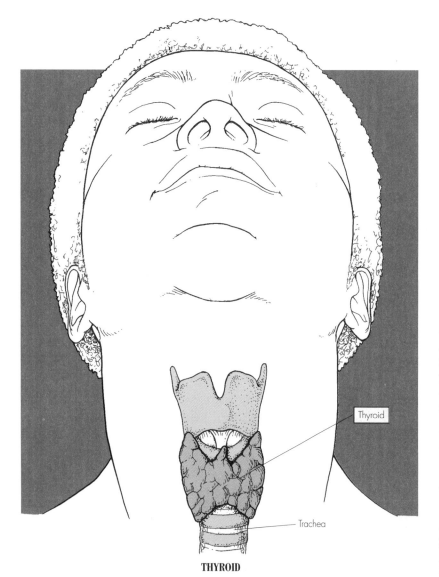

Thyroid

Trachea

**THYROID**

reveal high levels of calcium and parathyroid hormone.

## Treatment

In some cases, treatment is unnecessary and your doctor will just keep an eye on your condition. If hyperparathyroidism causes symptoms or gets much worse, surgery is done to look for and remove the tumor.

## Hyperthyroidism

- Nervousness or tremor
- Weight loss, usually with increased appetite
- Fast, irregular heart rate
- Increased sweating
- Muscle weakness
- Intolerance of heat and comfort in cold
- Emotional ups and downs
- Enlarged thyroid gland

*Hyperthyroidism* results from the increased production and release of an iodine-containing thyroid hormone called *thyroxine*. When too much thyroxine is in the blood, your metabolism increases and causes you to burn energy rapidly. This leads to weight loss, increased sweating, a fast heart rate and feeling anxious and jittery. *Thyroid-stimulating hormone* (TSH), a hormone made by the pituitary gland, then signals the thyroid to make thyroxine. Sometimes hyperthyroidism is caused by too much TSH. Hyperthyroidism may also have a number of other causes.

**Grave's disease.** In Grave's disease, the thyroid is stimulated by an antibody produced by the immune system. Overstimulation of the thyroid gland produces symptoms of hyperthyroidism. In Grave's disease, the eyes may also be affected. They may protrude or "bug out" of the eye sockets. This is called *exophthalmos.* Grave's disease is the most common cause of hyperthyroidism. It usually occurs in women, and it's hereditary.

**Multinodular goiter.** Small thyroid tumors, called *adenomas,* can replace much of the thyroid gland. They may make the thyroid look and feel enlarged, or "goitrous." Adenomas are benign tumors that may or may not secrete hormone. Adenomas lead to hyperthyroidism if they produce thyroxine. This condition is also called *Plummer's disease.*

**Thyrotoxicosis or thyroid storm.** Grave's disease and multinodular goiter can cause a sudden and severe increase in thyroxine—a condition called *thyrotoxicosis* or *thyroid storm.* Symptoms of thyrotoxicosis include fever, rapid pulse, confusion, agitation and extreme anxiety. Thyrotoxicosis is a life-threatening condition and must be treated right away.

### Testing

Blood tests can detect high levels of thyroxine and TSH. Your doctor will also examine your thyroid gland (at the base of the front of your neck). Ultrasound (p. 643) of the thyroid and a thyroid scan (p. 642) may be done. Blood tests to detect specific antibodies that stimulate the thyroid also are available.

### Treatment

Thyroid medicines (p. 626) may be used. In some cases, part of the thyroid gland is removed. Radioactive iodine can reduce the activity of the thyroid. This treatment is only used for people past their reproductive years. Eventually, these therapies can destroy thyroid function completely. When this happens, replacement hormones are needed. Sometimes surgical repair of the eye problems caused by Grave's disease is needed.

## Hypoglycemia

- Headache
- Feeling shaky and weak
- Excessive sweating
- Hunger
- Anxiety
- Sudden mood changes

*Hypoglycemia*, or low blood sugar, occurs when the sugar level in the blood drops below normal. When a large amount of sugar enters the bloodstream, more insulin is produced and the balance of sugar and insulin is more likely to be thrown off. Too much sugar may be absorbed by the cells, leaving low sugar levels in the bloodstream.

Anyone can experience hypoglycemia when they're hungry—even if they don't have diabetes. People who eat or drink large amounts of simple sugars rather than complex carbohydrates are at risk for low blood sugar. Drinking too much alcohol on an empty stomach can lead to hypoglycemia. Certain tumors can also cause hypoglycemia.

However, hypoglycemia most commonly occurs in people who have diabetes (p. 211). And hypoglycemia is most dangerous in people who have diabetes. People who have diabetes are at greater risk of low blood sugar when they're taking insulin or oral hypoglycemic medicine. People who have diabetes don't secrete enough insulin. They often need to take medicine or insulin to maintain the balance of sugar in the blood. If too much is taken, the blood sugar level may become too low, producing symptoms of hypoglycemia.

When hypoglycemia occurs in someone who has diabetes, possible consequences include coma and death. When hypoglycemia is severe and due to taking too much insulin, it's called "insulin shock."

### Testing and Treatment

Your doctor will probably be able to diagnose hypoglycemia based on your symptoms. A blood test may help confirm the diagnosis. Treatment may be as simple as eating something. People with diabetes may choose to keep a piece of candy or some fruit juice handy in case they experience hypoglycemia. It can be serious in people with diabetes, so should be addressed immediately.

### Prevention

The most effective prevention for dietary or stress-induced hypoglycemia is to change your diet. Try evenly spacing your meals and snacks throughout the day—eat six small meals or three smaller meals and three snacks. Avoid sugary snacks. A diet low in sugars and fats and high in complex carbohydrates and fiber can help prevent hypoglycemia. See page 13 for more information on nutrition. Combine good nutrition with stress reduction, regular exercise and plenty of sleep. If you have diabetes, follow your doctor's suggestions on keeping your blood sugar steady.

## Hypoparathyroidism

- Muscle aches or spasms
- Numbness of the throat, hands and feet
- Dry skin
- Vomiting, convulsion and headache in children

*Hypoparathyroidism* occurs when the parathyroid glands don't make enough parathyroid hormone. It causes low calcium levels and high phosphorus levels in the blood. Hypoparathyroidism is rare.

Hypoparathyroidism may be caused by damage to several parathyroid glands during thyroid gland surgery. It may also occur if the parathyroid glands are missing or have wasted away, but this is uncommon.

Hypoparathyroidism is diagnosed by low calcium and high phosphorus levels on blood tests.

Treatment involves correcting the calcium level. Your doctor will prescribe calcium and vitamin D supplements, which must be taken for life.

## Hypothyroidism

- Fatigue, weakness
- Dry, coarse skin
- Sweaty hands, face and feet
- Hoarseness of the voice
- Constipation
- Modest weight gain with less appetite
- Intolerance of cold and comfort in the heat
- Depression
- Enlarged thyroid gland

Low levels of thyroid hormones lead to a sluggish, tired, slow feeling, along with fluid retention. This condition is called *hypothyroidism.* The

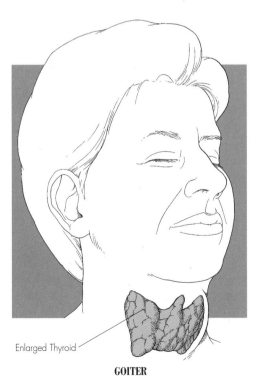

Enlarged Thyroid

**GOITER**

pituitary gland normally sends thyroid-stimulating hormone (TSH) to stimulate the thyroid gland to produce more thyroid hormones. Iodine is an important component of the thyroid hormone. If iodine is in short supply, the pituitary gland will send TSH to stimulate the thyroid gland to make more thyroid hormone. But the thyroid won't able to produce enough hormones to turn off the pituitary. The thyroid will enlarge under the stimulation of TSH, resulting in a *goiter.*

Hypothyroidism is often caused by *Hashimoto's thyroiditis.* In this disease, antibodies produced by the immune system slowly destroy the thyroid gland. But hypothyroidism isn't always associated with a goiter. This is called *secondary hypothyroidism.* One type of secondary hypothyroidism occurs when TSH levels are too low, so the thyroid isn't stimulated to produce thyroid hormones.

### Testing

Blood tests can detect low levels of thyroid hormones and measure the level of TSH. Your doctor will probably also examine your thyroid gland. A thyroid scan may be ordered. Blood tests to detect specific antibodies that destroy the thyroid gland also are available.

### Treatment

Hypothyroidism is treated by taking thyroid medicine (p. 626). To make sure you have a stable level of this thyroid hormone, it's usually best to use the same brand of thyroid hormone medicine all the time, because each brand is slightly different.

## Pancreatic Cancer

- Nausea and vomiting
- Abdominal pain
- Weight loss
- Jaundice (later)

### Subacute Thyroiditis

An infection of the thyroid gland, probably caused by a virus, leads to minor inflammation of the thyroid. The gland may be slightly enlarged and tender to touch. You may feel fullness or pain when swallowing. Thyroid hormone levels aren't usually affected. Treatment consists of taking corticosteroids (p. 622) to reduce the inflammation and analgesic medicines (p. 614) to reduce the pain and discomfort.

No risk factors for *pancreatic cancer* have been confirmed. But this cancer has been linked to heavy smoking, a high-fat diet and heavy consumption of alcohol. Pancreatic cancer is almost always fatal. It's one of the most common causes of death from cancer, after lung, colon and breast cancer. It causes about 5% of cancer deaths each year. It occurs more often in men than in women and, like many cancers, is more common after age 70. Your doctor will thoroughly investigate unexplained weight loss accompanied by abdominal pain of any sort to make sure this cancer isn't present.

### Testing

Although blood tests may provide some clues, a CT scan (p. 632) or ultrasound (p. 643) of the abdomen will be needed to look for cancer in the pancreas. Other tests may be done to search for the spread of the cancer.

### Treatment

If found early, the cancer can be removed surgically. Unfortunately, the cancer usually isn't found until it has spread into the surrounding tissues

and to distant organs. Radiation therapy (p. 225) and chemotherapy (p. 225) may slow the progress of the cancer, but these treatments aren't as effective with pancreatic cancer as they are with other types of cancer.

## Pancreatitis

- Severe abdominal pain, spreading to the back
- Nausea and vomiting
- Low-grade fever
- Shock (rare)

Inflammation of the pancreas, called *pancreatitis,* is uncommon and related primarily to two problems—alcohol consumption or blockage of the bile duct by a gallstone. For unknown reasons, drinking too much alcohol can lead to severe inflammation of the pancreas.

The *common bile duct* drains the pancreas. When this duct is blocked, the digestive enzymes back up into the pancreas, causing severe inflammation and destruction of tissue. Blockage of the bile duct may also cause jaundice (p. 205).

Other causes of pancreatitis include high levels of fat in the blood, high levels of parathyroid hormone, or an ulcer of the duodenum or stomach that erodes into the pancreas. Severe pancreatitis can lead to shock and death if not treated quickly.

In *acute pancreatitis,* abdominal pain builds over one to two days and is accompanied by nausea and vomiting, fever and shock if the condition isn't treated.

Repeated episodes of acute pancreatitis may cause scarring and the development of cysts in the pancreas, blockage of the bile duct and glucose intolerance or diabetes mellitus. After the pancreas has been damaged and scarred by recurrent episodes of

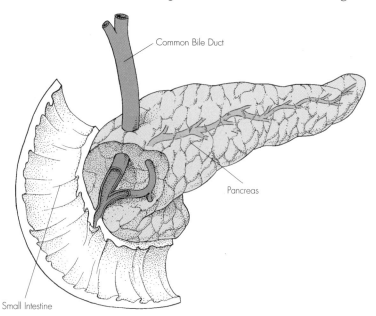

Common Bile Duct

Pancreas

Small Intestine

**PANCREAS**

pancreatitis, it produces fewer digestive hormones and less insulin. This is called *chronic pancreatitis.*

### Testing

Severe abdominal pain usually brings the person to the emergency room. The initial blood tests usually check for the pancreatic enzyme, *amylase.* If amylase levels are high, damage to the pancreas is suspected. Pain in the abdomen that spreads to the back, certain signs on abdominal x-rays, such as changes in the way the pancreas looks or swollen loops of bowel, along with a high amylase level, confirm the diagnosis.

### Treatment

Treatment of an acute bout of pancreatitis includes hospitalization, medicine for pain relief, intravenous fluid, antibiotics and withholding food and liquids by mouth so that your digestive tract and pancreas can rest. If you have chronic pancreatitis, you may have to take pancreatic enzymes by mouth and insulin by injection. Pain medicine may also be needed. Surgery to remove the damaged tissue may eventually be needed. Treatment for alcoholism can prevent recurrent bouts of pancreatitis.

### Prevention

Consumption of small amounts of alcohol—one to two drinks a day—hasn't been shown to cause pancreatitis, but large amounts of alcohol may be harmful. If you have trouble not drinking (alcoholism, p. 562), talk to your doctor for help before alcohol destroys the pancreas and other organs. Treatment of gallbladder problems may also prevent blockage of the bile ducts and pancreatitis.

## Pituitary Dwarfism

- Unusually slow growth and short height

If the pituitary doesn't produce enough growth hormone in children, a type of dwarfism, called *pituitary dwarfism,* results. Dwarfism is a symptom of a number of disorders that affect height. The word dwarfism commonly refers to the short height of people who have one of these disorders. Most cases of pituitary dwarfism are caused by a pituitary tumor.

Suspected pituitary dwarfism can be confirmed by blood tests. Children with pituitary dwarfism are treated with growth hormone replacement therapy.

## Thyroid Cancers

- Firm lump in the thyroid gland
- Hoarseness
- Trouble swallowing

Different types of cancer can occur in the thyroid gland. As with any cancerous tumor, the cells from the thyroid cancer can spread to distant areas of the body. Anyone who had radiation treatment for an enlarged thymus, acne or other skin disorders as a child or teenager has a higher risk for this type of cancer. Years ago, radiation was used to treat these conditions.

### Testing and Treatment

Fine-needle biopsy (p. 636), or removal of a small amount of the thyroid or tumor tissue, helps to identify the type of cancer.

Surgical removal of the thyroid, followed by radiation therapy (p. 225) or radioactive iodine, is the most common treatment for thyroid cancer. Hormone supplements are required to restore thyroid hormone levels and to help suppress any cancer cells that remain. If thyroid cancer is treated at an early stage, the chances for a complete recovery are good. Thyroid cancer has one of the highest cure rates of all types of cancer.

# CHAPTER 14

# IMMUNE SYSTEM

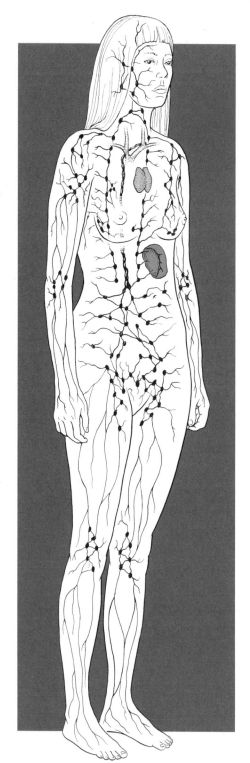

**LYMPH SYSTEM**

The *immune system* is your body's defense against germs such as bacteria, viruses or fungi. Your immune system also fights against cancer cells, any substance unfamiliar to your body and even transplanted tissues.

This defense system is complex and uses different kinds of cells to help you stay healthy. For example, your skin acts as a barrier to keep germs out. There's even a chemical in tears and saliva to help kill germs.

*Lymphocytes* are a type of white blood cell (p. 131) made by the bone marrow (p. 131), thymus and spleen. Lymphocytes travel throughout your body by way of the *lymph system,* which is made up of the *lymph nodes* and *lymphatic vessels.* The lymphatic vessels connect throughout different parts of your body much like your blood vessels do.

The lymph system is an amazing system that helps the body fight against infections. Some scientists have estimated that more than 99% of viruses, bacteria, fungi and foreign substances are attacked and killed by the lymph system before any signs of infection occur.

The lymph nodes are one of the most important parts of the immune system. They're strategically placed throughout the body to defend against germs. If an infection occurs, the lymph nodes swell and make extra lymphocytes to help fight the infection. When lymph nodes react to an infection, they begin to grow over a few days to a week. Once the lymph nodes finish fighting the infection—in one to three weeks—they return to normal size. In children, they may take one to three months to shrink.

The lymphocytes jump into action when an *antigen,* or something that's not recognized as a normal part of the body, is encountered. There are different kinds of lymphocytes. *B-lymphocytes* produce antibodies, or *immunoglobulins,* that fight the antigens. You normally have about 100 million trillion antibodies in your bloodstream. *T-lymphocytes* are divided into *helper cells,* which help identify antigens, and *killer cells,* which release chemicals that help destroy

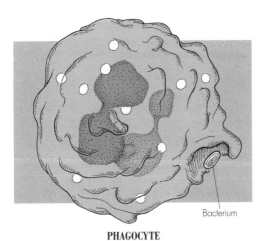

Bacterium

**PHAGOCYTE**

the antigens. Some of the lympho-cytes "remember" antigens so they can attack the antigens more quickly in the future.

Another type of white blood cell, called a *phagocyte,* surrounds bacteria. Phagocytes "swallow" the bacteria and then destroy them. Phagocytes come to the rescue when a site is swollen, or inflamed, from an infec-tion. This is part of the process called the *inflammatory response.*

Sometimes the immune system doesn't work properly. Some people are born with *immunodeficiency dis-orders.* In these disorders, part or all of the immune system fails. These people are extremely susceptible to certain infections and some kinds of cancer.

Other people may develop an immunodeficiency disease, such as AIDS (p. 325). People who have AIDS have very low levels of the helper T-cells, so they can't identify antigens and fight infections. Malnutrition, long-term steroid treatment, some types of cancer and the aging process can also make the immune system less efficient.

In some cases, medicine is used to intentionally suppress the immune system. For example, a person who receives an organ transplant takes spe-cial medicines to suppress his or her

## How Vaccines Work

Usually, you only get viral infections, such as chickenpox or mumps, once. That's because you develop antibodies against these diseases the first time you have the infection. When you're exposed to the viruses again, they're destroyed by the antibodies before they can make you sick. This is the principle behind vaccines, or immunizations.

A killed or modified form of the virus, which won't cause you to get the disease, is injected or swallowed, as with the polio vaccine. This causes your immune system to produce antibodies, protecting you in the future against the "real" viruses. Vaccines usually are taken as a series of shots or are taken periodically throughout your life. See page 11 for more information about immunizations. They're our best prevention against many viruses. Unfortunately, vaccines haven't been developed for all viruses.

immune system so it doesn't attack the new organ. The medicine helps reduce the chance that the body will recognize the new organ as foreign and reject it.

### Allergies

In an allergic reaction, your body's immune system identifies a usually harmless substance, known as an *aller-gen,* as dangerous. Antibodies come to the body's "defense" and call the *mast cells* to action. Mast cells are located in the skin and in the lining of the nose, lungs and gastrointestinal tract. They release chemicals such as *histamine.* Histamine is what causes the symp-toms of allergy, such as a runny nose.

## Allergic Contact Dermatitis

Sometimes an allergic reaction may occur on your skin. The result is an itchy, red rash. Poison ivy, poison oak and poison sumac are examples of plants that cause contact dermatitis. The allergic reaction is caused by the oils in these plants. Chemicals and other substances can also lead to allergic contact dermatitis. See page 277 for more information on allergic contact dermatitis.

### Allergic Rhinitis

- Sneezing
- Runny nose with clear discharge
- Itchy nose and eyes
- Watery eyes

*Allergic rhinitis* is what most people think of when they think of allergies. It's caused by an allergy to substances in the air. If you have symptoms year-round, you may be allergic to house dust (the culprit is actually a tiny mite that lives in house dust), molds and animal dander. If your itchy eyes and runny nose strike around the same time every year, you may be allergic to pollen from trees, grasses or weeds. This type of allergy is often referred to as "hay fever."

---

### Common Allergens

- Pollen from trees, grasses and weeds
- Dust mites (in house dust)
- Molds
- Feathers
- Animal dander

---

### Anaphylactic Shock (Severe Allergic Reaction)

- Wheezing or difficulty breathing
- Hives or itching
- Abdominal cramps or pain
- Swelling of the tongue or throat
- Vomiting

*Anaphylactic shock* is a type of allergic reaction that can occur suddenly and is life-threatening. It requires immediate medical attention. Anaphylactic shock usually occurs as a reaction to insect stings or medications.

### Drug Allergies

- Skin rash
- Hives
- Trouble breathing or wheezing
- Anaphylactic shock

Some people have allergic reactions to certain drugs. Penicillin (p. 625) is a common cause of such reactions. If you know you're allergic to any drugs, you should carry identification that states what drugs you are allergic to. Many pharmacies sell Medical Alert bracelets and tags.

Don't confuse the possible side effects of a medicine, such as nausea or diarrhea, with an allergic reaction. If you're in doubt, talk to your doctor.

### Food Allergies

- Runny nose and sneezing
- Swelling of the lips
- Rash around the mouth
- Nausea and vomiting
- Abdominal cramps
- Diarrhea

Food allergies are more rare than many people realize. They're particularly rare in adults. If you or your child is allergic to a particular food, you'll have to be extremely careful to read food labels and to ask questions when eating out.

In children under age three, the most common foods that cause reactions are milk, eggs, wheat products and peanuts. Older children and adults are most often allergic to fish, peanuts and shellfish.

Don't confuse food allergy with food intolerance. For example, lactose

---

### Bee Sting Kits

If you know you're allergic to bee or other insect stings, ask your doctor about a prescription for an emergency medical treatment kit that contains epinephrine, the drug used to treat anaphylactic shock. You may also want to ask your doctor about allergy shots (p. 619), or *desensitization*.

intolerance (p. 194) is actually not an allergy but an inability to digest milk and other dairy products.

## Testing

If your allergy is bad enough, your doctor will probably need your help in figuring out what you're allergic to. You may be asked to keep a diary of when your symptoms occur, what you eat and your activities. Do you always get a runny nose early in the fall? Ragweed may be the culprit. Do you start sneezing after playing with your neighbor's cat? Blame cat dander.

Skin tests (p. 641), although not 100% reliable, can help identify allergies. Skin patch tests (p. 641) are used to detect allergens in allergic contact dermatitis.

## Treatment

Although there's no cure for allergies, there are plenty of medicines to relieve symptoms. Medicines are available over-the-counter or with a prescription from your doctor. Talk to your doctor about what's right for you.

Most instances of allergic contact dermatitis and allergic rhinitis can be treated by an antihistamine (p. 615). There are more than 100 varieties of this medicine on the market. Unfortunately, many varieties cause drowsiness, but some of the newer products don't have this side effect.

Cromolyn (p. 623) nasal sprays and inhalants help block the chemicals that cause allergic symptoms. Corticosteroid (p. 622) nasal sprays and inhalants relieve inflammation without causing the side effects of oral corticosteroids. Your doctor can help you find the right regimen. Don't rely on over-the-counter decongestant nasal sprays, because using these products for more than a few days can cause a "rebound" effect. A rebound effect makes your symptoms worse than they were in the first place.

If your symptoms are severe, your doctor may recommend oral corticosteroids for a short period. Long-term use can cause a number of side effects.

The best treatment for food and drug allergies is to avoid what causes your allergic symptoms. Anaphylactic shock requires treatment in an emergency room. Don't delay if you suspect this type of reaction.

## Prevention

The tendency to develop allergies is inherited, so there's very little you can do to prevent them. But you can prevent the symptoms by avoiding what you're allergic to as much as possible. See page 144 for tips on how to reduce your exposure to allergens.

*Allergy shots* are an option for many allergy sufferers. Also referred to as *desensitization* or *immunotherapy*, these injections are given regularly and contain a tiny amount of the allergen. The injections help you build up a tolerance to the allergen, which lessens your allergic reaction. The drawbacks of allergy shots are that they may take several years and can be fairly expensive.

Some researchers believe that breast feeding in infancy may help prevent or

---

### Autoimmune Disorders

*Sometimes, the immune system starts attacking the body's own cells. The reasons for this aren't yet understood. Conditions in which the immune system attacks the body's cells are called autoimmune disorders. Some examples of autoimmune disorders are:*

- Insulin-dependent diabetes (p. 211)
- Rheumatoid arthritis (p. 231)
- Systemic lupus erythematosus (p. 252)
- Sjögren's syndrome (p. 250).

Medicines that block the action of the immune system, such as corticosteroids (p. 622), may be used to treat these conditions. Other treatments are available and can be explained to you by your doctor.

reduce the severity of allergies. Most doctors recommend starting babies on solid foods after they're four to six months old, and avoiding common allergens until babies are one year old.

## Cancer and Tumors

- Cough or hoarseness that won't go away
- Trouble swallowing
- Changes in a wart or mole
- Abnormal lump or swelling
- A sore that won't heal
- Any unusual bleeding or discharge
- Change in bowel habits

*Tumors* develop when abnormal cells start to multiply and grow out of control. The immune system can identify and eliminate most abnormal cells, but sometimes the immune system slips up, and a tumor forms.

Tumors may be close enough to the surface of the skin so you can feel them. They feel like a lump, swelling or thickening under the skin. Often, though, tumors are farther inside your body.

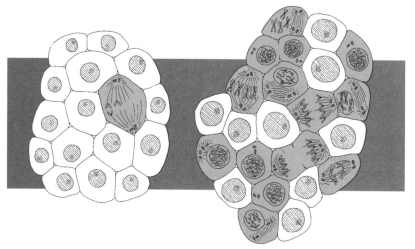

NORMAL VS. CANCER CELLS

Tumors can be either noncancerous (*benign*) or cancerous (*malignant*). How and why cancer occurs isn't yet completely understood. A number of factors seem to be at work. Your genetics, or what genes you've inherited from your parents, play a role. So does your environment. Your health habits and lifestyle are also factors.

While cancer usually begins in a specific area or organ of the body, it can spread, or *metastasize,* to another part of the body. Cancer that spreads is usually much harder to treat. This is why finding cancer early is so important.

Just thinking about cancer, in yourself or someone you know, can be scary. Years ago, some people would even avoid saying the word "cancer." That's because little was known about cancer—about what caused it and how it could be treated and prevented.

Doctors know much more about cancer today. Many cancers are treatable, particularly if they're discovered early. And we're much more aware of how to prevent cancer. Cancer isn't as scary as it used to be. Never let it scare you from seeing your doctor if you have unusual symptoms or notice anything unusual while doing self-exams.

### Types of Cancer

| | |
|---|---|
| Bone (p. 254) | Mouth (p. 100) |
| Brain (p. 47) | Ovarian (p. 416) |
| Breast (p. 408) | Pancreas (p. 217) |
| Cervix (p. 414) | Penis (p. 426) |
| Colorectal (p. 175) | Prostate (p. 428) |
| Eye (p. 75) | Skin (p. 290) |
| Esophagus (p. 184) | Stomach (p. 196) |
| Larynx (p. 105) | Testicle (p. 429) |
| Leukemia (p. 138) | Thyroid (p. 219) |
| Liver (p. 206) | Urinary tract (p. 159) |
| Lung (p. 151) | Uterus (p. 417) |
| Lymphoma (p. 139) | Vulvar (p. 422) |

## Testing

See the box on the next page for some of the tests that can be done to check for cancer. You can do some of these at home. You can help find breast cancer, testicular cancer and skin cancer by

## Exams That Can Detect Cancer

*Many types of cancer can be caught early if you check yourself for early signs. Self-exams can be very important in catching cancer early. Be sure to let your doctor know if you notice anything unusual. Further testing may be needed to check for cancer. Some of the tests that may be used to check for cancer are listed below.*

| Cancer | Exam | Cancer | Exam |
|---|---|---|---|
| Breast cancer | Breast self-exam (p. 408) | Oral cancer | Self-exam of mouth |
| | Doctor exam of breasts | | Exam by doctor |
| | Mammography (p. 638) | Prostate cancer | Rectal exam (p. 633) |
| Cervical cancer | Pap smear (p. 639) | | PSA (p. 640) |
| Colorectal cancer | Rectal exam (p. 633) | Skin cancer | Skin self-exam (p. 291) |
| | Test for blood in stool | | Doctor exam of skin |
| | (fecal occult blood test, p. 635) | Testicular cancer | Testicular self-exam (p. 429) |
| | Sigmoidoscopy (p. 640) | | Doctor exam of testes |
| Lymph node cancer | Self-exam of lymph nodes | Uterine cancer | Endometrial biopsy (p. 634) |
| | Doctor exam and testing | | |
| | if lump is found | | |

doing regular self-exams and reporting anything unusual to your doctor.

If a problem is suspected, tests such as x-rays, CT scans (p. 632), mammography (p. 638) and MRI scans (p. 637) can be used to look for tumors. Other tests are available to identify cancer. Some blood tests can show the growth of the tumor over the course of the disease. Sometimes, a biopsy is done to determine whether cancer is present.

### Treatment

If possible, tumors (especially if they're cancerous) are surgically removed. Radiation therapy or chemotherapy may be used depending on the location of the tumor, the type of cancer and how it has progressed.

Radiation therapy uses strong doses of carefully aimed x-rays to destroy the tumor cells. Sometimes, small radioactive pellets are inserted into the tumor. Radiation can be used alone, or before or after surgery. It can be particularly useful if the cancer hasn't spread to other parts of the body. If the cancer has spread, chemotherapy will probably also be needed.

Chemotherapy uses medicines that kill cancer cells or keep them from multiplying. These medicines may be given in a pill form or intravenously. Several different types of anticancer medicines may be given at the same time.

Unfortunately, radiation treatment and chemotherapy can have side effects, such as hair loss, nausea and vomiting. These side effects occur because the treatments affect the "good" cells as well as the "bad" tumor cells. These side effects usually go away after treatment is complete, and the severity of side effects can usually be controlled.

### Prevention

You can help prevent cancer. One of the main things you can do is not smoke. Smoking is the major cause of lung cancer. See page 31 for tips on quitting if you smoke. Any type of tobacco use is associated with cancer: smoking with lung cancer, and chewing tobacco with cancers of the mouth and throat.

Your diet may also play a role in your risk of cancer. Eat a variety of foods, and try to avoid high-fat foods and foods that are smoked or preserved with nitrites. Instead, focus on eating high-fiber foods, lean meats, grains, and plenty of fruits and vegetables. See page 13 for more information on nutrition.

Also avoid getting too much sun. Sun exposure is tied to skin cancer.

Limit how much alcohol you drink. Alcohol is connected with oral and liver cancer. Smokers who drink alcohol have a higher risk of oral cancers.

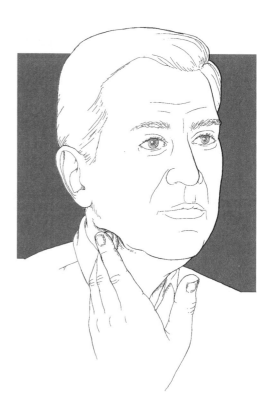

**ADULT CHECKING GLANDS IN THROAT**

## Swelling of the Lymph Nodes of the Neck

* Enlargement of one or more lymph nodes in the neck, often with some tenderness

Have your doctor check right away any lymph node larger than ³/₄ of an inch, a lymph node that keeps growing or a lymph node that's painful, hard or warm. If you're unsure about whether a lymph node is swollen or growing, have it checked by your doctor. There's a small chance it could be a serious problem, such as an *abscess,* or pocket of pus, or cancer.

### Testing and Treatment

If you go to your doctor because of a swollen lymph node, he or she will probably ask when you first noticed the swelling and whether you have other signs of infection. This information will help your doctor determine the severity of the problem. Knowing how your lymph nodes typically react to infection is also helpful, for example, whether you usually have a swollen node in your neck right before you get a cold. After feeling the size of the node and looking for other signs of infection, your doctor may suggest waiting to

see if the node becomes smaller while the infection is being treated.

If an infection isn't apparent, blood tests may show the cause of the enlarged lymph node. Large lymph nodes may need to be drained, tested or removed. X-rays, CT scans (p. 632) or other tests may be done to check the size of other lymph nodes, to identify infections or to look for cancer.

Treatment of the enlarged lymph node depends on the cause. Symptoms of viral infections can be treated with analgesics (p. 614), decongestants (p. 616), cough medicines (p. 616), expectorants (p. 616) and fever-reducing medicines (p. 616). Bacterial infections or fungal infections may be treated with antibiotics (p. 615) or antifungal medicines (p. 615). Abscesses may require drainage. If the enlarged lymph node is caused by cancer, such as leukemia or lymphoma, treatment for cancer will be started.

---

### Causes of Lymph-Node Enlargement

* Viral infections
* Bacterial infections
* Abscess in the lymph node
* Lymphoma (p. 139)
* Leukemia (p. 138)
* Spread of cancer
* Tuberculosis (p. 307)
* AIDS or HIV infection (p. 325)

# CHAPTER 15 BONES, JOINTS AND MUSCLES

The *skeleton* is a lightweight but rugged structure of 206 bones. It's the frame that protects some body parts, such as the heart and lungs. The skeleton provides a supporting structure for other parts of the body, such as the muscles.

*Bones* are made of strong protein strands, or fibers, that hold together a solid mixture of the minerals calcium and phosphorus. The calcium and phosphorus provide hardness and strength. Many bones contain a center cavity filled with *bone marrow.* Bone marrow is where red blood cells (p. 131) are made.

*Joints* occur where one bone meets another bone, such as at the shoulder, elbow, knee and ankle. The ends of the bones, where they join together, are smooth and coated with a slippery, fibrous substance called *cartilage.* Cartilage protects the ends of the bones and helps the joint move smoothly. Each joint is surrounded by a *synovial membrane.* The synovial membrane secretes a sticky fluid, called *synovial fluid,* that lubricates the joint surfaces, also allowing them to move smoothly.

*Ligaments* are tough, fibrous bands that hold joints together and connect bones and cartilage. They allow joint flexibility but also limit movement of the joint to provide stability.

*Tendons* are also fibrous bands of tissue. They're extremely strong. They attach and hold muscles tightly to the bones. Tendons are kept lubricated within a *tendon sheath,* a covering that allows smooth movement of the tendon.

Bones, joints, cartilage, ligaments and tendons are all types of *connective tissue.* As its name suggests, the major function of connective tissue is to connect and support other body tissues. Connective tissue is strong and flexible. It's made up of bundles of different types of protein fibers. *Collagen* is the primary protein in the white fibers of the bones, cartilage, ligaments and tendons.

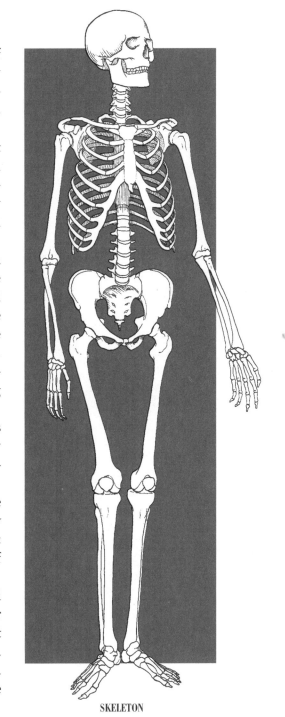

**SKELETON**

*Muscles* give your skeleton its ability to move. Movements of muscles are controlled by the brain and nervous system. The brain and nerves make muscles contract so that movement can occur. The muscle contracts, or shortens, and pulls on a tendon. The tendon then pulls on the bone, raising or lowering it.

*Striated*, or *voluntary*, muscles are under "conscious control," contracting

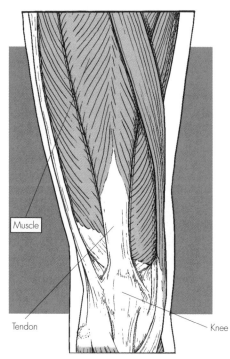

**MUSCLES AND TENDONS**

or relaxing only when you decide to move. Muscles of the skeleton are voluntary muscles. *Smooth*, or *involuntary*, muscles aren't under conscious control. They work automatically. Involuntary muscles are found in the digestive tract, where they control the movement of food through the esophagus, stomach and intestines. They're also present in blood vessels, where they control the flow of blood. Both voluntary and involuntary muscles respond to signals from your nervous system. Involuntary muscles also respond to chemical signals.

A third type of muscle is called *cardiac muscle*, or heart muscle. It makes up most of the heart. Cardiac muscle combines the properties of striated and smooth muscle—it's very strong striated muscle, but its movement can't be controlled in the way that movement of other striated muscles can be controlled whenever you want. Instead, cardiac muscle moves automatically in response to involuntary signals.

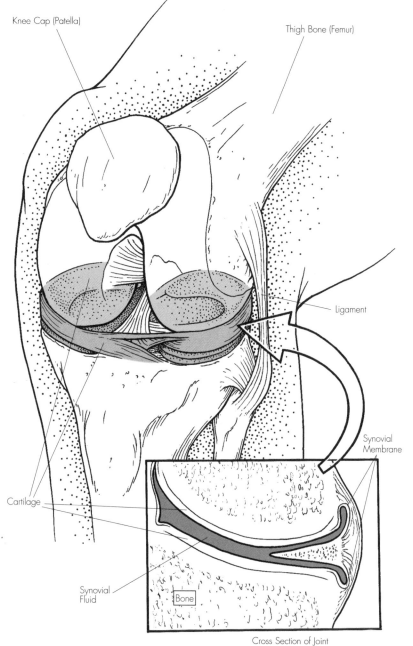

**KNEE JOINT**

## Arthritis

- Pain
- Loss of movement in joints
- Swelling of the joints

*Arthritis* is a type of connective tissue disorder (p. 235). For centuries, people have searched for the cause of arthritis and the means to prevent it. Although research during the past century has provided much information about arthritis, many questions remain unanswered. In most cases, the cause of arthritis is unknown.

Some forms of arthritis develop because of a problem with the immune system, the body's defense against infection. The problem with the immune system makes the body attack its own tissues. This is called an autoimmune disorder (p. 223). For example, if the immune system doesn't recognize the lining of a joint as its own tissue, it sends various cells to destroy the joint lining, causing the pain and swelling of arthritis. The reason for this reaction isn't known. Rheumatic fever (p. 304), which is caused by infection with streptococcal bacteria, can cause an autoimmune reaction. After the infection, the immune system may attack the linings of the joints, as it would the bacteria. As a result, the joints are damaged, sometimes leading to arthritis.

Causes of other forms of arthritis may include bacterial and viral infections, an inherited tendency toward the disease, nutritional deficiencies or being overweight. These are several major forms of arthritis.

**Ankylosing spondylitis.** Ankylosing spondylitis seems to be inherited. It affects men more often than women and sometimes is associated with inflammatory bowel disease (p. 178). The joints of the spine (the *vertebrae*) become painful and stiff. After a time, the vertebrae begin fusing together (*ankylosing*), creating a stiff, stooped posture. Breathing problems and inflammation of the iris are other effects of the disease.

Anti-inflammatory medicines (p. 615) are used to reduce the pain, stiffness and inflammation. Exercises may help slow progression of the disease. Sleeping on a thin mattress on top of a bed board may help maintain as normal a posture as possible.

**Infectious arthritis.** This form of arthritis isn't common, thanks to the use of medicine to treat infections. Infectious arthritis may be caused by the spread of bacteria through the bloodstream from an infection elsewhere in the body or from infection following injury or joint surgery. Lyme disease (p. 301), an infection spread through deer tick bites, can lead to infectious arthritis. Arthritis from Lyme disease most often affects the knee joints.

Bacterial infections of the joints can be serious and require prompt diagnosis and treatment. If a bacterial infection of the joint is suspected, some of the fluid may be removed from the joint with a needle and syringe. The fluid can then be examined with a microscope to identify the responsible bacteria.

When a bacterial infection is present, your doctor may prescribe an antibiotic (p. 615) to fight the infection. When the results of the fluid exam become available, the dose may be changed or a different medicine may be prescribed. Treatment usually lasts for three to four weeks. During this time, your doctor may prescribe exercises to help you recover full movement of the joint as it heals. In some cases, your doctor may need to drain the affected joint and remove any damaged or infected tissue.

**Juvenile rheumatoid arthritis.** Juvenile rheumatoid arthritis affects

---

### When should I see my doctor about joint aches?

- If your joints are red, swollen or warm.
- If only one joint is tender.
- If you have early morning joint stiffness.
- If joint stiffness and discomfort don't get better with over-the-counter analgesic medicines.
- If you have a family history of arthritis and your joints ache or are stiff.
- If you have a fever or rash along with joint swelling.

## Home Treatments for Mild Arthritis

- Over-the-counter anti-inflammatory medicines
- Moist heat—such as a damp warm towel—applied to the stiff joints
- Mild exercise of the affected joints, especially in a pool
- Massage of the tender joints

children, but it is rare and can be quite different from the adult form. In addition to a type of juvenile rheumatoid arthritis that resembles adult rheumatoid arthritis, there's a form in which one or only a few of the larger joints are mildly affected and eye inflammation occurs. There's another form in which the whole body is involved. The type that affects the whole body occurs along with a rash and fever.

Juvenile rheumatoid arthritis can fade as the child grows, but some children continue to have the disease as adults. The more severe it is in childhood, the more likely it will continue into adulthood.

Testing and treatment are similar to that for the adult disease. Splints may help you rest the joint. Physical therapy may be needed in severe cases. It's important to do the physical therapy exercises regularly to avoid long-term crippling effects. Surgical replacement of joints is an option after growth has stopped and when the disease is so severe that it destroys the joints or causes severe pain. Because juvenile rheumatoid arthritis may also lead to inflammation of part of the eye, including the iris, that may lead to partial or complete blindness, regular eye exams should be done during the first few years of the disease.

**Osteoarthritis.** Osteoarthritis is the most common form of arthritis in older people. Symptoms range from mild pain and stiffness to severe, disabling pain. In the beginning, the pain usually occurs after use of the joint and goes away when you rest. If the disease progresses, you may have joint pain even when you're resting.

Although osteoarthritis can affect almost any joint in your body, it most often affects finger and weight-bearing joints, such as the hips, knees and

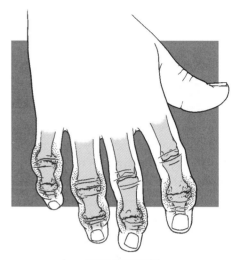

**OSTEOARTHRITIS**

ankles. Some people who have had a joint injury develop osteoarthritis in the damaged joint years after the injury. In addition to normal wear-and-tear or unusual trauma to joints, heredity seems to play a part in the development of the disease. Osteoarthritis, especially in the hips and fingers, tends to run in families. Being overweight may also bring on osteoarthritis, probably because the excess weight puts more stress on the joints, especially the knees.

Treatment for osteoarthritis is aimed at relieving pain. If you have signs of osteoarthritis on an x-ray or physical exam but you aren't in any pain, your doctor probably won't prescribe any treatment. Exercises to strengthen the area around joints and to maintain a normal range of motion can reduce symptoms. Simple lifestyle changes, such as changing your sleeping position or the way you carry heavy items may also help minimize symptoms. When the osteoarthritis is more severe, you may need to use a cane or walker.

If you need treatment for pain, your doctor will probably advise you to take nonsteroidal anti-inflammatory drugs (NSAIDs, p. 617). Acetaminophen (p. 614) may also be useful. Resting the affected joints, soaking in a warm bath or using a heating pad may also help.

In more severe cases of osteo-arthritis, treatment may include oral corticosteroids (p. 622) or injections of a corticosteroid, such as cortisone (p. 623), directly into the joint. But corticosteroid injections can only be used a few times a year for weight-bearing joints. The last line of treatment is joint replacement surgery for severely diseased joints. This surgery has a good success rate.

**Reiter's syndrome.** Reiter's syndrome is a form of arthritis found mainly in men. It results from an abnormal response to a variety of infections, especially urethritis due to chlamydia, which can be transmitted by sexual contact. Symptoms appear over several weeks and may include pain in the joints (especially the ankles, feet and fingers), sores on the palms of your hands and soles of your feet, and conjunctivitis (p. 71). Treatment may include antibiotics for the infection and NSAIDs or other analgesic medicines (p. 614) for the pain and swelling of the joints. The symptoms of arthritis often last after the other symptoms go away, and can continue off and on for a number of years.

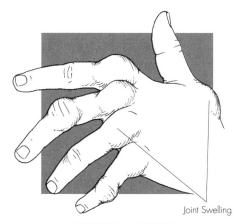

Joint Swelling

**RHEUMATOID ARTHRITIS**

**Rheumatoid arthritis.** This type of arthritis is less common than osteo-arthritis, but can be far more severe.

The cause of rheumatoid arthritis is unknown, but it's believed to be an autoimmune disorder. Rheumatoid arthritis tends to run in families.

Mild forms of rheumatoid arthritis are more common than severe forms. Severe cases can result in extreme disability, since rheumatoid arthritis is a progressive disease that has no cure. It affects women more often than men and adults more often than children. Rheumatoid arthritis often starts with swollen, red, stiff and tender finger joints in both hands or feet.

The disease usually develops in the smaller joints, but the elbows, wrists, knees and ankles can also be affected. Most often there is symmetry—the same joint is affected on both sides of the body. As opposed to the pain of osteoarthritis, pain from rheumatoid arthritis occurs during rest as well as during movement. Joint stiffness in the morning is common. The disease isn't limited to the joints. It can affect the entire body and cause general fatigue and problems in other body parts, such as the heart, kidneys and eyes.

Your doctor may diagnose rheumatoid arthritis after a physical exam. Other tests that may be helpful include x-rays of the painful joints and a blood test called the erythrocyte sedimentation rate (p. 634).

Treatment for rheumatoid arthritis may begin with high doses of aspirin, combined with exercises to maintain joint range of motion. If aspirin upsets your stomach, you may be given a medicine that'll relieve that side effect. NSAIDs may be used. Your doctor may prescribe gold salts (p. 620), penicillamine (p. 620) or, in more severe cases, a corticosteroid such as prednisone (p. 620). Corticosteroids may be injected directly into a joint up to three times a year.

*Home Remedies for Backaches*

- Lie on your back with your head on a pillow and another pillow under your knees.
- Use heat or ice packs on the tender area. (If you use heat, be careful not to burn yourself. Wrap a hot water bottle in a cloth or set your heating pad on low.)
- Massage the sore, spastic muscles.
- Gently stretch the muscles in the sore area.
- Use an analgesic medicine.
- Improve your posture when standing or sitting, especially in the car or at work.

These medicines may cause significant side effects, so anyone taking them must be checked regularly by a doctor. Another option for severe cases is use of a medicine that suppresses the immune system, such as methotrexate (p. 620). But this can leave the body susceptible to other infections.

## Back Pain

- Pain in the lower or upper back
- Aching, or sharp, shooting pains in the back
- Stiffness or loss of normal flexibility in the back
- Pain, numbness and tingling in the arms and hands
- Weakness in the legs, possibly with some numbness or tingling

Overuse of the back muscles at work, at home or during recreation is the usual source of spasms, aches and pain in the back. The muscles and ligaments of the lower spine and pelvis may be particularly susceptible to overuse. Overuse can be considered the cause of back pain if the pain begins within 24 hours after excessive use of the back. Poor posture at work, while watching TV or even during sleep may also bring on an episode of achy stiffness or muscle spasms.

Other problems can also cause back pain. Viral illnesses can cause tender areas in the neck or back. A herniated disk (p. 238), spinal cord tumors (p. 58), compression fractures of the spine (p. 234), and damage to muscles, ligaments or nerves after an injury can all put pressure on these nerves. Other serious causes of pain in the back include spinal cord trauma (p. 58).

### Testing and Treatment

If your doctor thinks your symptoms are due to overused muscles, home treatments will usually help relieve the

spasms and pain. Anti-inflammatory medicines (p. 615) may help reduce swelling and pain. If those medicines upset your stomach, acetaminophen (p. 614) may be helpful for pain relief.

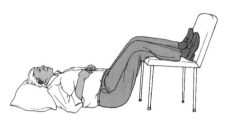

**EASING BACK PAIN: POSITION 1**

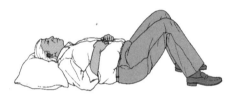

**POSITION 2**

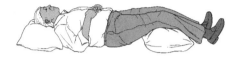

**POSITION 3**

If the pain is in your lower back, resting in bed with one pillow under your head and another under your knees may also help. You may also try lying on your back on the floor with pillows under your knees, with your hips and knees bent and your feet on a chair, or just with your hips and knees bent. This helps relieve the pressure on your back. While resting for one or two days may be helpful for an injured back, resting longer than two days can weaken your muscles and slow down your recovery. This is why it's important to try to walk a few minutes every few hours during your recovery.

You may also try ice packs (p. 243) for a few days and then a heating pad alternated with ice. To relax a spasm, gently stretch or massage the tender muscle.

When the pain is more severe or long-lasting, your doctor may prescribe stronger analgesic medicines (p. 618) or muscle relaxants (p. 625) to reduce spasms. Your doctor may also refer you to a physical therapist for further treatment.

If your doctor suspects a more serious cause for your back pain, he or she may order x-rays, a CT scan (p. 632), a MRI scan (p. 637) or sometimes a myelogram (p. 638) to diagnose the problem. If a pinched nerve is responsible, treatment includes bed rest and medicines taken orally or by injection for pain and swelling.

Sometimes *traction* or surgery is needed, depending on the cause of the pain. Traction involves putting the area under tension using a system of pulleys and weights. If surgery is needed, the surgeon will remove the structure that's pinching the nerve and then *fuse,* or join together, the vertebrae for stability.

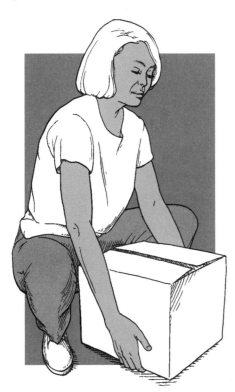

**PROPER LIFTING TECHNIQUE**

### Prevention

To help prevent back pain, learn proper techniques for lifting. Avoid lifting with a bent back. Instead, lift with your legs by bending your knees and squatting, keeping your back straight. Don't strain to reach for heavy objects. Push rather than pull when you must move something heavy.

Also, try to improve your posture when you stand, sit or work. When standing, keep your ears, shoulders and hips in a straight line, with your head up and your stomach pulled in. Use straight-backed chairs or chairs with low back support. Sit with your knees a little higher than your hips. Take frequent breaks from sitting or driving to stretch.

If you have low back pain, sleep on your side with your knees bent. Put a pillow between your knees. If you sleep on your back, put pillows under your knees and a small pillow under your lower back if you have low back pain. Avoid sleeping on your stomach unless you put a pillow under your hips.

Exercise on a regular basis to keep your back and stomach muscles in shape, which will help flatten the curve of the lower back. Your exercise plan should include regular back- and stomach-strengthening and back flexibility exercises to maintain good muscle tone. This helps reduce the number and the severity of repeated back pain episodes. Not all exercises are helpful for everyone, and some may be harmful. So be sure to talk to your doctor first for information about what exercises may be helpful for you.

## Bursitis

- Pain with motion, sometimes with redness and swelling over the joint

A *bursa* is the slippery, flat sac located over some joints. A bursa helps muscles and tendons glide over bones. When the bursa becomes irritated, it fills with fluid and becomes inflamed and painful. This is called *bursitis.*

---

### *Symptoms Requiring Medical Attention Right Away*

- Severe pain that leaves you unable to move
- Pain or numbness that travels from the back down to the knee or ankle
- Extremely intense pain that travels down an arm or leg, especially after sneezing or coughing
- A backache or neckache combined with weakness in a leg or arm
- A stiff neck combined with fever, headache and vomiting
- Sensitive eyes that hurt in response to normal light
- Inability to control bladder or bowels

The most common location of bursitis is the shoulder. Activities such as throwing, swinging or pushing may cause irritation of the bursa, resulting in pain with motion. Bursitis of elbow, knee and other joints may also develop.

A common condition is *housemaid's knee,* in which excessive kneeling irritates the bursa in front of the knee cap. Another problem, called *weaver's bottom,* involves inflammation of the bursa of the hip. It sometimes affects people whose work requires them to sit for long periods of time. Some episodes of bursitis are caused by an arthritis-like process or infection.

### Testing and Treatment

Your doctor will examine the sore area to find where it's tender or to determine if fluid has collected in the bursa. Rarely, your doctor may use a needle to get a sample of the fluid and check for infection.

Anti-inflammatory medicines (p. 615) and rest may be enough to treat a mild case of bursitis. Injections of corticosteroids (p. 622) into the bursa may offer more immediate relief, especially for more persistent episodes. Surgical removal of the bursa is reserved for cases that don't respond to oral or injectable medicines.

### Prevention

If you're starting a new activity, such as playing in a summer softball league, where you'll be using a particular joint often, start with a low level of activity and increase slowly to prevent overuse. If your activity involves kneeling or makes you susceptible to bumping your knees or elbows, such as skateboarding or roller-skating, wear protective pads.

## Compression Fracture of the Spine

- Intense back pain, sometimes extending into the arms, legs or buttocks

*Compression fractures* occur when a vertebra collapses, or *fractures.* Most compression fractures of the spine result from osteoporosis (p. 244) in elderly women. Bones weakened by osteoporosis are more likely to collapse when they're jarred from a fall or squeezed together during a movement of the spine.

Compression fractures of the spine can cause severe pain. If nerves are pinched between the collapsed vertebrae, the pain can spread from the back around to the front of the chest or abdomen. Because even minor stress on the back can cause compression fractures, most elderly adults are surprised to learn they've fractured a bone when they seek medical attention for back pain.

Compression fractures can occur with prolonged use of steroid medicines and prolonged inactivity due to an injury or other disease, both of which can reduce the calcium in bone. Cushing's syndrome (p. 210) can also lead to compression fractures. In Cushing's syndrome, the body's own steroid hormones are produced in excessive amounts by the adrenal gland.

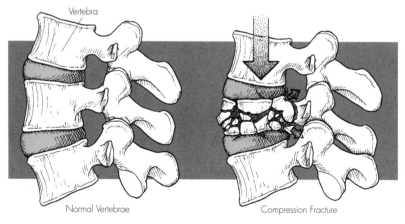

Vertebra

Normal Vertebrae

Compression Fracture

**COMPRESSION FRACTURE**

## Connective Tissue Disorders

The connective tissue is a network of tissue that supports and joins other body tissues and parts. Bones, joints, cartilage, ligaments and tendons are types of connective tissue. With connective tissue disorders, the tissue becomes inflamed. Connective tissue is rich in *collagen*, a fibrous protein found in your skin, bones, ligaments and cartilage. That's why these conditions are also called *collagen diseases*. But the characteristic common to all is inflammation of the connective tissue. Connective tissue disorders include arthritis (p. 299), polymyalgia rheumatica (p. 246), polymyositis (p. 246), scleroderma (p. 248), Sjögren's syndrome (p. 250) and systemic lupus erythematosus (p. 252).

### Testing and Treatment

An x-ray of the spine usually reveals the compression fracture.

Treatment depends on the amount of pain. Severe pain may require bed rest, injected pain medicine, heat, muscle relaxants (p. 625) and other supportive treatments. A back brace may be worn to limit movement of the spine so the fracture can heal. Sometimes, hospitalization and intravenous pain medicine may be needed. Minor pain may be relieved with rest, heat and analgesic medicines (p. 614). Pain usually improves over a period of weeks to months, but doesn't always go away completely.

### Prevention

Women at high risk for osteoporosis are also at a high risk for compression fractures of the spine. The best way to prevent compression fractures is to keep your bones healthy and strong. See page 245 for information on how to prevent osteoporosis.

## Dislocated Joint

- After an injury, a joint that's out of place, painful, difficult or impossible to move

Almost any bone can be pulled or knocked from its joint if enough force is applied. If a basketball player is hit on the end of the finger with a ball, the joint may "pop out of place." A football player may get hit on the arm while throwing the ball, and the force of the blow may dislocate the shoulder joint.

Dislocation usually affects joints that move, such as the ankles, knees, hips, wrists, elbows and, most commonly, the shoulders and fingers. Nonmobile joints, such as in the pelvis, can also be "separated" when a ligament that holds the joint together is stretched or torn.

Dislocation of a vertebra can be life-threatening if it damages nerves or the spinal cord. Dislocation of a vertebra sometimes occurs in spinal cord trauma (p. 605), which can cause paralysis.

### Testing and Treatment

After examining the affected joint, your doctor will order x-rays to rule out fractures or other damage that might have occurred with the dislocation. If a finger or shoulder joint is out of place, your doctor may be able to reposition it with simple motions. The larger the joint, however, the harder it is to stretch and relax the muscles so the joint can be put into place.

Treatment includes use of a splint or brace so the joint can't be moved. Putting an ice pack on the area and taking analgesic medicines (p. 614) may also be helpful. Surgery may be needed if the joint can't be repositioned because of a fracture, cartilage tear or other problem.

## Fasciitis

- Pain in affected area
- Swelling of the skin
- Redness over the painful area
- Weakness in affected area

The muscles and bones are supported and enclosed by thick sheets of fibrous tissues called *fascia*. These tough tissues surround groups of muscles, divide organs or muscles, and give strength to the deeper layers of the skin. *Fasciitis* occurs when the fascia become irritated. This can occur if the tissues inside the fascia, such as the muscles, swell. The tough, fibrous fascia surrounding the tissue doesn't stretch or expand as the contents swell. This results in pressure inside the compartment, which reduces the blood supply to the tissue and hinders its ability to heal itself. If the pressure keeps building, the tissues will eventually die from lack of oxygen and blood supply. When this is due to an autoimmune-like disorder, similar to scleroderma (p. 248), it's called *eosinophilic fasciitis.*

Symptoms usually come on slowly and result in limited movement of the limbs.

### Testing and Treatment

Your doctor will probably perform a physical exam. Blood tests may be done. If an area of the arm or leg is swollen or becomes weak or numb, the pressure of the area may be checked with a special device, and the need for surgery may be evaluated.

Fasciitis is usually treated with prednisone (p. 620) or other medicines. It will usually go away in time.

## Fibromyalgia

- Aches
- Pain
- Stiffness
- Fatigue
- Tender points on the body

*Fibromyalgia,* sometimes referred to as *fibrositis* or *fibromyositis,* is the name given a poorly understood set of symptoms. Fibromyalgia affects muscles, joints and other soft tissues. The cause is unknown, and no blood or tissue test has been developed to prove its presence. The disease is diagnosed by its symptoms—and the lack of any other disease. If affects women more than men.

Symptoms include aches in the neck, upper shoulders and back, along with fatigue and headaches. The muscles are most tender where they attach to the bone or where a ligament holds the muscle close to the bone. These areas are called "trigger points." They may be tender even to a light touch. Because of the pain, lack of sleep may become a problem, especially if you're experiencing emotional stress.

### Testing and Treatment

Pain at typical trigger points usually confirms the diagnosis of fibromyalgia. Because other, more serious, arthritis conditions have symptoms similar to fibromyalgia, your doctor will do several tests to exclude them. Exercise, a balanced diet and adequate rest are important. Because stress may increase symptoms, people with fibromyalgia should use relaxation exercises (p. 572) and other stress management techniques to relieve stress. Over-the-counter medicines, such as aspirin or ibuprofen, often have no effect. Small doses of antidepressant medicines (p. 619) are often effective in relieving the symptoms.

## Fracture

- After injury, pain in a leg or arm, sometimes with an open wound and exposed bone

Bones can be broken, or *fractured*, in many ways, including from strong blows to a bone or twisting or bending of the bone. Types of breaks, or *fractures*, include the following:

**Comminuted fracture.** This involves several breaks in the bone, creating numerous bone fragments.

**Compound fracture.** A broken bone that punctures the skin.

**Displaced fracture.** The break separates the bone so that the two pieces aren't lying next to each other.

**Greenstick fracture.** The bone is broken only on one side (the break doesn't go all the way through the bone).

**Oblique fracture.** A break that occurs at an angle.

**Simple fracture.** A broken bone that hasn't separated; the two broken ends are still next to each other.

**Spiral fracture.** The bone has been twisted, resulting in a spiral-shaped break.

**Stress fracture.** A break caused by repeated, long-term stress to the bone, primarily those in the feet.

**Transverse fracture.** This break goes straight through the bone (no angle).

The seriousness of a fracture depends on several factors: its location, other damage caused by the accident (such as torn ligaments), movement of the two broken ends (whether it's a simple or displaced fracture), and involvement of other vital structures (such as a nerve or the lung). If the skin is broken, as in a compound fracture, infection becomes a serious risk as well.

**Testing and Treatment**

During the exam, you'll need to give your doctor a detailed history of the accident. Knowing how the limb was stressed will help your doctor assess the possibilities of other damage.

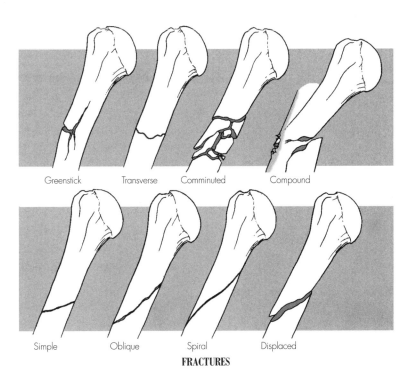

Greenstick    Transverse    Comminuted    Compound

Simple    Oblique    Spiral    Displaced

**FRACTURES**

X-rays of the injured area will be taken to identify the fracture.

If the break is a simple fracture, the injured limb will be placed in a splint or cast to help it heal. Stress fractures of the feet may be treated with a special type of shoe. With a displaced or compound fracture, surgery may be needed to place the two bone ends next to each other or to place a metal screw, pin or a plate into the bone to hold the broken bone in place.

The limb may be placed in *traction*, during which the affected area is put under tension using a system of weights and pulleys to hold the fractured bone in place or to bring displaced parts of the bone together. In the elderly, severe fracture damage to the hip or knee may require replacement of the joint with an artificial joint.

You may be given analgesic medicines (p. 614) to relieve pain and antibiotics (p. 615) to treat any possible infection. After a cast or splint is removed, your doctor may recommend physical therapy to strengthen the affected area.

It usually takes about four to 12 weeks for a broken bone to heal, depending on the type of fracture, the cause and your age.

## Gout

- Severe pain and swelling in joints, usually one joint at a time

The kidneys usually filter and excrete *uric acid*, one of the body's wastes, in the urine. But the body may make excess uric acid or the kidneys may become overwhelmed and not get rid of enough uric acid, so that crystals of uric acid form in the joints. This is *gout*.

The accumulation of these crystals causes severe pain and swelling, usually in one joint at a time. The big toe joints are often affected. But gout can occur in an ankle, knee, elbow, wrist or finger.

Gout is most common in older men and may be associated with the use of thiazide diuretics (p. 623), a type of medicine often used in the treatment of high blood pressure. Rich foods and alcohol may contribute to the rise in uric acid and, therefore, symptoms.

Gout attacks usually occur over a 12- to 24-hour period and, left untreated, may last as long as two weeks. After the attack, the joint may look and feel perfectly normal.

### Testing and Treatment

Your doctor may diagnose gout based on an exam of the inflamed joint, blood tests to check the level of uric acid, x-rays and, if needed, an exam of joint fluid removed with a needle and syringe.

If the arthritic symptoms improve after treatment with an antigout medicine (p. 619) called colchicine, the arthritis is almost certainly gout. If colchicine is used, your doctor will give it to you for only a short time because it can cause severe side effects

in the digestive system. Antirheumatic medicines (p. 620) are used more commonly than colchicine to help reduce the swelling and pain of a gout attack.

After the attack has subsided, future attacks may be prevented with long-term treatment with medicine such as allopurinol (p. 619), which reduces the amount of uric acid produced by the body. Drink lots of water, avoid alcoholic beverages and reduce rich food intake to help control a build-up of uric acid.

## Herniated Disk

- Pain and numbness in an arm, hand or leg
- Pain that travels into the buttocks or down the leg
- Shooting pain down the leg that worsens with coughing or sneezing

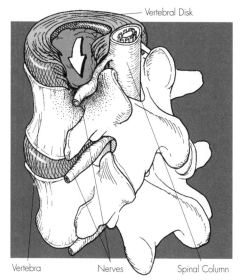

Vertebral Disk

Vertebra        Nerves        Spinal Column

**HERNIATED DISK**

Disks of cartilage are located between the bones of the spinal column (the *vertebrae*). These disks have a soft, rubbery core and a tougher, donut-shaped outer ring. The disks act as shock absorbers and allow the spinal column to bend in all directions.

If a disk has enough pressure placed on it or has a defect, it may *herniate*. This means the soft core is squeezed out and pushes against a nerve or the spinal cord. The pressure on the nerve leads to pain, numbness and weakness. Because the nerves extend to many areas of the body, the pain can travel to the neck, upper arm, hand, chest, abdomen, buttock or leg, depending on the location of the herniated disk.

A herniated disk, sometimes called a "slipped" disk, usually results from an injury or stress in the neck or back. People often suffer this kind of injury when they move heavy furniture or appliances.

### Testing

First, your doctor will probably examine your back and legs and test for strength and numbness. Then, he or she may order an x-ray of the back. In addition, tests such as a CT scan (p. 632) or MRI scan (p. 637) may be done to provide a more detailed picture of the disk. If surgery is necessary, a myelogram (p. 638) may be performed to show the exact location of the damaged disk. A myelogram is an x-ray taken after dye has been injected into the spinal column.

### Treatment

Usually, treatment of a herniated disk consists of bed rest until the pain has decreased (usually in two to three days). Prolonged bed rest isn't recommended. Analgesic (p. 614) and antiinflammatory (p. 615) medicines, heat, ice packs (p. 243), muscle relaxants (p. 625) and sometimes traction may be used. Ideally, the central portion of the disk will slip back into place. After the pain has improved, activity can be increased and exercises to strengthen the back and stomach muscles can be

started. Strengthening the back and stomach muscles helps hold the disks of the spine in place.

Most people improve without surgery. If improvement doesn't occur, surgery may be done to remove part or all of the herniated material or part or all of the disk.

### Prevention

Proper lifting is essential in preventing many injuries that lead to herniated disks. In addition, activity such as walking and certain toning exercises to strengthen the stomach muscles and the muscles that support the back are an important part of preventing a herniated disk.

## Hip Problems in Children

- Limping
- Knee pain, including swelling
- Difficulty flexing the leg

The hip joint is the largest joint in your body. It's a ball-and-socket type of joint. This means you can move it in every direction, unlike the knee, for example, in which the hinge-like joint allows motion only in two directions. The hip joint is made up of the rounded head of the thigh bone, or *femur*,

### *Could you have a "slipped" disk?*

- Do you have severe pain in your lower back?
- Does the pain travel down your leg past your knee?
- Do you feel shooting pain down your leg when you cough or sneeze?
- Do you have numbness or weakness in a leg or arm?
- Have you noticed any changes in your ability to hold your bowels or bladder?

*If you answered yes to two or more of the above questions, you may have a herniated, or "slipped," disk. See your doctor right away.*

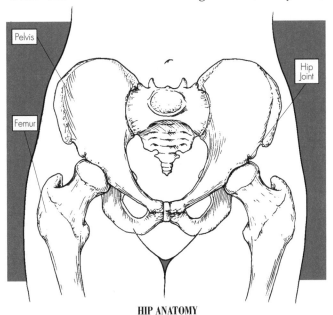

Pelvis

Femur

Hip Joint

**HIP ANATOMY**

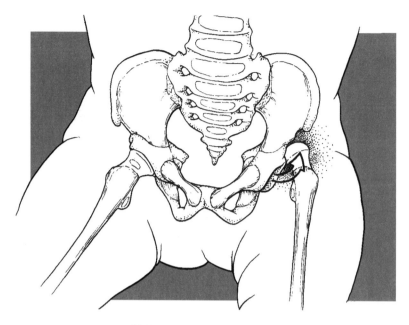

**CONGENITAL HIP DISLOCATION**

which fits into the cup-shaped socket of the hip bone, or *pelvis.*

**Congenital dislocation of the hip.** The top of the largest bone in the leg, the femur, fits into the socket of the hip much like a ball would fit in a cup. In some children, the ball is positioned partly or completely outside of the socket. This placement outside the socket is called *congenital hip dislocation.*

In a simple test performed during the baby's first exam in the hospital, your baby's doctor will listen and feel for a "click" when the baby's hips are moved. The doctor may order x-rays of the hips if he or she thinks that your baby's hip is dislocated.

Early treatment of hip dislocation helps the hip joint to develop normally. It's important to treat this problem before your child begins walking or your child will most likely walk with a limp.

**Legg-Calvé-Perthes disease.** This disease usually occurs in children between the ages of three and 10. The blood supply to the femur is reduced, causing the bone to collapse. A child with this disorder usually will limp and complain of knee pain.

X-rays may not show the changes in the bone, so your doctor must perform a careful physical exam and other tests to make the diagnosis.

Treatment may include having the child stay in bed to avoid stressing the hip joint or using crutches so the hip bears only partial weight. Many cases heal in two years or more without causing damage. Some children with chronic pain in the hip joint require surgery, or they may require hip replacement when they become adults or reach maturity.

**Slipped capital femoral epiphysis.** This condition generally occurs between ages 10 to 17. It's much more common in boys than in girls. The femur can slip out of the hip socket by itself or as a result of an accident. Damage can also occur to the growth plate of the bone, which is the area at the end of the bone where bone growth occurs. This may happen slowly, over weeks or months, or after a hip injury. Symptoms include a limp, combined with knee pain and difficulty moving the hip.

A physical exam and x-rays of the hip area usually provide information needed for a diagnosis. A sudden slip of the upper thigh bone should be treated immediately by your doctor. He or she will take steps to stop the movement of the affected hip. Pins may need to be inserted into the joint to prevent future displacement. With treatment, the hip may heal. But permanent damage of the joint cartilage can result if the hip doesn't heal properly. This can cause osteoarthritis (p. 230) and possibly require that the femur and pelvis be fused together.

## Knee Problems

- Pain, tenderness and swelling of the knee
- Bruising of the knee
- Trouble walking

Your knee joints are second only to your hip in size. But your knees are hinge-like joints, unlike your hips, which are ball-and-socket type of joints. Knee joints have cartilage inside them and ligaments inside and outside the joint that keep the joint from moving from side to side. The outside of the joint is bound by many ligaments, including the patellar ligament, the tibial collateral ligament, the fibular collateral ligament and the tibiofibular ligament. Inside, the cruciate ligaments join the femur to the tibia. Two oval-shaped pads of cartilage, called the *menisci,* cushion the shocks of walking and running, and help reduce friction of the bones.

Most knee problems result from injuries that occur in contact sports such as football. Hitting or twisting the knee can stretch or tear one or more of the ligaments or the cartilage within the joint. Pain, swelling, bruising, locked movement and inability to walk may occur with a knee injury.

A fairly common overuse syndrome is called *jumper's knee.* It's caused by overuse of the tendon just below the kneecap (which attaches the quadriceps muscle to the patella) and produces inflammation and pain. It often occurs in jumping sports. It's also called *patellar tendonitis.*

Many other injuries that can occur to the knee include a tear of the meniscus, usually caused by a twisting injury with the knee slightly bent. The patella can also be fractured, usually by a direct blow to the front of the knee.

A knee problem that may occur in adolescents is called *Osgood-Schlatter disease.* It's related to overextending the knee. The growth plate, also called the *epiphysis,* is the area at the end of the bone where bone growth

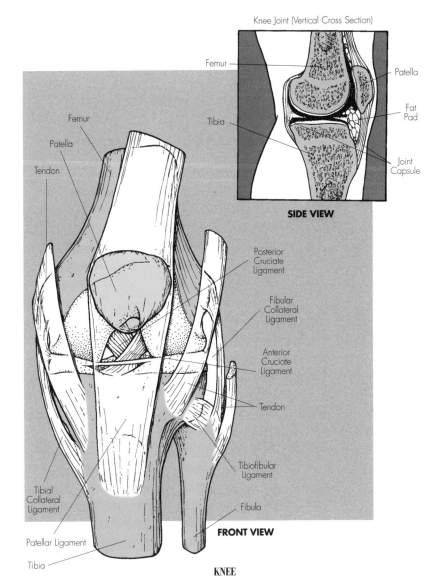

Knee Joint (Vertical Cross Section)

Femur

Patella

Tibia

Fat Pad

Joint Capsule

**SIDE VIEW**

Femur

Patella

Tendon

Posterior Cruciate Ligament

Fibular Collateral Ligament

Anterior Cruciate Ligament

Tendon

Tibiofibular Ligament

Tibial Collateral Ligament

Fibula

**FRONT VIEW**

Patellar Ligament

Tibia

**KNEE**

occurs. In Osgood-Schlatter disease, the growth plates in the top and front of the *tibia,* the larger of the two lower leg bones, don't grow together properly, causing pain and swelling under the knee. This also can affect the tendon of the knee cap, which attaches to this part of the growth plate.

**Testing**

If your knee pain is due to an injury, your doctor generally will make the diagnosis based on what you tell him or her about the injury, a physical exam and x-rays. Resting the leg for a few weeks usually brings relief of symptoms, but the problem can come back when physical activity, such as climbing stairs, is resumed.

In Osgood-Schlatter disease, your doctor will find a tenderness below the kneecap and will probably order x-rays to rule out any other skeletal problems.

### Treatment

Rest, ice and wrapping the knee in an elastic bandage are the first steps of treatment of a knee injury. Taking anti-inflammatory medicine (p. 615) may help the tendons and ligaments heal. A rigid support or hinged brace may be needed. Strengthening exercises may prevent another injury. Surgery, usually through an arthroscope (p. 628), may be needed to repair the damaged ligaments, tendons and cartilage so the chances of complete joint movement are improved. In some people, part of the cartilage has to be removed.

Osgood-Schlatter disease is usually outgrown and responds to treatment of the symptoms with analgesic medicines (p. 614), anti-inflammatory medicines and rest. Osgood-Schlatter disease may require splinting or casting if less aggressive measures fail. Surgery is rarely required. If healing isn't complete, the disorder may flare up in adulthood.

## Muscle Cramps, Pulls, Spasms and Tears

- Pain, swelling or bruising in a muscle after an injury
- Sharp, shooting pains

Muscles consist of many cells that can shorten, or *contract*, to move different parts of the body. A muscle can become overworked, strained or stretched beyond its elastic ability, producing a *pull* or *tear*. Weekend activities, such as fixing something at home or recreational sports, may cause strained, sore muscles on Monday mornings.

As with all injuries, the amount of damage depends on the degree of the injury and the force that caused it. Minor muscle pulls cause minimal swelling or tenderness. But a major tear of the muscle can produce bruising, swelling, extreme pain and the inability to move the affected part of the body. A direct blow to a muscle can cause bleeding within the deeper tissues, a *deep-muscle bruise*. Chronic pain and calcium deposits, called *calcification*, within the muscle may be consequences of a serious tear or deep bruise.

Muscle strain or injury can also bring on a muscle *spasm*, or *cramp*, when the muscle suddenly contracts on its own and stays tight. This can produce sharp, shooting pains that travel from the affected muscle. Muscle spasms often occur in the back, but may occur anywhere in the body, such as in the calf muscles. Spasms in the chest or shoulder muscles can cause stabbing-like pain around the chest or a feeling of pressure and pain similar to that of a heart attack.

### Testing and Treatment

Tell your doctor about the cause of the injury to help him or her make the diagnosis. A thorough exam will be done. For spasms occurring in the chest muscles, a chest x-ray (p. 631) may be needed to make sure the pain isn't due to lung damage, rib fractures or a collapsed lung (p. 146). If you have shortness of breath, severe chest pain, bluish lips or a gurgling sensation in the lung area, see your doctor right away. It could be a sign of a more serious chest injury.

First aid for pulled or torn muscles can be easily recalled if you remember the following formula: R-I-C-E (Rest,

Ice, Compression and Elevation). As soon as the injury occurs, stop the activity. Continued exercise forces more blood to the injured area. Next, apply an ice pack or ice wrapped in a towel to the area to keep swelling down. Keep the ice in place for at least 15 minutes and then alternate 10 minutes with the ice off and 10 minutes with it on.

Compression of the injured area using an elastic bandage keeps excess fluid from accumulating. But the bandage shouldn't be too tight, because it can interfere with blood flow. To make sure this doesn't happen, you should be able to put one or two fingers under the wrap without too much trouble. Finally, elevate the limb above the rest of the body. This also helps cut down on fluid buildup at the site of injury.

Over-the-counter analgesic medicines (p. 614) usually provide adequate pain relief. Continue to rest the injured area and apply ice for the first two to three days. You may then apply heat alternating with ice and slowly begin using the muscle again.

For a severe tear or a deep-muscle bruise, weeks or months of healing will be required. For torn or ruptured tendons, surgery may be necessary to reattach the tendon and regain function of the muscle.

If you have a cramped muscle, try to stretch the area. For example, if a calf muscle is cramped, sit down, straighten your leg, grab your toes and pull your foot in toward your body. This almost always causes the calf muscle to loosen up. Massage helps further relax the muscle. Heat also relaxes muscles in spasm.

### Prevention

Stretching and gentle warm-up exercises before a workout help prevent muscle pulls and strains. Avoid overstraining the muscles with too much activity too soon. Instead slowly build up your muscles' tolerance for each new physical activity. Include a cool-down period each time you exercise. Be sure to wear proper padding for contact sports to prevent direct blows to the muscles.

## Neck Pain

- Aching, or sharp, shooting pains in the neck
- Stiffness or loss of normal flexibility in the neck
- Pain, numbness and tingling in the arms and hands

Neck pain and back pain (p. 232) often have similar causes, including overuse of the muscles. Poor posture is a common cause of neck pain. Other problems that can cause neck pain include viral illnesses, such as meningitis (p. 302), and osteoarthritis of the neck, which can lead to bony growths or spurs. Whiplash (p. 254) can cause severe neck pain by pinching nerves of the spinal cord in the neck, even leading to shooting pain and numbness in the arms and hands.

### Testing and Treatment

Your doctor's assessment of your neck pain may begin by checking your range of motion. Your doctor will ask you to move your head into several positions and assess the ease of movement. If your doctor suspects a more serious cause for your neck or back pain, he or she will want to do x-rays, which are used to rule out certain possible causes of neck pain.

If your doctor thinks your symptoms are due to overused muscles, home treatments will usually help relieve the spasms and pain. Anti-inflammatory medicines (p. 615) reduce swelling and pain. If those medicines upset your

---

*R-I-C-E for Muscle Pulls or Tears*

R=Rest. Stop the activity right away.
I =Ice. Apply ice for 15 minutes, and then alternate ice on and off every 10 minutes.
C=Compression. Wrap the injured area with an elastic bandage, but don't wrap it too tight.
E=Elevate the injured part of the body.

stomach, try acetaminophen (p. 614) for pain relief. You may also try heating pads or ice packs, or a mix of both, on the affected area. To relax a spasm, gently stretch or massage the tender muscle.

When the pain is more severe or long-lasting, your doctor may prescribe stronger pain medicine or muscle relaxants (p. 625) to reduce spasms. A neck brace may be used to provide relief from neck pain. Your doctor may also refer you to a physical therapist for further treatment.

### Prevention

To help prevent neck pain, don't abuse your neck! Try to maintain good posture, and avoid holding the telephone between your cheek and shoulder, a common cause of neck pain. Also, don't sleep with too many pillows. This position can lead to a "crick" in the morning.

## Osteomalacia

- Pain in the bones of the arms, legs and spine
- "Bow-legged" appearance

Commonly called *rickets,* osteomalacia leads to pain in the bones of the arms, legs and spine. Children with rickets have a "bow-legged" appearance when they stand or walk. The disorder occurs when calcium of the bone is lost, usually because of a vitamin D deficiency. Vitamin D helps the body absorb calcium and phosphorus from foods. Rickets may also result if acids produced by the kidneys can't be excreted into the urine. The increased acid in the body begins to literally dissolve the bone. Since milk is now fortified with vitamin D, rickets is very rare.

X-rays of the bone, analysis of a bone tissue sample and blood tests to check calcium, phosphorus and vitamin D levels help your doctor diagnose osteomalacia. Simply taking calcium and vitamin D supplements may cure this disorder.

## Osteomyelitis

- Pain, swelling and warmth in the area
- Fever

Bones, like any other tissue, may become infected when bacteria are spread through the bloodstream. Bacteria may also enter the bones through a wound or fracture. The infected area becomes inflamed and pus forms. Movement becomes painful and eventually swelling appears. Infection of the bone is called *osteomyelitis.*

### Testing and Treatment

Infection of the bone is rare. People who have received serious wounds are often taken to surgery for cleaning of their injuries to help prevent infection. Intravenous antibiotics are also given. X-rays and a high white blood cell count will help diagnose a serious infection.

Osteomyelitis is a severe infection, so treatment with antibiotics (p. 615) can last for four to six weeks. Analgesic medicine (p. 614) may be needed until the antibiotics begin fighting the infection. Rest is required, and applying heat to the area may help reduce the discomfort. Surgically draining the infected site may speed healing.

## Osteoporosis

- Often no symptoms
- "Brittle" bones that fracture easily
- "Hunched" back or loss of height during or after menopause
- Back pain due to compression fractures of the spine

*Osteoporosis* almost always occurs in the elderly. Women are affected more than men. Loss of calcium from the bones makes them less dense, meaning more porous (osteoporosis literally means "porous bone") and brittle, and consequently easily damaged from minor injuries. The factors that combine to produce osteoporosis aren't all completely understood. But inadequate calcium in the diet in early life, an inactive lifestyle and decreased levels of hormones such as *estrogen,* a female sex hormone, all play important roles in osteoporosis.

Osteoporosis develops slowly. The condition may not have any symptoms until a fracture occurs. Compression fractures of the spine (p. 234) and hip fractures occur most often in people with osteoporosis.

### Testing

X-rays of the spine will show a loss of bone density and may reveal collapse of some vertebrae. Collapse of the vertebrae causes the typical hunch of the back and loss of height in old age. Other tests include single and dual photon absorptiometry (p. 627), dual-energy x-ray absorptiometry (p. 627) and CT scans (p. 632).

### Treatment

Although prevention of this disease should start early in life, there are treatments that may keep osteoporosis from getting worse once it has started. One treatment for women is hormone replacement therapy (p. 407), in which you begin taking hormone supplements during menopause and keep taking them beyond menopause. Estrogen keeps your bones from losing calcium. But your body stops making estrogen during menopause. Replacing estrogen will help prevent calcium loss.

Another treatment is calcitonin. Calcitonin, also a hormone, helps prevent further bone loss from

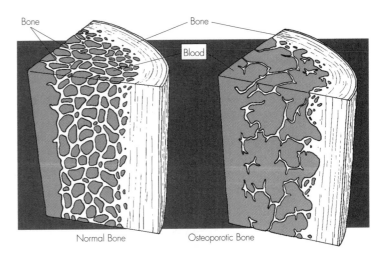

Bone                                    Bone

Blood

Normal Bone                    Osteoporotic Bone

**OSTEOPOROSIS**

osteoporosis. A new, nonhormonal treatment with a drug called alendronate also slows bone loss.

Another way to treat osteoporosis is to get enough calcium (p. 20) in your diet. Women need about 1,000 mg of calcium a day before menopause and after menopause starts, if estrogen is taken. If estrogen isn't taken, 1,500 mg of calcium a day is needed. Even though this won't stop the calcium loss, it may slow it down.

Eating plenty of foods that contain calcium and taking calcium supplements may help replace the calcium your bones are losing. Foods high in calcium include most dairy products, such as cheese, yogurt and milk. Skim milk and low-fat yogurt or cottage cheese are also low in fat and high in protein. Exercise is also important.

### Prevention

Until about age 35, people tend to produce more bone than they lose. Therefore, prevention of osteoporosis begins early in life by taking in enough calcium to build enough bone before the bone loss occurs. If you're at risk for osteoporosis, taking hormone replacement therapy when you begin menopause can help prevent the condition. Even if you've already gone

### Risk Factors for Osteoporosis

- Female
- Menopause before age 48
- Removal of ovaries before menopause
- Slender
- Small bone frame
- Fair skinned
- Sedentary lifestyle
- Smoking
- Alcohol abuse
- Family history of osteoporosis
- Hyperthyroidism (p. 215)

through menopause, hormone replacement therapy can help. Discuss the benefits and risks of this treatment with your doctor.

Maintaining a lifelong exercise program is also important to help reduce calcium loss from the bone and to keep bones strong and healthy. Exercises that put some stress on the spine and long bones of the legs and arms (weight-bearing exercises) are most beneficial. These include walking, aerobic dancing and bicycling. For more information on exercise, see page 2.

## Paget's disease

- Often no symptoms
- Headaches
- Bone pain

Normal bone is always being "remodeled" by the body—microscopic areas of the bone are removed and added constantly. In *Paget's disease*, this breaking down and reforming process happens too quickly, so the bones are hastily put together and never harden completely. Thus, the bones are fragile. The weakened bone may become deformed or even fracture under the normal stresses of walking or standing. Paget's disease usually affects people over age 50. Its cause is unknown.

Most people with Paget's disease don't develop symptoms. When they do, there may be bone pain, headaches and, if the skull is affected, hearing loss. Sometimes, the abnormal bone presses against the spinal cord or other parts of the nervous system, causing pain and muscle weakness. Paget's disease is difficult to diagnose, however, because the symptoms are found in many other disorders, such as arthritis.

### Testing and Treatment

X-rays or nuclear bone scans (p. 639) will show poor bone formation when Paget's disease is present. Blood and urine tests may be done to look for signs of bone formation or breakdown. Rarely, your doctor may need to analyze a bone tissue sample.

Paget's disease doesn't require treatment in many cases. If pain is a problem, treatment with analgesic medicines (p. 614) may be needed. Regular injections of calcitonin, a hormone that slows the rate of bone breakdown, may help decrease the rapid breakdown and formation of bone. Surgery may be needed to correct deformities, such as bowing of the long bones in the legs or joint problems due to osteoarthritis (p. 230), which often occurs with Paget's disease, and damage to nerves.

## Polymyalgia Rheumatica

- Aching pain and fatigue in shoulders
- Low fever
- Weight loss

*Polymyalgia rheumatica* is a type of connective tissue disorder (p. 235). It begins with aching pains and fatigue around the shoulders. Some people also have mild fever and weight loss. Polymyalgia rheumatica is more common in people over 60. It is a form of autoimmune disorder (p. 223) that appears to attack the blood vessels.

Polymyalgia rheumatica is diagnosed by a physical exam, blood tests, x-rays and other tests as needed.

Polymyalgia rheumatica often disappears after a few years. Oral corticosteroids (p. 622) usually relieve the pain.

## Polymyositis

- Weakness in the arms
- Aching in the shoulders and hips
- Rash on the face, arms or legs (sometimes)

*Polymyositis* causes an inflammation in the muscles or in the deeper layers of the skin. It's a form of connective tissue disorder (p. 235). Weakness of the arms and aching in the shoulders and hip muscles are usually the first symptoms. When skin irritation and rashes on the face, arms or legs occur, the disease is called *dermatomyositis.*

Blood tests, biopsy of skin and muscle, and electrical studies of the muscles, called electromyography (p. 634), may help your doctor diagnose this problem.

Corticosteroids (p. 622), such as prednisone (p. 620), are the most effective treatment. Many people who have polymyositis will have long periods without symptoms. But the disease affects the lung and heart in some cases, which can lead to severe symptoms and even death.

## Sciatica

* Sharp pain that runs from the buttocks and down the side of the thigh or to the knee or foot

*Sciatica* is an inflammation of the *sciatic nerve.* The sciatic nerve begins in the buttocks and travels down the back of the leg where it branches off into other nerves. The pain of sciatica follows this nerve—from the buttock, down the side of the thigh or sometimes to the knee or foot. Sciatica usually affects only one side of the body.

Sciatica is caused by pressure on a nerve, usually from a herniated disk (p. 238) and sometimes from tight muscles as a result of an injury or just sitting in an awkward position. It's also common during pregnancy, if the baby presses against the nerve.

*Spinal stenosis* is a less common form of sciatica found most often in middle-aged or elderly people. In spinal stenosis, the spine presses

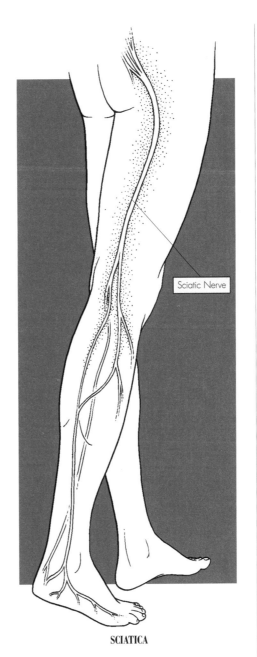

Sciatic Nerve

**SCIATICA**

against the sciatic nerve, causing pain in the buttock, thigh or calf. The pain can be eased by flexing the back, such as by bending over, or sitting still.

### Testing and Treatment

An exam and special tests will determine where the sciatic nerve is affected and what's causing the inflammation. These tests may include x-rays, a CT scan (p. 632), an MRI scan (p. 637) or a myelogram (p. 638).

If the pain of sciatica is mild and seems to go away after treatment with heat, rest and over-the-counter medicines, no further testing or treatment is needed. If sciatica doesn't improve with these measures, physical therapy is often helpful.

You should see your doctor if the pain is severe, worse when you cough or sneeze, or travels down your leg past your knee. These are signs of a herniated disk, which may require surgery.

**Prevention**

Avoid straining the muscles in your back when you lift heavy objects. See page 233 for tips on lifting. Exercises to strengthen the stomach muscles will help make your back stronger. To avoid sciatica, a pregnant woman shouldn't lie on her back for long periods of time.

## Scleroderma

- Tightening of the skin of the face and hands
- Thickening of the skin
- Trouble moving the fingers

*Scleroderma* is a fairly rare disorder that often begins with some tightening of the skin of the face and hands. Later, the skin thickens, and it becomes difficult to move the fingers. Other symptoms include swelling of the feet, joint pain and stiffness. In more severe cases, the kidneys, lungs and other organs can become involved.

Scleroderma is a connective tissue disorder (p. 235). It results from extra layers of collagen growing within the skin and other tissues, almost like a scar.

Your doctor can take a sample of skin to identify the problem. No effective treatment has been found to reverse this disease. Your doctor may prescribe corticosteroids (p. 622) to relieve pain and other symptoms.

Scleroderma may not worsen and may stay about the same for long periods.

If it involves the heart, lungs or urinary system, symptoms may become severe.

## Scoliosis

- A curvature of the spine causing one shoulder blade to be higher than the other

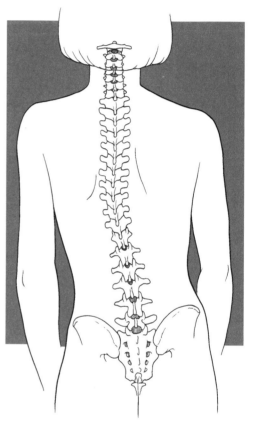

**SCOLIOSIS**

The spine is normally straight. With *scoliosis*, the spine is curved into an S shape, causing one shoulder to be higher and, sometimes, one hip to be higher and stick out further than the other. Bending forward at the waist tends to make the curvature more noticeable.

Most often, scoliosis begins developing during adolescence. It affects girls more often than boys. The reason scoliosis occurs is usually unknown. Most cases are mild and require no treatment.

Severe scoliosis can produce painful deformities of the upper and lower spine. The back may be so twisted that the rib cage presses on the lungs, reducing the ability of the lungs to expand and causing difficulty in breathing.

### Testing and Treatment

X-rays of the spine will help your doctor assess the angles of curvature and decide whether treatment is needed. Exercises or a spinal brace may be used to slow the curvature of the spine during adolescence. Surgery may be needed if these measures don't help and the curvature becomes much worse. With surgery for scoliosis, metal rods are placed on one or both sides of the spine to straighten it.

## Shoulder Problems

- Pain
- Limited motion of the shoulder

The shoulder joint is a ball-and-socket type of joint, which allows it to move in any direction. It provides even more movement than the hip, which is also a ball-and-socket type of joint. This is why the shoulder is so susceptible to dislocation and other problems. The joint occurs where the ball of the *humerus,* or upper arm bone, fits into the scapula. A fibrous capsule, called the *joint capsule,* surrounds the joint.

The shoulder joint can be affected by many problems, including tendinitis (p. 253) and bursitis (p. 233). Other problems are more specific to the shoulder joint.

When the joint capsule shrinks, movement of the shoulder becomes severely limited and produces extreme pain. This condition is called *frozen shoulder,* or *adhesive capsulitis.* Frozen shoulder seems to result from abnormal changes in the tissue of the joint capsule, particularly in the protein, or *collagen,* portion. This causes shrinking of the space. Frozen shoulder most often affects people in middle age.

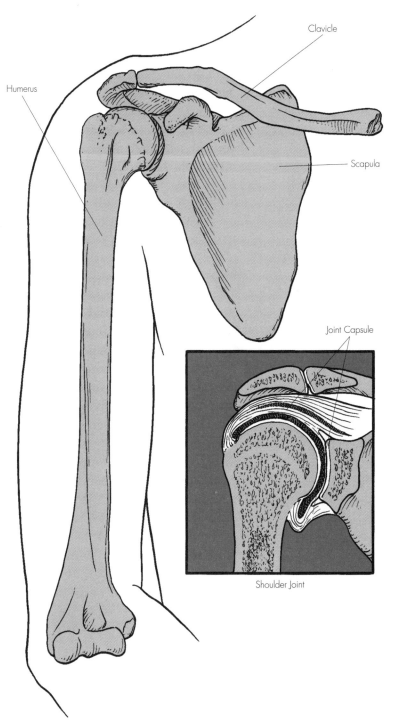

**SHOULDER ANATOMY**

Besides being related to age, frozen shoulder may develop after a shoulder injury if the shoulder joint isn't moved enough after the injury.

*Rotator cuff* injuries can cause symptoms similar to those of frozen shoulder. Rotator cuff injury means one of the tendons that surrounds

## Shin Splints

When an athlete has pain along the shin, the problem is known as *shin splints*. Athletes who run and jump a lot may get shin splints. They occur when the *fascia*, thick, fibrous connective tissue, and tendons fail to keep the muscles of the shin area attached to the bone. Activity may cause the muscle to pull the tissue away from the shin bone, producing pain. There's little or no swelling. Resting the leg, applying ice to the painful area, bandaging the area and taking over-the-counter pain medicine usually help relieve pain and speed healing. To reduce the chance of having shin splints, stretch your calf muscles before exercise and avoid running on concrete or other hard surfaces.

the joint is torn. When this happens, someone else can move your shoulder through its range of motion, but you can't do it by yourself. These tears may be small ones that occur over time with use, or a tear may occur as the result of an injury, such as falling and catching yourself with your arm or lifting something quite heavy.

### Testing and Treatment

Because pain and problems with moving the shoulder joint can occur in many conditions, your doctor probably will perform a complete exam and a few tests to rule these conditions out. An x-ray of the shoulder may show shrinkage of the joint capsule when frozen shoulder is present.

Besides analgesic medicines (p. 614) to control pain, the main treatment for frozen shoulder is physical therapy, including shoulder exercises to stretch the joint capsule. If improvement doesn't occur after weeks of exercise, your doctor may need to loosen your shoulder while you're under general anesthesia.

Small tears in the rotator cuff tendons may be treated with cortisone (p. 623) injection and by doing exercises to improve your range of motion. Surgery may be needed to repair a larger tear in the rotator cuff.

## Sjögren's Syndrome

- Dry, red, painful eyes
- Dry mouth
- Dry skin

*Sjögren's syndrome* is a type of connective tissue disorder (p. 235). It can occur by itself or in combination with rheumatoid arthritis or another connective tissue disorder. Symptoms include dry mouth and red, dry and painful eyes, and sometimes dry and scaling skin.

Sjögren's syndrome may be diagnosed based on your symptoms and some simple tests. Blood tests may be helpful, as may tests to measure the moisture in your eyes or mouth.

Your doctor may prescribe eye drops to relieve eye pain and dryness. To relieve the mouth dryness, try sipping fluids during the day, chewing sugarless gum or using special mouthwashes to replace your saliva. Avoid medicines that may cause further dryness, such as decongestants (p. 616) and antihistamines (p. 615). Take very good care of your teeth to help prevent decay and other problems that may arise due to the dryness. If symptoms are severe, a corticosteroid (p. 622) may be prescribed.

## Spondylosis and Spondylolisthesis

- Changes in how a person walks
- Back pain
- Stiffness of the back
- Numbness and weakness of arms or legs

*Spondylosis* is a narrowing of the spinal column, usually of the cervical spine, or neck. *Spondylolisthesis* occurs when two of the vertebrae in the spine become slightly out of line, narrowing the space for the nerves. This may be the result of a neck injury, changes in the cartilage between the vertebrae or the formation of bony spur-like growths. The bony growths sometimes occur with rheumatoid arthritis (p. 231) or osteoarthritis (p. 230). Spondylosis and spondylolisthesis may also affect the *lumbar* spine, or lower back. When the lumbar spine is affected, the problem is usually due to a minor birth defect.

In many cases, these conditions don't cause symptoms. When the narrowing pinches the nerves or the spinal cord, shooting leg pains similar to those of sciatica (p. 247) often occur.

You may have pain in other parts of the body, such as an arm or leg, depending on which vertebrae and nerves are involved.

### Testing and Treatment

The location of your pain can help your doctor figure out which area of the spine is affected. X-rays usually show the problem, but a CT scan (p. 632) or MRI scan (p. 637) may be needed as well.

Sometimes, the symptoms of spondylosis or spondylolisthesis go away on their own. Otherwise, you may need to wear a soft collar brace around your neck and have physical therapy to help relieve the pain and stiffness. If symptoms worsen, your doctor may recommend surgery to release a pinched nerve.

## Sprains

- Swelling and pain in and around a joint after twisting or stretching it too much
- Inability to use a joint after an injury

*Ligaments* are strong bands of tissue that connect bones together at a joint. A ligament is sprained when it's twisted, pulled or hit hard during motion. The damage occurs when the ligament is stretched too much. Ligament injury causes swelling, bruising, pain and an inability to move the joint.

A sprain can be just as serious as a fracture and requires just as long, or longer, to heal. Sprains of the knee and ankle can make it difficult to walk for days or months, depending on the severity of the injury. Sometimes a sprained ankle is put in a cast after the swelling goes down to reduce movement, prevent the swelling from returning and decrease the pain.

### Testing and Treatment

Swelling from a sprain should first be treated with ice packs. The joint

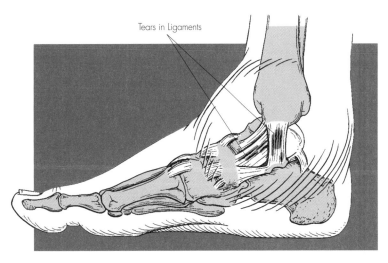

Tears in Ligaments

**SPRAINED ANKLE**

shouldn't be moved, and it should be elevated to reduce swelling. Wrap the joint in an elastic bandage to provide some support and help keep the swelling down. Resting the joint is essential until it's healed. A simple way to remember these treatments is the R-I-C-E formula (Rest, Ice, Compression and Elevation, p. 243).

See your doctor if you hear a "pop" when you injure a joint, if you're unable to walk or use the limb, or if the pain lasts for three days despite using R-I-C-E. X-rays of the joint or other tests may be needed to find out if a fracture or other problem is present.

Anti-inflammatory medicines (p. 615) may help relieve pain and reduce swelling. For an ankle injury, crutches and a cast may be needed so you can still walk while keeping pressure off the damaged joint. More serious sprains may require surgery to repair the torn ligaments.

### Prevention

Keeping muscles as strong as possible helps protect ligaments. During sports activities, wear high-top athletic shoes and protect joints with wraps, braces or athletic tape to help prevent a sprain. Try to avoid running or playing on fields that have holes or irregular surfaces.

---

### Grades of Sprains

*Grade I* — A mildly stretched ligament; may have microscopic tears

*Grade II* — A partial tear of a ligament with some joint looseness

*Grade III* — A complete tear of a ligament; with grade III sprains, other ligaments may also be stretched

## Systemic Lupus Erythematosus

- Butterfly-shaped rash across the nose and cheeks
- Joint pain and swelling
- Weakness and fatigue
- Weight loss
- Rash after sun exposure

*Systemic lupus erythematosus* is a connective tissue disorder (p. 235) that usually affects women from 15 to 35 years old. A rash across the nose and cheeks that is shaped like a butterfly is the usual symptom of systemic lupus erythematosus. Other symptoms include joint pain and swelling, weakness, fatigue, weight loss and a rash after being in the sunlight. Sometimes the heart, kidneys and brain become damaged.

Blood tests may help the doctor make a diagnosis. Corticosteroids (p. 622) and other medicines are used to treat both mild and more severe disease. Lifestyle changes are needed to avoid fatigue and reactions to sunlight. These may include getting more rest and staying out of the sun. Lupus can usually be controlled. Rarely, it can be fatal.

## Temporomandibular Joint (TMJ) Disease

- Pain in the jaw, sometimes spreading into the ear
- Stiffness of the jaw
- Headache

*Temporomandibular joint* (TMJ) disease causes pain with the movement of the jaw, or temporomandibular joint. TMJ occurs when the joint is worn down, becomes abnormal in shape or dislocated, or has been affected by arthritis-like changes.

The muscles of the jaw may also become stiff and tender, and opening the mouth may be difficult, especially after waking up in the morning. Headaches and other long-term pain may result from damage of the jaw joints and muscles.

People most prone to TMJ are those who have *malocclusion* of their teeth, which means their teeth don't meet when they bite. Other factors that cause TMJ disease include grinding the teeth during sleep, an overbite, a history of dental braces, chewing gum frequently or rheumatoid arthritis.

### Testing and Treatment

Your doctor may order special x-rays of the jaw to diagnose TMJ. Blood tests may reveal an underlying problem, such as rheumatoid arthritis (p. 231). In the early stages of TMJ disease, anti-inflammatory medicines (p. 615) can reduce the discomfort. Heat and muscle-relaxants (p. 625)

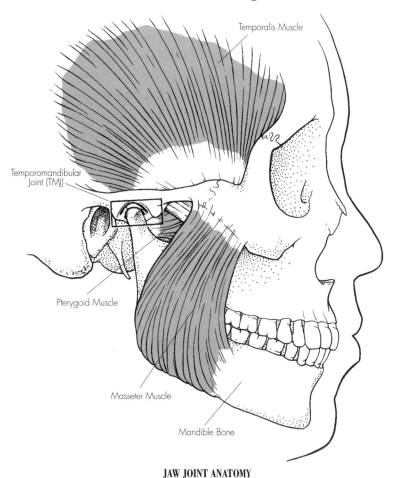

Temporalis Muscle

Temporomandibular Joint (TMJ)

Pterygoid Muscle

Masseter Muscle

Mandible Bone

**JAW JOINT ANATOMY**

may reduce the pain and tightness in the jaw muscles.

If malocclusion or an overbite is the cause of TMJ disease, your dentist or orthodontist may be able to correct it. If you grind your teeth at night, your dentist may suggest that you put a special bite plate in your mouth when you're sleeping. The bite plate is made of plastic and is molded to fit your mouth. It will keep you from grinding your teeth. Surgery to correct the jaw problem is reserved for cases of extremely painful and damaged joints that don't respond to the other treatments.

### Prevention

Stress appears to be a key factor in causing TMJ disease. Grinding your teeth at night is sometimes a symptom of stress overload during the daytime hours. See page 571 for information on how to deal with stress. Chewing gum can aggravate the problem and should be avoided.

## Tendinitis

- Pain with motion
- Inability to move the affected area
- Swelling along the path of the tendon

Any tendon can become inflamed. This is called *tendinitis*. Overactivity, infection or an inflammatory condition, such as rheumatoid arthritis (p. 231), gout (p. 238) or Reiter's syndrome (p. 231), can cause swelling of the *tendon sheath*, a tube-like structure that surrounds the tendon. The swelling causes pain whenever the tendon moves. If the tendon is also swollen, it may be unable to fit through the sheath, or it may move through the sheath with a "pop."

Common sites for tendinitis include the elbow (tennis elbow, see the box on the right), the shoulder (*biceps tendinitis*), and the knee (jumper's knee, p. 241). *Trigger finger* is the medical term for a form of tendinitis that affects a finger tendon. With trigger finger, a popping sensation occurs every time the finger is flexed or extended. The pain may disappear during rest and return after brisk activity. It may continue for many months, or it may come and go.

### Testing and Treatment

Your doctor will probably examine the muscle, tendon and joint for tenderness and possibly swelling along the course of the tendon. X-rays may be taken to make sure no bone disorder is causing the problem.

Anti-inflammatory medicines (p. 615), resting the injured area and applying ice (p. 243) are usually effective for reducing the inflammation.

A splint can keep the joint from moving for a few days to ensure proper rest of the inflamed area. Injections of corticosteroids (p. 622) into the tendon sheath or next to the tendon can reduce the pain and tenderness within a few days.

A warm, red, very tender area over a tendon may mean an infection is present. If these symptoms occur, see your doctor right away. Surgery is only rarely needed, but may be needed to drain infected tendons or tendon sheaths. Drainage helps get rid of the infection and stops an infection from spreading. Surgery may also be

---

### Self-Treatment for Tendinitis

- Reduce or stop the activity that's causing the irritation.
- Use an over-the counter anti-inflammatory medicine.
- Use ice on the painful area.

---

### Tennis Elbow

Repeated twisting motions of the arm, such as those used by tennis players, may irritate the muscles and tendons in the forearm. This produces pain in the elbow. The injury isn't limited to tennis players—it can occur in many other sports, including baseball and bowling. Overuse of undeveloped muscles and improper technique and equipment are usually to blame.

Treat the injury with rest, ice and anti-inflammatory medicine (p. 615). Tennis elbow may take some time to heal—it often returns because people resume activities too soon. To prevent future recurrence, learn the proper techniques for tennis strokes and other sports activities, use a flexible racquet with a large grip size and strengthen the forearm muscles with exercises.

needed when scar tissue has formed because of long-term tendinitis.

### Prevention

Perform stretching exercises and stay in good physical shape to help prevent tendinitis. Strengthening an area that seems prone to tendinitis may also prevent return of the problem.

## Tumors of the Bone

- A painless bump on a bone
- Pain in the leg that occurs for no apparent reason

Cancer that has spread from other organs, called *metastatic cancer,* is the most common cause of bone cancer. Cancerous tumors that can spread to bones include breast cancer (p. 408) in women and prostate cancer (p. 428) in men. Tumors directly from bone tissue are rare.

Noncancerous bone tumors don't usually cause pain unless they're hit or bumped. These painless tumors include *osteomas* (tumors of the bone), *bone cysts* (a sac-like growth on or in the bone) and *osteochondromas* (tumors made of bone and cartilage).

### Testing and Treatment

X-rays will usually show whether a tumor is cancerous. Usually treatment of noncancerous bone tumors is unnecessary, but osteochondromas may need to be removed for cosmetic or structural reasons.

In most cases, cancer produces pain *before* it causes a lump or mass to form on a bone. Cancerous tumors of the bone may cause fractures from little or no trauma. Cancer that has spread to the bones from elsewhere in the body may be treated with radiation. Two types of bone cancer, *osteogenic sarcoma* and *Ewing's sarcoma,* must be removed. These tumors usually develop in the arms or legs. Early removal of the tumor may save the person's life, but amputation is usually required. Treatments also include radiation therapy (p. 225) and chemotherapy (p. 225).

## Whiplash

- Neck pain
- Stiffness of the neck
- Tightness or tenderness of the neck after stretching or straining

When car wrecks occur and the car stops quickly, the neck is likely to be injured because of the jerking movement of the neck. *Whiplash* occurs when the ligaments and muscles in the neck are stretched, torn, pulled or damaged during the quick, forceful movement.

### Testing and Treatment

If you're involved in a car wreck, see your doctor to make sure you don't need tests and treatment. Usually x-rays are done to make sure the neck joints are stable and in proper line. Apply heat and creamy skin analgesics to treat a mild pull or "crick" of a neck muscle. Anti-inflammatory medicines (p. 615) may also help.

In a typical whiplash injury, the pain will get worse on the second or third day after the injury and then begin to subside. Severe injuries need to be treated with a neck brace, physical therapy or traction.

### Prevention

Pay attention while driving, wear a seat belt and avoid activities that stress the neck to help prevent whiplash. Some people have neck pain, headaches or neck stiffness on a regular basis. Strengthening the neck muscles by doing special exercises keeps them in better tone and reduces the chance of whiplash.

# CHAPTER 16 HANDS AND FEET

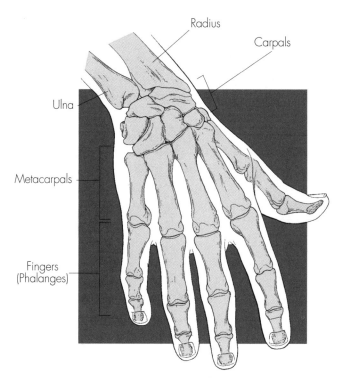

**HAND AND WRIST**

Radius

Carpals

Ulna

Metacarpals

Fingers
(Phalanges)

Your hands and feet are complex structures that take a great deal of abuse as you perform your daily activities. The hand is composed of 27 bones, called *carpal, metacarpal* and *phalangeal bones*. The metacarpal bones make up the palm of the hand, and the carpal bones meet the bones of the forearm (the *ulna* and *radius*) to form the wrist. The *phalanges* are the bones of the fingers. The bones that meet to form a joint are held together with tough bands of tissue called *ligaments*. Each joint is surrounded by a small joint capsule made of *connective tissue*, tough bands of tissue that support and bind the joint together.

The foot contains 28 bones, all held together by more than 100 ligaments. Like the hands, each joint in the foot is surrounded by a joint capsule made of connective tissue. The foot is joined to the bones in the leg, the *tibia* and *fibula*, at the ankle. The bones are called *tarsal* (hindfoot), *metatarsal* (midfoot) and *phalangeal* (toe) bones. The bones are arranged to form two arches, one that goes from the front of the foot to the back and another that goes from side to side. Along the bottom of the foot, the arches are strengthened by the *plantar fascia*, a tough, wide band of connective tissue. This reinforcement, combined with the two arches, gives the foot the strength to carry its heavy burden every day.

Few people give their hands and feet the care they deserve. Instead, we often wear poorly fitting, unsupportive footwear. We expect our hands to perform everything from intricate tasks to carrying heavy objects, all without the slightest thought—that is, until an injury occurs.

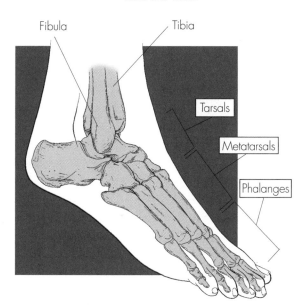

**FOOT AND ANKLE**

Fibula

Tibia

Tarsals

Metatarsals

Phalanges

255

## Athlete's Foot

- Red rash, especially between toes
- Itching
- Pungent odor

***See photo of athlete's foot, page 271.***

*Athlete's foot* is a fungal infection. The space between the toes makes an ideal environment for moisture-loving fungi to multiply and begin breaking down the skin. The fungi cause a red rash, itching and often a pungent odor. The most annoying part of athlete's foot is the constant itching.

### Treatment

Athlete's foot can be treated with an over-the-counter antifungal (p. 615) cream, spray or powder. Your doctor can prescribe a more potent antifungal (p. 619) cream or pills if the infection persists. Treatment is needed for at least a month to get rid of the infection.

### Prevention

To prevent athlete's foot, dry your feet thoroughly after bathing and use an antifungal foot powder. Avoid sharing the same bath towel or mat with anyone. Wear well-ventilated shoes, such as sandals or shoes with porous upper covering, and cotton or wool socks that absorb moisture. Change your socks at least once a day—more frequently if they become damp. At home, keep your feet dry and uncovered whenever possible. If your shoes are wet or damp, use a hair dryer to dry your shoes, or set them outside to air dry.

## Bunions

- A sore, bulging area where the big toe meets the foot

The three bones in the big toe normally form a straight line. But in people who have an inherited tendency toward bunions, the ligaments that hold the bones in line weaken. Because of the weakened ligaments, the bones begin to push sideways, forming a bump, or *bunion.* Sometimes the big toe becomes so crooked that it lies on top of the second toe.

Bunions are a result of continual pressure from walking and standing. Poorly fitting shoes and shoes with pointed toes or high heels worsen the problem by putting more pressure on the bone, and by not providing adequate support under the ball of the foot. The more deformed the toe becomes, the harder and more painful it is to wear shoes.

### *Home Care for Athlete's Foot*

- Keep the infected foot uncovered and dry whenever possible.
- Change socks whenever they are damp.
- Use only white socks to avoid any irritating dyes.
- Use a hair dryer to dry your shoes or leave them outside to dry.
- Don't wear shoes that are damp—wait until they're thoroughly dry inside.
- Use over-the-counter antifungal sprays, powders or creams.

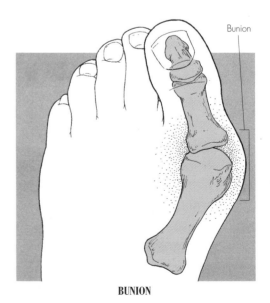

Bunion

**BUNION**

## Testing and Treatment

Your doctor will probably take an x-ray of your foot. The x-ray will reveal any changes in the alignment of the bones where the bunion occurs.

If you have pain and swelling, oral anti-inflammatory medicines (p. 615) may be useful. Surgery to realign the bones and repair the ligaments is reserved for people with such severe pain and deformity that they can't perform routine daily activities.

## Prevention

Wear comfortable shoes that don't cramp your toes. Your shoes should also provide good support across the ball of the foot.

## Carpal Tunnel Syndrome

- Tingling and numbness in the hand
- Loss of strength
- Pain

*Carpal tunnel syndrome* is a common and painful problem of the wrist and hand. The *carpal tunnel* is a thick, fibrous channel that runs through the wrist and holds the *median nerve.* The median nerve carries signals to and from the nerves in the thumb, index and middle fingers. When the tunnel swells, usually because of overuse, it puts pressure on the median nerve.

The pressure leads to numbness, tingling and pain in the thumb, index and middle fingers. Carpal tunnel syndrome sometimes leads to weakness in the thumb and pain that shoots from the hand into the forearm and shoulder. Carpal tunnel syndrome is one of a group of nerve problems that are caused by compression of a nerve (p. 48).

Repeated movement of the wrist, especially from using a computer or typewriter, can cause swelling in the carpal tunnel. Hobbies that involve lots of wrist movement and certain sports

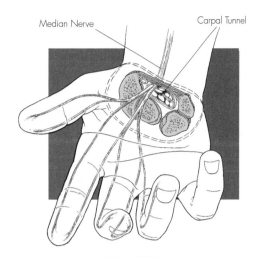

**CARPAL TUNNEL**

can cause the swelling. Pregnant women and people with certain thyroid disorders are also prone to carpal tunnel syndrome. Without treatment, the pressure on the nerve can damage it over time, slowing or stopping the signals sent to or from the nerves in the hand.

## Testing and Treatment

Your doctor will probably diagnose carpal tunnel syndrome based on your description of pain, tingling and numbness. When the cause of the symptoms is uncertain, nerve conduction studies (p. 638) can help determine the cause.

Carpal tunnel syndrome may clear up simply by resting the wrist. Reducing the amount of repeated wrist movement can allow the nerve to heal. This can be accomplished by changing habits or positions or using a wrist splint. A wrist splint is often the most helpful treatment. It keeps the wrist still and stops the pressure on the nerve.

Oral anti-inflammatory medicines (p. 615) may be helpful. In severe cases, corticosteroid (p. 622) injections in the wrist or surgery to open the tunnel is needed to prevent nerve damage.

## Prevention

The first step in preventing carpal tunnel syndrome is being aware of the

*Workers Most
Likely to
Develop
Carpal Tunnel
Syndrome*

- Assembly-line
  workers
- Carpenters
- Keyboard operators
- Meat processors
- Mechanics
- Musicians,
  especially those
  who play stringed
  instruments

damage that can occur from repeated motions of the wrist. If you have symptoms, wearing a supportive bandage or splint when you resume the activity may help.

Learn the proper techniques to protect your wrist. And make sure that your equipment, such as your computer keyboard, is properly placed in relation to your height. This can limit the amount of stress placed on your wrist and hand. Wrist supports may help take stress off the carpal tunnel. Wrist supports are flat, rectangular pieces of foam that attach to the keyboard or sit on the desk to support the wrist and keep it flat.

### *Preventing Carpal Tunnel Syndrome*

- Take regular breaks from activities that require repetitive wrist movements.
- Occasionally change how you do the movements, if possible.
- If you type or do data entry, adjust your chair so that your forearms are level with your keyboard. Try using a wrist support.

## Corns and Calluses

- Patches of thickened, hard skin on the feet or hands
- Occasional tenderness or pain in the area

When a shoe doesn't fit your foot properly, it puts pressure on the bony parts that rub against the shoe. With days or weeks of this pressure, the skin over the bone thickens. If the pressure is over a small area, a *corn* is produced. If the rubbing and thickening occurs over a larger area, such as the ball of the foot, a *callus* is produced.

Calluses form on the hands when an activity causes the palms or fingers

to repeatedly rub against something such as a tool handle or steering wheel. Musicians who play stringed instruments get calluses on their fingertips from the continuous pressure of the strings.

### Treatment

Removing the thickened skin with a pumice rubbing stone is usually the only treatment needed. Softening the callus or corn first with an over-the-counter corn-remover solution (p. 616) or pad, or soaking in water, may speed the process of removing the thickened skin.

Corn pads are small, donut-shaped pads that can be placed over the bony area to take the pressure off the corn until the softening agents begin to work. If needed, the dead skin in the corn or callus can be trimmed away with a pair of small, sharp scissors. Cut small amounts of skin at a time and cut parallel to the skin surface. Start in the middle of the corn, cutting a little deeper with each pass. Be careful not to cut too deep. If that happens, apply pressure to stop the bleeding. Then cover the area with an antibiotic ointment and a bandage. Don't use a razor blade, which can be hard to control and may cut the skin too deeply.

### Prevention

Corns or calluses are usually caused by tight areas in a shoe. Properly fitting shoes reduce your chance of developing this skin irritation. Uncomfortable shoes, even if you wear them only for special occasions, can hurt your feet. Wear two pairs of athletic socks with tennis or basketball shoes. Wear supportive shoes for daily or routine tasks to help prevent calluses, corns and other foot problems. Soak your feet and use a pumice stone to prevent the buildup of thickening skin.

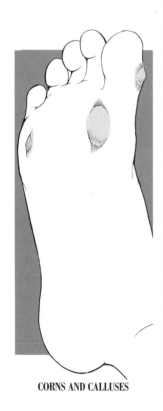

**CORNS AND CALLUSES**

## How to Safely Trim a Corn or Callus

- Use a pair of small, sharp scissors.
- Cut parallel to the skin surface.
- Start in the middle, cutting a little deeper with each pass.
- If the area is more comfortable when you press it with your finger, you have trimmed away enough skin.
- If you cut yourself, apply pressure to stop the bleeding. Then apply an antibiotic ointment and a bandage. Avoid this problem by being careful and not trimming too much at one time.

*If you have diabetes (p. 211), have your doctor or a* podiatrist, *a doctor who specializes in caring for the feet, remove calluses and corns to prevent damage or possible infection. People with diabetes are at increased risk for serious infection from foot wounds.*

## Deformed Toes

- Abnormally bent toe that causes pain

Weakness in the toe ligaments and other factors can cause toe deformities, including *hammer toe*. Hammer toe can develop on an extra-long second toe if it rubs the top of the shoe too much. A callus forms on the top of the toe and produces pain and discomfort. People with chronic nerve damage to the toes, including many people with diabetes, are more prone to hammer-toe deformities.

### Treatment

A cast can be taken of your foot and used to make an insole for your shoes. This ensures proper spacing and alignment of your toes. Surgery may be needed for deformities that are very painful and don't improve with other therapies.

### Prevention

Make sure when you buy shoes that they're comfortable and fit properly. If you have foot problems, consult your doctor about whether you should have your shoes or insoles custom-made. This can help prevent serious deformities of the toes.

## Flat Feet

- An arch in the foot that doesn't curve

*Flat feet* occur because of a defect in the way the bones in the arch of the foot connect to one another. People with flat feet are usually born with the condition. While most infants appear to have flat feet at first, the arch should begin to form at about two to three years of age. Flat feet usually aren't a problem and don't cause severe symptoms.

Your doctor will probably be able to diagnose flat feet with an exam. X-rays usually aren't needed, but can help identify which bones are involved.

Treatment usually isn't needed. Shoes with a built-in arch support can be worn if flat feet cause pain or limit activities.

## Ganglion

- A firm swelling in the wrist or ankle

A *ganglion cyst* is a growth under the skin, usually appearing on the wrist or ankle. The cyst is made up of the tissue that covers the nearby tendons. Some ganglion cysts become tight and hard and may be painful. Others stay soft, causing no pain or discomfort.

Usually, no treatment is needed, especially if the ganglion cyst causes no pain. Your doctor may drain the cyst with a large needle. Surgery can be done to remove the cyst if it's bothersome and won't go away.

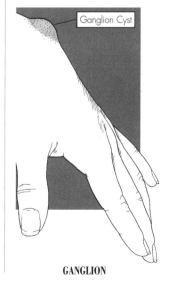

Ganglion Cyst

**GANGLION**

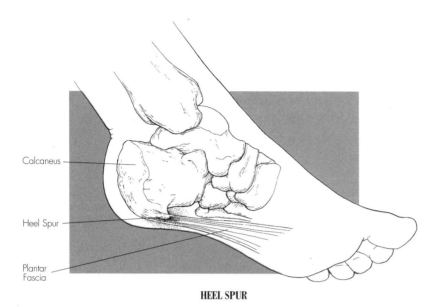

**HEEL SPUR**

spur. Blood tests may be done to rule out arthritic conditions.

Your doctor may inject the area of the spur with cortisone (p. 623) to relieve swelling. You may have to curtail your activities to prevent further damage. An *orthotic*, a shoe insert made from a cast of your foot, can be tailored to reduce the pressure over the area of the spur.

## Morton's Neuroma

- Pain over the ball of the foot
- Burning sensation in the ball of the foot

A *neuroma* is a small mass or gathering of nerve cells and nerve fibers on a nerve. *Morton's neuroma* is located in the ball of the foot, usually between the third and fourth toes. It's most common in people between 15 and 55 years old, especially women. It may be caused by tight-fitting shoes or some other irritation to the nerve.

Your doctor will diagnose the problem by examining your foot. Treatment may involve injections of lidocaine and corticosteroids (p. 622). Shoe pads

## Heel Spur

- Increasing heel pain when walking

A *heel spur* is a bony growth on the bottom of the heel bone. Jumping on the heel, carrying heavy weights and playing various sports can damage the heel. Calcium may then build up on the heel bone, the *calcaneus*, forming a hard growth. Depending on its size, the spur may cause irritation and inflammation of the *plantar fascia*, the cushion-like connective tissue that runs along the bottom of your foot. This inflammation, plantar fasciitis (p. 263), may cause pain when you walk.

### Testing and Treatment

The pain of a heel spur usually comes from irritation of the plantar fascia, so treatment usually is directed toward plantar fasciitis. The spur may grow in time and irritate the skin around it as well. Over-the-counter anti-inflammatory medicines (p. 615) may relieve pain and swelling.

Other helpful measures include using a shock-absorbing heel pad or a thick felt pad with a hole in it where the heel is most tender. If this doesn't relieve your discomfort, your doctor may want to do x-rays to identify the

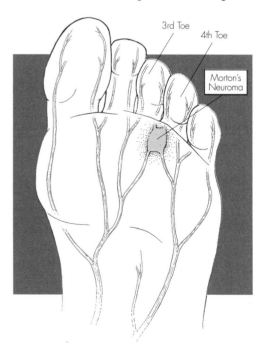

**MORTON'S NEUROMA**

may be helpful. If medicine doesn't help, surgery may be used to remove the neuroma.

## Nail Problems

- Pits, ridges or splits in fingernails and toenails
- Thickened or otherwise deformed fingernails or toenails
- Change in color of the nail or of the skin under the nail
- A torn or ripped nail causing pain, bleeding and irritation
- Blood under the nail from pinching or slamming the finger

**Complications of artificial nails.** Artificial nails can damage the natural nails and the skin around them. The glue used to attach artificial nails may irritate the skin. It also interferes with the natural nails' access to moisture, causing them to become dry and brittle. When the artificial nail comes off, it may take part of the natural nail with it, possibly causing injury and creating a breeding ground for infection. Even if the artificial nail comes off without causing injury, you may find that the natural nail beneath has become more brittle and weaker than before.

The weakened condition of the natural nails beneath the artificial nails makes it easier to get an infection. If a nail becomes injured, clean the area and treat it with antibiotic ointment (p. 615). A bandage may be useful to protect it from further damage.

If you decide to get artificial nails, go to a reputable salon and let a professional apply them rather than trying to do them yourself. Someone who's experienced will probably do a better job securing the nails and will be less likely to injure your real nails.

**Deformed nails.** If you smash your finger in a car door you may see a ridge or other mark on the nail weeks later, when the finger is no longer in pain. Injury to the cuticle or to the *nail bed*, where the nail is formed, is the usual reason for a nail deformity. Infections or disease may also cause nail deformities.

Pits on the nail may be caused by injury or a disease, such as psoriasis (p. 288), severe lung disease or heart disease. For example, when oxygen to the tissues is reduced, the tips of the fingers, along with the nails, can take on a club-like appearance.

Any nutritional deficiency or serious illness may temporarily reduce nail growth, causing ridges or splits in the nail. When the illness ends or the deficiency is corrected, the nail usually resumes normal growth and the ridges eventually grow out.

**Discolored nails.** The most common cause of discoloration is a pocket of blood, called a *hematoma,* under the nail after it's been smashed or partly torn off. Depending on the size of the hematoma, the nail may or may not fall off in a few days or weeks. Your doctor may need to drain the blood to relieve pressure and pain. As the nail grows out, so does the discoloration. The nail will usually return to normal.

Nail discoloration occurs for other reasons as well. For example, smokers often have yellow nails on the fingers they use to hold their cigarettes. Exposing the nails to certain chemicals may change the color. Infections can cause discoloration as well. Anemia (p. 133) makes all the normally pink areas on your body turn pale or whitish, including the nail beds. Whitish spots embedded in the nail usually come from injury or changes in nutrition.

**Hangnails.** A tear in the skin of the *cuticle,* or the outline of the nail near the skin, is called a *hangnail.* This can cause redness and pain. Infection

---

*Helping Your Nails Be Healthy*

- Avoid using products, such as harsh detergents, that may weaken the nails.
- Eat right.
- Use hand and nail cream.
- Keep your nails trimmed and repair broken nails.

### First-Aid Tips for a Broken or Torn Nail

- Apply antibiotic ointment to the torn area.
- Use tape or a bandage to hold the loose nail down.
- Don't remove the nail unless it's about to fall off.

can also develop. Use nail clippers to trim the hangnail close to the skin surface, apply antibiotic ointment and protect the area with a bandage. Hangnails usually heal in a few days.

**Infected nails.** Infection with bacteria or fungi can cause nail problems that need treatment. A bacterial infection under the nail or of the skin around the nail may occur following nail injury or the removal of a hangnail. Signs include redness and pain in the area and a whitish-yellow to greenish discoloration under the nails. This discoloration is caused by pus. The area may need to be opened and drained. Treatment with an antibiotic, in the form of pills (p. 618) or skin ointment, usually takes care of the infection.

Symptoms of a fungal infection under the nail include a white, brown or yellow nail discoloration. The nail thickens and eventually softens and weakens. Sometimes, the nail may tear away from the nail bed or become deformed. Several nails may be infected at the same time. Fungal infection is often caused by infection from another part of the body. Infection of the skin around the nail can cause redness, pain and swelling in the area. A cheese-like pus may build up under the skin.

Treatment of fungal infections usually begins with an antifungal (p. 615) ointment applied to the infected area. You may need to take an oral antifungal medicine as well. These infections can be difficult to cure and may require treatment for four to six months for fingernails, or 12 to 18 months for toenails. Removal of the nail reduces the length of treatment. Nail removal can be done when only one to two nails are infected. Fungal infections tend to come back, so watch your nails closely.

**Ingrown toenail.** An *ingrown toenail* occurs when a corner of the nail gets trapped under the skin. It can cause pain, redness and swelling at the edge of a toenail. The most common cause of ingrown toenails is clipping the nail too short, so that its corner gets trapped under the skin fold. An ingrown toenail can also form when someone steps or jumps on your toe, smashing the nail into the skin edge. As the nail continues to grow, a broken or trapped piece pushes under the skin. Ingrown nails also may result when you stub your toe, have an infection around the edge of your nail, wear poorly fitting shoes or have a nail that regrows in a deformed shape following nail removal.

Soaking the toe in warm, soapy water or an Epsom-salt (p. 615) solution will help the area drain, as well as soften the nail. Antibiotic ointment or pills can heal most infections of the toe. Regardless of the treatment, the skin will stay red and irritated until the nail edge is removed from under the skin. This can be done in your doctor's office under local anesthesia. Chronic ingrown nails may need to be partly or completely removed.

To avoid ingrown nails, wear properly fitting shoes and don't cut your nails too short.

**Injured nails.** Whether on the finger or the toe, a torn nail can cause pain and discomfort. Nails are designed to protect the tips of the fingers and toes. When they're missing, fingers or toes are vulnerable and will be more tender if squeezed, pinched or hit. After a nail has been torn or damaged, you usually shed the torn pieces and grow a new, healthy nail to replace the injured one.

Soak the injured nail in soapy water or an Epsom-salt solution to reduce the chance for infection. If part of the nail is about to fall off and cutting doesn't cause discomfort, remove any pieces you can. Otherwise, apply antibiotic ointment to the area and use

## Home Treatments for Ingrown Toenails

- Soak the foot with the ingrown nail daily.
- Place a small piece of cotton under the nail edge on the tender side.
- Wear comfortable, loose-fitting shoes and two pairs of socks when playing sports such as basketball or tennis.
- If an injury breaks the nail, soak it and gently try to remove any broken pieces. You may need help from your doctor.
- Use an antibiotic ointment on an infected nail edge.
- Don't cut your nails too short. Cut the nail straight across to keep the newly cut edge from splitting off and growing into the skin.

tape or a bandage to hold down the loose pieces to prevent them from being torn off. Don't remove the nail unless it's about to fall off.

## Pigeon Toes

- Feet that point inward

When the feet point inward, the condition is known as *pigeon toes.* This can be caused by abnormalities in the foot bones, the thigh bone (*femur*) or the shin bone (*tibia*). It's very common. Most often it occurs in infants. The feet straighten without treatment by the time the child is two to three years old. Pigeon toes usually don't cause major problems. Calluses (p. 258) may cause some pain after the child begins to walk because the outer part of the foot may rub against shoes.

### Testing and Treatment

Your doctor will probably want to perform an exam and may want to take x-rays to find out which bone abnormalities are causing the problem.

Treatment usually isn't required, and the problem goes away on its own. Rarely, the feet will need to be immobilized in casts. If casting is used, the casts are worn on both feet for two to four months. The casts are changed periodically as the feet straighten. The abnormalities are usually corrected after two or three cast changes.

## Plantar Fasciitis

- Heel pain or pain on the bottom of the foot when weight is put on it

Jumping repeatedly or from an unsafe height can bruise the bones in the bottom of your feet and stretch or tear the connective tissue of the arch, called the *plantar fascia.* The strong fibrous bands of the plantar fascia hold the bones together. Repeated injury to the plantar fascia can cause inflammation, called *plantar fasciitis.*

## Club Foot

Club foot occurs when bones in a child's foot aren't properly formed, resulting in the foot being set at an unusual angle. The foot may appear deformed, either turning sharply inward, upward or downward. Club foot usually involves at least several bones. It won't go away on its own. Treatment should start as soon as the problem is discovered.

Treatment involves using casts to help correct the alignment of the foot and its bones. New casts replace old casts as improvement is made. Special shoes can also be helpful. Treatment times vary from six months to two years. The later the treatment is started, the longer it will take. Sometimes surgery is needed in addition to casting.

More gradual damage to the arch comes from wearing shoes with poor arch supports during a strenuous activity or when walking for long periods of time on hard surfaces. Pain and trouble walking sometimes occur after the activity is over. Heel spurs (p. 260) may sometimes be the result of plantar fasciitis.

### Testing and Treatment

X-rays of the foot aren't usually needed, but they may help determine the source of the pain and rule out other bone or joint problems. Treatment may include rest, ice packs, oral anti-inflammatory medicines (p. 615) and corticosteroid (p. 622) injections into the tender area. Keeping your foot raised when you're sitting may be helpful. You may also want to use a heel pad in your shoe.

### Prevention

Buy shoes that fit properly and provide good arch support. Special supports for your shoes can be designed to help reduce stress on the arch of the foot and thus reduce the occurrence of plantar fasciitis.

## Ulcer of the Foot

* A nonhealing but usually painless break in the skin

Foot ulcers are almost always found in people who have damaged nerves or blood vessels in the feet. For example, foot ulcers are common in people with diabetes (p. 211), which can damage the nerves and blood vessels in the feet, or when blood flow to the feet is reduced, such as may occur with atherosclerosis (p. 111).

This causes skin damage to heal very slowly or not at all.

### Testing and Treatment

The first step in treating foot ulcers is to search for any underlying health problems that might cause sores that don't heal well. If areas of the feet are numb but there are no signs of disease, then the ulcer may be related to nerve damage. Your doctor may recommend a variety of blood, urine and nerve conduction tests (p. 638) to determine the cause.

Treatment depends on the source of the problem. For example, keeping your blood sugar levels under control if you have diabetes will help. Surgery may be a last resort if medicine doesn't help.

### Prevention

If you have diabetes or if you have nerve damage to your foot or lower leg, it's important to practice good foot care. Wear properly fitting shoes and avoid damage or injury to your feet. Don't cut your toenails too short and cut them straight across. Ingrown toenails can become infected and cause ulcers. Examine your feet daily and promptly treat any sores. Inform your doctor when an infection lasts longer than a few days.

# Photographic Guide to Symptoms

## Eye Disorders

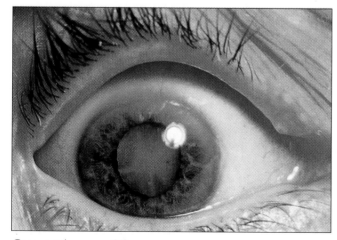

**Normal Eye** *(see page 62)*

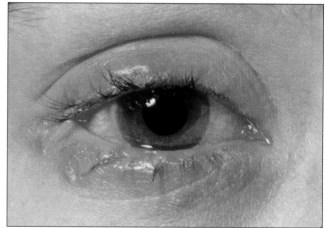

**Blepharitis** *(see page 64)*

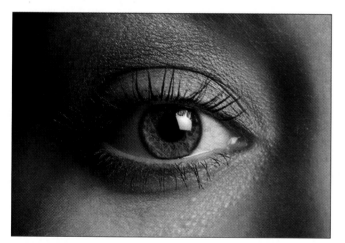

**Cataract** *(see page 64)*

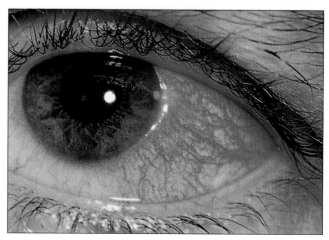

**Corneal Abrasion** *(see page 68)*

# EYE DISORDERS *(continued)*

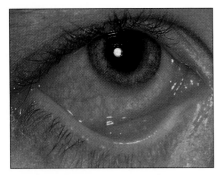

**Conjunctivitis** *(see page 71)*

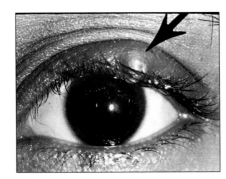

**Stye** *(see page 74)*

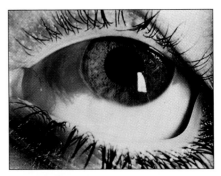

**Subconjunctival Hemorrhage** *(see page 74)*

## *Eyelid Lumps*

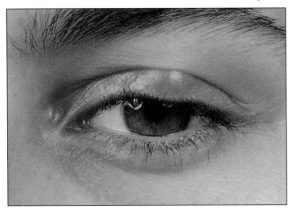

**Chalazion** *(see page 66)*

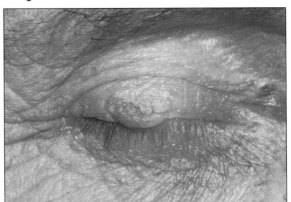

**Papillomas** *(see page 66)*

# MOUTH DISORDERS

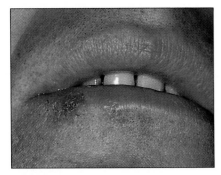

**Cold Sore** *(see page 94)*

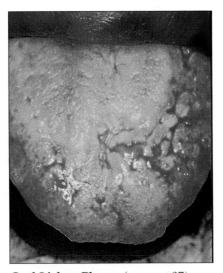

**Oral Lichen Planus** *(see page 97)*

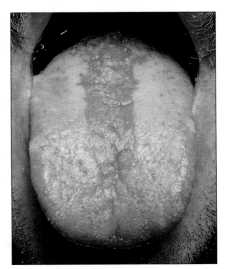

**Thrush** *(see page 98)*

# MOUTH DISORDERS *(continued)*

## *Infection of the Gums*

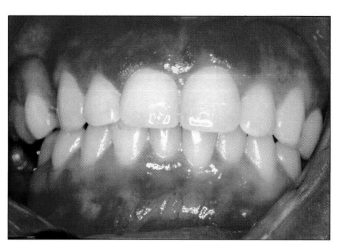

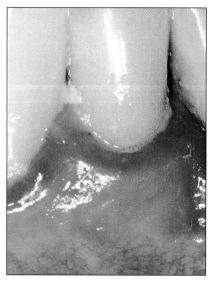

**Gingivitis** *(see page 96)*

**Periodontitis** *(see page 96)*

# SKIN DISORDERS

## *Birthmarks*

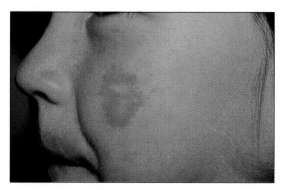

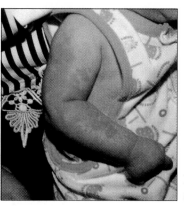

**Strawberry Hemangioma** *(see page 275)*

**Cavernous Hemangioma** *(see page 275)*

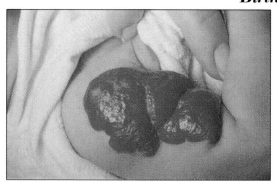

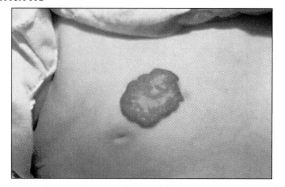

**Salmon Patch** *(see page 276)*

**Port-wine Stain** *(see page 275)*

# SKIN DISORDERS *(continued)*

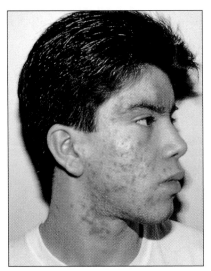

**Acne** *(see page 274)*

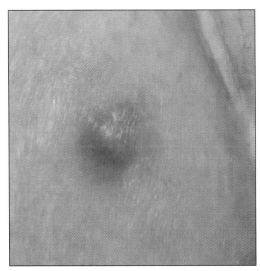

**Boil** *(see page 276)*

## *Dermatitis*

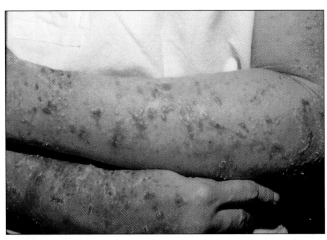

**Poison Ivy** *(see page 277)*

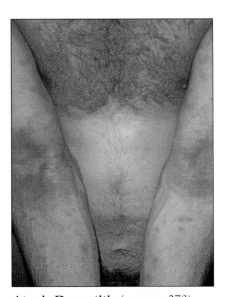

**Atopic Dermatitis** *(see page 278)*

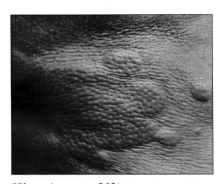

**Hives** *(see page 282)*

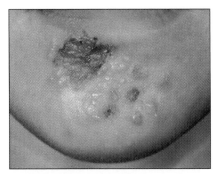

**Impetigo** *(see page 283)*

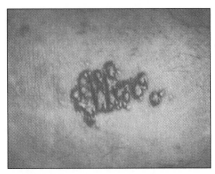

**Lichen Planus** *(see page 284)*

# SKIN DISORDERS *(continued)*

## *Lumps & Bumps*

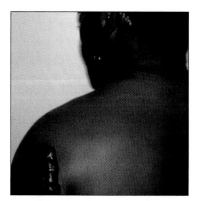

**Keloid** *(see page 285)*

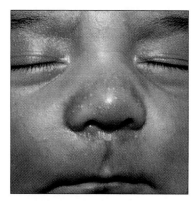

**Milia** *(see page 285)*

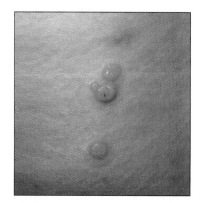

**Molluscum Contagiosum** *(see page 285)*

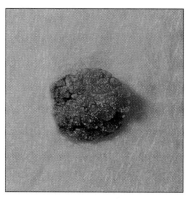

**Seborrheic Keratosis** *(see page 286)*

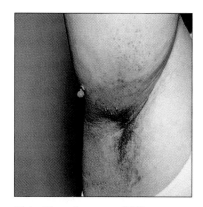

**Skin Tags** *(see page 286)*

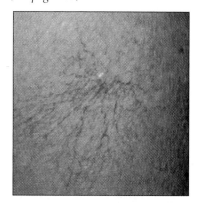

**Spider Angioma** *(see page 286)*

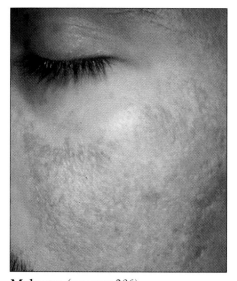

**Melasma** *(see page 286)*

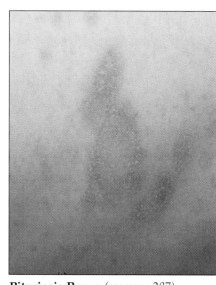

**Pityriasis Rosea** *(see page 287)*

# SKIN DISORDERS *(continued)*

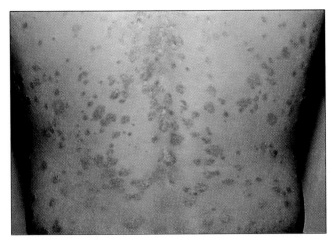

**Psoriasis** *(see page 288)*

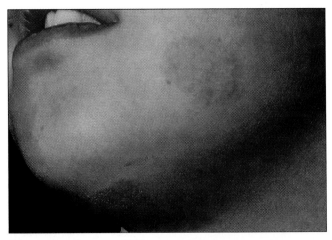

**Ringworm** *(see page 289)*

## *Skin Cancer*

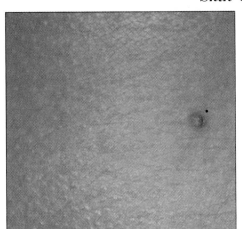

**Normal Mole** *(see page 287)*

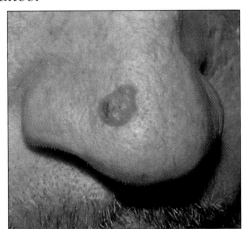

**Basal Cell Carcinoma** *(see page 290)*

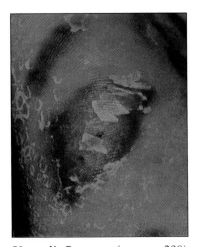

**Kaposi's Sarcoma** *(see page 290)*

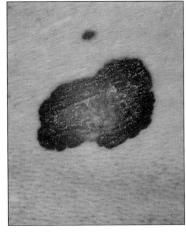

**Malignant Melanoma**
*(see page 290)*

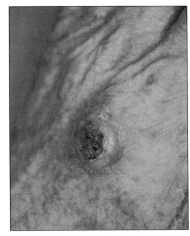

**Squamous Cell Carcinoma**
*(see page 291)*

# SKIN DISORDERS *(continued)*

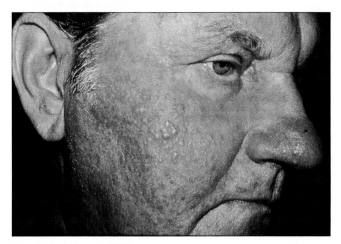

**Rosacea** *(see page 289)*

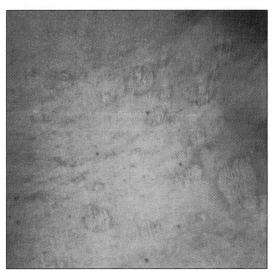

**Tinea Versicolor** *(see page 292)*

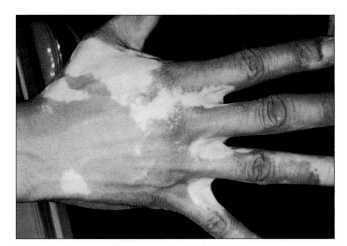

**Vitiligo** *(see page 293)*

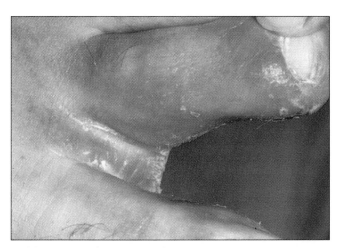

**Athlete's Foot** *(see page 256)*

# INFECTIONS

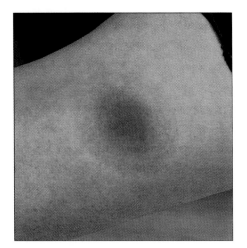

**Lyme Disease Rash** *(see page 301)*

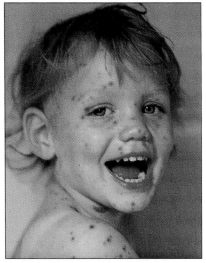

**Chickenpox** *(see page 321)*

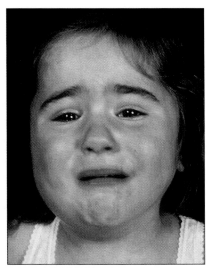

**Mumps** *(see page 329)*

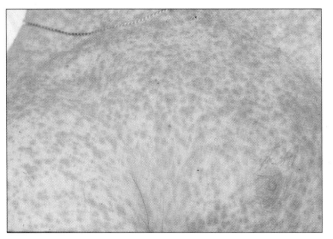

**Measles** *(see page 327)*

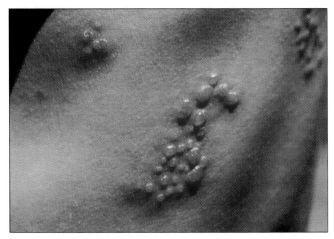

**Shingles** *(see page 331)*

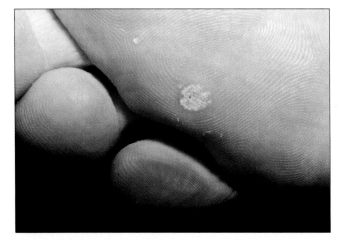

**Plantar Wart** *(see page 332)*

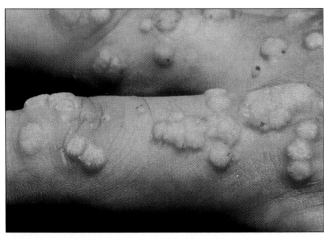

**Warts on Fingers** *(see page 332)*

# CHAPTER 17

# SKIN AND HAIR

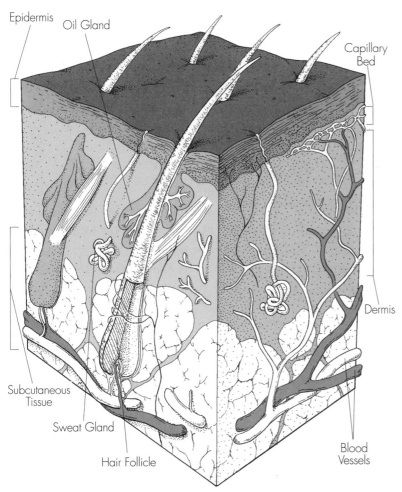

Epidermis
Oil Gland
Capillary Bed
Dermis
Subcutaneous Tissue
Sweat Gland
Hair Follicle
Blood Vessels

**SKIN (CROSS SECTION)**

Skin and hair aren't just for decoration. The skin is your body's largest organ and serves many essential functions. For example, it acts as the first line of defense against injury and invasion from bacteria, viruses, fungi and parasites.

The temperature of the body is partly controlled by the skin because blood vessels and *capillaries* (tiny blood vessels) in your skin expand *(dilate)* or shrink *(constrict)* in response to your body's need to reduce or raise its temperature. When you're hot, your blood vessels expand to give off heat, and you sweat. Then the moisture on your skin evaporates to make you cooler. When you're cold, the blood vessels shrink to slow down the flow of blood to your skin. This reduces your body's heat loss and saves the heat for the main part of your body.

The skin also conserves fluid and allows the fluid balance in your body to be maintained. Nerves in your skin give you the sense of touch by sending messages to your brain.

Your skin is made up of three layers of different types of cells. The top layer, the skin that we see, is called the *epidermis*. The middle layer is the *dermis* and the lower layer is *subcutaneous tissue*. The epidermis is made of fibers called *collagen* and *elastin,* which make your skin strong and elastic. Blood vessels, muscle cells, nerve fibers, hair follicles and glands are in the dermis. The epidermis is constantly making new skin cells to replace the old skin cells as they die and wash off or flake off.

The subcutaneous tissue is the layer of your skin closest to your muscles and organs. It's made mostly of fat. Blood vessels and nerves run through it, and the roots of your skin's oil and sweat glands are also there.

### Acne Quick List

- Wash your face twice a day with an acne soap.
- Use over-the-counter medicine to help acne heal.
- Don't squeeze, pick or pop pimples.
- Don't wear makeup that irritates the skin.
- Don't overdo sun exposure.
- See your doctor, who may prescribe medicines to help treat acne.

The hair on your body helps make your skin more sensitive and provides some protection for your body. For example, your hair helps protect you from sunburn. Hair grows from a hair *follicle* (a sac-like structure) that has roots in the subcutaneous tissue layer of your skin. Oil from the oil glands, which are also in the subcutaneous tissue, makes your hair somewhat glossy. The hair follicles are nourished by minerals, proteins, vitamins, fats and carbohydrates that are brought to them by the capillaries.

## Acne

- Pimples on the face, chest, neck and back, usually beginning in adolescence
- Blackheads
- Whiteheads
- Occasionally, large cysts

*See photo of acne, page 268.*

Hormonal changes that begin in adolescence are a major cause of *acne.* Levels of sex hormones, called *androgens,* increase in both sexes during teen years. The rise in the hormone levels makes the skin produce more oil, or *sebum.* This sebum can mix with skin cells to form a sticky plug that blocks the hair follicles. These blocked follicles can become infected with bacteria that live on the skin.

A *whitehead* forms when a follicle is plugged with sebum and skin cells. If the plug of sebum and skin cells comes to the surface of your skin and air touches it, it turns black. This is a *blackhead.* If the side of the follicle breaks near the surface of the skin, the area will turn red—a *pimple.* If the side of the follicle breaks further beneath the skin, a *nodule,* or *cyst,* may form. The pimples and nodules can become infected with bacteria that live on the

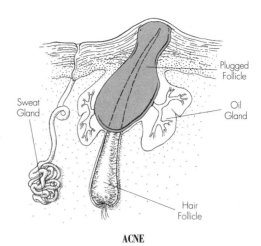

**ACNE**

skin. *Cystic acne* is the type of acne that's most likely to lead to scarring.

Acne usually begins during adolescence and may continue until the late teens or early 20s. Male hormone production may prolong the problem until the late 20s or longer.

### Treatment

A number of medical treatments are available for acne. Oral antibiotics have been used for years to prevent the infections that lead to facial scarring. Lotions, creams or gels with ingredients such as benzoyl peroxide, tretinoin and isotretinoin help prevent infection, dissolve the oily clogs in the hair follicles and speed up the healing process. Isotretinoin can be used for severe cystic acne but must not be used one month before pregnancy or during pregnancy, because of the risk of serious birth defects. Keep in mind that treatment will take about two months before you'll notice an improvement.

Acne is often made worse by our attempts to help the situation. Squeezing, popping or lancing pimples may spread or worsen the infection. Bacteria on your hands can easily spread the infection. Gentle washing with soap and water, use of over-the-counter acne preparations for cleaning and drying the skin, and keeping your hands away from your face are the best self-treatments and the best means of preventing further infections. Talk to your doctor for help with mild or severe acne.

## Bedsores

- Large skin ulcers in bedridden and paralyzed people that can become infected, most commonly on shoulders, elbows, lower back, hips, knees, ankles and heels

People who are bedridden, confined to a chair or paralyzed are most likely to suffer from *bedsores*, also called *decubitus ulcers*. They may not be able to turn frequently to relieve pressure on bony areas like the hips and heels. In addition, they may be thin and weak, with less fat and muscle padding the bones. Bedsores can develop on the shoulder blades, elbows, lower back, hips, ankles and heels.

Malnutrition, anemia and infection may contribute to the development of bedsores. Lying or sitting on wrinkled sheets and clothing, and wet skin from perspiration or urinary incontinence, add to the problem. An early warning sign of bedsores is redness of the skin where pressure is placed while sitting or lying in bed.

### Treatment
The pressure must be relieved before the sore can heal. You can help relieve the pressure by using a waterbed, air-filled mattress or egg-crate mattress, and changing positions at least twice an hour. After relieving the pressure, clean the sore frequently as instructed by your doctor and use topical or oral antibiotics (p. 618) as prescribed. Surgery may be needed to cover the sore with healthy skin.

### Prevention
If you care for someone who's bedridden and unable to move, be sure to change his or her position twice an hour. Help wheelchair-bound people change their position every 10 to 15 minutes. Put pillows between the knees and under the shoulders and use protective padding, such as sheepskin on the bed, to help relieve pressure. Certain types of mattresses or waterbeds may help. Wash the skin regularly and make sure that it stays dry.

Learn the early warning signs of bedsores and be sure to check the skin every day in good light. Look for red areas that stay red when the pressure is taken off. This is one of the first signs of bedsores.

## Birthmarks

- Discoloration of the skin present at birth

The skin of a newborn child may have areas of discoloration, called *birthmarks*. Birthmarks are common and often disappear as the child grows.

*See photo of hemangiomas, page 267.*

**Hemangioma.** This is a noncancerous tumor under the skin. The tumor consists of blood vessels. It's bright red and raised. A *strawberry hemangioma* appears on the face, back or chest. It may grow quickly after the child is about two months old, stay at one size for a while and then shrink. A *cavernous hemangioma* may be reddish-blue and deeper in the skin than the strawberry hemangioma. Large cavernous hemangiomas or those inside organs or on the neck may require treatment with lasers, surgery or radiation.

Another form of hemangioma is the *port-wine stain*. It consists of dilated capillaries, or tiny blood vessels. Port-wine stains usually appear as red or brown stains on the skin. They usually don't go away on their own. Laser therapy can be used to remove the color from the port-wine stain when a child reaches adolescence. Large areas of the body may be affected with this type of hemangioma.

*See photo of salmon patch, page 267.*

**Salmon patches.** Found on one-third of all newborns, these patches become brighter when the child is crying. They most commonly occur on the eyelids, between the eyebrows and on the back of the neck. Most will fade with time, although some on the neck persist. Treatment isn't usually needed.

## Boils and Carbuncles

* Large, red, tender lumps or swellings under the skin, often filled with pus

*See photo of boil, page 268.*

A *boil* is the result of your body's attempt to defend itself against an infection. The infection usually is caused by staphylococcal (p. 305) bacteria. A boil can grow rapidly, as white or yellowish pus collects under the skin. It usually will come to a "head," then burst, drain and heal. Boils are most commonly located on the neck, breasts, face, legs and buttocks. The good thing about boils: Your body is usually able to fight off the infection.

A cluster of boils that results in a deeper infection is called a *carbuncle.* Carbuncles are almost always found on the back of the neck below the hairline. They're more common in men than women.

### Treatment

Never squeeze a boil that isn't draining by itself. Most boils eventually drain on their own. You can speed up the process by applying warm, moist compresses or soaking the area in warm water for 20 minutes three or four times a day. After the boil has softened, gently scrub away the top of the boil. If it starts to drain, gently squeeze out the pus. Apply an antibiotic ointment after the boil has opened and is draining. Continue to soak the area or apply warm compresses three to four times a day.

See your doctor right away if the boil is on your face, if it's large and extremely tender or if redness increases around the boil. Never squeeze a pimple or boil on your face, because this can spread infection and make it worse.

An antibiotic (p. 618) taken by mouth isn't usually needed for small boils. When a large boil or carbuncle is present, an antibiotic may reduce the spread of infection into the surrounding tissues. Recurrent boils or carbuncles may be a sign of a more severe medical problem, such as diabetes (p. 211) or an immune-deficiency disorder (p. 221).

### Prevention

Good hygiene can reduce the chance of getting boils and carbuncles. Wash thoroughly after exercise and dry well after bathing or swimming. The germs that cause boils multiply in hot, sweaty environments. Be sure clothing, towels, linens and other personal articles are washed. Don't share unwashed items with anyone. Watch out, too, for chairs or benches in locker rooms that come in contact with bare skin.

## Cellulitis

* Red, tender, swollen areas of skin, often around a cut or scrape

Red, warm skin surrounding a cut, wound or bite may indicate the beginning of an infection of the skin called *cellulitis.* Once bacteria are introduced into the skin, they may spread through the tissues, destroying them. The warmth, redness and swelling are all part of the body's fight against the invading bacteria.

Diseases that lower your immune system's effectiveness, such as diabetes (p. 211), allow simple cuts, scrapes or puncture wounds to turn into life-threatening infections. If you have diabetes, any red, swollen or tender skin should be checked right away by your doctor.

Possible complications of cellulitis include the spreading of the infection into the bloodstream or the lymph channels, and death of the skin, called gangrene (p. 300).

### Treatment

Cellulitis can be very serious, spreading quickly into the deeper tissues. Heat and antibiotic lotions or ointments (p. 615) may stop a small area of infection. Larger areas of infection or rapidly spreading redness should be seen right away by your doctor. Oral antibiotics (p. 618) might kill the infection, but you may have to be admitted to the hospital for intravenous antibiotics to prevent gangrene or spread of the infection into the bloodstream. It's especially important to treat cellulitis around the eyes aggressively, usually with intravenous antibiotics in the hospital.

### Prevention

Treat any wound promptly. Carefully cleanse it with soap and water. Apply an antibiotic ointment. Cover the wound with an adhesive bandage if it's in an area that's likely to get dirty or be injured again. Puncture wounds, such as those caused by a nail, should be soaked for about 10 minutes in a soapy water solution. Your doctor may also recommend a tetanus shot (p. 11). When you first notice redness or tenderness around a cut or scrape, apply warm compresses and then an antibiotic ointment.

## Dandruff

- Flaking and itching of the scalp in spite of frequent shampooing

Skin cells are constantly growing and flaking off. You don't notice the shedding from most of your skin, but the flakes from your scalp tend to clump together and form *dandruff*. The flaking and itching of dandruff isn't a serious problem, but it can be a nuisance. If you get patches of scaly, itchy skin on your face or scalp despite using dandruff shampoos, you may have seborrhea (p. 289).

### Treatment

Over-the-counter dandruff shampoos (p. 616) can usually cure and prevent future dandruff problems. Switch shampoos if one product doesn't work or stops working after you have used it for awhile. Be sure to follow the directions on the bottle. Many products recommend that you lather twice and leave the second lather on your hair for five minutes before rinsing.

## Dermatitis

- Red, swollen skin
- Tiny blisters that leak moisture, then break and become crusted
- Intense itching

*Dermatitis* is a form of skin inflammation, or swelling. The skin turns red, swells, oozes, crusts and becomes scaly and itchy. There are many types of dermatitis. *Eczema* is a type of dermatitis.

**Allergic contact dermatitis.** Sometimes an allergic reaction may occur on your skin. The result is an itchy, red rash. The rash that follows exposure to poison ivy, poison oak or poison sumac is an example of an allergic reaction to the oil in those plants. Other common causes of allergic contact dermatitis include nickel (a metal used in jewelry),

---

*Signs of Spreading Infection*

- Fever, aches or chills
- Redness spreading to the surrounding skin
- Streaks of red going up the arm or leg
- Swelling

*See your doctor right away if you have any of these signs.*

fragrances, formaldehyde and other chemicals in detergents, shampoos and cosmetics. See page 221 for more information about allergies.

It can take up to 48 hours for contact dermatitis to appear after you've been exposed to something that makes you break out in a rash. You can often treat allergic contact dermatitis yourself. Over-the-counter antihistamines (p. 615) or anti-itch lotions (p. 615) can relieve your symptoms. Hydrocortisone cream (p. 616) may help, but read the label carefully—don't use it longer than recommended. If the rash doesn't get better, see your doctor.

*See photo of atopic dermatitis, page 268.*

**Atopic dermatitis.** This type of dermatitis causes intense itching. It's sometimes called "the itch that rashes," because it starts with itching and when you scratch the itch, the scratching causes the rash to appear. The rash often appears on the face, especially in infants and young children, in the folds of the inner elbow and behind the knee.

Atopic dermatitis often starts in childhood and is most common in people who have allergies or asthma, or a family history of these problems. Most children with atopic dermatitis outgrow it.

Food may play a role in causing atopic dermatitis. Some common possible food causes are eggs, peanuts, milk and fish. If you suspect a food may be causing your outbreak, avoid eating that food until the rash clears. Reintroduce the food into your diet later as a test. If you get a rash again, chances are good that food item is the cause of the rash.

**Dermatitis herpetiformis.** This form of dermatitis produces intense itching and recurring clumps of blisters on the buttocks, shoulders, elbows, knees and, sometimes, the face and neck. The cause is unknown. Treatment is possible with special medicines.

**Dyshidrotic dermatitis.** Dyshidrotic dermatitis is marked by deep itchy blisters that appear on the palms, the sides of the fingers and the soles of the feet. The cause is unknown. It's most common in people under age 40. It generally starts suddenly and lasts a few weeks, but it may occur again and again. High-strength prescription corticosteroid creams (p. 622) are usually used to treat it.

---

## Protecting Your Skin if You Get a Rash

- Keep fingernails clipped short so they can't damage your skin when you scratch. If needed, put mittens or gloves on young children at night, so they don't scratch while they're sleeping.
- Use a moisturizer frequently, at least once a day. Choose a product that doesn't contain fragrance, alcohol or lanolin, all of which can increase itching. Always apply the moisturizer after bathing or showering.
- Take lukewarm, not hot, showers or baths.
- Use a nonsoap cleanser (p. 615) or a gentle soap cleanser.
- Don't use a washcloth. It's abrasive and irritates the skin. Use your hands or a soft sponge instead.

- Take a shower or bath after swimming to remove all the chlorine and other chemicals from your skin and hair.
- Use a sunscreen with an SPF of at least 15 to protect your skin from sunburn.
- Avoid sudden temperature changes, which can irritate your skin.
- Be sure to wash new clothes before you wear them to remove any irritating chemicals.
- Use a mild laundry detergent and rinse clothes twice.
- Choose loose clothing made of breathable fabrics like cotton. Avoid wool or other scratchy materials.

**Irritant contact dermatitis.** This form of dermatitis causes an itchy, red rash that results from contact with a chemical or other substance. It isn't caused by an allergy, like allergic contact dermatitis is.

The two types of dermatitis look different. Irritant contact dermatitis has indistinct borders and a scaly looking rash. It often occurs on the hands because the hands most often come into contact with irritants. Allergic contact dermatitis usually has a distinct border and oozing blisters.

Although a single exposure to a substance may cause irritant contact dermatitis, this type of dermatitis more often occurs after prolonged and repeated exposures. Soaps, industrial solvents and topical medicines are some of the common causes. Chemical solutions used in the workplace can be a cause. Some people are so sensitive to workplace chemicals that they have to change jobs.

**Nummular dermatitis.** Nummular dermatitis is named for its coin-shaped patches of red, swollen blisters. "Nummular" means shaped like a coin. The blisters usually appear on the legs. It's most common in middle-aged people and is associated with dry skin.

### Testing

Your doctor will probably diagnose dermatitis based on the appearance of the rash and your medical history. A skin biopsy is rarely needed, but samples of your skin may be taken by scraping the area of the rash. The skin samples are examined under a microscope to make sure you don't have a fungal infection. You'll probably be asked about your exposure to possible allergens and irritants. Skin patch testing (p. 641) can be performed when contact with different substances appears to aggravate the rash. After the

> ### *Relieving the Itch*
> - Use cool compresses. Dip a clean cloth in cool water or even whole milk, and put the cloth on the rash for 10 to 15 minutes every hour. Use compresses only on a rash with weeping or oozing blisters to dry it out.
> - Take a soaking bath. Add a cup of baking soda or colloidal oatmeal bath treatment to lukewarm bath water.

irritating agent is identified, it can be avoided, or the skin can be protected from exposure to the substance.

### Treatment

Don't scratch! Scratching will only make dermatitis worse. Also, keep your skin moist. If you have dermatitis, your doctor may prescribe some type of corticosteroid cream. But long-term use of very potent corticosteroid creams may have side effects. Mild over-the-counter hydrocortisone cream should be safe for occasional use. Taking antihistamines can also help reduce the intense itching.

Don't use over-the-counter ointments or creams that have names that end in "-caine." These can make dermatitis worse and may cause an allergic reaction. So can antihistamine sprays or creams.

Unfortunately, when the skin is irritated by a rash, a bacterial infection may also start. If blisters form, if the rash gets very red or if you have a fever, you may have a secondary bacterial infection and need an oral antibiotic (p. 618).

### Prevention

Avoid exposure to harsh chemicals. Protect your skin from liquid chemicals or dry chemical dust. If possible, wear vinyl gloves when you work with chemicals—cotton liners will help absorb sweat.

## Dry Skin

- Itching, flaking and scaling of the skin

Itchy, dry skin can be miserable. It often gets worse during the cold winter months, and it gets worse as you get older.

### Treatment

Petroleum jelly (p. 617) is the most effective skin moisturizer, but you may not find it pleasant to use during the day. Choose a skin moisturizer that you like and will use frequently. Remember, just because a moisturizer costs more doesn't mean it works better. You're paying for packaging and marketing.

A moisturizer is most effective if applied just after showering or bathing. Pat, don't rub, yourself dry using a soft towel. Then apply the moisturizer while your skin is still damp to seal in moisture. Moisturizers with fragrance or color may irritate sensitive, dry skin.

Don't take long, hot showers or baths. Keep the water warm, not hot. Soap is extremely drying to skin, so use soap only where needed. For example, use soap on hands, face, armpits and groin area. But don't suds up your arms, legs and back to avoid drying.

Protect your hands from harsh household cleaners by wearing vinyl gloves when you're using cleansers and washing dishes. Be sure to wear gloves or mittens outdoors during cold weather.

## Excessive Sweating

- Sweating more than seems normal

Excessive sweating may be limited to the palms, armpits, groin or soles of the feet, or it can be all over the body. The cause can vary. Excessive sweating may be caused by a hormonal disorder, such as hyperthyroidism (p. 215), a central nervous system problem, a fever or being overweight.

Your doctor may want to check for a medical problem. If one is present, treatment may help relieve the perspiration problem. If no specific cause is found, antiperspirants with aluminum compounds may be helpful. Your doctor may prescribe a solution to rub on your palms and soles.

To prevent odor, stay clean. Shower or bathe often and use an antiperspirant that contains aluminum. Shaving the armpit hair can also be helpful.

## Folliculitis

- Small, boil-like sores on the skin around a hair shaft

The hair shafts or the oil glands around them may become infected with bacteria. Small blisters or pustules form near one or several hair shafts. It's an infection of the hair follicle and most often occurs on the chest, arms, thighs or buttocks. The usual cause is staphylococcal bacteria. This infection is called *folliculitis*.

### Treatment

Your body is usually able to heal mild infections of the follicles by itself. Clean the area and wash any clothing or equipment that comes in contact with the infected skin to prevent re-infection. An over-the-counter antibiotic ointment (p. 615) may be helpful. In severe cases, you may need an oral antibiotic (p. 618) prescribed by your doctor. If your skin becomes red or swollen, see your doctor.

### Prevention

Good hygiene, cleaning surfaces exposed to skin—such as benches, hot tubs and saunas—and not touching skin infections on other people will help prevent spread of the infection.

## Hair Loss

### Alopecia Areata

- Sudden loss of hair in round patches on the scalp or other areas of the body

Sudden hair loss on the scalp, often in large amounts, occurs in *alopecia areata*. The hair comes out in patches, usually in areas the size of a dime or a quarter. Sometimes the hair loss is also on the face, with the loss of eyebrows and lashes, or even all over the body. When all the body hair is lost, the condition is called *alopecia universalis*.

The cause of alopecia areata is unknown, but it's suspected to be an autoimmune disorder (p. 223). The condition is most common in people under age 25.

### Male-Pattern Baldness

- Loss of hair, starting with thinning of hair on temples and crown, leading to various degrees of baldness

This type of baldness affects the hair on the crown of the head. Blame your genes if you have male-pattern baldness. It's more common among whites, and more than 50% of white men will have lost part of their scalp hair by age 50.

Women may also suffer from *hereditary alopecia*. They seldom go entirely bald, but have thinning of the hair along the scalp edge. The hair loss progresses slowly with age.

### Thinning Hair

- Thinning hair that rarely results in baldness

Thinning hair is the second most common cause of hair loss, next to male-pattern baldness. Generally, people have 100,000 or more hairs on their head. At any time, around 85% of those hairs are growing, or are in the *anagen* phase, which lasts three years. Around 15% are in the resting, or *telogen* phase, which lasts 100 days. After 100 days in the resting phase, the hairs fall out.

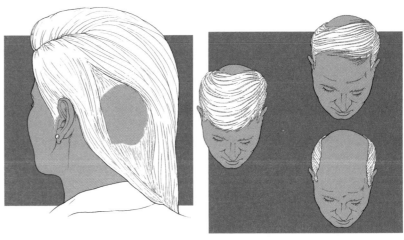

**ALOPECIA AREATA**    **MALE-PATTERN BALDNESS**

When something happens that upsets this balance, more hairs than usual enter the resting phase, and more than the normal 100 hairs a day are shed. Stress—physical or psychological—is the most common cause. Other causes include pregnancy, malnutrition, thyroid disorders, chemotherapy (p. 225), radiation therapy (p. 225) or medicines, such as birth control pills (p. 550), blood thinners (p. 619) and beta blockers (p. 621).

### Testing

If you suspect your hair loss is caused by something other than hereditary factors, talk to your doctor. You may be tested for possible disorders that could cause the baldness. Alopecia areata is diagnosed after other conditions are excluded. Your doctor may suggest a scalp biopsy to confirm the diagnosis.

Classic male-pattern baldness is the likely diagnosis in younger men who are becoming bald on the front and top of the scalp. Tests can be done to be sure a disease isn't present.

Older men and women can be reassured that their hair loss is probably genetic and not a medical problem. Testing is needed only if symptoms of a disease are present, or if the hair loss isn't typical.

### Treatment

Treatment depends on the cause of the hair loss. In alopecia areata, steroid creams or steroid injections into the scalp may speed the regrowth of lost hairs. Long-term steroid use should be avoided because of side effects. Recovery is hard to predict. In some cases, the disease disappears within five years, but it may occur again.

Thinning hair is often reversible once the underlying cause is discovered and treated.

There's no cure for hair loss due to male-pattern baldness, although one medicine, minoxidil (p. 625), promotes hair growth on the top of the scalp in some people. It's most effective in young men whose hair loss is recent, but months of treatment may pass before the hair growth begins. Minoxidil must be applied daily to maintain the hair growth and it's expensive. In some men, the medicine may not cause any hair growth.

There are no other medicines for baldness, so don't be taken in by false advertising claims. Millions of dollars are wasted each year on unproven remedies.

If you wish, you may conceal your hair loss with hairpieces, hair weaving or *hair transplants*, which involves moving parts of the scalp with hair to cover the areas without hair.

### Hirsutism

• Excessive hair growth, usually on the face and chest

This condition is often caused by an imbalance in hormones. It may appear at menopause in women, or in people who've been taking

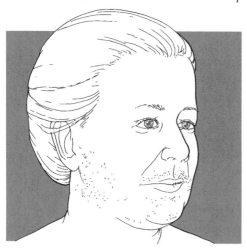

**HIRSUTISM**

steroids (p. 626) or certain antihypertensive medicines (p. 619). Hirsutism can also be caused by an ovarian tumor (p. 416) in women, but this is less common.

### Treatment

If possible, your doctor will treat the disorder that's causing the hair growth. Plucking, shaving, waxing and bleaching are temporary solutions that might be adequate. Electrolysis permanently removes the hair, but it's expensive and time-consuming.

### Hives

• Intense itching
• Raised or swollen bumps or patches on the skin

*See photo of hives, page 268.*

Hives can itch like crazy, but they're not like a rash. Instead, you'll notice swollen areas, or "wheals," which may be smaller than a dime or as large as a dinner plate. Each hive, or wheal, only lasts a few hours, but new ones constantly form until the cause of the reaction is treated or removed.

Hives are the result of blood plasma leaking into the skin. Just about anything can cause this reaction. Allergies (p. 221), especially to foods and medicines, may cause them. But so can stress, sunlight, cold, heat, exercise and fever. In many cases, you may not be able to figure out what triggered an outbreak of hives. Some people have outbreaks that last for months, or even years, or recur frequently.

### Testing

If you have long-lasting or recurring hives, your doctor may recommend allergy testing. Following a diet to identify possible food causes may help eliminate any foods that cause hives. Some common triggers are chocolate, shellfish, strawberries and nuts.

## Treatment

You can relieve some of the itching and misery of hives with home treatment. Don't scratch! Wear gloves to bed if you're afraid you'll scratch while sleeping. Antihistamines (p. 615) may be helpful. Put an ice pack on the affected area for five minutes, three to four times a day. Or try a wet cloth soaked in cold water or milk. Put it on the skin for 10 to 15 minutes. Add a cup of baking soda or oatmeal to lukewarm bath water and soak yourself in the tub. You can use a special oatmeal preparation that you can buy at the pharmacy or grind cooking oatmeal up in the blender so it'll dissolve better. Over-the-counter hydrocortisone cream (p. 616) generally doesn't make hives go away, but may relieve some of the itching.

Severe hives or recurrent attacks need a doctor's attention and treatment with prescription corticosteroids (p. 622) or antihistamines (p. 615). If the hives are part of anaphylactic shock (p. 222), you need to get medical attention right away. In rare cases, hives may be a symptom of another disease, such as a thyroid disorder, hepatitis (p. 204), systemic lupus erythematosus (p. 252) or some cancers.

## Prevention

If you know what causes the hives, avoid it. If stress is responsible, learn some stress-reduction methods (p. 572). The cause of hives is discovered in only 25% to 50% of cases.

## Impetigo

- Small, honey-colored, crusted sores around the nose, mouth or other areas of the skin

*See photo of impetigo, page 268.*

*Impetigo* is very contagious and is easily spread from one person (usually a child) to another. The honey-colored, crusted spots are caused by streptococcal (p. 306) or, rarely, staphylococcal (p. 305) bacteria that invade the skin. Impetigo isn't a serious medical problem if it's treated properly. Impetigo shouldn't be treated without consulting your doctor first.

## Treatment

Tests can be done on skin underneath one of the crusty spots to make sure the sores are impetigo. Testing isn't needed, however, when the sores have the typical appearance of impetigo. Early treatment with antibiotics (p. 618) can prevent impetigo's possible complications, which include swelling of the heart and kidney.

## Prevention

Regular hand washing can help prevent the spread of impetigo. Keep children with impetigo away from others, especially in a school or nursery setting. Because impetigo is usually very contagious, keep children out of school, day care or nurseries until the sores are dry and healed. Avoid sharing towels and washcloths with someone who has impetigo. Sometimes, a family pet can spread the infection if the pet has the bacteria in its mouth.

## Ingrown Hair

- A growing hair that's turned into the skin, causing swelling, pain or infection

Adults with thick, curly hair may get ingrown hairs on their scalp. Men can get them in their beard area as well. Ingrown hairs can also occur on shaved parts of the body, so they can be a problem for women who shave their legs as well as men who shave their faces. After the hair is shaved or cut, the stubble grows back into the skin because

---

### Get Medical Help

*Sometimes hives signal anaphylactic shock (p. 222), a rare but life-threatening allergic reaction. If you have the following symptoms, see your doctor or go to the emergency room right away:*

- Swelling of your face and throat
- Trouble breathing
- Hoarseness
- Red, itchy skin
- Dizziness
- Sense of impending doom

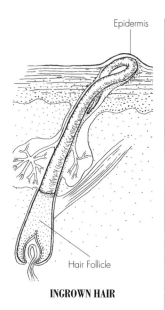

Epidermis

Hair Follicle

**INGROWN HAIR**

of a curl. Once in the skin, the tissue begins to swell, creating small lumps. Ingrown hairs occur more commonly among black people, especially in the beard area of black men.

### Treatment

Use tweezers to pluck the hair out of the skin. Leave the hair long enough so it can't grow back into the skin. Apply antiseptic to help prevent infection.

### Prevention

For men who have many ingrown facial hairs, growing a beard will usually prevent the problem. The beard also hides some of the scars caused by previous ingrown hairs. Removal of an ingrown hair may still be needed.

## Lichen Planus

• Purplish bumps with white lines on the back of the wrist, mid-back, lower legs and genitalia
• Lacy white spots in the mouth

***See photo of lichen planus, page 268.***

This is a mysterious rash. Doctors don't know what causes it, why it comes during the middle-aged years, why it lasts for weeks and why it leaves a brown mark on the skin after it disappears. Lichen planus occurs most often on the back of the wrists, the mid-back, the lower legs and the genitalia. It can affect the inside of the mouth and the fingernails as well.

Many cases of lichen planus are related to certain medicines, such as oral gold (p. 620) taken for rheumatoid arthritis, streptomycin and antimalarial medicines (p. 620). Other culprits include heavy metals and the chemicals used to develop film. When the irritation fades, a darkened area is left. The more you scratch the rash, the more discoloration will remain in your skin after the irritation leaves.

### Testing and Treatment

If needed, a skin biopsy can confirm the diagnosis. The rash may be treated with corticosteroid (p. 622) cream to reduce irritation and itching. Even with the cream, the rash may not improve or it may come back. Try to avoid the irritants that cause lichen planus.

## Lumps and Bumps

Swellings and lumps are a common reason for a child or an adult to see the doctor. The great majority of these bumps and lumps on the skin are noncancerous. They may have started with a skin infection that left a small, hard nodule. Some lumps are soft and movable, attached to the middle layers of the skin, and grow slowly for years. Other lumps are swollen lymph nodes under the jaw or on the sides of the neck that arise in response to a throat infection.

How can you tell if lumps are a serious problem? What are the warning signs of a dangerous lump or growth? A few simple guidelines can be followed. If the swelling comes and goes in a few hours or days, it's usually not serious and not cancer. If the lump is red, swollen and tender, an infection may be present that may need to be treated or drained by your doctor. The lump may be cancerous if it's firm, painless, strongly attached to the surrounding tissues, doesn't move when you press on it and continues to grow.

If you have an infection, a lymph node near the infection may swell. Lymph nodes swell in response to any infection, including viral infections. They may stay swollen for one to two weeks, then shrink back to their normal size. The faster a noninfectious lump grows, the sooner it should be checked by your doctor. All persistent, growing or tender lumps should be examined by your doctor.

Different types of lumps, bumps, skin tags and thickened or crusted areas may appear anywhere on your body. Many of these, like warts (p. 332), are noncancerous and can be left alone. But some of them may be early signs of skin cancer (p. 290).

Some of the most common noncancerous growths on the skin are described here.

**Actinic keratoses.** These are scaly, pink, gray or tan patches or bumps that appear on your face or scalp, or on the back of your hands. They appear mostly on people who have light skin that has been damaged by the sun. The patches start out feeling like sandpaper, then become hard and wart-like. Actinic keratoses are benign but may be an early warning of precancerous conditions on your skin.

See your doctor right away. Your doctor can freeze or burn away the patches, or use a cream, ointment or surgery to remove the patches. A piece of the patch may be tested for cancer.

*See photo of keloid, page 269.*

**Keloid.** A *keloid* is a scar that grows much larger than expected. It doesn't take much of a cut or puncture wound to produce enlarged scars in some people. A pierced ear, a small cut requiring two or three stitches or the scar of a surgical incision may be the beginning of these lumps. For an unknown reason, the scar heals but continues to produce extra scar tissue, creating a lump where a flat scar should be. Keloids aren't cancerous, but they're a cosmetic problem for many people. They're most common in blacks.

Laser surgery to remove the keloid can be tried, and injectable corticosteroids (p. 622) can be used during healing to reduce the formation of new keloids. But there's no guarantee that the keloid won't form again. In fact, the new one may be worse than the one removed by laser surgery.

**Lipoma.** This is a noncancerous growth that's soft and rubbery. It's usually made of mature fat cells and grows from the subcutaneous layer of your skin. Lipomas occur more often in women than men, and most often develop on the trunk of the body, the nape of the neck or the forearms, although they can crop up anywhere. Treatment isn't usually needed, but if a lipoma is bothering you, your doctor can remove it with surgery.

*See photo of milia, page 269.*

**Milia.** These small white bumps appear on the face of an infant in the first few weeks after birth. Milia has also been called "baby acne." The bumps disappear within a few weeks and don't need any treatment.

*See photo of molluscum contagiosum, page 269.*

**Molluscum contagiosum.** This is caused by a virus similar to the one that causes warts. The bumps are small, firm and round, with pits in the center. They're contagious and are most common in children and teens. Early treatment will help prevent the spread of these harmless but annoying bumps. Your doctor may drain the tiny white, hard center, which often allows the lesion to heal completely. Or your doctor may want to remove the bump surgically or by freezing it with liquid nitrogen.

**Sebaceous cysts.** These form when the oil gland at the base of a hair follicle becomes blocked with a thick, waxy material, preventing the oil from reaching the skin. As the oil continues to be produced, it collects in a cyst, or pocket, under the skin, forming a soft or hard knot that may have a whitish dome. These cysts are often found on the scalp, the nape of the neck and the upper back.

During the months or even years of blockage, the oil thickens and becomes waxy or cheesy. The cyst may rupture on its own, releasing a whitish material and irritating the skin. Although these cysts can be an unsightly problem, they don't become cancerous. To be safe, though, any change in a cyst should be checked by your doctor. If a cyst becomes large, inflamed or tender, grows rapidly or bothers you because it rubs against clothing, your doctor can remove it with surgery.

*See photo of seborrheic keratosis, page 269.*

**Seborrheic keratoses.** Also called senile warts, seborrheic keratoses may be smooth or warty-looking and often occur in middle-aged and elderly people. Their size varies, and they grow slowly. They may be flesh-colored, brown or black, and often arise on the trunk or temples. They aren't harmful and don't need treatment. If they itch, get irritated easily or bother you because of the way they look, your doctor can remove them with surgery or by freezing them with liquid nitrogen.

*See photo of skin tags, page 269.*

**Skin tags.** These small, soft, fleshy growths are found primarily on the face, neck, armpits and groin. They may be flesh-toned to dark brown. They usually cause no symptoms, but if they get irritated (from clothing, for example) or are bothersome because of appearance, your doctor can cut them off or freeze them with liquid nitrogen.

*See photo of spider angioma, page 269.*

**Spider angioma.** This bright red lesion has a center with thin, spider-leg-like branches. Women may develop them during pregnancy or while taking birth control pills (p. 550), but children and men may get them as well. If the way they look bothers you, your doctor can remove them using a technique called *fine-needle electrodesiccation.* This involves using an *electrocautery* device, which uses electricity to generate heat, with a very fine tip to scar the blood vessel.

**Xanthelasma.** These yellowish patches, or *plaques,* under the skin often appear in or near the eyelids. They are fatty deposits and can be removed by freezing them.

## Melasma

- Dark brown symmetrical patches on the forehead, cheeks and nose

*See photo of melasma, page 269.*

*Melasma,* or *chloasma,* is sometimes also called the "mask of pregnancy" because it can occur during pregnancy.

---

### See Your Doctor About a Skin Lump

- If the lump is red, swollen and tender. It may be infected and needs to be treated or drained by your doctor.
- If a nearby lymph node swells. Lymph nodes swell in response to any infection, including viral, and may stay swollen for several weeks.

- If the lump is firm, painless, strongly attached to the surrounding tissues and continues to grow or forms an ulcer.
- If the lump persists, grows or is tender.
- If the lump or bump ulcerates and won't heal or won't remain healed.

The dark-colored blotches may merge into a butterfly-shaped mask around the eyes. Melasma is most common during pregnancy, although women taking birth control pills (p. 550) or going through menopause (p. 407) may also get it. Changing the brand of birth control pills sometimes helps. Sun exposure can make it worse.

If you have melasma during pregnancy, it often goes away or fades after the baby is born. If not, your doctor may prescribe hydroquinone, which bleaches skin.

## Moles

- Roundish growths of pigmented skin that are darker than surrounding skin
- May be flat or raised, smooth or rough
- May contain hair

*See photo of a normal mole, page 270.*

A mole, often called a "beauty mark" when it's on the face, is a collection of cells that produce *melanin*, the pigment that gives your skin color. You probably weren't born with any moles, but by adulthood you might have 20 or more of them. Most moles aren't dangerous. Only a very few become cancerous. See page 290 for information on skin cancer.

### Treatment

Your doctor can surgically remove a mole that bothers you or that's unsightly. If skin cancer is suspected, the mole will be tested. See your doctor if you notice that a mole changes, grows, bleeds without reason or scabs over.

## Pityriasis Rosea

- Small, flat, tan or red circular patches that may appear all over the abdomen, chest, upper arms and legs

- A single large "herald" patch that usually appears a few days to two weeks before the other patches

*See photo of pityriasis rosea, page 269.*

The specific cause of *pityriasis rosea* is unknown, but it may be a virus. The condition goes away by itself without treatment. It occurs most often in adolescents or young adults. There may or may not be itching.

This peculiar rash often begins with a tan or red, slightly scaly patch, which is followed in a few days to two weeks by many more patches. The new patches are small, round to oval and red, have little scaling, and arise on the abdomen, back, upper arms and thighs. They may last from weeks to months. No treatment seems to shorten the duration of the rash. Most people have little or no itching with the rash.

### Treatment

Your doctor will look at the rash to be sure it's pityriasis rosea. A few tests may be needed to rule out other diseases that can cause a similar rash.

Oral antihistamines (p. 615), along with hydrocortisone cream (p. 616), can be used to relieve any itching. A cool compress or a soothing cream containing aloe can also help relieve the itch.

## Prickly Heat

- Itchiness
- Tiny blisters
- Redness

If your sweat ducts get blocked, sweat is trapped in your skin. This can cause irritation and itching—called *prickly heat*. It's most common in warm, humid weather. It usually lasts only a few days unless conditions that led to it aren't changed.

To relieve prickly heat, cool off. Wear light clothing that doesn't constrict movement. Stay dry. If needed, use an over-the-counter hydrocortisone cream (p. 616) for relief of itching.

## Psoriasis

* Pink, red or purple, raised, firm patches with silvery-white scaling and sharp edges, most often on elbows, knees or scalp
* Itching
* Pits and yellowish areas on the fingernails

*See photo of psoriasis, page 270.*

Of all the common skin rashes, psoriasis may be the most despised. It's uncomfortable and causes thickly scaled-over areas that range in color from pink to purple. These spots, which are called *plaques,* are usually found on the elbows, the nape of the neck, the scalp, the back, the knees and the elbows.

The cause is unknown. Psoriasis occurs when the skin cells—which normally grow, die and fall off—start to grow very quickly at the site of a psoriasis plaque. The more quickly the skin cells form, the thicker the lesion becomes. Stress or illness may make psoriasis worse.

By itself, the skin rash of psoriasis usually isn't serious. But in a few patients psoriatic arthritis can accompany the skin rash. The more severe the psoriasis, the more severe the arthritis can become.

Psoriasis is hereditary. About half of people who have psoriasis have a family history of the disease. It can appear at any age, but around one-third of people who have psoriasis develop it by age 20.

### Testing and Treatment

A skin biopsy (p. 640) can confirm psoriasis if the diagnosis is uncertain.

There's no cure for psoriasis, but treatment can decrease the severity of the disease. Hydrocortisone cream (p. 616) may help reduce swelling and redness, and may help slow the rapid growth of cells, but long-term use can cause side effects. Coal-tar creams and shampoos (p. 616) also seem to help. If over-the-counter products don't help, talk to your doctor about other options.

Some people who have psoriasis say they get better during the summer. Your doctor may recommend sunbathing in moderation, but a sunburn will only make psoriasis worse. Artificial ultraviolet light used at home or at a tanning salon in moderate amounts, as prescribed by your doctor, is another option.

PUVA is another treatment for psoriasis. With PUVA, a medicine that increases your sensitivity to the sun, called a *psoralen,* is combined with ultraviolet-A (UVA) rays. The UVA rays are longer than the ultraviolet-B (UVB) rays and can cause cataracts, skin cancer and premature aging of the skin. But used carefully, UVA light seems to slow the growth of skin cells and help control the plaques, especially when it's used with a psoralen.

Researchers are looking for new treatments. One medicine that has recently been approved is calcipotriene (p. 621). People with severe psoriasis may need to be hospitalized for intensive ultraviolet light therapy. Chemotherapy (p. 621) medicines may also be useful in treating psoriasis. After the psoriasis improves, treatments can be continued on an outpatient basis.

## Purpura

* Purplish-red marks on the skin that don't turn white when you press on them
* Any bruise in areas where the skin has been traumatized or injured

*Purpura* is the general name for bruises caused by blood under the skin.

Most of us have experienced bruises of various sizes, shapes, locations and tenderness. They usually heal without treatment or problems.

Other types of purpura that aren't caused by trauma occur in a few serious medical disorders. For example, a severe allergic reaction may destroy the body's ability to form blood clots, and bleeding into the skin occurs. This is called *thrombocytopenic purpura*. In this case, purpura may be caused by a serious blood disorder. If you notice that you get a lot of bruises for no reason, you should see your doctor right away for diagnosis and treatment.

## Ringworm

• Circular rash with raised borders

*See photo of ringworm, page 270.*

Ringworm, or *tinea capitis,* is caused by a fungal infection of the skin, not by a worm burrowing in a circle. It can occur anywhere on the skin, including the scalp, arms, abdomen, back and legs. The areas of ringworm are usually small.

Ringworm is contagious and can be passed from one person to another. Ringworm also can occur from touching a surface that has the fungus on it. For example, wrestlers may get ringworm from mats that have the fungus on them. Dogs and cats can carry the fungus from one family member to another.

Over-the-counter antifungal creams (p. 615) can treat small areas of ringworm. See your doctor if ringworm occurs on the scalp, in severe patches or if you've never seen this type of infection before.

## Rosacea

• Facial acne
• Flushed appearance of the face
• Visible blood vessels around blisters

*See photo of rosacea, page 271.*

Just when you thought you had reached the age when acne would never blemish your complexion again, along comes "adult acne," or *acne rosacea*. Rosacea may persist for months or years. Some people believe alcohol or spicy foods make this condition worse. Vitamin deficiency or immune-system deficiency might be the culprit. Rosacea seems to be most common in people with a fair complexion.

The rash occurs more often in women, but the complications occur primarily in men. The most frequent complication is a condition called *rhinophyma*—a bulbous red nose.

### Treatment

Your doctor can usually tell that the problem is rosacea simply by looking at the rash. Most moderate or severe cases are treated with the same antibiotics that are used to treat teen acne. Soaps or washes may be suggested by your doctor when the cause of the rash is confirmed.

## Seborrhea

• Reddish, scaling, greasy patches of irritated skin on the face, near the nose, on cheeks, eyebrows or the edge of the scalp

You may have *seborrhea* if the skin of your eyebrows is greasy and peels, itches or even bleeds, or if you have patches of itchy, scaling skin on the scalp that come back again and again, despite the use of dandruff shampoos.

Seborrhea is a form of dermatitis (p. 277). It's an irritating, itchy rash that has no specific cause. It runs in families. In adults, the rash is confined to the face, often in folds, such as the fold between the nose and the cheek. It recurs often. Certain foods in the diet, sun exposure, stress and other factors may stimulate seborrhea to return. In babies, the rash usually stays on the head and sometimes the face. This is called *cradle cap.*

### Treatment

Prescription corticosteroid creams (p. 622) may control the swelling, redness, itching and scaling of seborrhea, but they don't permanently cure the problem. Long-term use causes side effects. Another treatment is selenium sulfide (p. 616) shampoo. See your doctor if your problem persists.

## Skin Cancers

### Basal Cell Carcinoma

- Usually a flesh-colored, pearly lesion that may form an ulcer, most frequently on the face near an eye or the nose
- Less commonly, can occur on the arms, chest or back

*See photo of basal cell carcinoma, page 270.*

This is the most common type of skin cancer. It's a very slow-growing tumor and will only rarely spread, or *metastasize,* to a distant site in the body. As with all skin cancers, exposure to the sun or to irritating chemicals on a routine basis is the probable cause.

Basal cell cancer begins with a flesh-colored growth that typically appears on the eye area or nose, although it can occur elsewhere. As it grows, it becomes a scaly sore that won't heal. It may scab but never heals and continues to grow.

Who's most likely to get this form of skin cancer? Middle-aged and elderly people who have been exposed to sunlight on a regular basis. Black and Asian people are seldom affected.

### Kaposi's Sarcoma

- Reddish-purple to brownish-blue lesions anywhere on the body that resemble a growing birthmark
- First spots may be on arms and legs, then on hands, ears and nose

*See photo of Kaposi's sarcoma, page 270.*

These dark tumors were very rare before AIDS (p. 325). They were associated with other cancers and immune-deficiency disorders, and occurred most frequently in people living in Africa. The immune deficiency produced by HIV allows this cancerous growth to get started. Further growth of these tumors into the deeper tissues and organs is likely if they aren't treated.

Symptoms of HIV infection may help your doctor make the diagnosis. If blood tests for HIV are positive, they confirm the diagnosis of Kaposi's sarcoma. A biopsy of the lesion can also confirm the diagnosis. If the HIV test is negative and the biopsy is positive for Kaposi's sarcoma, your doctor will probably look for another reason for the immune deficiency.

Treatment may include removal of the tumor, radiation therapy (p. 225) and chemotherapy (p. 225). Prevention of Kaposi's sarcoma involves the same measures as prevention of HIV infection (p. 325).

### Malignant Melanoma

- A black or spotted growing mass or lump in the skin
- A mole that changes in appearance, grows, is ulcerated, bleeds or is scabbed and doesn't heal

*See photo of malignant melanoma, page 270.*

This is the fastest growing and most serious type of skin cancer.

Melanomas can spread early to distant parts of the body (a process called *metastasis*). These types of skin cancers can be found in adolescents and young adults, especially in areas of skin that were affected by severe sunburns in the past. However, they can occur on any skin surface—face, chest, back, arms and legs—and have even occurred between the toes or on the soles of the feet. They can also form inside the eye. Some malignant melanomas start in a mole (p. 287). If you have a dark, growing skin growth, see your doctor to have it checked. He or she will remove it or test it to make sure it isn't cancerous.

## Squamous Cell Carcinoma
- A firm, fleshy mass that sometimes ulcerates
- A mass or lump usually located on skin that has been regularly exposed to the sun

*See photo of squamous cell carcinoma, page 270.*

This is another cancer related to sun exposure. The usual site for this type of skin cancer is on the face, below the mouth or on the lip, and on the hands and forearms. It may look like a wart but continues to grow and may ulcerate. People in middle to later life, especially men and those with long-term sun exposure, are most likely to get this cancer. It's often preceded by an *actinic keratosis*, a precancerous growth—a small, scaly red spot—that doesn't go away.

### Testing
See your doctor if you suspect you have skin cancer. He or she can do a biopsy to rule out cancer or diagnose what type it is.

### Treatment
Depending on the size and type of your skin cancer, your doctor will remove it surgically or destroy it with a chemical or liquid nitrogen.

If the lesion is large, skin grafting can fill in the place where the cancer was removed and reduce scarring. Early diagnosis and removal are important for the best survival rate and the least disfigurement.

When basal cell carcinoma or squamous cell carcinoma is caught in the early stages, spread to other organs is rare. See your doctor if you notice a skin lesion that doesn't heal in two to four weeks. Removing the lesion almost always cures a localized skin cancer. Other treatments to remove the lesion, such as freezing or radiation therapy, can also be used. Chemotherapy and radiation may be needed if the cancer has spread.

Removal of a malignant melanoma in its earlier stages may cure the problem. After the cancer has spread to other parts of the body, such as the lymph nodes or the brain, the chance of recovery is poor. Radiation therapy or chemotherapy may be tried after the cancer has spread, but it's usually not very successful. Several experimental treatments are available.

If you have a lesion removed or treated, regular follow-up visits for 24 to 48 months may be recommended. Some types of skin cancers return and must be treated again.

### Prevention
Regularly examine your skin to help detect skin cancer early. Do it after a bath or shower and use both full-length and hand-held mirrors.

Look at your body, front and back, and note the moles, freckles and other colored areas. Be sure to examine your scalp, your palms and the soles of your feet, and the spaces between your fingers and toes.

You may want to make a "map" of your skin, marking the locations of large moles. Use the sample body map

---

## Preventing Skin Cancer

- Wear a hat to protect your face from the sun.
- Wear long sleeves and long pants when in bright sunlight.
- Avoid being outdoors from 11 a.m. to 3 p.m., when the sun's rays are strongest and most damaging to your skin.
- Use a sunscreen with an SPF of 15 or higher.
- Reapply sunscreen often if you're swimming or perspiring heavily.
- Examine your skin regularly.
- Have any suspicious skin lesions checked right away.

## Warning Signs of Skin Cancer

- One half of the mole isn't like the other half.
- Border is irregular, blurred or ragged.
- Color changes from one part of the mole to another.
- Diameter seems to be growing or is larger than a pencil eraser.
- The mole is raised above the skin surface.

below to keep track of where your moles are so you'll notice any new ones.

## Sunburn

- Red, swollen skin, hot to the touch
- Blisters, in a more serious burn

The pain of a sunburn is brought on by a low-level, superficial, first- or second-degree burn of the skin. This injury occurs when the skin is overexposed to the ultraviolet rays of sunlight. Blisters are the result of a deeper, more serious second-degree burn that destroys the top skin layers.

### Treatment

First, get out of the sun! Unfortunately, sunburn isn't always noticed until an hour or more after exposure ends. Second, take a mild pain reliever such as aspirin or acetaminophen to reduce the pain.

You can cool the burning sensation by taking cool showers or baths, or by applying cool compresses to the sunburned areas. Be careful not to over dry the skin. Don't use ice, because you can damage the skin. Be careful about applying topical anesthetics. Many of them can cause allergic reactions. Ointments containing hydrocortisone or aloe are helpful.

Be sure to protect the sunburned skin when you go back outdoors. Apply a sunscreen with a sun protection factor (SPF) of 15 or higher before you go outside and reapply it often if you're swimming or perspiring. Long sleeves, pants and hats can further protect you.

Young children with large areas of sunburn or a large blistered area should be seen by the doctor.

### Prevention

The best way to avoid a sunburn is to stay out of the sun and not use tanning booths. If you're planning on being outside, wear a hat and protective clothing. Avoid the sun from 11 a.m. to 3 p.m., when the sun's rays are the strongest and most likely to cause sunburn. If you must be in the sun, use a sunscreen. The SPF is a guide to how much sun is blocked. For example, an SPF of 8 means eight hours of sun exposure equal one unprotected hour. Sunscreens that have SPFs of 15 or higher protect the skin better than those with lower SPFs.

## Tinea Versicolor

- Patches of lighter-colored or darker-colored skin, usually on the upper back, abdomen or chest

*See photo of tinea versicolor, page 271.*

This mild fungal infection is often noticed in the summer because the affected areas don't tan, appearing as various-sized white spots on the skin. The infection causes the outer layer of the skin to peel off, exposing the paler

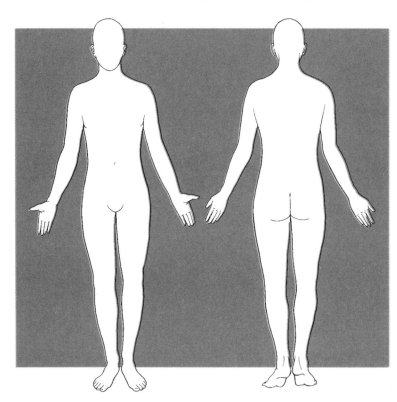

**SAMPLE BODY MAP**

## The Dangers of Tanning

A suntan is actually a sign that the skin is trying to protect itself from damage. When exposed to ultraviolet rays of the sun, the body produces *melanin*, the pigment in the upper layers of the skin that gives the skin its color and serves as a defense mechanism. The more sun exposure, the more melanin, and the darker the tan.

Repeated exposure to the sun damages some of the deeper layers (connective tissues), eventually causing the skin to wrinkle and age prematurely. It also increases the risk for skin cancer.

skin underneath. Your doctor may recommend applying selenium sulfide shampoo (p. 616) to affected areas or prescribe an antifungal cream (p. 619). Even after treatment with antifungal cream, the skin must be exposed to the sun before the color will again match the rest of the skin.

## Vitiligo

- Pale, irregularly shaped patches on the skin, often with very distinct borders
- Usually on the face, neck, hands, arms or knees

*See photo of vitiligo, page 271.*

The cells within the skin responsible for producing *melanin* (the pigment that gives the skin color) can, without warning, stop working in certain areas. The reason for this condition is unknown. There may be an inherited tendency to develop *vitiligo*. It may also be related to an autoimmune disorder (p. 223). The discolored areas aren't harmful.

There's no treatment or cure for vitiligo. Your doctor can help you find special makeup that helps disguise the patches. Sometimes drugs called psoralens are used. They're either taken by mouth or applied to the skin, but the results vary. Your doctor will make sure you don't have any other medical problems that might be causing vitiligo.

If you have any kind of pigment disorder, it's extremely important to protect yourself from the sun's ultraviolet rays as much as possible (p. 292) by wearing sunscreen with a sun protection factor (SPF) of at least 15.

## Wrinkles

- Fine lines around the eyes and mouth
- Deep creases on the face, especially the forehead

The underlying layer of the skin, the *dermis*, is made up of connective tissue. As you age, this connective tissue loses thickness and elasticity, resulting in wrinkles.

How much your skin wrinkles as you age depends on two primary factors—your inherited tendency toward wrinkling and the amount of sun exposure you've had in your lifetime. The sun's long rays (ultraviolet-A light) are most damaging to the skin. Cigarette smoking also prematurely ages the skin.

**Treatment**

There's no cure for wrinkles. Using a moisturizer can disguise fine lines, but dry skin doesn't cause wrinkles. New products make "anti-aging" claims. Some of these products contain glycolic acid, which helps plump up the skin and hide lines. Tretinoin, which is available by prescription only, may help

## Warts

Warts are raised lumps on the skin. They are caused by a group of viruses, called *papillomaviruses*. The viruses make the skin produce skin cells at a faster rate. This leads to the development of warts. Warts can develop just about anywhere. They commonly appear on the hands and feet (p. 332). They can also appear in the genital area (p. 318).

reduce some of the damage caused by the sun, but it may be most effective only for people in their 20s and 30s.

Plastic surgery, including facelifts, dermabrasion (removing imperfections through a process that "sands" the top layer of skin) and collagen injections, can change the appearance of your skin and help minimize wrinkles. A plastic surgeon can review the pros and cons of these techniques with you.

**Prevention**

Protecting your skin against the sun is the only thing you can do to prevent wrinkles. See page 292 for tips on protecting your skin from the sun.

# PART 3

# INFECTIONS

# INFECTIONS

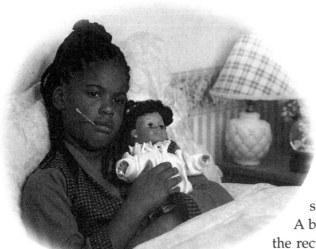

I llnesses caused by *germs* are called *infections*. Germs can be bacteria, viruses, fungi or parasites. They're responsible for infections ranging from minor annoyances like the common cold to fatal diseases like AIDS.

Fever is a common symptom of infection. It's your body's natural response to invading germs. As your body temperature rises, the spread of the infection slows down.

A baby's or young child's temperature is taken in the rectum or under the armpit. But remember, temperatures taken in the armpit are about 1° lower than temperatures taken rectally. Add 1° to the temperature if you use an armpit thermometer or a "fever strip."

To take a rectal temperature, use a rectal thermometer. Coat the tip in petroleum jelly (p. 617). Insert it half an inch into the rectum. Hold it there for two minutes. Don't let go of the thermometer.

Temperature can be taken orally in adults and children over four years old. (Don't take your baby's temperature orally if your child is younger than four. There's a danger that the thermometer will break if the child bites it.) But never leave your child alone while taking his or her temperature. Put the thermometer in the mouth under the tongue for three minutes. Wait about 10 minutes after drinking before checking the temperature, since cool or hot liquids can affect the thermometer reading.

What qualifies as a fever and how you treat it depends on the age of person with the fever, how high the fever is and if there are other symptoms.

**Baby under one month old.** A rectal temperature above 100.4°F is considered serious in babies younger than one month old and merits a call to your doctor. That's because infections can spread rapidly in very young babies. Your baby can quickly become dehydrated (p. 179) with a fever. If your baby is crying but has no tears or only a few wet

---

### Symptoms of a Fever

- Chills
- Flushing
- Hot and cold sensations
- Achiness
- Elevated body temperature

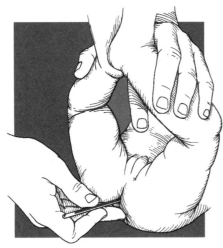

**BABY HAVING TEMPERATURE TAKEN RECTALLY**

296

## Warning Signs: Call Your Doctor If Your Child Has Any of These

| | |
|---|---|
| Behavior changes | Severe headache |
| Dry mouth | Skin rash |
| Earache or pulling at ears | Sore or swollen joints |
| Fever that comes and goes over several days | Sore throat |
| High-pitched crying | Stiff neck |
| Irritability | Stomach pain |
| Limp or unresponsive | Swelling of the soft spot on the head |
| Not hungry | Vomiting and diarrhea that won't stop |
| Pale | Wheezing or trouble breathing |
| Seizures | Whimpering |

diapers, he or she is becoming dehydrated. Vomiting and diarrhea bring on dehydration even more rapidly. Call your doctor if your baby has any of the warning signs in the box above.

**Baby one to three months old.** A rectal temperature above 101.4 °F in babies from one to three months old merits a call to your doctor. Even a temperature of 100.4 °F that has lasted more than 24 hours merits a phone call. Also call your doctor if your baby has any of the warning signs in the box above.

**Baby or child over three months old.** Babies between three months and two years old are usually better able to handle infections and fever. A mild viral infection may raise temperatures to 102 °F or 104 °F without making your child very ill. If your child's temperature reaches 101.4 °F, watch him or her. Call your doctor if the fever rises or lasts for more than three days, or if your child has any of the warning signs in the box above. If the temperature reaches 103 °F, call your doctor even if your child is acting fine.

**Children over two years old.** Look for other symptoms in addition to the fever if your child has a fever of 101.4 °F. If there are no other symptoms and your child is uncomfortable, give your child acetaminophen to reduce the fever. Never give a child aspirin to bring down a fever because of the risk of Reye's syndrome (p. 370). Call your doctor if the fever rises, stays high for three days, or if your child has any of the symptoms in the box above.

**Adolescents and adults.** Adults generally have a fever that's a bit lower than in children. If you feel uncomfortable due to the fever or if your temperature is up to 104 °F, take fever-reducing medicines. Call your doctor if you have a fever that lasts more than three days with no other obvious symptoms or if you have other symptoms, such as pain when urinating, pain or swelling in or near the testicles, abdominal pain, a stiff neck, a rash, trouble breathing or a severe sore throat.

A fever isn't necessarily bad. It's one of the body's ways of fighting infection. Bacteria, viruses and fungal organisms grow more slowly when the body's temperature is elevated.

It's important to try to figure out what's causing the fever. If it's a virus, such as a cold (p. 322) or the flu (p. 326), antibiotics (p. 618) won't help because antibiotics fight bacteria, not viruses. On the other hand, if it's a bacterial infection, such as strep throat (p. 306), antibiotics are needed.

## When is a fever serious?

Fever above 105 °F can cause damage to the nervous system. Seizures (convulsions) can also occur with a rapidly rising temperature, usually above 102 °F. Call your doctor right away if your child has a persistent fever over 102 °F or convulsions.

## What can I do to feel better when I have a fever?

- Take fever-reducing medicines.
- Use sponge baths with lukewarm water, not alcohol. They're particularly useful if the person with fever is vomiting and can't keep medicine down.
- Don't overdress or use heavy blankets that trap the heat.
- Avoid taking hot showers or baths—they may relieve your achy joints but they'll increase your temperature.
- Drink plenty of liquids to prevent dehydration.

# BACTERIA

*Bacteria* are a kind of germ that cause infections. Bacteria are single, living cells. They reproduce by dividing into two cells, which divide again and again, building up large numbers in a very short time. Your immune system will try to fight off bacterial infection, but it's not always successful. That's when you get sick. Many illnesses caused by bacteria can be treated with antibiotics (p. 615).

## Bacteremia

- Nausea and vomiting
- Diarrhea
- Feeling too weak and ill to get up
- Skin rash
- Fever (may come and go)
- Chills

*Bacteremia* means that bacteria are present in the bloodstream. The condition sometimes follows surgery, labor and delivery or use of intravenous catheters or urinary catheters. It can also be due to infections, such as tonsillitis (p. 104).

Bacteria in the bloodstream can cause an infection of the lining of the heart (endocarditis, p. 115). It can also lead to blood poisoning or septic shock, which can be life-threatening. Symptoms that *septic shock* is developing may include irregular heartbeat and breathing, low blood pressure, bluish fingertips and confusion.

Blood tests can show if bacteremia is present and what type of bacteria is the cause.

Hospitalization is often required for bacteremia. Anyone with septic shock may need to be in the intensive care unit because of the seriousness of this condition.

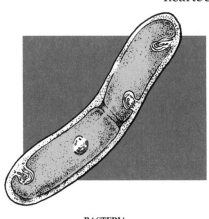

**BACTERIA**

Intravenous antibiotics (p. 618) and other medicines may be given. Life-support measures, such as oxygen and intravenous fluids, may be needed.

## Cat-Scratch Fever

- Headache
- Swollen lymph nodes in an area near where a cat or other animal scratched the skin
- Rash
- Fever

*Cat-scratch fever* may occur a week or two after a cat scratch or bite. Most cases occur in children. At first, the scratch has some swelling and pus-filled bumps around it. Within two weeks, the lymph nodes nearest the scratch begin to swell, and a fever develops. The lymph nodes often affected are those in the armpit, following a scratch on the hand or arm.

Don't worry about the health of the cat who gave you cat-scratch fever. Cats that pass along this disease to humans are healthy.

A sample of tissue may be taken from the swollen lymph node. It will be examined under a microscope to make sure that a more serious problem, such as a lymphoma (p. 139) or leukemia (p. 138), isn't present. A skin test can also diagnose whether you have cat-scratch fever, but this test may not be available in your area.

Fever-reducing medicines (p. 616) can help your fever and headache. Your doctor may drain a lymph node or blister that's infected. He or she may also prescribe antibiotics (p. 618) to fight the infection.

## Cholera

- Diarrhea

*Cholera* is a type of bacterial infection often transmitted through contaminated water, or unwashed or unpeeled fruits and vegetables from areas where hygiene is poor. Fortunately, cholera is rare in the United States.

The bacteria that cause cholera burn the inside of the intestine, forcing it to secrete large amounts of water in an attempt to flush out the bacteria. Two to four gallons of fluid may be lost each day. The main treatment is to replace the lost fluids, salts and sugars by drinking juices, water and other liquids, or by intravenous fluids if you are severely ill.

## Diphtheria

- Sore throat, husky voice
- Fever
- Breathing trouble

*Diphtheria* starts with a sore throat and fever. It causes a grayish film to form in the throat, which can block the air passages. Other complications, such as heart failure or throat paralysis, can cause death.

Hospitalization, often in intensive care, may be needed. A medicine known as an antitoxin should be given as soon as possible. It's important to check first to make sure the person doesn't have an allergy to the antitoxin. Antibiotics (p. 618) are also given.

Immunization against diphtheria has made this often fatal disease almost nonexistent in the United States. The DTP vaccine (p. 11), which protects against diphtheria, tetanus and pertussis, is given to children. If you're not sure you've been immunized and you're planning to travel to a country where diphtheria may be present, talk to your doctor.

## Epiglottitis

- Sore throat
- Hoarseness

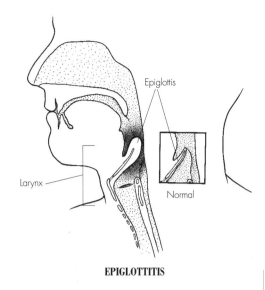

**EPIGLOTTITIS**

- High fever
- Noisy breathing
- Drooling

The *epiglottis* is a flap that covers the top of the windpipe, or *larynx*. It keeps food from going down the windpipe when you swallow. It can become infected with a type of bacteria called *Haemophilus influenzae* and cause a life-threatening disease called *epiglottitis*.

This illness is most common in children three to eight years old. It starts suddenly. Your child may have trouble breathing and may lose consciousness or turn bluish from lack of oxygen. Symptoms may be like those of croup (p. 323), although the barking cough typical of croup won't be present. A type of pneumonia, also caused by *H. influenzae*, may occur at the same time.

If your child has a sore throat and begins to have trouble breathing, call your doctor or go to an emergency room. Antibiotics (p. 618) and other medicines may be given intravenously. A surgical procedure known as a tracheostomy may be done so your child can breathe.

Your child can be immunized against *H. influenzae*, which will help prevent epiglottitis. It's known as the HIB vaccine (p. 12).

## Food Poisoning

Many types of bacteria can be transmitted in food. This can occur if food is prepared incorrectly. Most types of food poisoning are accompanied by diarrhea. Usually, symptoms will resolve on their own. Dehydration (p. 179) is a major risk when diarrhea and vomiting are present. If symptoms are severe, fluids may need to be given along with other treatments.

To prevent food poisoning, wash your hands carefully before preparing any food. Cook all meats, other foods and dishes properly, then cool them right away in the refrigerator after serving. Leaving them out at room temperature can lead to food poisoning. Meats, egg dishes and mayonnaise are particularly susceptible to growth of staphylococci, while canned foods and fish are susceptible to growth of clostridia.

**Botulism.** This type of food poisoning is caused by the *Clostridium botulinum* bacteria. Abdominal cramping, diarrhea and vomiting, along with blurred vision, muscle weakness and even paralysis, are possible symptoms. Symptoms usually occur 12 to 48 hours after eating the contaminated food. These bacteria can contaminate the food during preparation. If contaminated food isn't refrigerated properly, these bacteria multiply. They produce a toxin in the food that isn't destroyed, even if the food is reheated. Over 90% of cases are from improper home canning. The toxin prevents the nerves from functioning. Botulism must be treated with an antitoxin to reverse these symptoms.

***Clostridium perfringens* infection.** This type of food poisoning is caused by the *Clostridium perfringens* bacteria. Symptoms include abdominal pain and diarrhea. Symptoms may appear eight to 22 hours after ingestion. Food sources include improperly prepared or reheated meats. If symptoms are severe, penicillin (p. 625) may be needed.

**Salmonella.** Salmonella bacteria can cause a common kind of food poisoning. Symptoms include diarrhea, vomiting and possibly fever. The diarrhea and cramps can be mild to severe. Babies, young children and the elderly are most at risk. So are people with immune deficiencies. Rarely, infected people can carry the bacteria for months, infecting others and reinfecting themselves. Symptoms appear 12 to 36 hours after you've eaten contaminated food and may last several days or longer. Undercooked poultry and eggs are common sources for salmonella infection. Treatment involves plenty of fluids to prevent dehydration. In most people, the infection clears on its own. But in some people with severe infection, antibiotics (p. 618) may be needed.

**Shigella.** Illness caused by shigella bacteria is relatively rare in the United States. It's more common in areas where sanitation is poor. Shigella bacteria cause cramps and diarrhea that usually contains blood and mucus. Symptoms may appear one to seven days after contact with the bacteria and last indefinitely, depending on if you receive treatment. Foods that may harbor shigella include beans, potatoes, tuna, shrimp and turkey. You may need antibiotics if the symptoms are severe and include fever.

**Staphylococcal food poisoning.** Food contaminated with the staphylococcal bacteria may produce a toxin that leads to severe cramping and diarrhea. Symptoms may occur one to six hours after ingestion and last two to four days. Foods that may carry staphylococcal bacteria include improperly prepared custards, dairy products, potato and other salads, hollandaise sauce, gravies, reheated foods and many meats. Treatment with intravenous fluids may be needed if dehydration occurs.

## Gangrene

- Body tissues turn grayish to black
- Tissues lose sensation

*Gangrene* is the death of body tissue such as the skin, underlying muscle, fat layer and even bone. It usually occurs when blood can't reach an area of the body to nourish it. There are two forms of gangrene.

**Dry gangrene.** With this condition, no infection is involved. Dry gangrene can result from a blood clot, atherosclerosis (p. 111), poor circulation, frostbite (p. 652) or as a complication of diabetes (p. 211).

**Wet gangrene.** After the tissue dies because of a lack of blood, it becomes infected with bacteria. Without a blood supply, the area has no way of fighting the infection. The bacteria that invade the area keep it moist and produce a foul smell.

Antibiotics (p. 618) are usually prescribed to help the surrounding tissues fight off infection. The doctor will remove the dead tissue. If the damage is extensive, a portion of the limb or the entire limb may have to be *amputated*, or removed.

Another treatment involves a *hyperbaric oxygen chamber,* which is a machine that contains a high pressure of oxygen. A person with gangrene is put inside the oxygen chamber. Oxygen at high pressure penetrates the skin from the outside. This sometimes allows the area to fight off infection. If the area is small enough, it may be able to heal itself.

Factors that affect your circulation, such as smoking, diabetes, high blood pressure and infection, also affect your risk of gangrene. Stop smoking, start exercising, control conditions like diabetes and high blood pressure and treat any infection early to reduce your risk of gangrene.

Tests such as Doppler ultrasound (p. 644), angiography (p. 628) or a digital subtraction arteriogram (p. 628) can

help show areas at high risk for gangrene. It may be possible to improve the blood flow to that area before it's too late.

## Leprosy

- Sores on the skin
- Loss of feeling
- Reduced sweating

Although *leprosy*, or Hansen's disease, isn't common in the United States, there are cases in Hawaii, California, Texas, Louisiana, Florida and New York. The majority of people with leprosy are born outside of the U.S.

Leprosy is much less contagious than once believed. It's caused by bacteria and spread through droplets of nasal mucus. You're only at risk of catching the disease if you're in close contact with someone who's in the early stages of leprosy.

The disease causes sores on the skin, with extensive scarring. It also damages nerves, resulting in numbness and paralysis. It can invade bone, cartilage and the eyeball, leading to disfigurement and blindness if not treated.

A number of different medicines can either cure or keep leprosy under control. It may be necessary to take these medicines for years or for a lifetime. Plastic surgery can correct disfigurements. Nerve and tendon transplants can help restore use of arms and legs.

## Lyme Disease

- Red, target-like rash at the site of a deer tick bite
- Headache
- Chills
- Fever
- Achy joints

*See photo of Lyme disease rash, page 272.*

### Listeria Bacteria

Listeria bacteria can cause a number of different infections. The most common is meningitis (p. 302). Listeria infection is most common in babies and older adults. The bacteria can be found in foods, such as dairy products and raw vegetables.

### Haemophilus Bacteria

Haemophilus bacteria are one of the leading causes of meningitis (p. 302), bacteremia (p. 298), pneumonia (p. 154), ear infections (p. 79) and sinus infections (sinusitis, p. 89). The HIB immunization (p. 12), which should be given in childhood, can help prevent many of these infections.

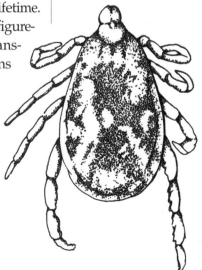

**DEER TICK**

*Lyme disease* is caused by a type of bacteria that enters the body from the bite of a deer tick. The tick must usually be attached for at least 24 hours to transmit the bacteria. A deer tick is smaller than the common dog tick. A deer tick is about the size of a small sesame seed, while the dog tick is about three or four times larger.

The first sign of the disease is a rash surrounding a tick bite, followed by flu-like symptoms, such as fever, aches, chills and headache. If the infection goes untreated, other symptoms appear within a few weeks or months, including heart problems, numbness or other nerve disorders, arthritis, swelling and even paralysis.

Although blood tests can help diagnose Lyme disease, they can't prove you have the condition. Your symptoms and possible exposure to deer ticks help your doctor make the diagnosis.

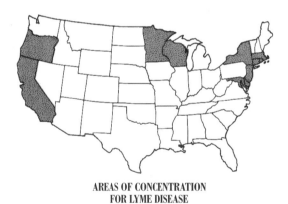

☐ Found throughout United States from May to October

■ Concentration found on East and West coasts (and especially in Minnesota and Wisconsin)

**AREAS OF CONCENTRATION FOR LYME DISEASE**

Antibiotics (p. 618) may stop the infection and treat the symptoms. They may be given by mouth or intravenously. Antibiotics and anti-inflammatory medicines (p. 615) will reduce the swelling and pain in the joints. Oral corticosteroids, such as prednisone (p. 620), may be given for heart problems caused by Lyme disease.

To help prevent Lyme disease, avoid tick-infested areas. When you go into woods or fields, wear long pants and long-sleeved shirts and use tick repellent. Check yourself at least every five to 12 hours for tick bites. See page 313 for information about removing a tick.

Although you can have your dog vaccinated against Lyme disease, that won't stop ticks from attaching to your pet, who in turn brings them into your home.

## Meningitis

- Severe headache
- Sensitivity to light
- Stiff neck
- Nausea and vomiting
- Fever
- Lethargy and irritability

*Meningitis* is an infection of the tissues that cover the brain and spinal cord, called the *meninges*. Meningitis can be caused by a virus or by bacteria. The infection is usually carried through the bloodstream from another infected area of the body. It may spread to the meninges from the sinuses or ears. Meningitis can also result from an injury that penetrates the skull or, rarely, from brain surgery. The infection spreads throughout the *cerebrospinal fluid*, the fluid covering the brain and spinal cord.

The symptoms of meningitis start suddenly. Within a few hours, the person will have fever, headache, nausea and vomiting, a stiff neck and a low tolerance to light (*photophobia*). Sometimes a purplish skin rash occurs. If the infection is left untreated, drowsiness and eventual loss of consciousness occur.

In children, this type of infection may be difficult to detect because headache, nausea, vomiting and fever are also symptoms of other less serious viral infections. Don't ignore your child's complaints of either a stiff neck or headache. The degree of illness and how quickly your child becomes ill may be the best clues that this serious infection is present.

Your doctor will take a sample of blood for examination. Your doctor will also take a sample of spinal fluid through a procedure called a spinal tap (p. 641) to confirm the diagnosis and help identify what's causing the infection.

Viral meningitis can't be treated with antibiotics but, fortunately, it's generally a mild infection.

Bacterial meningitis usually requires treatment with intravenous antibiotics (p. 618). The brain has a natural barrier that makes it more difficult for drugs to penetrate, so brain infections can be harder to treat than infections in other parts of the body. The earlier the treatment, the less chance of permanent damage, such as deafness, blindness or paralysis, and death.

Meningitis sometimes occurs in epidemics, spreading from one person to another. Preventive treatments will be offered if you or your child has been exposed.

An immunization called HIB (p. 12) is now given to young children as part of their immunization program to prevent meningitis caused by *H. influenzae*, a rare, but potentially fatal, form of bacterial meningitis.

## Pertussis

- Cough

*Pertussis* is also known as "whooping cough." It's named for the whooping sound that often comes at the end of the coughing spasms. It's a highly contagious disease and can be fatal, especially in babies and young children who haven't been immunized.

The disease occurs seven to 14 days after exposure to the bacteria. It lasts around six weeks. Whooping cough begins with sneezing and cold symptoms, but rarely fever. After 10 to 14 days, the cough gets worse.

Babies and young children may have to be hospitalized for supportive care. Don't use cough medicines or sedatives; they can be dangerous for someone with whooping cough.

Pertussis can be easily prevented by getting your child immunized with the DTP immunization (p. 11), which also protects against diphtheria (p. 299) and tetanus (p. 306).

---

**Could your child have meningitis?**

- Does your child have a stiff neck?
- Does your child also have a headache or does light hurt his or her eyes?
- Does your child have a fever, nausea or vomiting?

*If your child has these symptoms, take him or her to your doctor or to a local emergency room right away.*

---

### Pneumococcal Bacteria

Pneumonia (p. 154) is the most common serious infection caused by pneumococcal bacteria. It's most likely to occur in people who have AIDS (p. 325), certain cancers or other illnesses that affect the immune system. Anyone who has had chronic bronchitis (p. 145) or other respiratory disease may also be more susceptible.

Pneumococcal bacteria can also cause ear infections (p. 79), sinus infections (sinusitis, p. 89), meningitis (p. 302), bacteremia (p. 298) and infection of the lining of the heart (endocarditis, p. 115).

A vaccine against pneumococcus is recommended at least once for nursing home residents, the elderly and people with heart disease, lung disease, diabetes and immune and metabolic disorders. Some doctors recommend a second vaccination after three to five years, especially for people at high risk—including those who have had their spleen removed or whose immune systems are suppressed.

## Rheumatic Fever

- Arthritis
- Heart rhythm problems
- Rash
- Fever
- Bizarre motions

In the past, parents worried when their children had strep throat (p. 306), because the sore throat was sometimes followed in two weeks by a more serious disorder called *rheumatic fever.* Thanks to antibiotics (p. 618), rheumatic fever is much less common now. Rheumatic fever is caused by the streptococcal bacteria (p. 306), the same bacteria that causes strep throat.

If an antibiotic is prescribed for you or your child to treat strep throat, make sure the entire prescription is taken. This helps make sure the infection is completely cured, helps prevent bacteria from becoming resistant to antibiotics and can prevent rheumatic fever.

Why is rheumatic fever so dangerous? It causes inflammation and damage to tissues throughout the body, including the lining of the joints and the nervous system, kidneys and heart. Some middle-aged or elderly people have heart valve damage that was caused by rheumatic fever during their childhood. In some people, heart valves damaged by rheumatic heart disease are replaced with artificial heart valves.

The classic pattern of rheumatic fever includes an untreated sore throat or upper respiratory illness. Most children affected are between five and 10 years old. Blood tests and cultures, including white blood cell counts and a strep test (p. 642), will help your doctor confirm the diagnosis. An electrocardiogram (p. 634), along with a chest x-ray (p. 631), can reveal any possible effects on the heart.

Treatment for rheumatic fever includes bed rest, intravenous penicillin (p. 625) and oral anti-inflammatory medicines (p. 615), such as aspirin (p. 615) or corticosteroids (p. 622). The movement disorder, called *chorea,* may be suppressed with sedatives or tranquilizers. If heart damage has occurred, specific treatments for the heart problems can be given. Once the child has recovered, any throat infection should be treated right away with an antibiotic. Antibiotics should be given during surgery or dental work to people who have a history of rheumatic fever. This will help prevent the spread of bacteria to the heart.

## Problems Associated with Rheumatic Fever

**Arthritis.** The pain, swelling and redness of arthritis may occur in multiple joints. See page 299 for more information on arthritis.

**Chorea.** A child with rheumatic fever may make bizarre, involuntary movements of the arms, legs and face and waver erratically while walking. This behavior is called chorea and occurs because the infection has affected the central nervous system.

**Endocarditis.** This inflammation of the heart injures heart valves, leading to murmurs (abnormal sounds heard with a stethoscope) and pain in the chest. See page 115 for more information on endocarditis.

**Glomerulonephritis.** Kidney damage occasionally occurs as a result of the body's immune response to the streptococcal organism. See page 161 for more information on glomerulonephritis.

**Rash.** A faint, purple-colored rash appears in irregular blotches on the arms, back, chest, abdomen and legs.

**Skin nodules.** Small, hard lumps can be felt under the skin on the back of the forearm, hand and near the elbow.

## Rocky Mountain Spotted Fever

- Severe headache
- High fever (up to 105 °F)
- Aches and chills
- Spotted rash

*Rocky Mountain spotted fever* is

caused by a *rickettsia*, which is similar to a bacterium. Rocky Mountain spotted fever is transmitted to humans by a dog tick bite. The tick that causes Rocky Mountain spotted fever lives on rabbits, dogs and other animals. Dog ticks are larger than the deer ticks that can spread Lyme disease (p. 301). The infection is more likely to develop if the tick stays attached for hours or even days. If not detected, the disease can damage the liver, lungs and kidneys.

The symptoms begin 48 hours or more after the tick bite. The rash begins on the palms of the hands and soles of the feet, then progresses up the arms and legs to the chest, back and abdomen. High fever may lead to confusion and even coma.

Possible complications linked to Rocky Mountain spotted fever are middle ear infection (p. 80), inflammation of the salivary glands (p. 97), pneumonia (p. 154), blood clots, nerve damage and paralysis. Some cases are fatal.

Despite its name, Rocky Mountain spotted fever has occurred throughout the country, most frequently in the southeastern United States. It's most common in late spring and summer.

To prevent Rocky Mountain spotted fever, avoid tick-infested areas. Wear protective clothing (long pants and long-sleeved shirts) and use tick repellents if you must enter a tick-infested area. When you've been bitten by a tick, gently grasp it with a pair of tweezers and slowly and steadily pull until the tick releases. The sooner the tick is removed, the less likely it will pass any infection. Apply an antiseptic (p. 615) and hydrocortisone cream (p. 616) after removal of a tick.

Your doctor may diagnose Rocky Mountain spotted fever by the rash on your palms and soles. Blood tests and a skin biopsy may be needed to confirm the diagnosis.

The infection is often treated with intravenous antibiotics (p. 618). People with high fever, intense headaches or confusion are kept in the hospital for supportive care and further antibiotic treatment.

## Scarlet Fever

* Sore throat
* Bright red rash that begins on the trunk and spreads over the body within a few days of illness
* Fever
* Dry, flaky skin that peels once illness is over

In *scarlet fever*, or *scarlatina*, streptococcal bacteria (p. 300) first invade the tonsils and *pharynx*, or throat, causing a fever and sore throat. Later, the bacteria produce a *toxin*, or poison, that causes the skin to develop a very fine, bright red (scarlet) rash that feels like sandpaper. The rash appears first on the trunk and in skin creases,

### *Staphylococcal Infections*

The staphylococcal bacteria, or "staph," can cause folliculitis (p. 280), boils (p. 276), impetigo (p. 283), cellulitis (p. 276), food poisoning (p. 300) and wound infections. Infections around ingrown toenails (p. 262) or of the eyelid or mucous membranes of the eye, called a stye (p. 74), also can be caused by staphylococcal bacteria. In infants and children, these bacteria can produce a toxin that causes a peeling reaction that looks like scalded skin. In rare cases, staph causes more serious types of infection, such as pneumonia (p. 154), abscesses in the abdomen, bones and joints, and infection of the lining of the heart (endocarditis, p. 115), the kidneys, the brain or the spinal cord.

Many staphylococcal infections are resistant to penicillin and require stronger, more expensive antibiotics (p. 618). Staphylococcal pneumonia can be fatal. You may have to be hospitalized in order to get intravenous antibiotics and supportive care.

Help prevent staphylococcal infections by washing your hands before handling food, refrigerating food promptly and washing wounds, cuts or scrapes.

## Streptococcal Bacteria

Streptococcal bacteria, or "strep," normally live in the gastrointestinal tract, on the skin and in the ears, nose, mouth and rectum. Most of the time, they don't cause any trouble, because they're in balance with the body's natural defenses against bacterial invasion. Infection may occur when the balance is interrupted. This can happen if your body's resistance is lowered by a viral infection, for example. The infections caused by this type of bacteria include strep throat (below), impetigo (p. 283), cellulitis (p. 276) and pneumonia (p. 154).

Many types of streptococcal infections can still be treated with penicillin (p. 625). Some streptococcal bacteria are resistant to antibiotics, which means they must be treated with stronger, more expensive antibiotics (p. 618). Serious infections, such as pneumonia, may require treatment with intravenous antibiotics.

*Why is it so important to take all of the antibiotic prescription?*

Ten days of antibiotic treatment for a streptococcal infection has been proved to prevent almost all cases of rheumatic fever and some kidney damage (glomerulonephritis, p. 161) related to streptococcal bacteria. These streptococcal infections include strep throat, impetigo (p. 283), cellulitis (p. 276) and pneumonia (p. 154). Taking the full course of antibiotics prescribed by your doctor can also help prevent bacteria from becoming resistant to antibiotics.

and then spreads to the arms, legs and face (except around the mouth). The tongue becomes red and swollen. By the sixth day the rash begins to fade, but the skin peels for up to two weeks.

In mild cases, an antibiotic (p. 618) will destroy the streptococcal bacteria. More serious cases of scarlet fever may be treated in the hospital with intravenous antibiotics. Prompt treatment prevents complications, such as rheumatic heart disease and kidney damage (glomerulonephritis, p. 161).

### Strep Throat

- Headache
- Sore throat
- Fever

The typical symptoms of *strep throat* are slightly different from the common cold (p. 322) or the flu (p. 326). While the sore throat of a strep infection is sometimes accompanied by headache and fever, it usually doesn't include the cold symptoms of a runny nose, cough or sinus drainage.

Before the discovery of antibiotics in the 1940s, many people with a simple strep-throat infection developed rheumatic fever (p. 304), with heart damage, joint pain and kidney damage. Now, widespread testing for strep throat and treatment with penicillin have virtually eliminated rheumatic fever.

When you get a sore throat, treat the symptoms with analgesic medicines (p. 614) and fever-reducing medicines (p. 616) for two days. If the sore throat doesn't go away, see your doctor for a strep test. If your child has a sore throat, fever and headache but no runny nose, he or she should be checked for strep throat.

Your doctor will probably swab the throat to get a sample for a strep test (p. 642). The rapid antibody test looks for the body's immune reaction to the bacteria and can be read in 10 minutes. It takes 24 hours, on the other hand, to get the results of a throat culture (p. 642). A culture takes longer because the bacteria need time to grow so they can be identified in the culture. The culture takes longer, but is more accurate than the rapid strep test.

Taking antibiotics (p. 618) for 10 days will generally cure strep throat and prevent complications like rheumatic fever or kidney damage. If your doctor decides your child's symptoms are due to a viral infection, no antibiotics will be given, since these medicines aren't effective against viruses.

### Tetanus

- Severe, painful spasms of the muscles

*Tetanus,* or "lockjaw," is caused by bacteria, called *Clostridium tetani,* that live in the soil. Usually, the bacteria enter the body through a puncture wound, such as that caused by stepping on a nail. Once these bacteria enter the body, they produce a toxin that attacks the nerves that control the muscles. As a result, the muscles lose control and go into spasms. This infection is serious and may lead to death—40% of people who develop tetanus die.

Tetanus is rare in the United States because of the tetanus vaccine. Children are immunized with a combination vaccine called DTP (p. 11), which protects against diphtheria, tetanus and pertussis. Older children can be immunized with a vaccine called Td (p. 11), which also immunizes against tetanus and diphtheria. Adults should get a tetanus shot (p. 11) every 10 years.

If you or your child has a cut with dirt in it, make sure the cut is cleaned thoroughly in running water before bandaging. Some doctors recommend washing the cut with soapy water and applying an antiseptic (p. 615) before bandaging. If you have a puncture wound, such as from a nail, go to your doctor's office to get a tetanus shot if you haven't had one in the last 10 years or if the wound shows signs of infection, such as swelling, redness or pus.

Treatment of tetanus infection includes antibiotics (p. 618), intravenous fluids, injections of an antitoxin, muscle relaxants (p. 625) and an artificial respirator if breathing is affected.

## Tuberculosis

- Flu-like symptoms at first
- Dry cough
- Night sweats
- Weight loss
- Tiredness

*Tuberculosis* is often called "TB." It's spread when people who have active TB in their lungs cough or sneeze and the droplets come in contact with another person. Before the days of pasteurization, it was also spread by drinking "raw," unprocessed milk. TB has become more common in the past 10 years. People whose resistance to infections is lowered by other conditions, such as alcoholism (p. 562), diabetes (p. 211) or AIDS (p. 325), are more susceptible to infections, including TB.

Your greatest risk of getting TB comes from living around others who have TB. A few cases result from casual contact at work or with a friend. Tell your doctor if you know you've been exposed to TB. Adequate prevention includes knowing the symptoms of TB and having a skin test every few years if you've been around someone who has TB.

The slow-growing bacteria that cause TB can spread from the lungs to other parts of the body, such as the bones, the kidneys, the lymph nodes and even the brain.

If you're infected with TB, you may only have simple flu-like symptoms at first. The bacteria are either destroyed or lay dormant in the lungs. Years later, if your immune system is weakened by age or disease, TB may progress to the second stage.

The second phase of TB, which used to be known as "consumption" (see box), can occur many years after a person has been infected. The second phase occurs if the disease hasn't been treated. In this phase, the bacteria spread to other areas of the lungs and body. Death from TB occurs when vital tissues, such as the lungs, become so damaged from the infection that they no longer function.

If you have a fever, dry cough, unexplained tiredness, night sweats and weight loss, you should be checked for TB. Your doctor will probably do tuberculin skin test (p. 642)

### Why was TB called "consumption?"

TB was once known as "consumption" because the disease seemed to "consume" the victim. The second phase of TB leaves large scars in the lungs. These scars reduce the amount of oxygen the lungs can deliver to the rest of the body. As a result, the victim's normal body weight can't be maintained. The weight loss creates the impression that the person is wasting away, as if he or she is being *consumed* by the illness.

## Untreated Infections: Warning

If a fungal infection is untreated or doesn't respond to over-the-counter anti-fungal medicines (p. 615), a bacterial infection may develop. If an antibiotic ointment (p. 615) doesn't help, see your doctor.

and chest x-ray (p. 631), and may take samples of your saliva.

Early treatment can cure TB, and proper follow-up visits to the doctor for a few years can prevent relapses. TB is treated with medicines that must be taken for six to nine months. More than one medicine may be needed to make sure the bacteria don't build up resistance to the medicines.

## Typhoid Fever

- Headaches
- Nausea and vomiting
- Diarrhea
- Fever

*Typhoid fever* is a form of infectious diarrhea caused by eating or drinking contaminated food or water. It also can be caught through contact with an infected person. During floods, typhoid fever can be a problem because of contact with contaminated water. High fever, headache, nausea, vomiting and bloody diarrhea start quickly and may continue for a few weeks. Confusion may develop because of prolonged high fever and dehydration (p. 179).

If your symptoms suggest typhoid fever, your doctor may do tests on your blood, urine or stool to confirm the diagnosis. Antibiotics (p. 618) can be helpful in reducing the severity of symptoms. Immunization against this infection is available in certain circumstances.

## FUNGAL INFECTIONS

*Fungi* are all around us—in our offices, homes, yards and basements. They tend to grow in moist environments, such as old food, dirty sweat socks or parts of the body. While fungi seldom cause serious disease in people with normal immune systems, anyone whose immune system is impaired, such as someone with AIDS (p. 325), is at increased risk for serious fungal infections.

The Latin term *tinea*, meaning "grub" or "worm," is used to describe a number of fungal skin infections. For example, *tinea pedis* is another name for athlete's foot (p. 256). *Tinea cruris* is the fungal infection in the groin that's commonly called jock itch (p. 430). *Tinea capitis* is a fungal infection, or "ringworm," of the scalp. *Tinea corporis* describes single or multiple patches of fungal infection on the body. Another fungal infection is *tinea versicolor*, in which patches of lighter skin are on a background of darker, more tanned skin (p. 292). Fungi can also produce irritating vaginal yeast infections (p. 421).

## Candidiasis

- Redness
- Itching

*Candidiasis*, also referred to as a *yeast infection*, is caused by a germ called *Candida albicans*. *C. albicans* is present on the skin, in the gastrointestinal tract and in the vagina. It usually causes no harm. But sometimes it grows and results in an infection of the mucous membranes of the mouth (thrush, p. 97), diaper rash (p. 335) or vaginal yeast infections (p. 421).

Keep candida-prone areas, such as the diaper area in babies and the vaginal area in women, as dry as possible to help prevent yeast infections. Periodically, leave the area exposed to the air if you can. For adults, use a drying powder for external skin infections. But avoid cornstarch, which actually encourages the growth of yeast organisms. (It may be best not to

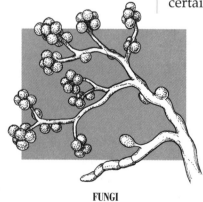

**FUNGI**

use talcum powder on babies and young children unless you're very careful not to let your child breathe in the powder dust.)

An antifungal (p. 615) cream or lotion may be needed to get rid of the skin infection.

Vaginal yeast medicines are made differently than skin creams and are available over-the-counter and by prescription. If you think you have a vaginal yeast infection, check with your doctor first to make sure that's what you have before treating it yourself.

## Fungal Infections of the Lungs

- Shortness of breath
- Cough
- Increase in mucus, or phlegm
- Chest pain
- Mild fever
- Aches
- Night sweats
- Weight loss

Some fungi can cause lung disease when they are breathed into the respiratory tract. Most fungal lung infections only cause a flu-like illness and an occasional scar, or "spot," that appears on a chest x-ray.

Rarely fungal infections spread to other areas of the body, including the brain. Persistent fungal infections of the lungs lead to scarring of the lungs and, years later, to reduced ability to breathe. People with immune problems, such as people who have AIDS (p. 325), are at risk for serious fungal infections.

**Aspergillosis.** This type of fungus is found on farms and in old buildings. It's a rare infection, mainly affecting people with lowered resistance to infection, older people and people whose lungs are scarred from smoking. Allergic reactions and inflammation of the lung may be a complication of an aspergillosis infection.

**Blastomycosis.** This is also a rare infection. This fungus is found in wood and soil in the eastern United States and Canada. Once it's breathed into the lungs, this fungus may spread to other areas of the body, such as the skin or bones.

**Coccidioidomycosis.** This infection is also known as San Joaquin Valley fever. The arid western desert and parts of California are the most common areas of the country where this infection occurs. A few people with this infection in the lung will also break out in a rash similar to measles (p. 327).

**Cryptococcosis.** People who breed pigeons and chickens may contract this fungal infection. The birds' droppings are extremely fertile for the growth of cryptococcal fungi. The infection can cause coughing and breathing problems, blurred vision, headache or meningitis. Most cases occur in people with lowered resistance to infection, such as people who have AIDS, Hodgkin's lymphoma (p. 139) or those being treated with immunosuppressants (p. 624).

**Histoplasmosis.** This fungal infection is most common in the eastern half of the United States, especially along the Ohio and Mississippi river valleys. The fungus is found in soil contaminated with droppings from birds and bats. The infection affects the lungs and lymph nodes. It can be fatal.

### Prevention and Treatment

To help prevent fungal infections of the lung, wear a mask or other protective breathing device when working around dusty areas, old barns, decaying dwellings or dried bird droppings.

Fungal lung infections that require treatment aren't common. Sometimes, oral medicines can be used to treat the infection. People who have medical problems, such as AIDS, diabetes (p. 211) or chronic lung disease, may require hospitalization and intravenous medicines, along with other supportive medical care.

## Sporotrichosis

- Small ulcer at the site of a puncture wound

This type of fungal infection is common among people who garden. When the skin is punctured by a thorn or splinter, fungi are introduced into the tiny wound. An infection then develops. A small crusted sore slowly grows at the splinter site. The infection may spread in the skin or to the lymph nodes in the area. An oral antifungal medicine, potassium iodide, will usually clear up the infection.

## PARASITIC INFESTATIONS AND INFECTIONS

A *parasite* is an organism that lives in or on another organism. Parasites may be tiny creatures, such as the single-celled protozoa that can't be seen without a microscope, or large creatures, such as worms and ticks.

Parasites can affect different parts of the body and cause different types of diseases. Giardia and many types of worms infest the intestinal tract. The protozoa that causes malaria attacks the red blood cells. *Pneumocystis carinii*, another protozoa, causes pneumonia and is common in people who have

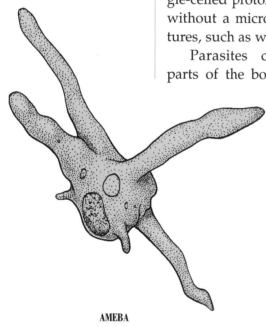

**AMEBA**

AIDS (p. 325) or other immune-deficiency disorders.

## Amebiasis

- Diarrhea, may be bloody
- Cramping abdominal pain
- Gas

The large intestine, or *colon*, can become infected with a type of *ameba*, a single-celled organism. *Amebiasis* is spread by drinking contaminated water and eating fruits and raw vegetables contaminated with the organism. Many cases of amebiasis result from travel to foreign countries where sanitation is poor. It's possible the infection won't cause any symptoms or a person will have mild diarrhea. Some people will suffer from *amebic dysentery*, a severe diarrhea with bloody stools. In the most severe cases, abscesses form on the walls of the intestine and even the liver. The disease can be fatal.

To help prevent amebiasis, wash your hands frequently, especially after going to the bathroom and before handling food. If you're traveling to an underdeveloped country, drink bottled water only. Be sure you're the one who opens the bottle, too. Wash fruits and vegetables with bottled water or eat fruits and vegetables that you must peel first.

To diagnose amebiasis, your doctor may examine a stool or tissue sample to see if ameba are present. It may take several samples to identify the ameba.

It's important to prevent dehydration (p. 179) if you're losing a lot of fluid through diarrhea. If your diarrhea is severe, your doctor may hospitalize you. Several medicines are available to treat amebiasis, but you need to be closely monitored while taking them.

## Fleas

- Severe itching, bite-like rash on the lower legs or in other areas

These small, jumping insects are usually picked up by a pet and brought into the home. The fleas then hide and breed in the carpet or in furniture, waiting for the animal—or a human—to pass by. Once in the house, fleas lay eggs in the carpet. The young, when hatched, will bite humans or pets for a meal. Some people may have more severe reactions to the flea bites, with hive-like spots lasting for days. Fortunately, serious diseases are almost never passed by fleas to humans in the United States.

The flea bites its host, then jumps off within seconds or minutes. In the fur of animals, fleas can be seen scurrying to hide while waiting for another meal or climbing to the top of a hair to jump off.

Ridding the household of fleas is the major treatment. Flea collars may prevent fleas in pets, but won't get rid of fleas once an infestation has started. Treating the infested area (the house and lawn) and using a flea powder or spray on your pets will help to free your pet—and you—from this uncomfortable pest.

## Giardiasis

- Abdominal pain
- Diarrhea
- Gas

*Giardia lamblia* is a protozoa that causes *giardiasis*, an infection of the small intestine. It's one of the most common parasites in America. It's become more prevalent among young children, especially those in day-care centers and preschools, in people living in institutions and in homosexual men.

Many people with giardiasis have no symptoms. Others experience violent attacks of diarrhea and gas, with abdominal swelling and discomfort and loss of appetite. In some people, the disease becomes chronic, causing periodic flare-ups.

Giardia can be spread by direct personal contact (either hand-to-hand or sexual contact) and by contaminated food or water. Many mountain streams harbor *G. lamblia.* To prevent giardiasis, don't drink untreated water, use good hygiene, wash your hands before handling food and follow guidelines to prevent sexual transmission (p. 32) if you're sexually active.

Samples of your bowel movement can be examined with a microscope for the protozoa Giardia. A biopsy of tissue from the intestine is another way to diagnose giardiasis.

Medicines, such as metronidazole (p. 618), can be given to treat the infection. Some cases may be resistant and require additional treatment. People in close contact with the infected person may need treatment to prevent the spread of the illness.

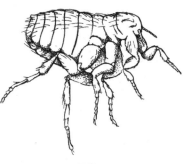

**FLEA**

## Lice

- Intense itching in the scalp, genital area or other areas of the body

These small, wingless blood-sucking insects look like small crabs. They can infest the head, the body or the pubic area. Lice lay eggs on the hair shafts and multiply rapidly. Within a few days of infestation, the itching becomes intense. The insects are large enough to see on the skin, where they climb the hair shaft and lay their eggs, called nits.

**LOUSE**

## Lice: Three Types

- Head lice—easily spread by children at school
- Pubic lice—spread by intimate contact, infested bedding and other sources
- Body lice—spread by close contact with an infected person

## How long can malaria last?

If not treated, the fevers, aches and sweats can come every third day for six months to four or more years. Some cases of untreated malaria can be fatal.

Head lice can be easily passed by sharing combs or hats. They're a common problem in children. Head lice are commonly spread among elementary school children through hand-to-hand contact. While the lice usually stay in the scalp area, they may also get into the eyebrows and eyelashes.

Body lice aren't very common among people who take regular baths. Pubic lice can be passed during sex. Lice can also be passed by contact with infested clothing or upholstered furniture, through intimate contact, or by sharing personal articles such as a comb or brush. And once you have lice, they can be difficult to get rid of.

Pubic lice, or "crabs," are usually spread by intimate sexual contact. But they can also be contracted through infested bedding and other sources.

You can help prevent head lice infestation by not sharing combs and brushes. Wash combs and brushes regularly with a disinfectant. Hand washing can also help prevent the spread of lice from one child to another. Reinfestation can be prevented by washing all towels, clothes and bedding in hot water (above 140°F) or having them dry-cleaned. Combs and brushes should be cleaned thoroughly. Those items that can't be cleaned should not be used for at least two weeks. This will allow time for all the eggs of the lice to die.

The treatment for head lice is twofold. First, go to the drugstore and buy an antilice treatment (p. 615). Shampoo with the medicated shampoo, let it stay on the hair for five minutes, then rinse. After shampooing, look through the hair for the eggs, or nits.

Remove all these nits with a fine comb. If you remove them with your fingers, you risk spreading the nits to others, unless you thoroughly scrub your fingernails afterward. All family members should be checked. If the infested family member is a child, the school should be contacted. The itching can be controlled with hydrocortisone cream (p. 616) or oral diphenhydramine (p. 615).

The shampoo also is used for pubic lice. A lotion can be used to get rid of body lice.

Sometimes, treatments you buy at the store may not work and you may need to see your doctor for prescription antilice medicine (p. 619).

## Malaria

- Chills
- Fever
- Sweating

*Malaria* is caused by any one of four parasites. Mosquitoes carry the parasites. Although the disease is common in tropical climates like Africa, Central America and Asia, it's rare in the United States because the Anopheles mosquito, which spreads the malaria-causing parasite, has been controlled with spraying.

Malaria is spread when a mosquito sucks in blood from a malaria sufferer and then passes the parasite when it bites another person. Once in the bloodstream, the parasite travels to the liver, matures, then infects red blood cells. The parasite multiplies inside the red blood cells until the blood cells break and release new parasites into the bloodstream. These cycles occur every two to three days. The symptoms—fever, chills and rigors or shakes—are produced by the breaking of red blood cells.

Before traveling to a malaria-prone area, discuss antimalarial treatments with your doctor. You can take some medicines to help prevent infection. Avoid mosquito bites. Stay indoors during peak mosquito feeding hours, from dusk until dawn. Put mosquito netting around your bed to prevent being bitten while you sleep. Use mosquito repellents.

If your doctor suspects you have malaria, he or she will probably take a blood sample to check for malaria under a microscope.

Chloroquine (p. 620), an antimalaria medicine, or another preventive medicine is given routinely to people traveling to malaria-infested areas of the world. But because some malaria parasites are now resistant to chloroquine, other medicines may be needed to prevent or get rid of the infection. All of these medicines have serious side effects.

## Scabies

- Itching in the webbed spaces between the fingers, at the wrists or at the belt line, often worse at night
- Small, red lines in the skin
- Rash that spreads from the hands or pubic area to the abdomen and other areas

Although the mite that causes scabies is too small to see without magnification, the rash, itching and discomfort it creates may be very large and intense. A mite is a small, burrowing insect that sucks blood after attaching to the skin. Sites usually affected by the bites include the webbed spaces between fingers, around the waist and at the armpits, elbows and wrists.

Scabies can be passed through contact with shared clothes, towels, bedding, furniture, sexual contact, or even by the family pet. Some cases affect whole families and can be difficult to cure.

Scabies infection is unlikely if clothing and bed linens are kept clean. Sleeping on a dirty couch or bed raises your chance of an infection. Intimate contact with an infected person, or his or her clothing, bedding or towels, can also pass the infection.

If the mite is found or the characteristic pattern of bites, burrows or rashes is seen, your doctor may prescribe an antiparasitic lotion (p. 620) to kill the mite. The lotion is spread over the entire body, except the head, and is left on overnight to allow the mite to absorb the active ingredient. All bedding and any clothing worn during the infestation should be washed in hot water to remove any living mites or kill any remaining eggs. The hair may need to be washed with the same medicine in shampoo form.

The itching usually persists for quite a while, even after the scabies are gone. Hydrocortisone cream (p. 616) may help relieve this. The continued itching doesn't mean treatment must be repeated.

## Ticks

- Irritation of skin where tick bite occurred

A tick is a flat insect that attaches to the skin to obtain its food. Ticks are picked up from grasses or bushes, where they sit, waiting for a meal. Then they jump on and embed their heads into the skin, usually after crawling around for a while first. The tick bite itself is usually painless.

When you're out in the fields and forests, wear long pants and long-sleeved shirts. Check yourself and your children for ticks after being outdoors in areas that may be infested. Tick repellents help prevent the problem, but don't guarantee that you will have no tick bites.

It's important to remove a tick as soon as it's discovered. Gently grasp the body close to the head with a pair of tweezers. Pull gently but firmly until the tick releases. The sooner it's removed, the less likely the tick will pass any infection. If you're not sure whether it's a deer tick or a dog tick,

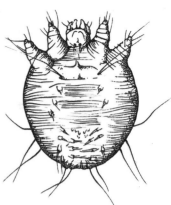

**MITE**

*Scabies Quick List*

*Scabies are spread by:*
- Intimate contact with an infected person
- Sleeping on unwashed sheets used by an infected person
- Wearing unwashed clothing containing the scabies mites
- Contact with pets that might carry the scabies mites

## Tick Quick List

*How to remove a tick:*
1. Grasp the tick close to the head with flat-tipped tweezers.
2. Pull gently, evenly and firmly until the tick releases.
3. Apply antiseptic or hydrocortisone ointment, as needed.
4. Do not use fire to remove ticks.

save the body of the tick for identification by your doctor.

Apply an antiseptic (p. 615). If you suspect that parts of the tick's head are still embedded, save the rest of the insect and take it to your doctor. He or she can remove the rest of the tick.

A few serious diseases can be passed by tick bites, such as Rocky Mountain spotted fever (p. 304) and Lyme disease (p. 301). Both require the tick to be attached for hours or longer. Rocky Mountain spotted fever is passed by dog ticks, which are larger than the deer ticks that pass Lyme disease.

Another disorder, called *tick paralysis*, causes weakness and inability to walk and can also be introduced by a longer bite. Removal of the tick will reverse the paralysis and is essential in slowing the course of Rocky Mountain spotted fever.

The diseases from tick bites can be confirmed by special antibody tests that confirm the body's response to the infecting agent, although some of these tests aren't very reliable.

Consult your doctor if you notice redness or swelling at the site of a tick bite, so that any infection can be properly diagnosed and treated. The small ticks that cause Lyme disease are only the size of a speck of pepper, so are rarely noticed until a reaction appears, or they're swollen with blood.

## Toxoplasmosis

• Fever
• Tiredness

In most people, *toxoplasmosis* is a mild illness, sometimes causing no symptoms at all. It's caused by a protozoa called *Toxoplasma gondii*. It's spread by eating undercooked meat, raw eggs and unpasteurized milk that's infected with the parasite. It's also spread through the feces of cats.

Pregnant women who get toxoplasmosis during the first six months of pregnancy can pass the infection to their unborn babies. This can result in miscarriage, stillbirth and birth defects such as mental retardation, blindness and hearing loss. Anyone who has an immune-deficiency disorder, such as AIDS (p. 325), will be more seriously ill if infected with toxoplasmosis.

Because toxoplasmosis is dangerous in pregnant women and people with immune deficiencies, medicine can be given to treat the infection. Your baby may also be treated after birth.

If you're pregnant, avoid contact with your cat's litter box or feces. Have someone else empty the litter box. Be sure to store meat at the proper temperature and cook it thoroughly. Don't eat raw eggs or drink unpasteurized milk.

## Worms

If you have children or pets, someone in the family is likely to have a case of worms. Pinworm is especially contagious in children, and worms are easily passed to adults in the house. Although many people are disgusted at the thought of having such a "beast" in their intestinal tract, worms often don't cause severe health problems. Worms may cause no symptoms at all or may cause only weakness. Effective treatments are widely available for worm infestations.

**Ascariasis.** Of all the round worms, Ascaris is the largest. Infection with Ascaris worms is called *ascariasis*. The larvae are found in soil where human waste is used for fertilizer. Once the larvae enter a human through contaminated water or food, the larvae travel from the intestine to the bloodstream and then to the lungs. The larvae move from the lungs and are swallowed. They then travel to the small intestine, where they grow into worms.

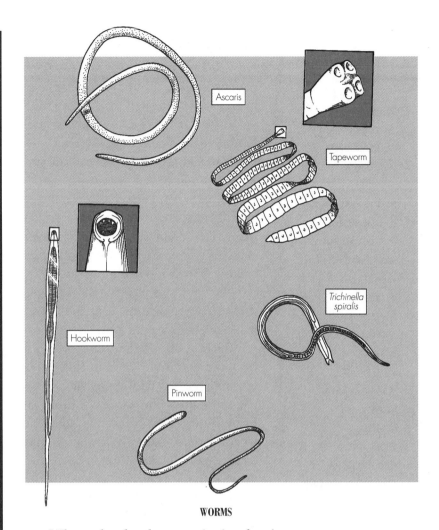

**WORMS**

## Types of Worms and Symptoms They Cause

**Ascaris**
Dry cough
Wheezing or shortness of breath
Stomach pain
Bloating
Diarrhea

**Hookworm**
Cough
Loss of appetite
Intestinal irritation
Weakness
Itchy rash on the feet or other
  areas of skin where the
  worm entered

**Pinworm**
Itching near the anal opening that
  worsens at night

**Tapeworm**
Stomach discomfort
Loss of appetite
Weakness
Worm segments in the
  bowel movement

***Trichinella spiralis***
Stomach discomfort
Cramps and diarrhea
Muscle pain and tenderness

**Hookworm.** The hookworm larvae are found in moist soil infected with human waste, usually in countries with warm climates. The hookworm attaches to any part of the skin that touches the contaminated soil, such as the feet. Once it enters the bloodstream through the skin, the hookworm travels to the lungs, up to the throat and is swallowed. Then it hooks itself to the wall of the small intestine and sucks blood. This journey may take up to two weeks, and it causes irritation along the way.

When the hookworm is in the bloodstream, symptoms of fever and weakness develop. When it's traveling through the lungs, the irritation may produce shortness of breath or a dry cough. Once hookworms reach the intestine, loss of appetite, weakness, diarrhea and abdominal pain may occur. Large numbers of hookworms cause anemia, due to blood loss. Most hookworm infestations cause no symptoms.

**Pinworm.** Pinworms, also known as threadworms, are about $1/4$ to $1/2$ inch long. They live in the intestines and lay their eggs at night. The female travels to the rectum and lays eggs in the anus while the infected person, usually a child, is sleeping. The child may be awakened by intense itching in the anal area. Pinworm eggs are picked up in the fingernails and passed to other children's fingers directly or by toys, for example. Fingers then go into the mouth and the cycle of infestation is repeated in another child.

**Tapeworms.** Tapeworms sometimes live inside animals, such as cattle, pigs and fish, and are passed to humans when the infected meat is eaten. Rarely, a tapeworm can be passed from a dog or cat to its owner. Children are infected more often than adults because their hands are washed less frequently and end up in their mouths more often.

The first symptom is finding the square-shaped segments of the worm in a bowel movement.

**Trichinosis.** Eating undercooked pork can lead to *trichinosis*. Like most worms, the adult *Trichinella spiralis* worm resides in the intestines of hogs. But instead of laying eggs, the worm larvae enter the muscles and form cysts. If the animal dies and decays, the worms die as well. If the muscle is eaten by a person, the larvae attach themselves to the human's intestines and form larvae that get into the human's muscles.

Symptoms of trichinosis usually occur in the larval stage, when the muscles are invaded by the larvae. Muscle pain, swelling or aching occurs within two weeks after eating the infected meat.

Testing of meat to prevent human infestation is usually done at the meat-inspection stage, where meat containing cysts is thrown away.

### Treatment

Your doctor may examine a sample of your bowel movement to look for Ascaris worms or hookworm. To check for pinworms, put a piece of clear adhesive tape across the anus first thing in the morning, before bathing or having a bowel movement. The tape will pick up any eggs that have been deposited during the night. The tape can then be examined by your doctor under a microscope. If you find a segment of a worm in your bowel movement, take it to your doctor to see if it's tapeworm and what type (dog, beef, pork, fish or rodent). A muscle biopsy may be needed to diagnose trichinosis.

Your doctor can prescribe medicines to take by mouth that kill most types of worms. The medicines for ascariasis may produce abdominal bloating, cramping and diarrhea as your body gets rid of the worms.

Mebendazole (p. 620) is highly effective in treating pinworm. It's wise to treat all children and adults in the household when anyone in your family has pinworms. Pinworm eggs can be transferred to toys, food and other people.

Taking medicine will kill a tapeworm within 24 hours, but the segments, or worm parts, may be seen in the bowel movements for days or weeks afterward. Although medicines are available to treat hookworm and trichinosis, both of these may eventually go away on their own.

## SEXUALLY TRANSMITTED DISEASES (STDs)

*Sexually transmitted diseases* (STDs) are bacterial, viral or protozoan infections that grow in the sexual secretions or on the skin, generally in the genital area. The infections are passed from an infected person to others through sexual contact. The infection enters the body through the moist membranes of skin in the genital area.

It's important to get tested and treated if you suspect you have an STD. If these diseases aren't treated, they can have serious consequences. Some can cause infertility in women.

Syphilis (p. 319) can permanently damage the major organs in the body and cause paralysis, insanity and even death. HIV (p. 325), which can be spread by either homosexual or heterosexual contact, results in AIDS, which is fatal.

Abstinence is the best way to make sure you don't catch an STD. If you're sexually active, it's safest to stay in a one-on-one *(monogamous)* relationship with someone who doesn't already have an STD.

If you have more than one sex partner or if you're not certain about whether your sex partner is having sex with anyone else, you may be at risk of catching an STD. The risk increases with the number of sex partners you have. You can reduce your risk of catching or passing STDs by practicing what's known as "safer sex" (p. 32).

Part of the safer sex guidelines include using male latex condoms. Condoms can greatly *reduce* the chances of passing or catching an STD, but they don't *eliminate* the risk. Condoms can break and they don't protect all of the skin in the genital area. See below for tips on how to use condoms to help prevent STDs.

## Chlamydia

- Discharge from the penis in men
- Vaginal discharge in women
- Abdominal pain in women
- Painful urination
- Frequent urination

The most common STD in the United States is *chlamydia*, which is caused by organisms called *Chlamydia trachomatis*. This infection is easily spread because it often causes no symptoms and may be unknowingly passed to sexual partners. Up to one in two men and one in four women with chlamydia don't have any symptoms.

When symptoms occur, men may have small amounts of clear or cloudy discharge from the tip of the penis and painful urination within three weeks after becoming infected. Women may have a vaginal discharge, irregular periods, abdominal pain with fever and painful sexual intercourse.

If untreated, chlamydial infections can damage the delicate fallopian tubes, causing pelvic inflammatory disease (p. 417) or infertility, and increase the risk of ectopic pregnancy (p. 393). Chlamydia may be passed

---

## *Using a Condom*

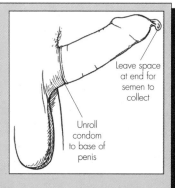

Leave space at end for semen to collect

Unroll condom to base of penis

- Use latex condoms. Condoms made of animal skin may not protect against tiny viruses, such as HIV (p. 325). These viruses may be able to pass through the porous animal skin.
- Make sure the condom has a teat, or reservoir, at one end to hold semen. Don't use a condom past its expiration date or one that looks like it's defective.
- Be sure to put the condom on before sexual contact.
- Unroll the condom over an erect penis. Leave about half an inch of space at the tip to hold the semen.
- Squeeze the tip to get the air out. Unroll the condom to the base of the penis.
- Use the *spermicide* (sperm killer) nonoxynol-9 (p. 617) with condoms. It may help kill some of the germs that can cause STDs.
- Don't use petroleum-based products, such as petroleum jelly, baby oil or lotion as a lubricant. These products can cause the rubber in the condom to break down. Instead, use water-based vaginal lubricants (p. 617).
- Pull out right after ejaculating and before the penis gets soft. Hold the rim of the condom at the base of the penis before pulling out.

along from the mother to her infant during childbirth, causing a minor eye infection or pneumonia in the infant.

Both men and women, particularly in the tropics, may suffer from *lymphogranuloma venereum* (LGV) as a result of the chlamydial infection. This condition causes blisters or ulcers on the genitals and causes lymph nodes in the groin to swell. The blisters may form abscesses.

There are several different tests your doctor can use to check for chlamydia. He or she will probably take a sample from the urethra in men or from the cervix in women. Your doctor may also check for gonorrhea (below), another STD. Some people with chlamydia also have gonorrhea.

Oral antibiotics, such as doxycycline (p. 618) or erythromycin (p. 618), should be taken by both partners if chlamydia is diagnosed in either partner. Women with severe infections may require hospitalization, intravenous antibiotics and analgesic medicine (p. 618).

## Genital Herpes

- Painful sores and blisters on the genitals

This infection is caused by the *herpes simplex virus*, which is also responsible for cold sores (p. 94). It results in painful sores and blisters on the genitals that disappear and then return. When a rash appears, it may be accompanied by headache, fever, enlarged lymph nodes in the groin and a feeling of being sick.

Unfortunately, you may be infectious even when no blisters or sores are visible or when you don't have symptoms.

A cesarean section may be needed if a pregnant woman gives birth during an outbreak of herpes. A C-section will prevent the baby from becoming infected.

Women with genital herpes should have Pap smears (p. 639) every year or two to check for cervical cancer. The risk of cervical cancer (p. 414) may be increased by genital herpes.

No medicine is available to cure the infection, but acyclovir (p. 621), an antiviral medicine, may help reduce the number, duration and pain of these episodes. Acyclovir comes as a pill or as a cream.

## Genital Warts

- Small, wart-like bumps on the genitals or anal region

Warts (p. 332) are caused by viruses and can appear anywhere on the body. Those that show up in the genital area are caused by the *human papillomavirus* (HPV) and are known as *genital*, or venereal, *warts*. They may form on the penis, the labia, vaginal walls or cervix or around the anal region. They aren't always visible.

The virus that causes genital warts can be easily spread through sexual contact. Condoms don't always prevent infection because they may not cover all affected areas. HPV is now recognized as a significant risk factor in cervical cancer (p. 414) and in cancer of the penis (p. 426).

No treatment gets rid of the virus that causes the warts. Your doctor can remove the warts with laser therapy, freezing or chemicals applied to the warts. Recurrences are common. Your doctor may want to see you every year because genital warts increase your risk of cancer of the cervix or penis.

## Gonorrhea

- Greenish-yellow discharge from the penis or vagina
- Burning when urinating

Also called the "clap" or "drip," *gonorrhea* is caused by a bacterial infection carried by semen and vaginal fluids. Some people have no symptoms, which can delay diagnosis. Women suffer the most serious consequences of untreated disease—they can end up with pelvic inflammatory disease (p. 417), infertility or a greater risk of ectopic pregnancy (p. 393).

After a culture from the affected site confirms the diagnosis, oral or injectable antibiotics (p. 618) cure the infection in most cases.

---

### Human Immunodeficiency Virus (HIV)

HIV is a virus that is often sexually transmitted. But it can also be transmitted by needles shared by infected drug addicts, from infected mothers to babies during delivery and by contact with infected blood. See page 325 for more information about HIV infection.

---

## Syphilis

* A single, painless sore (*chancre*) on genitals during the first stage of infection
* Headache
* Fever
* Aches and chills
* Swollen lymph nodes

*Syphilis* is a bacterial disease that has existed for centuries, but treatment has only been available for the past 50 years. Syphilis has three distinct stages in an untreated person.

During the first stage, a painless, open sore, called a *chancre*, appears on the genitals within a few weeks after infection. Usually just one shows up, although more are possible.

Within six weeks, fever, aches, chills, headache, swollen lymph nodes and usually a rash occur. The rash may look like grayish spots on the skin and may appear inside the mouth as well. Eventually the rash heals, but the bacteria remain active.

The second stage is called the "latent" period. There may not be any symptoms initially. In this stage the person isn't infectious, but continued damage occurs. Eventually, the victim may develop symptoms of the third stage of syphilis, which can include brain damage, blindness, paralysis and confusion. The blood vessels may become damaged, allowing aneurysms (p. 108) to form in larger vessels, such as the aorta.

Oral or injected antibiotics (p. 618) destroy the bacteria and cure the disease. If the latent stage is suspected, a blood test can help make the diagnosis. The disease can be cured at any stage but damage can't be reversed. Early treatment is important to reduce later problems.

About 50% of the people treated for syphilis have a reaction to the toxins released by the bacteria when an antibiotic is used. Symptoms of this reaction, which occur two to seven hours after receiving the antibiotic, include headache, fever, chills, aches, rapid heartbeat and slightly lowered blood pressure. This reaction can be treated with aspirin (p. 615) and bed rest.

## Trichomoniasis

* Greenish-yellow, frothy vaginal discharge
* Painful urination
* Vaginal itching and irritation

*Trichomoniasis* is caused by small protozoa called *Trichomonas vaginalis*. These organisms are especially irritating to the moist membranes of the vagina.

Women are most often affected by this condition, although men can become infected and pass Trichomonas to women through sexual contact. Men frequently have no symptoms and may not know they're infected until their partners need treatment.

Your doctor can take a sample of vaginal secretions and examine it for Trichomonas. Trichomoniasis is also sometimes diagnosed by a Pap smear (p. 639).

Both partners need to be treated. Usually, an oral medicine called metronidazole (p. 618) is prescribed. Tell your doctor if there's any chance you may be pregnant, since this medicine could harm the fetus.

## Urethral Infection

- Discharge from the opening in the penis
- Pain and burning sensation during urination

The *urethra* is the tube through which urine from the bladder passes out of the body. Symptoms of urethral infections, called *urethritis*, are often less obvious in women. Women may show few, if any, symptoms.

Most urethral infections are sexually related. Chlamydial infection is a common cause, although gonorrhea is also a possible cause. Urethral infections usually aren't dangerous by themselves, but may lead to scarring and constriction of the urethra if not treated.

Your doctor can take a sample of the secretions for a culture or antibody test. These tests can confirm the infection and help your doctor decide which antibiotic to use.

If you're diagnosed with urethritis, tell your sex partner so he or she can be treated, too, even if he or she has no symptoms.

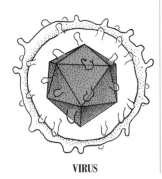

**VIRUS**

# VIRUSES

Many infections are caused by viruses. The infections range in severity from the common cold (p. 322) to more dangerous infections, such as HIV (p. 325). Viruses are the tiniest germs that can cause illness. They're much smaller than bacteria.

Does it matter if an infection is caused by bacteria or by a virus? A viral infection can't be treated with antibiotics. And a child or teenager with a viral infection should never take aspirin when a viral illness is present because doing so has been associated with Reye's syndrome (p. 370), a potentially fatal illness.

## Bronchiolitis

- Starts with a cold
- Severe cough
- Shortness of breath

*Bronchiolitis* is an infection of the *bronchioles,* the tiny air tubes in the lungs. It mainly affects children younger than two years old. Bronchiolitis is more common in the winter and spring. It's caused by different viruses, most often the *respiratory syncytial virus.* The virus first infects the nose and throat, causing cold symptoms. Then it moves to the lungs.

In some ways, bronchiolitis in children is similar to bronchitis (p. 145) in adults. Differences are due to the size of the airways in children, compared to the airway size in adults. Young children have smaller airways than older children and adults. As a result, secretions develop faster and shortness of breath occurs more quickly when a young child has an infection in the airways. In addition to secreting mucus, the lining of the airway swells, restricting the airflow into the lungs. This makes bronchiolitis more serious than most cases of bronchitis in older children or adults. Heart or respiratory failure and spread of the infection are possible when a child has bronchiolitis.

If your baby or young child has increased coughing, with shortness of breath or a bluish tinge to the skin, take him or her to the doctor's office or hospital right away.

Blood tests, cultures and x-rays can confirm the diagnosis. Treatment includes medicines to open up the airways. An oxygen/mist tent gives the child the oxygen he or she needs and makes breathing easier. Because bronchiolitis is caused by a virus, antibiotics (p. 618) can't help, but antibiotics may be given to prevent a secondary bacterial infection from developing in the respiratory tract.

Hospitalization is sometimes needed. Your child may need oxygen or a respirator to breathe. Procedures to help clear the mucus out of the lungs may be needed. Intravenous fluids may be given to prevent dehydration.

Some viral infections that cause bronchiolitis are spread by contaminated hands or respiratory droplets (produced in coughing or sneezing). When you have an upper respiratory infection, take precautions to avoid spreading the infection to your child. Wash your hands carefully and promptly dispose of tissues used for sneezing and blowing your nose.

## Chickenpox

- Fever
- Cold symptoms
- Tiredness
- A very itchy rash, including red, raised blisters that crust

*See photo of chickenpox, page 272.*

*Chickenpox* is a common childhood disease, but the new chickenpox vaccine, available since mid-1995, will make it much less common in the future. Chickenpox is caused by the *varicella-zoster virus,* the same one that causes shingles (p. 331) later in life. You can't get shingles unless you've had chickenpox, but anyone who has had chickenpox can get shingles.

Chickenpox is highly contagious. It's spread by infected droplets from the nose and throat. The characteristic rash doesn't show up until 10 to 21 days after exposure to someone who has chickenpox. Fever, aches and irritability may begin a day or two before the rash. Children (and adults) with chickenpox are contagious until the last bumps have crusted over.

The pale red bumps are filled with clear or light yellow fluid. The bumps are itchy and can appear anywhere on the body, including the scalp, ears, mouth and genital area. New bumps form for up to five days after the first bumps appear, and then begin to dry and crust over. Some children itch continuously and may scratch the bumps until they become infected.

Possible complications include scarring of the skin, pneumonia (p. 154), inflammation of the brain (encephalitis, p. 324) and skin infections. Chickenpox is often more serious in adults than in children. Birth defects may result if a pregnant woman has chickenpox.

You can't cure chickenpox, but you can help make your child more comfortable. Acetaminophen (p. 614) can relieve fever and achiness. Don't use aspirin in a child who may have chickenpox because it can lead to Reye's syndrome (p. 370). Your doctor may prescribe an antihistamine (p. 619) in liquid or tablets to help relieve the itching.

You can also soothe the itching by applying cool, wet cloths to the itchy areas. Or apply calamine lotion (p. 615) to the itchy bumps. Cool oatmeal baths are also soothing. You can buy oatmeal bath preparations at the pharmacy. Keep your child's fingernails clipped short to cut down on scratching.

Use only medicine or lotion recommended by your doctor to relieve the itching. Treating infected lesions with an antibiotic ointment (p. 615) may prevent scarring. If large areas of redness are observed, consult your doctor. He or she may prescribe antibiotics for a skin infection or for a complicating infection of the respiratory tract.

Acyclovir (p. 621), an antiviral prescription medicine, has been used to treat chickenpox when the infection becomes severe or when complications develop.

If you haven't had chickenpox, stay away from children or adults who are infected. Because chickenpox is extremely infectious even before the person breaks out with blisters, try to avoid anyone who's been exposed to others with chickenpox.

A chickenpox vaccination (p. 12) is available to prevent chickenpox.

## Chronic Fatigue Syndrome

* Forgetfulness or problems concentrating
* Headaches
* Sore throat
* Extreme fatigue
* Tender lymph nodes
* Muscle pain
* Joint pain

*Chronic fatigue syndrome* (CFS) was recognized in 1988 by the Centers for Disease Control and Prevention, which set guidelines for diagnosing the disease. CFS is controversial. Some doctors believe it's real, while others don't.

At one time, doctors believed that CFS might be caused by the Epstein-Barr virus, which also causes mononucleosis (p. 328). But the cause of CFS remains a mystery. Many researchers think it's likely to be due to some type of virus.

People with CFS suffer from extreme fatigue over a long period of time. The illness often starts suddenly, frequently after what was thought to be a bout with the flu or a cold. The fatigue doesn't get better, even after adequate rest. Other symptoms include headaches, sore throat, problems with memory or concentration, tender lymph nodes in the neck or armpits, muscle pain, pain in several joints and extreme tiredness after exertion.

CFS can be difficult to diagnose. There's no test to confirm the condition. It's important that your doctor rule out other possible causes of symptoms, such as hypothyroidism (p. 000). If you have extreme fatigue and at least four of the symptoms described above have been present for six months or longer, you may be suffering from CFS.

There's no cure for CFS and no proven treatment. If you have CFS you should get plenty of rest, eat a well-balanced diet and exercise. Treatment is aimed at relieving symptoms, like taking fever-reducing medicines (p. 616) and analgesic medicines (p. 614) for muscle and joint aches. Some people are helped by low doses of antidepressants (p. 619). Experimental treatments are being studied.

## Cold

* Headache
* Runny nose and sneezing
* Sore throat
* Coughing
* Fever
* Aches and chills
* Tiredness

Colds are caused by a group of several hundred viruses that infect the mucous membranes of the nose and throat. Viruses destroy the cells in the lining of the nose and throat, producing redness, pain, irritation and congestion. Within a few days, the immune system usually begins to recognize the virus and starts to fight it.

Most colds occur in the fall and winter. Colds are less likely to occur in spring and least likely to occur in summer. Colds are spread by touching someone or something contaminated with the virus or by breathing in the virus from droplets when someone coughs or sneezes. The older you are, the fewer colds you get, because you've become resistant to more and more cold viruses over the years.

You don't catch a cold as the result of being cold or having wet feet. But you're more likely to get a cold when your resistance is low, such as if you're tired or stressed.

Most colds last about a week and cause no lasting problems. Antibiotics don't cure a cold. Don't take an old antibiotic (p. 615) if you're suffering from a cold. If you get a bacterial infection, such as a sinus infection (p. 89) or ear infection (p. 79), bronchitis (p. 145) or pneumonia (p. 154), your doctor may prescribe antibiotics. Decongestants (p. 616) and other self-treatments that relieve congestion may help prevent these bacterial complications.

There's no cure for the common cold. Antibiotics and cold medicines won't get rid of it. But you can help yourself feel better while your body fights off the virus.

Get plenty of rest and drink plenty of liquids. Warm, not cold, drinks help break up the congestion in your nose. Chicken soup is an old-time home remedy that has been shown to help. Use a humidifier (the cold-mist humidifiers are recommended for children) and menthol rubs to help you breathe a little easier. Salt-water gargles can make a sore throat feel better.

There are plenty of over-the-counter medicines to help relieve your symptoms. Pick the product that matches your symptoms. Read labels to know what you're taking. Fever-reducing medicines (p. 616) can reduce fever. Analgesic medicines (p. 614) may help relieve aches. Decongestants (p. 616) may help relieve congestion.

Because colds are often spread by hand-to-hand contact, frequent hand washing is one of the best ways to protect yourself against the common cold. This gets the viruses you pick up from contact with infected people off your hands before you can rub your eyes or nose and infect yourself. If you have a cold, hand washing helps prevent spreading it to other people.

Get exercise, proper nutrition and enough sleep so your immune system is better able to fight off colds. Many people believe high doses of vitamin C help fight a cold, but vitamin C hasn't been proved to stop a cold from starting. Read label instructions and check with your doctor before taking higher-than-normal doses of vitamin C.

## Croup

- Cough that sounds like a bark or honk
- Shortness of breath
- Wheezing, squeaking, grunting or whistling sound while breathing
- Cold symptoms
- Fever
- Problems eating or swallowing

*Croup* is a common illness in infants and children. Children with croup tend to have a cough that sounds like a bark or honk. They may develop a squeaky sound in their throat when they're breathing. This sound is called *stridor*. Croup often develops at the same time as a viral respiratory infection, such as a cold.

---

### Reye's Syndrome Warning

Never give aspirin (p. 615) to a baby, child or teenager with the flu (p. 326) or chickenpox (p. 321) because of the risk of Reye's syndrome (p. 370), a rare but possibly fatal condition. Because the flu may seem to be a cold at first, it's probably best to avoid aspirin with colds as well.

---

### See Your Doctor

Sometimes a bacterial infection develops as the result of a cold. See your doctor if you or your child have any of the following symptoms:
- Pain in the face
- Earache
- Sore throat
- Increasing hoarseness
- Trouble breathing
- Wheezing
- Cough with fever and yellow or green phlegm
- Persistent fever

---

### Seven Don'ts for Colds

- If you have a fever, don't wrap up in too many blankets or stand in a hot shower, because the treatment may push your temperature to high levels.
- Don't smoke or breathe irritating fumes.
- Don't "starve" or dehydrate yourself. Your immune system won't be as efficient.
- Don't make salt-water gargle solutions too strong ($\frac{1}{2}$ to 1 teaspoon in 8 ounces of water is enough). They could irritate your throat.
- Don't overexercise when you have a cold. Overdoing your exercise regimen stresses your immune system, possibly prolonging or worsening the cold.
- Don't overdo the vitamin C. Large doses could lead to diarrhea or kidney stones.
- Don't overuse over-the-counter decongestant nasal sprays (p. 616). Use them three days at the most. They may cause a "rebound" effect if used longer, making congestion worse and causing you to continue to need them. Plain saline nasal sprays are okay to use whenever you need them. They can help relieve the dry, itchy feeling in your nose.

---

Croup develops when the tissues of the voice box, or *larynx*, and windpipe, or *trachea*, swell. The child often has symptoms of an upper respiratory infection, such as runny nose, sneezing and just generally not feeling well. Because of the smaller size of airways in children, shortness of breath is often more severe when children have respiratory illnesses.

Take your child to your doctor if you notice shortness of breath or squeaky breathing. Squeaky breathing may be a sign of croup or epiglottitis (p. 299). Your doctor may want to do blood tests and cultures and chest x-rays (p. 631).

Treatment of croup depends on the severity of the illness. Most children with the "barky" cough need cold medicines. Using a cool-mist vaporizer or humidifier at night may be helpful. Sitting in the bathroom with your child and letting the hot water run to fill the room with steam will help your child breathe better. If croup occurs during late fall or winter, taking your child out briefly into the cool, moist air may help the blood vessels in the throat constrict, or shrink, allowing for easier breathing.

Because croup is a viral illness, antibiotics can't cure it. Even though antibiotics can't cure croup, your doctor may prescribe an oral antibiotic to prevent a secondary bacterial infection. If croup becomes severe, your child may need to be admitted to the hospital. An oxygen/mist tent may be used, along with intravenous fluids and antibiotics. Most children recover within a few days. Sometimes, though, the symptoms last up to a week or more.

You can help prevent croup by preventing viral infections like colds from spreading through hand-to-hand contact. Wash your hands often. Throw away used tissues.

## Encephalitis

- Headache
- Fever
- Behavioral changes
- Extreme fatigue
- Seizures

*Encephalitis* is inflammation of the brain. It's a potentially serious condition and is usually caused by a viral infection, such as measles (p. 327), mumps (p. 329), chickenpox (p. 321) or herpes (p. 325). There's also an extremely small risk of some vaccinations causing this type of reaction.

Encephalitis usually doesn't cause lasting damage. In mild cases, it may cause flu-like symptoms and be hardly noticeable. In more severe cases, symptoms may include irritability, drowsiness, loss of nerve function, delirium or loss of speech or sight.

Encephalitis can be difficult to diagnose. Your doctor may need to do tests such as a CT scan (p. 632), MRI scan (p. 637) and electroencephalogram (p. 634). A spinal tap (p. 641) may also be done to examine the spinal fluid for infection.

Medicines can help relieve symptoms and pain. Some forms of viral encephalitis can be treated with acyclovir (p. 621), an antiviral medicine. Hospitalization and other supportive or life-preserving care may be needed.

## Fifth Disease

- Bright red rash on cheeks at first
- Lacy rash on arms and trunks later
- Low-grade fever
- Tiredness

Fifth disease, or *erythema infectiosum,* begins with a red, warm rash on the face, along with some paleness around the mouth. It usually affects children and occurs most often in spring. The cause is a respiratory virus spread by hand-to-hand contact, sneezing, coughing and sharing food or utensils.

The rash may last for up to a week, but may recur when the child is warm and flushed, such as when he or she takes a bath. No complications are known. Bed rest and plenty of fluids are the best treatment.

Although erythema infectiosum is usually a mild disease, it can cause significant problems in children with certain types of blood disorders (hemolytic anemias, p. 133) and to

fetuses. Keep a child with Fifth disease away from other children and pregnant women until the rash fades.

Make sure your child gets plenty of rest and fluids. Acetaminophen (p. 614) may reduce fever and aches. Never give aspirin to a child with a viral disease because of the risk of Reye's syndrome (p. 323).

## Human Immunodeficiency Virus

- Yeast infections of the mouth
- Swollen lymph nodes
- Fatigue
- Fever
- Night sweats
- Weight loss
- Frequent infections
- Shortness of breath
- Easy bruising and bleeding
- Memory loss and confusion (late)

HIV, the *human immunodeficiency virus,* is a virus that slowly destroys the immune system. The virus infects certain white blood cells, called *T4 helper cells,* which help regulate the immune system. When those cells are destroyed, the body can't fight infections or some forms of cancer, such as lymphoma or Kaposi's sarcoma (p. 290). Death is usually due to these diseases.

When first infected with HIV, adults may not have any symptoms for as long as 10 years. Children infected at birth may not have symptoms for two years. Before symptoms appear, a person may be described as "HIV-positive." Once the signs of immune system destruction show up, the person has AIDS, the *acquired immunodeficiency syndrome.* Everyone infected with HIV will eventually develop AIDS, though it may take as long as 10 to 15 years in some people.

HIV can be passed by sexual contact or by sharing infected intravenous needles or syringes. Babies born to

### Herpes Virus

The herpes virus has a number of different forms and leads to a number of different infections. Herpes simplex can lead to chickenpox (p. 321), cold sores (p. 94), genital herpes (p. 318) and roseola (p. 330).

### You're at Risk for HIV Infection If You . . .

- Are a man and have sex with other men.
- Have many sex partners.
- Have had sex with a prostitute.
- Use illegal injected drugs.
- Have had sex for drugs or money.
- Have had an STD.
- Have lived or were born in an area where HIV infection is common, such as Haiti.
- Received a blood transfusion between 1977 and April 1985.
- Have had or currently have a sexual partner with the above risk factors.

## HIV is NOT spread by:

- Insect bites or stings
- Shaking hands
- Sharing drinking glasses or eating utensils

infected mothers may be infected with HIV when they're in the womb or they can get the virus from their mother's breast milk. HIV is now rarely spread through blood transfusions. Screening of the blood supply used for transfusions started in April 1985. Before that time, many people who had hemophilia (p. 136) were infected with HIV because of tainted transfusions.

You can protect yourself against HIV infection by not having sex (*abstinence*) or by only having sex with someone who is only having sex with you (*mutual monogamy*) and who isn't at risk for HIV infection. Practicing what's known as "safer sex" can help protect you if you're uncertain about whether your sex partner is having sex with anyone else or is at risk for HIV. See page 32 for information about STD prevention and page 317 for further tips on how to use a condom to prevent STDs. Also, don't share intravenous needles.

The standard test currently used to detect HIV is an antibody test. This means the body has to produce *antibodies*, which fight the virus, before the test is positive. Most people test positive three months after they've been infected with the virus. Someone who is tested sooner may initially have negative test results. Even though the test may be negative in the early stage of infection, HIV could still be passed to others.

There is as yet no cure for AIDS. But early testing and diagnosis improve the outlook for anyone with HIV. Treatment with zidovudine (AZT, p. 621), an antiviral medicine, sometimes slows the progress of the disease. Other medicines may be used instead of zidovudine, or they may be used in combination with zidovudine. Antibiotics (p. 618) may prevent some of the AIDS-related infections such as PCP, or *Pneumocystis carinii* pneumonia (p. 154).

## Where to Go for Confidential HIV Testing

- Your doctor's office
- The local health department
- A local hospital
- The office of a specialist in infectious diseases

It's important to see your doctor as soon as possible if you suspect you have HIV. If you're HIV-positive, see your doctor regularly and whenever you detect any warning signs of infection.

A healthy lifestyle helps maintain a stronger immune system, which may delay the onset of symptoms. Don't smoke. Get enough exercise and rest. Eat balanced and nutritional meals. Limit stress.

## Influenza

- Headache
- Runny nose
- Sore throat
- Hacking cough
- Loss of appetite
- Fever
- Aches and chills
- Tiredness

The "flu" is caused by one of the influenza viruses and it affects both children and adults. The flu is spread by hand-to-hand contact or by breathing in the virus-containing droplets that are sneezed or coughed into the air. Symptoms may resemble those of the common cold, but the flu is much worse than a cold. With the flu, you may feel so sick that you don't want to get out of bed. Although nausea and vomiting can accompany the flu, what's often referred to as the stomach flu (gastroenteritis, p. 186) is a different infection.

The most common type of flu is type A, which usually infects people from November until March. Type A and type B can both cause epidemics, but type A is most often the culprit.

In infants, children and healthy adults, flu symptoms usually last from three to seven days, but cough or weakness may last up three weeks. Most people recover without problems. But the flu can lead to pneumonia, especially in the elderly or people who have immune-deficiency disorders. It can also lead to bacterial complications, such as a sinus infection (sinusitis, p. 89), bronchitis (p. 145) or ear infection (p. 79). Type B influenza can also lead to complications in young children, including Reye's syndrome (p. 370) and meningitis (p. 302).

All children younger than three months old should be checked by your doctor if they have a fever and cough—all common symptoms of the flu.

See your doctor right away if your child develops a headache, vomiting or diarrhea that won't stop, a coarse, moist cough or is extremely tired after the flu has run its course. These could be signs of a more serious problem.

There's no cure for the flu except time. Treatment is aimed at relieving symptoms. Rest and stay in bed, especially if you have a fever. Drink plenty of fluids to help loosen congestion, or mucus, and to prevent dehydration. Hot tea with honey and lemon, and chicken soup are two home remedies for flu. The honey in the tea can be soothing to your sore throat.

Use a vaporizer or humidifier to add moisture to the air. Gargle with warm salt water ($^1/_2$ to 1 teaspoon of salt to 8 ounces of water) to relieve a sore throat. Over-the-counter throat sprays or lozenges can also soothe a sore throat. Cough lozenges or hard candies can help reduce coughing. Be careful that you don't give a small child a lozenge that could cause choking.

Some people refuse any medicine unless it's "absolutely necessary." Treating your symptoms won't make the flu go away any faster, but will probably make you feel better and may prevent a bacterial infection, such as a sinus infection, if you reduce congestion.

Fever-reducing medicines (p. 616) and analgesic medicines (p. 614) may help relieve the fever, aches, chills and discomfort of the illness. A decongestant (p. 616) can help relieve congestion. Decongestant nasal sprays (p. 616) will open clogged nasal passages, but don't use these products for more than three days. They can cause a rebound effect and make your symptoms worse.

While cold medicines can help relieve symptoms, be sure to read labels. Don't take a product with a decongestant, for example, and then take another decongestant. Be sure any medicines you give children and teens don't contain aspirin because of the risk of Reye's syndrome.

Amantadine (p. 621), a prescription medicine, has been used during epidemics of type A influenza. If started early, amantadine can reduce the severity of an infection or help prevent illness in other family members who are at risk. Amantadine isn't effective against type B influenza.

The only known way to prevent flu and flu complications is by having a yearly "flu shot" in October, November or December. This is especially important for those who have immune system problems and for health care professionals. In the elderly, viral pneumonia can be fatal, so flu shots are recommended. The flu vaccine provides good protection against certain strains of type A and type B flu for that year, but won't protect against all other strains of the flu or other viral illnesses. See page 13 for more information about the flu shot.

## Measles

- Cold symptoms
- Sore throat
- Dry, hacking cough
- High fever
- Red rash starting on the face and moving down the body

*See photo of measles, page 272.*

*Measles* is a highly contagious viral infection spread by coughing or hand-to-hand contact. Measles begins with a fever and sore throat and usually lasts two to four days. This is followed by a rash of small, bright red bumps that starts on the face and spreads down the rest of the body. The rash spreads over two or three days.

Measles lasts 10 to 14 days before the rash fades away. It also takes about 10 days from being exposed for the measles to develop.

Once the child has the infection, medicine won't stop it. Fever may be relieved with acetaminophen (p. 614). Cough medicine may also be helpful. Rest, liquids, chicken soup, throat lozenges and cool compresses can make the child more comfortable.

If the cough becomes worse or there's shortness of breath, be sure to check with your doctor. Although pneumonia is rare with measles, these symptoms could mean the illness has led to pneumonia (p. 154), which can be fatal. Measles can also lead to an inflammation of the brain (encephalitis, p. 324). Your doctor may prescribe an antibiotic (p. 618) for any bacterial infections that develop with measles.

Although most children are immunized against measles, epidemics of measles are now occurring because some of these vaccinations were given before children were 15 months of age or not given at all. Make sure your children get the MMR immunization (p. 11) at 15 to 18 months old and again after age five.

If your child has the measles, keep him or her away from others for about five days after the rash appears to help prevent the spread of measles. The child is most infectious between the time of exposure to the disease and before the rash appears.

## Mononucleosis

- Cold symptoms
- Sore throat
- Profuse sinus drainage
- Large swollen glands
- Abdominal pain
- Fever
- Aches
- Excessive fatigue for weeks
- Weight loss

The old-fashioned term for *mononucleosis* was "kissing disease," because young couples seemed to contract and pass the disease to each other. "Mono" is actually a viral disease caused by the Epstein-Barr virus. It's not spread in waves or epidemics. The incubation period may be up to 60 days. People usually affected are from ages five to 35, with the peak number of cases occurring in the teen years.

Antibody testing has shown that 80% of college students have been exposed to the Epstein-Barr virus, yet only a small percentage—about 5%—have a history of mono. This means a large number of people have had the infection, but it wasn't severe. They probably thought they had the flu.

See your doctor if you have symptoms of mono. It can be diagnosed with a blood test. Return for follow-up exams during the illness, especially if you have any bacterial complications, such as strep throat (p. 306), bronchitis (p. 145) or a sinus infection (sinusitis, p. 89).

Antibiotics (p. 618) don't cure viral infections, including mononucleosis, but they may be prescribed if you have a complicating bacterial infection. Rest, fluids, pain relievers, throat lozenges, menthol rubs and other home remedies help relieve symptoms. Anti-inflammatory medicines (p. 615) may reduce the pain and swelling of the throat. Corticosteroids (p. 622) by injection or by mouth can also shrink swollen, tender throat tissues.

Mono symptoms may last for two to eight weeks. Getting plenty of rest and withdrawing from activities are wise. If no improvement is seen two weeks after the onset of the illness, strict rest should be enforced. Discuss with your doctor the need for rest and what, if any, medicines to take.

The possible complications of mono include an enlarged spleen, bacterial infection of the throat and inflammation of the liver. Enlargement of the spleen can make the spleen more vulnerable to injury. Minor bumps can cause it to rupture in some cases. That's why it's a good idea to tell your doctor about any abdominal pain, especially in the left upper abdomen, and to check with your doctor about avoiding contact sports for two months after mono.

To prevent mono, don't share food, drinks or utensils with other people and avoid passing saliva or respiratory secretions through other actions. You don't always know who's sick, so it's best just to avoid this kind of contact with everyone. Do your best to keep as fit and healthy as possible. Proper nutrition and adequate rest and exercise are essential to maintaining health.

## Mumps

- Swollen salivary glands in the back part of the cheek
- Sore throat
- Swollen lymph nodes
- Cold symptoms
- Fever
- Swelling and tenderness of the testes or ovaries

*See photo of mumps, page 272.*

The classic swollen cheeks of a child who has *mumps* are often comically compared with a chipmunk whose cheek pouches are full of nuts. Yet there's really nothing funny about this viral childhood disease. The swelling of the salivary glands causes pain and tenderness in the cheeks and neck.

The virus is spread by droplets, usually from saliva. A person with mumps is most infectious for seven days before the start of symptoms and nine days after symptoms appear. He or she should be kept at home and away from other nonimmunized people during this time.

There are a few serious complications of mumps. In males who contract mumps after puberty, painful swelling of the testes (usually just one testicle) can occur. This sometimes, but rarely, leads to sterility later in life. Abdominal pain in an adolescent girl may mean that the ovaries are inflamed.

Inflammation of the brain (encephalitis, p. 324) is the most serious complication of the mumps. It can occur before, during or after the salivary glands in the cheek become swollen. Headache, vomiting and lethargy may be symptoms of encephalitis.

Acetaminophen (p. 614) or ibuprofen (p. 617), bed rest and over-the-counter medicines or self-treatments can be used to relieve the symptoms of the mumps. If you're concerned that complications have developed, check with your doctor.

Have your children immunized with the measles, mumps, rubella (MMR) vaccine (p. 11). This should prevent them from contracting mumps.

## Polio

- Cold symptoms
- Muscular weakness and paralysis

*Polio* is caused by a virus that destroys the fatty substance that covers the nerves, called *myelin sheath*. Because the affected nerves control muscles, the illness can lead to paralysis.

> *Possible Complications of Mono*
>
> - Bacterial infection of the throat
> - Inflammation of the liver
> - Ruptured spleen

Before the first polio vaccine (p. 11) was developed in the 1950s, this frightening disorder was common. Cold symptoms, such as sore throat, headache and fever, appear first. Later, back pain and muscular weakness progress until the person is unable to walk or sometimes even unable to breathe without assistance.

Children are usually immunized against polio at ages two months, four months and 18 months and sometimes also at six months and five years. The rare cases that now occur in the United States are almost always in people who haven't been vaccinated. There *are* areas of the world where polio is still occurring. If you're traveling overseas, talk to your doctor about a booster immunization.

Analgesic medicines (p. 614) and bed rest are prescribed for polio. Physical therapy can help prevent muscle damage. If breathing is impaired, a surgical procedure to open the airway through the front of the throat, called a *tracheostomy*, and a ventilator will be needed.

## Rabies

- Pain or tingling at the site of an animal bite
- Headache
- Intense thirst but unable to drink (hydrophobia)
- Fever
- Paralysis
- Coma

*Rabies* is an extremely serious viral disease passed to a human by a rabid animal's bite, most often a rabid dog. Left untreated, the rabies virus attacks and destroys the nervous system and brain, usually causing death.

Dogs, cats, bats, skunks, foxes, raccoons, rats, mice and other rodents can carry the disease and pass it to a human through their saliva. The biting animal shows severe neurological damage, with drooling, choking, fits of rage, convulsions and paralysis.

Any animal that bites a human should be confined, if possible, and observed by a veterinarian for seven to 10 days. If the animal is in the wild or can't be caught, it should be assumed to be rabid. A series of injections stops the infection and also prevents its spread to the brain and nervous system.

## Roseola

- High fever at first
- Cold symptoms possible
- Swollen lymph nodes
- Fine, red rash

*Roseola* is a childhood viral disease caused by one of the herpes viruses, which are also responsible for chickenpox, shingles and cold sores. Typically, a child with roseola has a high fever (up to 105°F) for several days without feeling or acting as ill as would be expected. When the fever falls, a fine red rash usually appears and lasts from several hours up to three days. The illness usually affects children over six months old. The fever may cause seizures (p. 56).

Medicines, such as acetaminophen (p. 614) and ibuprofen (p. 617), and sponge baths (with lukewarm water, not alcohol) can lower fever. Make sure the child rests. Cold medicines may help, too. No complications, other than febrile seizures (p. 56), are known to occur from a roseola infection.

## Rubella

- Rash starts on face in butterfly pattern
- Swollen lymph nodes
- Mild fever
- Joint aches

*Rubella* has been nicknamed "German measles" because it's similar to measles, though much less severe. The rash starts on the face and spreads to the trunk and arms and legs. It lasts around three or four days. There's no treatment or cure for rubella. Acetaminophen (p. 614) can reduce fever and aches.

Rubella is of concern when a pregnant woman has the illness during the first four months of her pregnancy. Rubella can infect the fetus, causing miscarriage or birth defects such as deafness, heart and eye disorders, mental retardation, purpura (p. 288) and cerebral palsy (p. 346).

The MMR vaccine (p. 11) can be given to help prevent rubella. If you're considering pregnancy and don't know if you've been immunized, ask your doctor. A simple blood test can check whether you're immune to the disease. Don't get pregnant for at least three months after your immunization.

If you're pregnant and know you haven't been vaccinated, it's very important to avoid being around anyone who might have rubella. Get immunized after you've delivered your baby.

## Shingles

• Intense burning pain with a red, blistering rash

*See photo of shingles, page 272.*

Many people who have *shingles,* or *herpes zoster,* compare the pain with that of passing a kidney stone or giving birth. In other words, the pain is extreme.

Age affects the body's ability to handle this infection. The older you become, the more common and more severe the shingles. It usually strikes the elderly. If your immune system is weakened by a disease such as diabetes (p. 211) or by medicines such as those used in chemotherapy (p. 621), the infection can be more severe and prolonged.

Shingles is an infection of nerves to the skin. It usually begins with mild pain or tingling sensations, confined to the area served by the affected nerves. Within a few days the pain worsens, and red blisters appear on the skin in the area of the pain. The most common sites for shingles are on the face (which may cause paralysis or eye damage), under the arm, on the chest, on the back and on the buttocks.

The pain becomes intense because the virus is irritating and infecting the nerve in that area of the skin. Sometimes it takes three weeks or more for the blisters and rash to dry up and for the skin to return to normal. Pain may return for months or years to the same area where the shingles infection occurred. This is called *postherpetic neuralgia* and it afflicts almost half of people over age 60 who have had shingles.

Other complications of shingles include scarring and secondary bacterial infections of the skin from scratching. Headaches, inflammation of the eye or paralysis of the face may last for some time.

Your doctor will probably diagnose shingles by simply examining the painful, red, blistering rash.

Analgesic medicines (p. 614), cool compresses and time are the usual treatments for shingles. More severe cases may require acyclovir (p. 621), an antiviral medicine, or stronger medicines. Pain-relieving creams and aspirin may help put out the "fire" of postherpetic neuralgia.

Shingles around or in the eye require immediate medical attention to prevent scarring and vision loss.

You can prevent shingles by not getting chickenpox. The new chickenpox vaccine (p. 12) helps prevent chickenpox. There's no known way to prevent shingles if you've had chickenpox. Keep your immune system as healthy as possible through proper nutrition, exercise and stress reduction.

## Warts

- Hard knot in the skin, often with a rough, round surface
- Usually small lesion, the same color as the skin surrounding it
- Red or black dots in center of firm, raised lumps

*See photos of warts, page 272.*

Warts are caused by a group of viruses called *papillomaviruses.* There are two common types of warts. *Verruca warts* are the usual small, hard lumps with irregular surfaces. *Flat warts* are clusters of flat, slightly raised, smooth lesions.

Common locations for warts are the soles of the feet, on the hands or on the knees. Those found on the soles of the feet are called plantar warts (p. 272). Warts may also be located on the genitals (p. 318). Genital warts should be treated by your doctor.

A wart begins when a virus invades the skin cells. The skin cells then begin reproducing at a faster rate than the nearby tissue. This results in a growth. Warts often contain many small blood vessels, which can be seen as black dots in the wart. Warts don't hurt because they don't have nerves in them. But the skin next to the wart can become tender when the wart's destroyed or when pressure is placed on the wart.

The wart virus is spread by contact with someone who carries the virus. Warts can occur at any age and are especially common in school-age children, teenagers and young adults.

Adults should never assume a skin lesion is simply a wart. Some early skin cancers look very much like warts.

Many warts, especially flat warts, will disappear by themselves within a few months or years. Warts on the hands, soles of the feet or wherever they seem unsightly may be removed for cosmetic or comfort reasons. However, if a scar is left by the wart's removal, it may be larger or more noticeable than the wart was. A small pad or bandage worn over the wart may help relieve minor discomfort caused by clothes or shoes.

You can easily treat the wart yourself. (If you have diabetes, consult your doctor first.) Use an antiwart (p. 617) cream or ointment on a regular, daily basis. When a layer of dead skin forms, soak and soften it before removing the skin with a rubbing stone. The more often you treat and remove the dead skin, the more likely you are to get to the bottom of the wart for a complete removal. Don't treat warts on the genitals or on the face with these over-the-counter medicines.

If self-treatment is unsuccessful, your doctor can use one of several methods to remove the wart. He or she can use a stronger medicine, or can scrape, freeze or burn the wart off. A numbing agent can be injected into the area.

Warts can be deep and may recur in the same location after treatment. If you treat them while they're small, removal will more likely be successful and less painful.

Avoiding the viruses that cause warts may be difficult or impossible. You can help protect the soles of your feet by wearing rubber sandals in a public shower. Treat small warts early to prevent larger, more uncomfortable ones.

# PART 4

# SPECIAL GROUPS

| CHAPTER | | PAGE |
|---|---|---|
| 1 | NEWBORNS | 334 |
| 2 | INFANTS AND CHILDREN | 357 |
| 3 | ADOLESCENTS | 373 |
| 4 | WOMEN | 380 |
| 5 | MEN | 423 |
| 6 | ELDERLY | 433 |

# CHAPTER 1

# NEWBORNS

The first time you hold your new baby you may feel overwhelmed. You may feel as if you're not ready for the responsibilities of parenthood. How will you bathe, diaper and feed your baby? What if your baby gets sick? How do you raise a child to be a happy, well-adjusted human being?

Common sense will help you through some problems. When you have questions, you can get advice from your doctor, from this book and from other people you trust, such as friends and family. Parenting classes are also helpful. Your doctor or hospital may have information about parenting classes.

The following section will answer many of your questions about how to care for your baby during the first six weeks of his or her life.

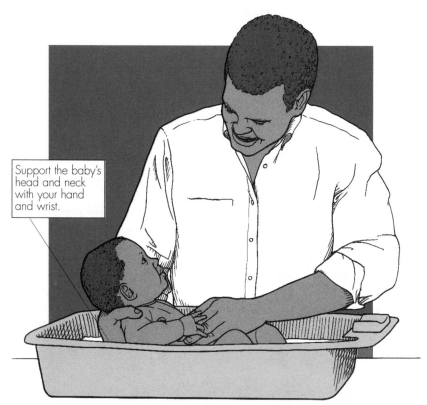

Support the baby's head and neck with your hand and wrist.

**HOW TO HOLD YOUR BABY FOR A BATH**

## Caring for Your Newborn

All the warnings about proper health care, toy safety, dangerous cribs and other dangers can be frightening if you've just become a parent. You may be reassured to find that many parenting skills come naturally as you bond and interact with your infant. But many parents don't feel instantly attached to their new baby. You and the baby need time to build a relationship. Don't let the fear of failure or of making a mistake keep you from using common sense when dealing with a problem.

### Bathing Your Newborn

Giving a baby a bath is a frightening task for many new parents. Don't worry if you don't know how to do this right after you get home. Only time and experience can tell you which things your baby likes and doesn't like during a bath and what kind of soap or shampoo is best for your baby's skin and hair.

While the diaper area needs to be cleaned at each diaper change, you only need to bathe your baby every other day, and often once a week is enough. When you bathe your baby, make sure the room is warm. You can use a portable heater, but keep it far away from the water. Have everything ready before you begin—soap, shampoo, washcloth, towel, cotton balls and, if needed, lotion. Lay out a fresh diaper and clean clothing.

Until the umbilical cord, or belly-button, is healed, give your baby sponge baths. To give a sponge bath, undress the baby from the waist up, and then bathe, dry and dress your baby in clean clothes. Then do the same from the waist down. Save the diaper area for last.

After the umbilical cord has healed, you can give your baby a tub bath. Don't bathe your baby in the adult tub. It's too big and it will be hard for you to hold on to your baby. Instead, use a sink or a baby bathtub. A dishpan will also work. Put an inch of water in the bottom of the tub. The water should be just warm to your touch (90°F to 100°F). Test the water temperature with your elbow or wrist. (The skin on your hand is much less sensitive to heat than your baby's skin.) If the water feels too warm on your elbow or wrist, wait a few minutes for it to cool.

Support your baby's head and upper back with one hand during the bath. Keep your wrist under the baby's head and neck and put your hand under the baby's armpit.

Wash the face first with a wet washcloth. Don't use soap on the baby's face. Use wet cotton balls to clean the eyelids. Rub baby soap over the rest of the body with your hand and rinse with a wet washcloth. Use a mild or "no tears" soap. If your baby's skin is dry, use soap once or twice a week or not at all. Instead of using soap and water, a moisturizing cleanser can be rubbed on and wiped off to clean your baby. Soap isn't really needed for newborns. Hypoallergenic soap may be good for some babies who have eczema (p. 277), since soap tends to worsen any dry-skin problem.

You may use a baby shampoo once a week, although it's not really needed. Lather your baby's hair, then rinse with a wet washcloth. Don't pour water over your baby's head.

Dry your baby right away by patting with a towel or receiving blanket. You may use lotion on dry skin. Talcum powder isn't recommended for newborns, who may inhale the fine powder. Cornstarch powder isn't a good idea either because it can encourage diaper rash to develop. If your baby has diaper rash, apply a cream that contains zinc oxide (p. 616) to any raw areas. The cream will protect and heal the skin on your baby's bottom better than powder.

*Never leave your baby alone in the bathtub.* If the phone rings or someone knocks at the door, ignore it or wrap your baby up in a towel and take him or her with you.

### Car Seats

Car seats protect infants and young children when they ride in a car, van or truck. Most states require that children under a certain weight ride in an approved car seat.

Never hold an infant or child in your lap when riding in a car. If a child is sitting on your lap in a car accident, the force of the crash will force the child from your arms and throw him or her against the dashboard or front seat. Use the safety seat *every* time the child is in the car, even on short trips.

Make sure the seat you buy has been approved by the Consumer

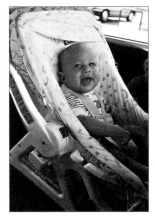

**CHILD CAR SEAT**

Product Safety Commission of the U.S. government and favorably reviewed by *Consumer Reports* magazine. Follow the instructions for installation and use. For infants who weigh less than 20 pounds, place the back of the car seat toward the front of the car for more protection.

If you can't afford to buy a car seat, check with the local hospital or other organizations. Some places sell or rent car seats at reduced prices or loan them out. Be sure that whatever seat you obtain is in working condition and is easy to use.

### Circumcision Care

*Circumcision* is a minor surgery done to remove the *foreskin,* or the flap of skin that covers the head of the penis.

Circumcision provides minor hygiene benefits. The medical benefits of circumcision are a reduced risk of urinary tract infection during the first year of life, prevention of *posthitis* (infected foreskin) and a reduced risk of cancer of the penis (p. 426) in later years. All of these health benefits probably can also be achieved with good hygiene—initially by the parents and later by the child. Circumcision doesn't

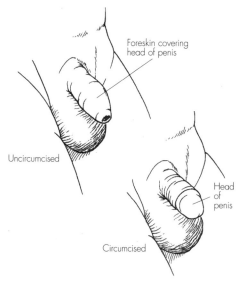

Foreskin covering head of penis

Uncircumcised

Head of penis

Circumcised

**CIRCUMCISED AND UNCIRCUMCISED PENIS**

reduce the risk of getting or passing sexually transmitted diseases (STDs, p. 316).

If you decide to have your baby boy circumcised, talk to your doctor about it before you leave the hospital. Many, if not most, circumcisions are performed for religious reasons or personal preferences. After circumcision, an antibiotic ointment (p. 615) may be used. The penis will be covered with gauze to keep the skin from sticking to the diaper for the first few hours after the circumcision. It takes one to two weeks for the penis to heal. During the time, carefully clean the penis using only water. Report any bleeding, swelling, redness, pus or other change to your doctor.

### Clothes

Your baby will grow very quickly during the first few months of life. It's best to buy clothes for your newborn in sizes such as three months and six months. It's more economical, and fit isn't that important to the baby. Also, your baby will grow into them. Keep the seasons in mind when you buy bigger clothes—it won't do any good if your baby "grows into" the winter snowsuit in the middle of summer.

Sizes on labels are different from brand to brand. The label on a pair of pants may say that the pants are for a 12-month-old baby but the pants may fit your baby at six or eight months. Don't worry if your baby's age doesn't match the label in his or her clothes.

Look for clothing that makes changing diapers easy, such as pants with snaps in the crotch or sweat pants that pull on and off quickly. Cotton clothing often seems most comfortable to many children and is easy to take care of. Some babies are irritated by synthetic fabrics and dyes.

Babies can lose a lot of body heat if they're not properly dressed, especially in cool or cold weather. Sixty percent of a baby's body heat is lost through the scalp, so always put a hat on your newborn in cold weather. Also remember that a baby's skin is very sensitive to sunburn, so make sure your baby is covered when you go outdoors, and include a sun hat. Don't overdress your baby, though. In general, your baby's clothes should provide as much warmth as yours. For example, if you aren't wearing a heavy coat to go outside, don't put one on your baby.

**Crib Safety**

The side rails of a crib should extend at least 26 inches above the mattress, and the slats in the sides should be no more than $2^3/_8$ inches apart. The crib shouldn't have posts that stick up above the side rails of the crib.

The mattress should fit snugly. A bumper pad should cover the slats on all sides so babies can't bump their heads on the side rails. No sharp edges should be exposed.

Don't use a crib that was built before 1960. Before 1960, paint used on furniture and houses contained lead, which can poison your child. Babies often chew on their cribs and sometimes swallow paint chips.

Never leave a pillow or other soft objects such as stuffed toys in the crib

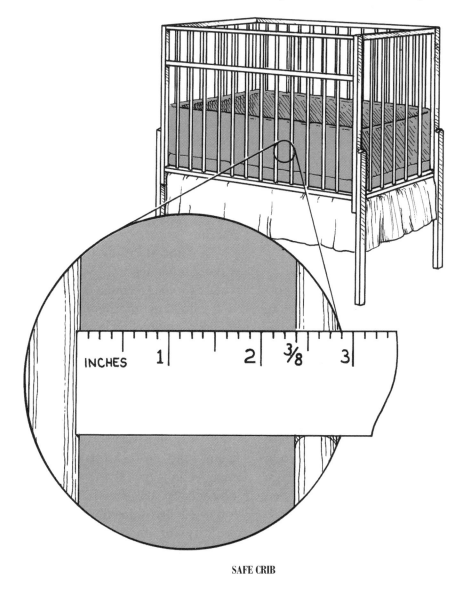

**SAFE CRIB**

when your baby is unattended. These could suffocate the baby.

### Crying

At first your baby's cries will all probably sound the same to you. But after a while, you'll be able to tell the difference between a cry of hunger and a cry for attention. Hunger is probably one of the most common reasons that babies cry. Babies cry because their diaper needs to be changed or because they're tired, scared, don't feel well or need to be held and comforted. Babies can't speak so they cry to communicate. When your baby cries, don't assume that he or she is "spoiled." If you're not already holding the baby, pick him or her up and try to find out the reason for the crying.

Some crying is to be expected. Some babies cry more than others. The average baby cries a total of three to four hours a day.

It's important to notice when your baby's cry sounds different. Check your baby's temperature. Does your baby look different? Does he or she have a runny nose, cough or loose bowel movements? If so, call your doctor.

### Diapers

Deciding whether to use disposable or cloth diapers, and whether to wash the diapers yourself or use a diaper service, can be a difficult decision. Usually, the choice you'll make will depend on what you can afford, how much time you have and your feelings about the environment and pollution.

The cheapest option—and the best for the environment—is to buy two to six dozen cloth diapers and wash them yourself. When the baby soils a diaper, flush the contents down the toilet, rinse the diaper and store it in a covered pail until you do laundry. When washing diapers, set the washing machine so it rinses the diapers at least twice. You may want to use disposable diapers when you travel with your baby.

Disposable diapers are more convenient than cloth diapers, but they're more expensive. Also, if you live in an area where the cost of trash pickup is based on the amount of trash you have, it may cost you more to get rid of the used diapers.

A diaper service delivers clean cloth diapers and picks up dirty ones on a regular basis, usually once or twice a week. A diaper service can be expensive, but it relieves you of washing the diapers.

When you change the baby, wipe the diaper area from front to back with a disposable wipe or a washcloth. If you use a washcloth, use soap and water and dry the area before putting on a clean diaper. Change your baby's diaper often, at least after each feeding. Frequent changes prevent rashes and yeast infections (diaper rash).

Don't leave your baby unattended on a changing table or bed. He or she could roll off and get hurt.

### Feeding

The first decision you'll have to make about feeding your baby is whether to use formula or breast milk. The following information will help you decide which is best for you and your baby.

**Breast feeding.** Breast milk is better for babies than formula. It's easier to digest than formula, it contains antibodies that help your baby fight infections and it doesn't cost anything. Babies who are breast-fed have fewer ear infections (p. 79) and urinary tract infections (p. 162) than babies who are bottle-fed. Breast feeding may prevent or delay certain conditions, such as allergies (p. 221), celiac disease (p. 194) and diabetes (p. 211). Mothers who breast-feed are less likely to develop osteoporosis (p. 244), breast cancer (p. 408) and ovarian cancer (p. 416).

Because breast milk is digested more easily than formula, your baby may get hungry more often. Breast-fed babies may need to nurse every two or three hours.

Good breast-feeding technique isn't second nature. You'll probably have to put some effort into getting started. It's important to start breast feeding the correct way to avoid problems with your nipples. These problems are easier to avoid than to treat. See page 404 for information on how to start breast feeding.

**Formula.** If you decide to bottle-feed your infant, use the type of formula recommended by your doctor. Premixed formula is more convenient, but it's also more expensive than dry formula. If you use formula that requires mixing, follow the instructions carefully. Make the formula in the correct proportions for proper nutrition.

Most babies aren't picky about the type of bottle or nipple that you use. However, you may find that your baby seems to prefer a certain kind. Bottles that use sterile, disposable liners may keep your baby from swallowing too much air. Burp your baby often by patting him or her on the back.

A two-week-old infant will drink about 15 to 20 ounces of formula each day. By the time your baby is one month old, he or she will probably be eating less often and consuming more formula at each feeding.

## Sleeping

The average newborn sleeps a total of $16^{1}/_{2}$ hours a day. Your baby may sleep more or less, from 10 to 23 hours a day. Don't be surprised if your baby seems to have day and night confused and is awake at night and asleep during the day. This is normal for babies. Keeping track of time isn't important to them. Don't expect your baby to sleep through the night. It's normal for babies to wake every few hours until they're at least several months old.

## Swaddling

Some babies are comforted by being *swaddled*, or wrapped snugly in a blanket. Swaddling can sometimes soothe a colicky baby.

To swaddle your baby, lay him or her diagonally on a receiving blanket or other small blanket with the top corner folded down about 6 inches. Wrap

### Spitting up

Some babies spit up after every feeding, other babies don't spit up at all. Spitting up is different from vomiting. Vomiting is a forceful removal of the liquid. Spitting up is when liquid oozes out of the baby's mouth. If your baby spits up often, try burping him or her more often during feedings.

### Burping

Babies often swallow air when feeding and need to be burped. Bottle-fed babies usually swallow more air than breast-fed babies. When you feed your baby, hold the bottle so that formula fills the nipple. Your baby may need to be burped once or twice during a feeding and again at the end, or not at all. You'll soon learn what your baby's patterns are.

There are several ways to burp a baby. One way is to hold your baby upright against your shoulder and gently pat his or her back. Put a towel or diaper on your shoulder to protect your clothes in case your baby spits up.

Another way to burp your baby is to put him or her face down on your lap when you're seated. Turn the baby's head to the side and support it with your hand. Or you can hold your baby in a sitting position. Support the baby's head and back and lean him or her forward a little.

one side of the blanket around your baby, and tuck the blanket under him or her. Then bring the bottom of the blanket up over the baby's body. Finally, take the other side of the blanket and pull it over the baby, tucking the blanket under your baby.

Don't worry if your baby kicks off the blanket. Not every baby likes to be swaddled. Older babies tend not to like this technique because they like to have room to move around.

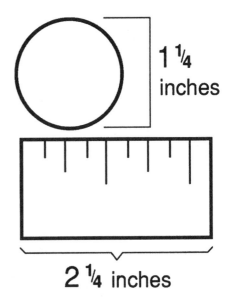

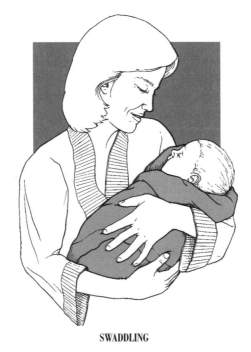

SWADDLING

### Toys

Toys that make sounds and toys that have different shapes, patterns, textures and colors are good choices for newborns. Mobiles, especially musical ones, provide sight and sound stimulation. But try to keep the crib from becoming cluttered with too many toys.

Most toys are now graded by what age children can safely play with them. Read the label on the box or package if you're not sure whether your baby is old enough for a certain toy. Even when a toy is recommended for a newborn, check it carefully for sharp edges or loose pieces before buying or using it.

**1 ¼ inches**

**2 ¼ inches**

SAFETY GUIDELINES

Babies put almost everything in their mouths. Keep very small toys out of your baby's reach so he or she doesn't choke on a toy. Toys that have parts smaller than 1 ¼ inches in diameter or 2 ¼ inches long shouldn't be given to a child younger than three years old. Don't be fooled if it seems like a part is secure. It could fall off or be chewed off and your baby could choke.

### Umbilical Cord Care

The "stump," or remnant, of your baby's umbilical cord will dry out and fall off after about two weeks.

Keep the stump dry to help it fall off. Don't cover it with the top of the diaper. To avoid infection, clean the stump two or three times each day with a cotton ball soaked in alcohol.

If small pieces of the cord remain in the bellybutton, they can produce a foul-smelling drainage. Your doctor may have to remove these pieces, especially if there's any redness around the bellybutton.

### Well-Baby Visits

Your baby's doctor will probably want to see your baby when he or she is one week old. Your baby will probably be expected to return to the doctor at ages two, four, six, 12, 15 and 18 months. At these visits, called well-baby visits, your baby will be weighed, measured and examined. Vaccines are usually given during well-baby visits. See page 11 for information about which vaccines your baby will need.

Well-baby visits offer a chance for you to talk to your doctor about any problems or concerns you have. Make a list of things to talk about with your doctor.

## Potential Problems in Newborns

During the first six weeks of your baby's life, several things may happen that will probably worry you. Some symptoms, such as fever (p. 296), are more severe in a newborn than in an older child. Other problems may seem severe but may actually be normal. Any time you're in doubt, call your doctor.

---

### Birthmarks

*Birthmarks* are areas of discoloration on the skin at birth. Birthmarks are fairly common. Many types of birthmarks occur. They range from faint marks that go away to dark marks that are permanent. See page 275 for more information about birthmarks.

---

### Colic

*Colic* is a condition that occurs in infants and causes them to cry excessively. If you've tried everything you can think of to stop your baby from crying, such as changing the diaper, feeding or putting him or her down for a nap, and nothing seems to help, your baby may have colic. Infants who are colicky cry after feeding, are irritable, eat poorly and may draw their legs and arms up toward their stomachs. Crying may be loud and may last for hours at a time. More than likely you will feel exhausted and frustrated by not being able to help your baby feel better. Colic can last for weeks or occasionally months, but usually ends by the time babies are about six months old.

The cause of colic is unknown. It was once believed to be caused by the baby swallowing too much air during feeding, causing intestinal gas, which produces pain. Although this cause has recently been questioned, doctors still aren't sure what causes colic. Babies with colic seem to need more attention than other babies. They also seem to be more sensitive to their environment.

After listening to a description of the baby's symptoms, your doctor may want to examine your baby. If your baby is growing normally and has no signs of other illness, the doctor may suggest that you burp your baby more often. Although medicines are available for colicky babies, don't use any medicine unless you've talked it over with your doctor.

Colic can be very difficult and frustrating. Pay attention to your feelings

---

### Suggestions for Soothing a Colicky Baby

- Burp your baby after feedings.
- Hold your baby in an upright position while feeding.
- Don't overfeed your baby. Overfeeding may cause your baby's stomach to be overfull, which can be painful.
- If your baby eats formula, try switching to a different brand. A formula that contains hydrolyzed protein may also help.
- To soothe your baby, try an automatic baby swing or take your baby for a car ride. Sometimes the noise from running a vacuum cleaner, dishwasher or clothes dryer is calming.
- Wrap your baby in a blanket.
- Put a warm-water bottle on your baby's stomach (make sure it's not too hot).
- Give your baby a pacifier.

about your baby and his or her crying. It's normal to feel frustrated, and even angry, in this situation. If you get frustrated, take a break. Find someone to watch your baby for you so you can get away for a while. If you feel extremely frustrated or can't get away and think you may hurt your baby, call your doctor or a friend to talk about how you feel.

### Drug Withdrawal

Mothers who are addicted to drugs, whether the drug is legal or illegal, may give birth to babies who are also addicted. When the baby is born, he or she will begin to have symptoms of drug withdrawal within a week after delivery. These symptoms may include shaking, seizures, convulsions, vomiting, diarrhea, sweating and irregular breathing. Treatment is available for babies who have severe drug withdrawal. Not all of the long-term effects of drug exposure and withdrawal are known, but they include problems with learning and physical development.

### Failure to Thrive

If your doctor tells you that your baby is *failing to thrive,* that means the baby isn't growing at an expected rate. Infants who don't gain weight or who gain weight too slowly probably aren't getting proper nutrition. Their formula may be incorrectly mixed or they may not be getting enough to eat. If the baby is breast-fed, he or she may not be nursing long enough or often enough.

Other things can also cause failure to thrive. Certain birth defects or heart problems can cause a baby to not grow enough.

Your doctor will probably talk to you about your baby's eating habits and may perform certain tests to find out what's causing your baby's slow growth. Treatment of failure to thrive will depend on the cause.

### Fetal Alcohol Syndrome

Women who drink alcohol during pregnancy may give birth to babies who have *fetal alcohol syndrome* (FAS). This term refers to a collection of birth defects believed to be caused by alcohol. The exact amount of alcohol that can be consumed before risking FAS isn't known, though the risk does increase as consumption increases.

Mental retardation is the most serious of these defects. Babies with fetal alcohol syndrome may have a smaller than average brain, cleft palate (p. 347), heart defects and joint abnormalities. Certain abnormalities of the face are also common, or the head may be too small for the body.

Babies with fetal alcohol syndrome may go through alcohol withdrawal shortly after birth. Serious withdrawal, if untreated, can be fatal.

To prevent fetal alcohol syndrome, don't drink alcohol while you're pregnant. If you're pregnant and you can't stop drinking, seek help. See page 562 for information about alcoholism.

### Jaundice

*Jaundice* is a yellow discoloration of the skin and may be noticed a few days after birth. Although many newborns develop a yellow tinge to their skin within a few days after birth, this is rarely related to a serious disease.

Almost 50% of all infants become mildly jaundiced. The discoloration is caused by a build-up of bile. The bile contains a reddish-yellow pigment called *bilirubin.* Too much bilirubin in the bloodstream makes the skin turn yellow. Jaundice usually clears in seven to 10 days without any treatment.

When a baby is born with yellow-colored skin, or when a baby rapidly develops high levels of bilirubin in the bloodstream, he or she may have a more serious kind of jaundice. One serious type of jaundice is caused by an incompatibility of the mother's blood and her baby's blood, called Rh factor incompatibility (p. 132). Other reasons for jaundice include infections of the blood or internal bleeding.

If your baby's skin looks yellow, your doctor may take a sample of blood from the baby's heel to check the level of bilirubin in the bloodstream. Other tests may also be done. If the blood test shows that there's a high level of bilirubin in your baby's blood, the baby may be placed under a "bili light," a treatment that uses light to speed the breakdown of excess bilirubin.

More serious causes of jaundice may require blood transfusions, intravenous antibiotics (p. 618) if an infection is causing the problem or intravenous fluids.

### Low Birth Weight

Because two out of three infants who die in the U.S. weigh less than $5\frac{1}{2}$ pounds at birth, ensuring a proper growth rate during pregnancy is important. Babies who have a low birth weight have been shown to have more health problems later in life than babies who have a normal birth weight. When you become pregnant, there are some things you can do to help your baby grow at a normal rate before he or she is born. Get prenatal checkups, eat a well-balanced diet, gain an appropriate amount of weight and don't smoke, drink or use illegal drugs. Talk to your doctor about taking prenatal vitamins.

### Prematurity

Pregnancy usually lasts about 40 weeks, although babies born after 38 weeks of gestation are considered full-term. Many infants born prematurely, or before 38 weeks, don't have any problems. But the earlier a baby is born, the more likely problems can occur. Even babies who are born just a few weeks early can develop problems.

In general, infants born after 26 weeks have a good chance of surviving. The baby's weight at birth may be the most important factor. Babies who weigh less than $5\frac{1}{2}$ pounds at birth are more likely to have health problems than babies who weigh more. Infants with a very low birth weight (less than two to three pounds) have an increased risk of death during the first year of life.

**Anemia.** The amount of iron a baby has stored in his or her body is used up faster in a premature infant. Babies who are born early may need iron supplements or blood transfusions. Iron-deficiency anemia (p. 133), caused by not having enough iron, makes it difficult for the blood to carry oxygen. Vitamin E is routinely given to premature babies because a deficiency can contribute to anemia.

Hemolytic anemia (p. 133), another type of anemia, isn't caused by iron deficiency, but by antibodies in the bloodstream that destroy red blood cells. If your baby has anemia, your doctor may do blood tests for hemolytic anemia.

**Apnea of prematurity.** *Apnea* means brief stops in breathing. Apnea of prematurity is most common in babies born very early. It usually begins two to three days after birth. Apnea of prematurity may be, but isn't always, a sign of another problem, so a baby with apnea of prematurity should be checked for other problems. Apnea spells can sometimes be reduced by making sure your baby sleeps on his or her back in a flat, straight position. Lowering the room temperature may also help. Medicine may be needed. If the apnea doesn't improve, your doctor may talk to you about at-home monitoring.

### Postmaturity

*Postmature* babies, or babies who are born after 42 weeks, may also have health problems. The placenta, which is the source of nutrition and oxygen for the fetus, begins to lose some of its ability to function after about 42 weeks.

**Asphyxia.** When a baby is born, he or she breathes air for the first time. *Asphyxia* occurs when the baby doesn't begin breathing after birth. In newborns who are affected by asphyxia, the message from the brain to the lungs to start breathing doesn't get through. The baby may make an effort to breathe at first, but becomes less active as little oxygen is obtained. If breathing doesn't start, the brain can be damaged after a few minutes, and the baby will die after about 10 minutes.

Fortunately, hospitals are prepared for the possibility of asphyxia. Equipment is present in the delivery room to clear the baby's throat of secretions, to push oxygen into the lungs or even to pass a tube into the lungs to help the baby breathe.

Sometimes, an infant can have too little oxygen while still in the womb. Monitoring the baby's heart rate with a stethoscope or a fetal monitor lets the doctor know if the baby is in trouble and if an emergency cesarean section (p. 403) is needed. Rapid treatment of this complication can prevent brain damage.

**Hypoglycemia.** In the first few days of life, premature infants, very sick newborns and babies whose mothers have diabetes are especially prone to *hypoglycemia*, or low blood sugar (p. 124). This causes babies to be lethargic, less responsive and to have difficulties with feeding. These babies can be given glucose intravenously.

**Pneumonia.** Pneumonia (p. 154), an infection of the lungs, may occur in premature infants because their lungs aren't fully developed. Your baby's doctor will probably use intravenous antibiotics to treat the infection.

**Respiratory distress syndrome.** Symptoms of *respiratory distress syndrome* include shortness of breath, a blue coloring of the skin, flaring of the nostrils and grunting sounds.

During birth, a baby's body must do several things in a very short period of time so the baby can survive outside the womb. For instance, babies must switch from the blood supplied by the umbilical cord to their own blood, lungs and heart as their sources of oxygen. The baby's life depends on his or her own circulating blood, and the lungs must expand and fill with air. Most babies have no problem doing this. However, when this process doesn't go smoothly, respiratory distress syndrome develops.

One type of respiratory distress syndrome is *hyaline membrane disease*. In mature infants a substance called *surfactant* coats the inside of the lungs to keep the lungs from collapsing. Premature infants may not have enough surfactant to keep their lungs open. A mother in premature labor is often given medicine that speeds up the lung maturation in a premature infant. Treatment involves placing a tube into the baby's lungs to help keep them expanded.

Depending on the size and age of the infant, the lungs will eventually produce their own surfactant and stay open by themselves. The baby will probably stay in the neonatal intensive care until he or she is out of danger. Artificial surfactants have recently been developed and may also be used.

Another, less serious, form of respiratory distress is *transient tachypnea*. The baby begins to breathe rapidly for no apparent reason. This problem usually goes away in a few days without treatment.

**Retinopathy of prematurity.** The retina of the fetus normally develops throughout the pregnancy. When a baby is born too early, this development is disturbed and abnormalities in the retina may occur. This is called *retinopathy of prematurity*. The condition can also result from oxygen use, which may be needed for premature infants. The smaller the newborn, the more likely this problem will occur. Most of the time, retinopathy of prematurity will heal. People who have had retinopathy of prematurity may have a greater risk of some vision problems and of retinal detachment (p. 74) later in life. In a small number of newborns with this problem, the retina will detach and vision will be lost.

**Sepsis.** Premature infants pick up infections very easily, and an infection can spread quickly throughout the bloodstream. This condition is called *sepsis*. It needs to be rapidly diagnosed and treated with intravenous antibiotics. Infections can be fatal in premature infants.

### Rh Factor Incompatibility

People who have *Rh positive* blood have the Rh factor antigen on the red blood cells. People who have *Rh negative* blood don't. This difference between the two groups can cause problems if an Rh negative woman is pregnant with an Rh positive fetus. This situation is called *Rh factor incompatibility*.

Pregnant women whose blood is Rh negative make antibodies against the Rh positive blood of the fetus. If the antibodies cross the placenta, they'll destroy the baby's red blood cells, which may cause the fetus to have hemolytic anemia (p. 133). This anemia can be so severe that the fetus dies before birth.

The first time an Rh-negative woman is pregnant, her body doesn't make the antibodies against the Rh-positive blood of the fetus. Therefore, first pregnancies are rarely affected by the Rh factor. After the first pregnancy, the risk increases with each pregnancy because the mother begins making antibodies against the Rh-positive blood.

All women are now screened for the Rh factor during prenatal visits. If a woman is Rh negative, the baby's father should be tested for the Rh factor. If the father's blood is Rh positive, the baby may be Rh positive.

Injections of antibodies can be given to the mother after her first delivery so her body won't make antibodies in future pregnancies. The antibodies that the mother receives won't destroy the red blood cells of infants in future pregnancies. Often, a doctor will simply give the Rh shot to all of his or her pregnant patients during their first pregnancies.

When a woman who is Rh negative doesn't get the Rh shot and the fetus she's carrying is Rh positive, the baby might need blood transfusions while in the womb to prevent problems such as hearing loss, mental retardation or even death.

## Birth Defects

Some babies are born with birth defects. Some defects are common and some are rare. Many birth defects have no known cause. Sometimes, problems are inherited. Inherited, or *genetic*, problems can occur when something goes wrong in how the *chromosomes* divide or grow. The chromosomes carry the *genes*, where the genetic information is stored. The genetic information is like a map, or blueprint, that the body follows as it develops. If something is wrong with the map, it could result in problems in how the body develops.

Birth defects can also be caused by problems during labor and delivery. Also, in some cases, drug use by the mother or father may cause birth defects.

Many parents feel guilty when their baby is born with a birth defect. Mothers may believe that something they did during the pregnancy caused or contributed to the birth defect. In most cases, nothing could have been done to prevent the birth defect and feelings of guilt only make the parents feel worse.

If you have a baby with a birth defect, you can work with your doctor to provide proper care and follow-up treatment for your baby. Your doctor may suggest genetic counseling if your child has a disease that may occur in future children you might have.

If you have a child with special needs, or you'll be caring for a child with special needs, you'll probably need more information and support than you can get from a book. Talk with your doctor and contact a social worker at your local health department for further information about the problem.

## Abnormalities of the Genitalia

In rare cases, a child may be born with abnormalities of the genitalia. One birth defect of sex organs in boys is called *hypospadias*. With hypospadias, the *urethra*, or the tube that carries urine out of the penis, opens on the upper or lower side of the penis instead of on the tip of the penis. Even more rarely, a child is born with external sex organs that aren't clearly male or female, a condition called *ambiguous genitalia*.

Surgery can repair deformities of the genitalia, or make them less of a problem. If the sex of a child is in doubt, chromosome or genetic studies will be done to determine the baby's sex. In children with ambiguous genitalia, surgery is usually performed by about age two.

## Anencephaly

*Anencephaly* is rare. Infants with anencephaly are born either without a part of their brain or without the whole brain. Most of these infants are born dead or die before the birth process is complete. Tests, such as an ultrasound (p. 643) and amniocentesis (p. 628), can detect anencephaly during pregnancy. A few newborns live for a short time after birth, but die within days.

## Biliary Atresia

In *biliary atresia*, the infant is born without a *bile duct*. The bile duct is the connection between the liver and the small intestine. Usually the bile duct and the gallbladder drain a secretion, called *bile*, from the liver into the intestines. Without this connection, toxic waste products build up in the liver and the bloodstream, causing jaundice (p. 342).

In some children, doctors are able to correct this problem with surgery. For other children who have no duct at all in the liver, a liver transplant may be the only option.

## Cerebral Palsy

*Cerebral palsy* is a disorder characterized by problems with movement. In most cases, cerebral palsy is caused by brain damage that occurs before delivery, during delivery or after birth. In some cases, cerebral palsy may be caused by a genetic disorder.

One of the most common reasons for brain damage is lack of oxygen for more than four to five minutes. Lack of oxygen can be the result of diseased lungs, such as in respiratory distress syndrome (p. 344), neonatal pneumonia (p. 344) or an injury during delivery that leads to internal bleeding. Encephalitis (p. 324) and meningitis (p. 302), which are infections of the brain or spinal cord, can also damage the brain and cause cerebral palsy.

The amount and cause of brain damage determines what kind of problems the child will have as he or she gets older. Some degree of mental retardation is possible, along with difficulty with movement, seizures and speech problems. However, children with brain damage aren't always totally disabled. The degree of brain damage varies from person to person, and numerous people with cerebral palsy have average or above-average mental abilities despite their physical limitations.

Different types of cerebral palsy have been identified. A thorough exam by a neurologist can identify the type and extent of cerebral palsy. Physical therapy, surgery, exercises, stretches, mechanical aids and special educational programs may all be used to help the child fully develop his or her potential.

### Cleft Lip and Palate

When a fetus is growing inside the womb, the skull begins to grow at the back of the head. The sides of the skull grow forward to meet at the place just under the tip of the nose. Sometimes, the two sides of the lip or the two sides of the roof of the mouth don't grow completely together. A *cleft lip*, or split lip, may have what looks like a notch in the upper lip, or it may be a more serious deformity, with the split extending to the nose. In a child with a *cleft palate*, the roof of the mouth (*palate*) may be partly or completely split. Sometimes a cleft lip and cleft palate occur together.

Cleft lip or cleft palate can cause feeding problems for the baby and may cause psychological discomfort to the parents and, later in life, to the child if not corrected. Also, speech difficulties may arise if a cleft palate isn't corrected. Plastic surgery can correct most facial deformities. Often the lip surgery is done when the child is two to three months old. In some cases, several surgeries may be needed over the years to correct cleft palate.

### Club Foot

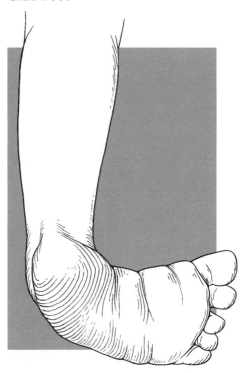

**CLUB FOOT**

*Club foot* is a common deformity, occurring in one in 1,000 births. With club foot, the baby is born with a foot that's abnormally bent or twisted. There are several different types of club foot. When several members of a family have club foot, it's thought to be hereditary.

Treatment for club foot should begin soon after birth. Massage and

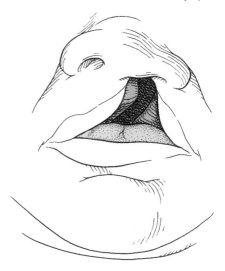

**CLEFT LIP AND CLEFT PALATE**

manipulation of the foot and ankle, along with special shoes, splints or plaster casts can help push the foot back toward its normal position. If the deformity is severe, surgical repair can be done. Surgery is usually best performed before the age of two.

A deformity that involves the hip, called congenital dislocation of the hip, is discussed on page 240.

### Cystic Fibrosis

*Cystic fibrosis* is an inherited disease that affects the respiratory and digestive systems, and the exocrine glands of the body. The exocrine glands release chemicals through a tube or duct. The pancreas, salivary glands, sweat glands, mucous glands and sebaceous glands are exocrine glands.

Cystic fibrosis causes the lungs to produce large amounts of thick, sticky mucus. People with cystic fibrosis may have trouble breathing and frequent lung infections. Sometimes, mucus can block the bowel, causing constipation, abdominal pain and vomiting. In people who have cystic fibrosis, the pancreas doesn't make an enzyme that's needed to digest fats and certain nutrients,

which can result in large, greasy-looking bowel movements. Also, children with cystic fibrosis often don't grow normally.

Cystic fibrosis can be so mild that it's not diagnosed until later in childhood or even adulthood. Two-thirds of people who have cystic fibrosis are diagnosed during the first year of life. But cystic fibrosis can also be so severe that it's life-threatening. About 10% of cases of cystic fibrosis are discovered just after birth, when the child is unable to have a bowel movement.

Treatment may include medicines that aid digestion and special breathing treatments to keep the lungs clear of mucus. You'll be taught how to use *postural drainage,* which involves placing your baby in various positions and vibrating or gently pounding his or her chest to loosen secretions and help clear the lungs. It's important to quickly treat infections with antibiotics. Your doctor can help design a daily exercise and treatment regimen.

### Down Syndrome

A baby born with *Down syndrome* has an extra chromosome in each cell. Chromosomes carry the genetic material.

The facial characteristics of a child with Down syndrome are the most recognizable signs of the condition. The ears are small. The nose is usually short with a flattened bridge. The eyes are slanted upward and outward. Heart problems, intestinal blockage, immune problems and mental retardation may also occur.

Although women who become pregnant after the age of 35, and especially after age 40, are more likely to have a child with Down syndrome, the majority of Down syndrome children are now born to women under 35. If you're over 35 and pregnant, your doctor may recommend that you have

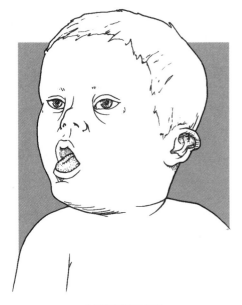

**DOWN SYNDROME**

a test called amniocentesis (p. 628). The results of amniocentesis can usually tell whether the baby will be born with Down syndrome. An alpha-fetoprotein test (p. 627) can also tell you if the fetus has Down syndrome.

Down syndrome can't be treated. The long-term expectations for the child depend on the level of mental retardation and other health problems. The family, doctor and social worker should openly discuss all the issues involved, including how the family and child are affected, finances and day care if it's needed.

Children with Down syndrome can be happy, loving members of families. As adults, people with Down syndrome are often able to work. Several agencies, organizations and support groups are available to help parents and families of children with Down syndrome. Look in your local phone book for phone numbers

### Dwarfism

*Dwarfism* is a symptom of a number of disorders that are genetically related. The word dwarfism commonly refers to the short height of people who have one of these disorders. The different types of genetic disorders that include dwarfism as a symptom also have other related symptoms. These symptoms may include an unusually large forehead, short forearms and a snub nose. As with other genetic disorders, genetic counseling can help identify couples who may be likely to have a child with dwarfism.

### Esophageal Atresia

In babies with *esophageal atresia*, the esophagus doesn't join the stomach. A portion of the tube is missing, causing food that's swallowed to end up in a part of the body where it doesn't belong. In some cases, the esophagus is connected to the windpipe.

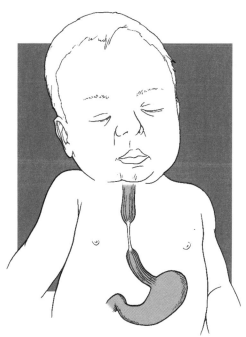

**ESOPHAGEAL ATRESIA**

Babies with esophageal atresia can't swallow saliva or milk. They drool and spit up constantly. If the esophagus leads to the windpipe, fluids may end up in the lungs, causing coughing and breathing problems.

A barium swallow (p. 629) can diagnose esophageal atresia. Surgery is needed to correct the problem. Many times the two ends of the esophagus can't be joined because they're too short. In that case, a section of the bowel may be used to lengthen the esophagus so it joins the stomach.

### Heart Defects

The heart is a muscle made up of chambers and valves. Normally, blood flows through the heart so that blood carrying oxygen to the body never mixes with blood that has already delivered the oxygen. For more information about how the heart works, see page 107.

Sometimes a defect occurs in a vein or an artery in the heart or in the heart muscle itself that causes "fresh" blood to mix with "used" blood. This problem can cause trouble breathing, heart

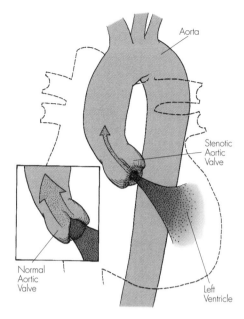

**AORTIC VALVE STENOSIS**

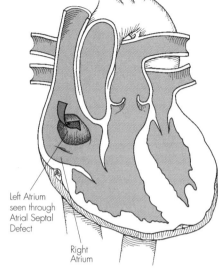

**ATRIAL SEPTAL DEFECT**

rhythm abnormalities or problems with physical activity.

While some heart defects are severe, most are minor and either don't require treatment or can be treated with surgery. If your doctor suspects that your baby has a heart defect, he or she will talk to you about the tests and treatments.

**Aortic valve stenosis.** This problem is characterized by *stenosis,* or narrowing, of the valve between the left ventricle and the aorta. This valve is the aortic valve. See page 122 for information on aortic stenosis. Most children with aortic valve stenosis don't have any symptoms and develop normally. Symptoms can include fatigue, dizziness and fainting.

The defect may be suspected when a heart murmur is heard during a routine physical exam of the heart. Surgical repair of the valve in children with symptoms prevents further heart damage as the child grows. The need for repair depends on the degree of narrowing.

**Atrial septal defect** (ASD). This birth defect consists of a hole in the wall, called the *interatrial septum,* that

separates the upper two chambers of the heart, or the *atria.* This allows the mixing of blood from the oxygenated (left) to deoxygenated (right) side of the heart. While most children with ASD have no symptoms, some may tire during brisk activities or may have recurrent bouts of pneumonia.

Surgery to close the hole will prevent damage to the heart and lungs. Surgery may not be needed for a small defect.

**Coarctation of the aorta.** A number of abnormalities may occur in the blood vessels around the heart. *Coarctation of the aorta* is a narrowing of the aorta after it leaves the heart. Symptoms of coarctation of the aorta include high blood pressure in the arms compared with lower blood pressure in the legs, with cold feet and absent or diminished pulses in the legs and feet.

Mild narrowing may not be detected until adulthood. Surgery to repair the defective vessel may be needed.

**Fallot's tetralogy.** Four defects make up this complex heart malformation. It causes babies to have *cyanosis* (turning blue from lack of oxygen) by

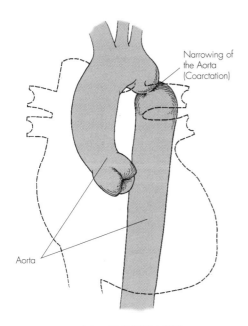

**COARCTATION OF THE AORTA**

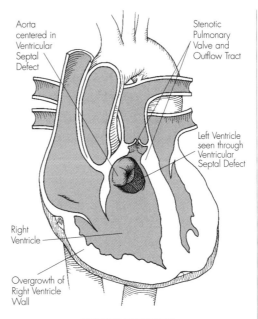

**FALLOT'S TETRALOGY**

age one. These babies may also have serious breathing problems, slowed growth and spells where the heart can't get enough oxygen.

Surgery can correct the defects or at least improve the function of the heart. It should be done by age five.

**Patent ductus arteriosus.** Before and just after birth, there's a normal opening between the aorta and pulmonary artery. This opening is called the *patent ductus arteriosus.* If it remains open after birth, oxygenated and deoxygenated blood are allowed to mix, making the heart work extra hard. Medicine is available for treatment if the opening can be identified in the first few days after birth. Surgery may be needed if medicines don't close the opening.

**Pulmonic valve stenosis.** *Stenosis* is the narrowing of the valve between the right ventricle and the pulmonary artery, the blood vessel that carries blood to the lungs. The valve is the *pulmonic valve.* Pulmonic valve stenosis may produce no symptoms at first. Later, shortness of breath and blue skin (*cyanosis*) can develop.

The need for surgical repair of the valve depends on the amount of

narrowing. This condition can be associated with a number of other heart defects so careful evaluation is needed.

**Transposition of the great vessels.** This defect is the *transposition,* or reversal, of the aorta and the pulmonary artery, the main vessels that carry blood away from the heart. When the aorta and pulmonary artery are reversed in their positions, the blood leaving the heart and going out to the body hasn't gone through the lungs to pick up any oxygen.

A baby with transposition of the great vessels will die immediately unless there's also an opening between the right and left sides of the heart, allowing oxygenated blood to mix and providing small but life-sustaining amounts of oxygen to the body. Emergency surgery is needed to save the life of an infant born with this defect.

**Ventricular septal defect** (VSD). This defect accounts for about one-third of all heart defects in newborns. A hole in the wall of the heart that divides the two ventricles, the *ventricular septum,* allows oxygenated blood to be driven into the right ventricle, leading to mixing of the blood and

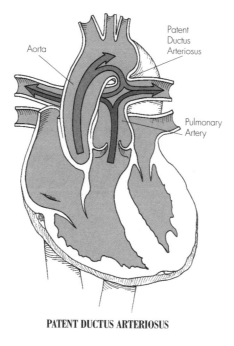

**PATENT DUCTUS ARTERIOSUS**

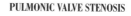

**PULMONIC VALVE STENOSIS**

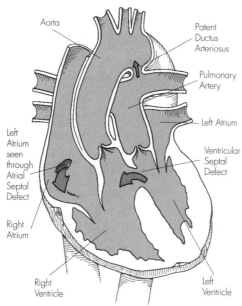

**TRANSPOSITION OF GREAT VESSELS**

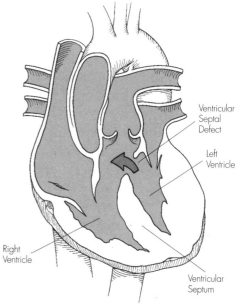

**VENTRICULAR SEPTAL DEFECT**

enlargement of the right side of the heart. Most are small defects that cause no symptoms and are usually found during a routine physical exam.

Shortness of breath, bouts of pneumonia and heart failure are symptoms of a large VSD. Larger holes may need to be patched by surgery. This is often delayed, if possible, until the child is between five and 10 years old because the holes tend to become smaller as the child grows.

## Hernias

Abdominal hernias are defects in the wall of the abdomen. The most common congenital hernia is an *umbilical hernia,* a defect near the umbilicus, or bellybutton. A soft mound is seen on the baby's abdomen when the baby cries or strains during a bowel movement. This type of hernia usually doesn't need to be fixed or treated. This hernia usually goes away by the time the

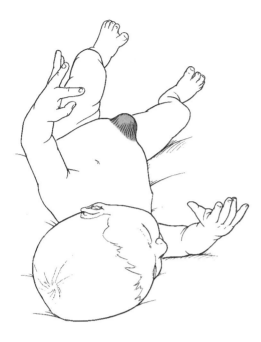

**UMBILICAL HERNIA**

child is two years old. If it doesn't, it can be repaired with surgery.

A *diaphragmatic hernia* is rare. With a diaphragmatic hernia, the intestines are pushed into the chest through a defect in the diaphragm, which stretches across your midsection underneath the lungs. The intestine presses on the lungs, and the child has difficulty breathing. Emergency surgery is usually needed to correct the problem. See page 191 for information on hiatal hernia and information on inguinal hernia.

### Hirschsprung's Disease

Rarely, a baby is born with a problem in the nerves of the intestinal tract. These nerves help control the muscles in the intestines that contract and relax. This action, called *peristalsis*, moves food and stool through the digestive tract.

In children with *Hirschsprung's disease*, the nerves that control the muscles aren't connected to the lower part of the intestine. As a result, stool doesn't pass through and builds up in the large intestine. The baby has constipation, a swollen abdomen and vomiting. In some babies, constipation may alternate with diarrhea. Children with Hirschsprung's disease may not grow normally.

Treatment for Hirschsprung's disease requires surgery.

### Hydrocephalus

Spinal fluid circulates around the brain and spinal cord, and is then reabsorbed into the blood by special membranes. In newborns, the flow of this fluid can become blocked or the fluid is poorly absorbed by the membranes. Fluid keeps forming and pushes on the brain, compressing the brain tissue. This causes increased pressure in the brain. The increased pressure and fluid causes the soft skull of the newborn to swell where the bone would normally begin to fuse together. This condition is *hydrocephalus*, which is sometimes also called "water on the brain."

If the pressure isn't treated, brain damage can result. A drainage tube can be surgically inserted into the brain to drain the fluid away from the brain so the pressure is relieved.

### Imperforate Anus

In children who have *imperforate anus*, the part of the anus that connects

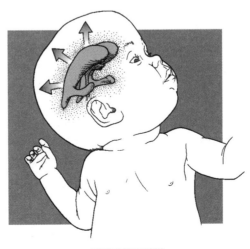

**HYDROCEPHALUS**

the intestines to the outside of the body is missing.

Most newborns pass a dark greenish stool, called *meconium,* within eight to 12 hours of birth. If this doesn't happen, the baby may have an imperforate anus. Often there's an abnormal opening into the vagina or the urinary tract.

Surgery can be done to create a more normal opening. Constipation or bowel-control problems may persist after surgery, depending on how high into the intestine the problem extends.

### Intestinal Atresia

A baby can be born with sections of the intestines that are very small, thin and underdeveloped (a condition called *stenosis*) or that have no connection to the next portion of the intestine (called *atresia*). Because no fluid can move through the intestines, the fluid backs up and causes vomiting. The vomit is often dark green.

Small areas of atresia or stenosis can be corrected with surgery. If large sections of the intestine are absent, the condition may be fatal.

### Muscular Dystrophy

*Muscular dystrophy* is the name given to a group of rare, inherited disorders that affect how the nerves communicate with the muscles. The result is muscle wasting and weakness.

The most common form of this disease is called *Duchenne's muscular dystrophy.* It affects boys almost exclusively because it's transmitted through the mother's X *chromosome.* The chromosomes are structures that carry genetic information. Girls don't get the disease because they receive another X chromosome from the father, which overrides the abnormal X chromosome from the mother. Boys receive a Y chromosome from the father, so the X chromosome from the mother must be used.

Early symptoms include difficulty walking or running, enlargement of the calves and the inability to rise to a standing position without "pushing off" from the thighs (called *Gowers' sign*). The weakness begins before age five and progresses until the child is completely crippled. Most children die before they reach adulthood due to pneumonia, respiratory trouble or heart failure from extensive physical deformities.

A muscle tissue sample, blood tests and medical history help to make the diagnosis. The disease can't be prevented, and current treatments offer little more than limited symptom relief. There is no cure.

For a woman who has a child with muscular dystrophy, the chances are one in two that future male children will have the same disorder. Genetic counseling may be helpful in deciding whether to have more children.

### Phenylketonuria (PKU)

Some babies are born without an enzyme that's needed to digest phenylalanine, an *amino acid* that's one of the building blocks of protein. Excessive amounts of this amino acid will eventually cause mental retardation.

Newborns are routinely screened for PKU. Children who are diagnosed with PKU must follow a special low-protein diet. This diet must be followed until at least age five, although some doctors recommend it until adulthood. A woman who was born with PKU must return to a low-protein diet during pregnancy to protect the fetus.

### Pyloric Stenosis

Blockage, or narrowing, is a fairly common deformity in the *pylorus.* The pylorus is the muscular valve at

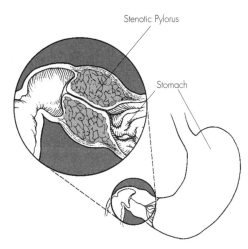

**PYLORIC STENOSIS**

the bottom of the stomach that controls the passage of food into the intestines. When it's narrow, the condition is called *pyloric stenosis.* In some infants, the muscle around the bottom of the stomach may be overdeveloped.

While pyloric stenosis isn't usually a problem at birth, symptoms begin to develop over the first few weeks. The infant will vomit and be unable to keep down milk. An ultrasound (p. 643) is used to find this thickened muscle. A simple operation can be performed to cut the fibers of the muscle. This allows the stomach contents to move normally into the intestines.

### Spina Bifida

Normally, the lower part of the spine grows together over the spinal cord after the rest of the nervous system has finished growing. If this process of growing together is interrupted, an opening is left at the lower end of the spinal cord. This is called *spina bifida.*

Small openings of the spinal cord covering usually don't put the spinal cord or other nerves in danger and may be surgically corrected without risk of nervous system damage.

Larger openings, however, may result in damaged nerves, causing paralysis or problems with bowel or bladder control. Damage to the spinal cord is permanent. Physical therapy, braces and other devices can help build the child's mobility and self-esteem.

Spina bifida may be prevented if pregnant women take adequate amounts of folic acid during the first nine weeks after conceiving. If you're planning to get pregnant, take 0.4 milligrams (mg) of folic acid every day. If you're pregnant, or if you have a family history of spina bifida, take 1.0 mg of folic acid each day. Folic acid is found in vitamins and food. Talk to your doctor about taking prenatal vitamins, which contain extra amounts of folic acid.

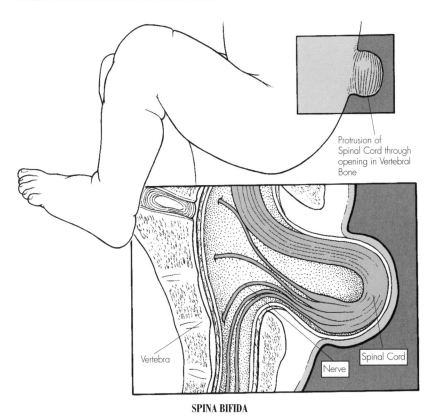

Protrusion of Spinal Cord through opening in Vertebral Bone

Vertebra

Spinal Cord

Nerve

**SPINA BIFIDA**

### Undescended Testicle

An *undescended testicle* is a testicle that hasn't come down from the

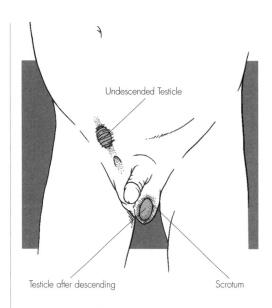

Undescended Testicle

Testicle after descending

Scrotum

**UNDESCENDED TESTICLE**

abdomen into the scrotum. Testicles are formed in the abdomen of an unborn baby boy. They usually descend into the scrotum before birth. Sometimes, one or both testicles remain within the abdomen and don't descend into the scrotum. This occurs in 3% of newborns and 20% of premature baby boys.

Once the testicles have descended into the scrotum they won't go back into the abdomen. There are normal reflexes that may pull the testes high in the scrotum for short periods of time. If a testicle hasn't descended by the time a boy is three to five years old, it can be surgically released and lowered into the scrotum. If the testicle is left in the abdomen, it will become infertile. There is an increased risk of testicular cancer in undescended testicles.

# CHAPTER 2

# INFANTS AND CHILDREN

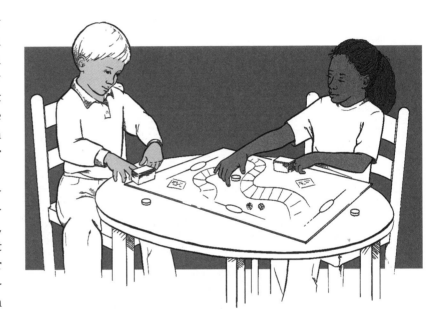

Every child is different, and many people will give you advice on how to raise your child. Even child-care experts don't agree on how to handle such challenges as toilet training and not sleeping through the night. Get advice and learn as much as you can—and then trust your instincts as a parent.

If you need advice about parenting, community resources are available. These include parenting classes, parent-support groups, single-parent support groups and others. Ask your doctor, counselor, local health department, hospital, local YMCA or church for information.

## Emotional Dos and Don'ts of Parenting

**Dos**

- Do set limits.
- Do show affection to your children.
- Do take time to have fun with your children.
- Do listen to your children.
- Do praise your children when they've been well-behaved.
- Do teach your children responsibility, such as picking up and taking care of their toys, earning an allowance or helping with chores at home.
- Do guide them in making decisions, giving pros and cons, while sharing your values.
- Do support those in authority, such as teachers and baby-sitters, when your child's behavior is wrong. Give appropriate punishment.

**Don'ts**

- Don't degrade your children after they disobey by telling them they're worthless or stupid.
- Don't openly criticize your spouse in front of your children.
- Don't spoil your children and let them nag endlessly about what they want.
- Don't make all of their decisions for your children or solve all of their problems for them.
- Don't protect your children from the consequences of bad behavior.

# Caring for Your Infant and Child

Parents or caregivers of newborns are often overwhelmed by the physical demands of caring for an infant. But as children grow older, many parents soon believe that the hardest part of raising their children relates to the emotional well-being of children and how to teach them values and good behavior. For example, how do you teach a child right from wrong? How do you get a three-year-old to follow rules? How do you get a two-year-old to go to bed—and stay there all night?

This section offers some advice on the issues you'll be facing. For more information, ask your doctor or read books on childrearing.

## Five Factors for Raising Healthy Kids

- **Consistency.** Parents and caregivers act cooperatively. Limits should be enforced consistently.
- **Discipline.** Children learn the consequences of their actions.
- **Encouragement.** Positive encouragement builds self-confidence. Belittling destroys self-esteem.
- **Love.** Love and affection are shown between parents and caregivers, and between the parents or caregivers and children.
- **Modeling standards and values.** In all areas, parents and caregivers set a good example by following the standards and personal values they hold.

## Discipline

Most people think of punishment when they think of discipline. Child-care experts say that's the wrong way to view discipline. Instead, think of discipline as a way you can teach your child to behave, follow rules and get along with others.

How you discipline your child depends on your child's age and level of understanding. For example, you can often distract a baby. If your baby wants to play with your purse, find something else to interest him or her. Then move the purse out of sight. However, disciplining an older child requires more than distracting the child's attention.

You can control your child's environment by trying to reduce the things your child can get into and the number of times you discipline your child. For example, if you have a toddler, put breakable items away until your child is older. This is easier than having to tell the child "no" all the time.

As children get older, be sure they understand what kind of behavior you expect of them. Set a good example. Your behavior will teach your values to your children better than anything you say. Be consistent in the rules you set. Your child should realize that when you say "no" you mean it. Children will test the rules you establish, and it's important for them to know the limits.

Reward or praise good behavior. When your son sits still during dinner at a restaurant, for example, tell him you're proud of him.

On the other hand, bad behavior should be punished. Punishment is a part of discipline. Spanking has been a common way to punish children, but today child-care experts disagree about its value. Some say spanking teaches children to be violent, because it's an example of a parent being violent to a child. It seems inconsistent to say, for example, "Don't hit your brother!" but for you to spank your child. Yet a light slap on the hand or bottom may teach a curious toddler not to poke his or her fingers into the electrical outlet.

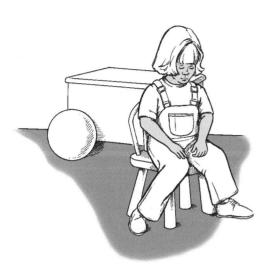

**TIME OUT**

You must make your own decisions about whether spanking is going to be a part of the way you discipline your child.

*Time out*, or standing or sitting in a quiet place away from the activity, is an effective method of punishment. Sending a child up to his or her room may not be much of a punishment if the room contains toys or a television. Taking away a privilege, such as watching TV or playing TV video games for an evening, may be an effective punishment for older children. Remember, too, that your displeasure when you're scolding your child is a form of punishment.

Don't let yourself fall into the habit of nagging or making empty threats. If you find yourself saying "no" or "don't" all the time, try to figure out why this is happening. Don't tell your child he or she is stupid, lazy or bad as part of punishment. Children need to know you expect them to behave well, not badly.

### Feeding Changes

Talk to your doctor about starting solid foods when your infant is four to six months old. When it's time to start solids, your child should be able to hold his or her head up well. The *tongue thrust reflex*, which involves pushing things out of the mouth, should be gone. Don't add salt or sugar to your baby's food.

If there's a history of allergies in your family, your doctor may recommend waiting to start solid foods until your baby is a little older. Add one new food at a time. The first solid food is usually an infant cereal, such as rice.

Don't start solid foods too early just because you've heard they'll help your baby sleep through the night.

Getting toddlers and preschoolers to eat can be a challenge. If you're concerned about the amount of food your child is eating, watch to see if he or she is filling up on milk, fruit juices or other foods between meals. If your child is growing and healthy, your child is getting enough to eat.

Be sure to give your child nutritious foods like fruits, vegetables and whole grains. Watch out for foods that contain a lot of sugar and fat. For more information on nutrition, see page 13.

### Growth and Development

It's difficult to know how to help your children grow and develop properly. Some parents are concerned about physical development. What should your child be able to do at two months?

## Sick Kids and Food

Children who are sick may not want to eat. In some children, loss of appetite may be the only sign that they're ill. They may want only liquids, not food. If your child has a poor appetite, check for a fever (p. 296) and give your child clear liquids. Don't give milk to a child with diarrhea, because diarrhea often strips away the layer in the intestines that contains the enzyme that digests milk sugar. This will make it hard for your child to digest the milk. Call your doctor if loss of appetite or diarrhea lasts longer than 24 hours. Call sooner if any other signs of infection, such as fever, appear.

At six months? Here are some guidelines to help you with some of the questions you'll face as your child grows.

Every child grows and develops at a different pace. Your 10-month-old may have taken his first step, while your neighbor's 14-month-old is just starting to walk. The chart below gives the average age that certain milestones occur. If you're concerned about your child's development, talk to your doctor.

| Developmental milestone | Typical age |
| --- | --- |
| Roll over | 2 - 5 months |
| Sit | 5 - 7 months |
| Crawl or creep | 7 - 12 months |
| Stand | 9 - 12 months |
| Walk | 9 - 15 months |
| Say first word | 10 - 12 months |
| Use two-word phrases | 15 - 18 months |
| Use three-word sentences | 18 - 24 months |

**Allowance.** Opinions differ on whether giving a child an allowance is a good practice. Generally, children learn how to handle money from having an allowance. A child can be given an allowance by age six or seven, if not earlier. Some experts believe an allowance should be tied to doing chores, while others say an allowance shouldn't be given in connection with chores because chores are a part of the child's responsibility as a member of the family. A middle ground may be to let your child earn money by doing extra or unusual chores.

**Chores.** Once your child is two and a half to three years old, he or she is old enough to do simple tasks. Children can put their dirty clothes in a hamper, help set or clear the table and put away their toys. It's important to start giving children some responsibilities when they're about three years old.

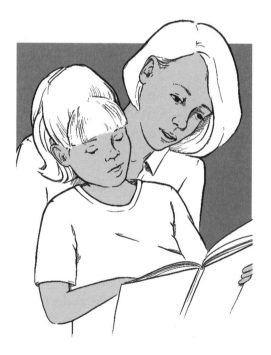

**Reading.** Read to your child every day, if possible. Experts recommend reading at least half an hour a day, even to babies. Young babies may not care what you read to them—they just like the sound of your voice. Take your children to the library. The librarian can suggest books appropriate for their ages.

**Separation anxiety.** Babies usually go through a period when they cry when their mother leaves the room. This is called *separation anxiety* and is a normal developmental stage. It usually starts when they're about a year old.

**Television.** While TV may make a handy baby-sitter, keeping your kids quiet and out of trouble, you need to monitor what they're watching. Is it violent? Too scary? Children under age four can't tell the difference between fantasy and reality. Remember, time spent watching TV is time that the child could spend reading, exercising or playing with friends. That's why it's best to limit your child's TV watching to one or two hours a day.

**Toys.** Make sure your child has toys that are interesting. Some of the best toys don't cost much money. A wooden spoon and a pan make a great drum. An oversized cardboard box can be a playhouse. Measuring spoons and cups and bowls of water can be messy but fascinating. Crayons and paper are another favorite.

## Self-Esteem in Your Children

Self-esteem starts early in life. A child learns what kind of person he or she is by the interactions he or she has with other people. Children decide how they feel about themselves by their parents' reactions to them. For this reason, it's important for parents and caregivers to help children feel good about themselves. Don't constantly criticize, shame, reject or scold your child. Don't set unrealistic standards and don't predict that your child will fail at something.

Instead, show your child constant, unconditional love and acceptance, even though sometimes you disapprove of your child's behavior. Be affectionate. Let your child know you love him or her and that he or she is a valued part of the family. Some parents proudly display birth certificates and family trees to help their children see they're part of a larger family. You can help build self-esteem and self-respect in your child by creating and sharing stories about your family's history or by allowing your child to participate in family decisions.

Encouragement is another crucial part of building your child's self-esteem. In today's competitive society, children need to learn that it's okay if they aren't number one, as long as they do their best. Foster self-confidence in your child by showing that you believe in his or her unique potential.

## Sleeping

Parents generally wish their children would sleep through the night or at least sleep a lot longer. How much sleep a child needs varies. Infants usually sleep as much as they need, although they may not always sleep when you want them to sleep. By age two, though, your child may not be getting enough sleep if he or she stays awake too late at night. Too much excitement or fear of bad dreams may make it hard for a child to fall asleep. A child between four and six years old usually needs 11 to 12 hours of sleep each night, although anywhere between eight to 14 hours is normal.

**Bedtime.** Children often try to put off going to bed. For a toddler, wanting to delay going to bed may be related partly to separation anxiety. Make sure late-afternoon or long naps aren't keeping your child from being sleepy at night. Avoid any roughhousing or other stimulating play before bedtime.

Set a time for bedtime and stick to it. Establish a night-time routine to help your child wind down and relax. A bath relaxes some children but stimulates others. The nightly routine of going to bed can include eating a light snack, reading a story, singing lullabies or saying good-night to the dolls and stuffed animals. Having a nightlight and leaving the bedroom door open can help your child feel less alone in his or her bedroom. Sometimes you may have to sit out in the hallway quietly so your child can see you—and so you can make sure he or she stays in bed.

**Family bed.** The idea of keeping your baby in the same room or even the same bed at night is controversial in this country, although it's not unusual in other cultures. Having your baby sleep with you does make night feedings easier. But the older your child is when you try to switch to sleeping separately, the harder it will be for your child to adjust to sleeping alone. Starting the switch by the time your baby is two to three months old may make it easier for your baby to sleep alone.

**Naps.** Don't try to keep the noise level down during nap time. It's good to let your baby learn how to sleep during normal background sounds. Older babies will take two naps a day. By the time a baby is 18 months old, the number of naps should be reduced to one a day.

**Nightmares.** Comfort your child when he or she has a bad dream. Ask what happened in the dream. Explain that dreams aren't real.

**Night terrors.** With night terrors, your child will scream out in the middle of the night and look frightened. Comfort your child, but don't try to wake him or her. Children don't remember having night terrors. If night terrors occur often, talk to your doctor.

**Sleeping through the night.** A few infants may sleep through the night by the time they're two months old, while others won't do so until they're two or three years old.

Experts have different theories about handling night-time waking. You have to decide what's right for you and your child. In general, though, don't make night-time wakings too much fun for your baby or child.

Respond right away to a cry to make sure nothing is wrong. Sometimes children cry without waking up. If your baby's hungry, feed him or her, but don't talk or sing. Be very matter-of-fact.

Once a child is between six and 12 months old, he or she shouldn't need to eat at night. That's when some experts recommend letting a child "cry it out" to teach them to sleep through the night.

**Sleepwalking.** Boys are more prone to sleepwalking than girls. Sleepwalking usually occurs in children five to 12 years old. The child wakes up and walks around, even going up and down stairs, but the child doesn't remember the incident after waking. With sleepwalking, all you can do is prevent your child from going outdoors. Sleepwalkers very seldom hurt themselves.

### Toilet Training

Theories abound on the "right" way to toilet train a child. You can find a number of books and videos on the subject.

Experts agree that most children aren't ready for toilet training until they are 18 to 24 months old, and many children may not be ready until age three. Signs of readiness include staying dry for several hours at a time, wanting a dirty or wet diaper changed, showing a desire to be clean and being able to follow simple commands.

One of the most popular theories emphasizes the need to do toilet training at your child's pace. First, let your child gradually become used to the potty chair. It's okay for him or her to sit on it fully clothed. Later, explain what the potty chair is for. Your child may understand from having seen a friend or older sibling use a potty chair. You may want to leave the urine guard off a boy's potty chair because it can hurt him.

The next step is to put your child on the potty chair without a diaper. After your child's had a bowel movement in a diaper, explain that he or she could have sat on the potty chair and put the bowel movement in the potty. Try putting your child on the potty chair when you think he or she is about to have a bowel movement. Be sure to praise your child if he or she goes to the bathroom in the potty chair.

Finally, let your child play without a diaper or other clothing on from the waist down. Put the potty chair in the same room, which will make it easier for your child to use the potty chair if he or she has the urge to urinate or have a bowel movement.

Training pants can make toilet training easier. They may not catch all the urine, so you may be mopping up a few accidents. Disposable training pants absorb more urine, but they stay drier so your child doesn't feel as wet. Wetness can be an incentive to use the potty chair.

Bowel control may occur before bladder control. It's easier for a child to hold a bowel movement than to hold back urine. Bladder control during the daytime will generally come next, followed by night-time bladder control. Most children will stay dry at night when they're around three years old (bedwetting, p. 364), but many children continue to wet the bed until they're five or six.

Once your child is toilet-trained, be ready for some of the consequences. Carry a portable potty on car trips. Know where the public restrooms are in the places you frequently go, such as the grocery store or shopping center. Your child is likely to decide that it's time to go to the bathroom when you're in the middle of grocery shopping.

## Potential Problems

The problems your child faces will change as he or she grows. Most children will have many of the usual childhood diseases as well as their fair share of colds and stomachaches.

### Anal Itching

Itching around the anus, a condition called *pruritus ani*, can be due to pinworms (p. 315), which often occur in children. Pinworms can be treated with an oral medicine prescribed by your doctor.

---

*Vaccinations and Immunizations*

Infancy is the time in your child's life when most of his or her vaccinations are due. You can help protect your child from a number of illnesses by making sure he or she gets properly immunized. See page 11 for more information on the vaccinations and when they should be given.

---

## Tips for Toilet Training Your Child

- Never scold or punish your child for not using the potty chair or for having an accident.
- Don't show disgust or complain about how nasty or dirty urine or bowel movements are.
- Praise your child when the potty chair is used, but don't praise too lavishly.
- For children younger than two and a half years old, flush the toilet after the child has left the room. Some children are scared by the sound of the toilet flushing.
- Teach the child how to wipe when he or she is interested in learning. Teach girls to wipe from front to back, which may help prevent urinary tract infections (p. 162).

Other common reasons for anal itching include not wiping completely after a bowel movement, fungal infections, irritation from dyes in toilet tissues and bubble bath, and laundry detergent residue on underwear.

### Bedwetting

The medical term for bedwetting is *enuresis*. This term applies to children who wet the bed only at night when they're sleeping, not during the day. Boys are more prone than girls to bedwetting. Exact causes for this problem haven't been identified. One important factor seems to be a family history of enuresis.

Bedwetting is usually not caused by a medical problem. When it is, it's often due to a bladder infection or diabetes (p. 211). Bedwetting also can be a young child's response to stress, such as the birth of a new baby or separation from parents.

Bedwetting usually isn't treated until a child is at least six years old. Your doctor may want to obtain certain tests to make sure a medical illness isn't causing the problem.

An effective treatment for bedwetting uses behavior modification techniques. One successful method is the wetting alarm. As urine touches the bed, an alarm sounds that wakes the child. Cutting down on liquids after the evening meal may help some children, but studies don't show that this method is effective overall, especially if fluid restriction gets to be a source of battle between the child and parents. Medicines can be used for enuresis, but because of side effects and general low effectiveness, they aren't usually recommended.

Although bedwetting may stop with the use of behavioral modification, it isn't conscious behavior on the part of the child. If your child wets the bed, always be positive. Never scold or spank your child for bedwetting. Punishment tends to make the problem worse. Without any treatment, bedwetting almost always stops by the time the child is a teenager.

### Breathing Trouble

Infants often have a runny nose or seem to have some trouble with breathing without actually being sick. Clearing the nose of secretions very gently with a bulb syringe is often all that's needed.

If your baby gets a cold, call your doctor. You may be advised to give your infant an over-the-counter cold medicine or a medicine prescribed by your doctor.

Sometimes trouble breathing is a sign of croup (p. 323), epiglottitis (p. 299) or asthma (p. 142). If you suspect your child has one of these illnesses, call your doctor.

### Warning: Shortness of Breath in Young Children

If your child has trouble taking a breath, coughs a lot and appears short of breath, or makes wheezing, whistling or grunting sounds while breathing, take him or her to the nearest emergency room right away. These symptoms could be signs of a severe infection, such as croup (p. 323) or epiglottitis (p. 299).

### Constipation

Not having a bowel movement every day doesn't mean your child is constipated. Constipation occurs when bowel movements are infrequent or produce hard stools, or bowel movements. It can have a number of causes, including not enough fluids or fiber (bulk) in the diet. See page 177 for more information about constipation in adults.

Iron added to infant formula may cause very hard, dry bowel movements. If the bowel movements are hard, increase the amount of liquid in your child's diet. Some water can be given by bottle, but no more than three or four ounces a day. Breast-fed infants often have a change to firm stools when they're three to four months old. This change shouldn't be mistaken as constipation.

If your child is constipated, make sure he or she drinks plenty of liquids. Add more fruits, vegetables and whole grains to your child's diet. Don't give your child a laxative without talking to your doctor. See your doctor if constipation continues, if it's severe or if blood or mucus is present in the bowel movement.

## Cradle Cap

*Cradle cap* appears as yellow, scaling patches on an infant's scalp. It's actually a form of seborrhea (p. 289) and usually occurs in infants between two and 10 weeks old. The cause is unknown.

The crusting, slightly red, scaling patches seem to come and go. Despite the way these areas of skin look, they rarely become infected.

Apply baby oil to your baby's scalp to help soften the crusts and scales. *Very gently* scrub your baby's scalp each day with mild soap and water. This should remove most of the scales. Gently brushing and combing your infant's hair may help, too. Your doctor may recommend 0.5% hydrocortisone cream (p. 616) or advise you about other treatments. Cradle cap generally clears up without any treatment by your baby's first birthday.

## Crossed Eyes

Crossed eyes, or *strabismus,* can sometimes occur in infants. The sooner the problem is detected and treated, the faster and more successful the treatment. See page 65 for more information about crossed eyes.

## Diaper Rash

Diaper rash begins as redness and sometimes progresses to peeling of the skin, open sores or even infection. The most common source of the irritation is urine.

Once the skin becomes irritated from urine, other things can make the irritation worse. A baby's skin can be sensitive to many fabrics, liquids, powders and detergents. Soaps, perfumes, the diaper itself (especially a disposable diaper) or a poorly rinsed cloth diaper that has detergent in it may cause the irritation to become worse. If sores develop on the skin, they may become infected, which leads to a severe case of diaper rash.

The first step in treating or preventing diaper rash is simple: Change your baby's diaper often to keep the skin from being irritated by urine. Wash and dry your baby's skin thoroughly when the diaper is changed. Apply a cream that contains zinc oxide (p. 616) to the skin to protect and soothe any raw areas. The cream will protect and heal the skin on your baby's bottom better than powder. Leave the diaper off for short periods and expose the skin to the air to dry.

If the rash doesn't go away, see your doctor. If the diaper rash appears to be caused by yeast, your doctor may prescribe a topical antifungal cream (p. 619).

## Diarrhea and Vomiting

The most common cause of diarrhea and vomiting in infants and

## Signs of Dehydration

- Crying without tears
- Dry mouth
- No wet diaper for six hours in an infant or toddler, or no urination for more than eight hours in an older child
- Lethargy

children is gastroenteritis (p. 186), also known as the "stomach flu." It may cause fever, cramps and some cold symptoms, such as a runny nose, cough or sore throat. The usual cause of gastroenteritis is a viral infection of the digestive tract.

Most of the time, gastroenteritis lasts between two and five days. But it may last up to two weeks.

Diarrhea and vomiting can have other causes besides stomach flu. Mild food poisoning (p. 300) may cause vomiting, diarrhea and abdominal pain. Food poisoning can occur if the baby's bottle isn't clean. Bacteria and yeast can grow under the nipple, and these organisms may cause food poisoning. Vomiting or diarrhea with severe abdominal pain should be checked right away by your doctor to make sure your child doesn't have appendicitis (p. 171) or some other abdominal problem.

Prolonged or severe bouts of diarrhea and vomiting may require tests to find the cause.

The most serious complication of diarrhea and vomiting is dehydration (p. 179). Infants can become dehydrated quickly, and dehydration in infants can be life-threatening. If you suspect your child is dehydrated, take him or her to your doctor or to an emergency room right away.

See page 179 for information on how to help prevent dehydration in your child, including whether you should continue breast-feeding or feeding formula during bouts of vomiting and diarrhea, and how to give an oral rehydration solution.

If vomiting lasts for more than a few hours, call your doctor. Be sure to note if your child has a fever or any other signs of illness before you talk to your doctor. See page 297 for information about how to take your child's temperature and for information about when to call your doctor if your child is ill.

Rest and antifever medicines, such as acetaminophen (p. 614), may help relieve the achy symptoms in children. Because of the risk of Reye's syndrome (p. 370), never give aspirin to your child.

If the diarrhea and vomiting are severe and your child becomes dehydrated, hospitalization may be needed so your child can be given intravenous fluids to treat the dehydration.

As your child feels better, begin to let your child eat simple, plain foods, such as gelatin, toast, broth and cooked cereals. For younger children, try the BRAT diet (p. 182).

You can help prevent viral illnesses, such as the stomach flu. These illnesses are spread by hand-to-hand contact, so washing your hands is important in preventing these infections. Wash your hands carefully before preparing food for yourself and your family, especially after visiting a sick friend.

### Encopresis

*Encopresis* is the term used for the soiling of underpants with bowel movement in toilet-trained older children. It may be due to severe constipation and leakage of looser stool around the firmer stool. Sometimes anal fissures (p. 171) make bowel movements painful and the child delays going to the bathroom, which may lead to constipation. Encopresis can also be a fairly normal adjustment to changes, such as a family move, or emotional problems in the child and the family as a whole.

Talk to your doctor if your child begins having bowel movements in his or her underpants. If other conditions are ruled out, your doctor may suggest that you begin a regimen to try to restore regular bowel movements. This may involve giving your child mild laxatives or enemas and changing your child's diet so he or she eats plenty of fruits, vegetables and other high-fiber foods.

### Hemorrhoids and Anal Fissures

Rarely, children may have painful bowel movements and bright red blood in the stool from a hemorrhoid. A *hemorrhoid* is a bulging vein in the anal opening.

If your preteen child has symptoms of hemorrhoids, have your doctor examine your child. Because hemorrhoids in children are rare, it's important to find out if there's an underlying cause of the hemorrhoids. Your doctor may recommend hemorrhoid suppositories to reduce the discomfort and swelling. Don't use these products in children without first talking to your doctor. (See page 189 for information about hemorrhoids in adults.)

An *anal fissure* is a split that occurs in the skin of the anus. It causes pain with bowel movements and bright red blood in the bowel movement or toilet. Your doctor may suggest using hemorrhoid suppositories, glycerine suppositories or a stool softener to help relieve symptoms and allow the skin around the anus to heal. Use these only on the advice of your doctor. (See page 171 for information about anal fissures in adults.)

### Hydrocele

*Hydrocele* is an accumulation of fluid in the scrotum (the sac around the testes). A hydrocele can cause swelling and enlargement of the scrotum.

This condition is sometimes confused with a hernia. Your doctor can make the diagnosis. A *congenital hydrocele*, or one that's present at birth, may not need treatment if it disappears on its own. If it doesn't go away, surgery may be needed.

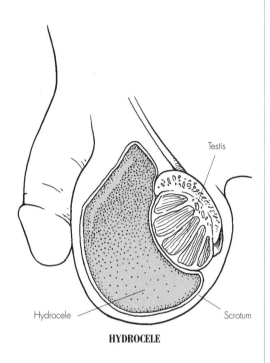

**HYDROCELE**

### Hyperactivity

*Hyperactivity* is hard to define because it depends greatly on the perception of the person observing the child. Some people are more tolerant than others of the activity level of children. But if a child is highly active to the point of being hard to control, hyperactivity may be the diagnosis.

Hyperactivity may be related to emotional problems or a problem with the central nervous system. It may run in families. Tolerance is the key to handling hyperactivity. Punishing the child won't help. If the hyperactivity is extreme, it may be a symptom of a more serious disorder that may require treatment. For example, hyperactivity may accompany attention deficit disorder (p. 369), which is a learning disorder. This problem can often be treated.

### Infections in Children

Infections occur more often in children than in adults, because children haven't been exposed to the many different types of viruses and bacteria that cause infections. Exposure to these germs is how the immune system develops a strong immunity to fight them off. Another reason for infections in children is that children don't wash their hands regularly, and many infections are spread by hand-to-hand contact.

See page 297 for information on how to take a temperature, when you should call your doctor, and warning signs of serious problems when a child runs a fever.

| Childhood Diseases | | | |
|---|---|---|---|
| Bronchiolitis | p. 320 | Mumps | p. 329 |
| Chickenpox | p. 321 | Pink eye | p. 71 |
| Common cold | p. 322 | Rheumatic fever | p. 304 |
| Croup | p. 323 | Rubella | p. 330 |
| Ear infection | p. 79 | Scarlet fever | p. 305 |
| Encephalitis | p. 324 | Sore throat | p. 103 |
| Fifth disease | p. 325 | Strep throat | p. 306 |
| Measles | p. 327 | Thrush | p. 97 |
| Meningitis | p. 302 | Tonsillitis | p. 104 |

### Kawasaki Syndrome

*Kawasaki syndrome,* or *mucocutaneous lymph node syndrome,* is a childhood illness that was first described in Japan in the 1960s. It now occurs throughout the world. It's most common in children under five years old. Kawasaki syndrome typically occurs following a respiratory illness. No one knows what causes it, and it's difficult to diagnose.

Kawasaki syndrome usually starts with a fever, sometimes with abdominal pain. In a few days, the child may develop *conjunctivitis,* or pink eye (p. 71), a rash, swollen lymph nodes and swelling and redness of the fingers and toes. During the recovery period, the skin on the fingers and toes may peel. Kawasaki syndrome can last from two to 12 weeks.

If the disease affects the heart and the blood vessels around the heart, it can be fatal.

Your doctor may need to do some blood tests to help diagnose the disease. Acetaminophen can help relieve symptoms. An echocardiogram (p. 633) can show whether damage to the heart or blood vessels has occurred.

### Lead Poisoning

Lead poisoning usually occurs gradually and typically because a child has been eating or licking old paint that contains a high lead level. However, lead from paint can get into house dust, especially after sanding for remodeling or repair, and can leak into the soil around the outside of a home. Houses built before 1980 are most likely to have lead-based paint. Another source of lead poisoning is drinking or eating food stored in pottery with lead-based glazes or inhaling fumes from burning materials containing lead. Lead accumulates in the body and can lead to brain damage and even death.

Unborn babies, infants and children are at the highest risk for lead poisoning. Symptoms may start slowly. The child may initially be irritable and tired-acting. The next symptoms may include vomiting, clumsiness, seizures and coma.

Blood tests can show whether lead poisoning is present. If so, your child may need to be admitted to the hospital. *Chelation therapy* can help remove lead from the body. In chelation therapy, medicines are used that attach to the unwanted metals, like lead, in your body and carry them out in the urine.

## Sources of Lead Poisoning

- Lead-contaminated dust and soil
- Paint chips
- Swallowing a lead object, such as a fishing weight, curtain weight or lead shot
- Contamination of acidic foods and beverages from lead-glazed ceramic ware
- Burning lead-painted wood or battery cases in home fireplace or stove
- Folk medicines that contain lead
- Lead-glazed ceramic ware and leaded glass

If your child is diagnosed with lead poisoning, it's extremely important to find the source of lead and remove it immediately.

### Learning Disorders

**Attention deficit disorder (ADD).** *Attention deficit disorder* was once called hyperactivity (p. 367). But hyperactivity is only one possible symptom of ADD. Children with ADD have a short attention span, are easily distracted and may be more active than other children.

The cause of ADD is unknown. It seems to run in families, and it's more common in boys than in girls. Treatment of ADD may include counseling and enrolling the child in a special classroom.

Food dyes, additives and sugar in the diet have been blamed for causing ADD, but scientists haven't been able to prove any link between diet and ADD. But some doctors recommend eliminating certain foods for a few months' trial.

**Autism.** *Autism* is a severe, chronic disorder that may have biochemical origins. It affects a child's ability to form relationships with parents, siblings and others. The signs of autism include repetitive movements, such as rocking or head-banging, and problems interacting with people.

Signs of autism are usually first noted by age two and a half. An infant may not smile at his or her parents. In fact, he or she may seem to "look right through them," as if they weren't there. Feeding may become a problem because the child appears uninterested in his or her surroundings, including food. As the child grows, speech may be absent or defective. Facial expressions are usually flat. Episodes of extreme irritation, frustration and anger occur for little or no reason. The child may seem to be deaf or mentally retarded, yet neither deafness nor mental retardation is present.

A child psychiatrist will need to examine the autistic child and recommend treatment. Some of the special treatments now available may help the child break through his or her shell and be able to function normally.

**Dyslexia.** A child with *dyslexia* has trouble learning to read because letters in words are reversed. It's as if the brain sees the letters backwards. But not all of the letters are reversed all of the time. For example a "b" may look like a "d" part of the time but also sometimes look like a "b." Reading becomes frustrating for the child, who may do well in other subjects. If your child has reading problems, he or she should be examined to rule out other problems before dyslexia is diagnosed. Dyslexia often becomes apparent when a child first begins to learn how to read. Frequent letter reversal is the best clue that your child needs help.

**Mental retardation.** An estimated 3% of the population has a lower level of intelligence, or *mental retardation.*

Mental retardation can be caused by a number of problems, including chromosomal abnormalities, such as Down syndrome (p. 348); genetic metabolic disorders, such as PKU (p. 354); infections that affect the fetus during pregnancy, such as rubella (p. 330), or the use of drugs or alcohol during pregnancy. Low in birth weight babies and premature babies have an increased risk of mental retardation. After a child is born, mental retardation can be the result of encephalitis (p. 324), meningitis (p. 302), lead poisoning (p. 368), head injuries (p. 50) and severe malnutrition.

### Rashes

Rashes can vary greatly—they may or may not itch. They may be dry, red patches of skin or they may be tiny blisters that pop and crust over.

There are many causes of rashes. In some cases, a rash is a symptom of an illness like measles (p. 327) or Fifth disease (p. 325). Other causes include bacterial and fungal infections, such as impetigo (p. 283), ringworm (p. 289), allergies (p. 221), fever or a reaction to medicine.

Infants and children have sensitive skin that's easily irritated. Diapers, powder, urine, perfume, soap, foods, clothing, plants and other objects that touch the skin may be responsible for a rash. Dry skin can make it worse.

Some detective work may be needed to identify the cause of a rash. If only one area of the body is affected, consider any substance that touches that particular area of skin. Eliminating exposure to the offending agent often leads to rapid clearing of the rash.

Any rash that looks unusual, lasts longer than a few hours or is associated with other symptoms like fever or vomiting should be checked by your doctor. Treatment may include an over-the-counter or prescription medicine.

To help prevent rashes, dress your baby in all-cotton clothing, use gentle unscented soaps and bath oils and don't bathe your child too often because this will dry the skin and may cause the rash to worsen.

### Reye's Syndrome

*Reye's syndrome* is a rare but possibly fatal condition that generally occurs as a complication of the flu (p. 326) or chickenpox (p. 321). Symptoms of Reye's syndrome occur seven to 10 days after the onset of flu or chickenpox. Symptoms include excessive vomiting, drowsiness, confusion and headache. Reye's syndrome causes swelling of the brain and damage to the liver and kidneys.

Children and adolescents who are given aspirin for fever during flu or chickenpox have a greater risk for Reye's syndrome, although the majority of children who take aspirin don't develop it. Don't give your child aspirin if he or she has symptoms of influenza or chickenpox.

If your child develops vomiting, headache and signs of confusion after having the flu or chickenpox, see your doctor right away. If you suspect your child may have Reye's syndrome, take him or her to your doctor or an emergency room right away.

In early or mild stages of Reye's syndrome, watchful waiting in the hospital, to make sure no other problems develop, may be all that's required. But some cases can be severe.

### Seizures

Many factors play a role in seizures or convulsions. There are different types of seizures. Some of the most common types of seizures in children are the following:

**Febrile seizures.** Febrile seizures occur in about 5% of children, usually when a fever is rapidly rising. Many children have a shaking spell, or convulsion, during an illness with a fever. Neither permanent damage nor a long-term seizure disorder is likely to result from febrile seizures.

**Infantile spasms.** Infantile spasms occur in infants older than three months and cause them to make jerking motions or to curl up in a ball. The episodes only last for a few seconds, then the child relaxes. Most children with this type of seizure disorder stop having it by age three, then may develop another type of seizure disorder.

**Epilepsy.** Epilepsy (p. 56) is defined as repeated convulsions or seizures. A single convulsion with a fever in a child shouldn't be considered epilepsy. If your doctor suspects that your child has epilepsy, further testing will be performed, including blood tests, a CT scan (p. 632), MRI scan (p. 637) or an electroencephalogram (p. 634).

The better the control of seizures with medicine, the more normal your child's life will be. Periodic blood tests are usually needed to check medicine levels in the blood to make sure enough medicine is in the system to stop the seizures.

A severe concussion (p. 50) or head injury (or repeated head injuries) can lead to seizures. Talk with your doctor about limiting your child's participation in sports after a severe concussion. Children (and adults) should wear head protection when doing anything that could result in a head injury, including bicycling, skating, playing football and other activities.

**Stomach Pain**

Sudden and severe abdominal pain is a symptom that shouldn't be ignored. It could indicate a serious problem.

Stomach symptoms are usually due to a stomach flu (gastroenteritis, p. 186). Although appendicitis (p. 171) is rare in very small children, the risk increases as children get older. In appendicitis, fever and abdominal pain are usually the first symptoms. Within a few hours, vomiting, diarrhea, a higher fever and an increase in the abdominal pain occur. The appendix may rupture if it isn't removed in the first 24 to 48 hours.

Another rare cause of sudden and severe abdominal pain in children is intussusception (p. 173), in which one section of the intestine telescopes inside another section. Intussusception tends to occur in children six months to one year old. It cuts off the blood and oxygen supply to the intestine and blocks food from moving through the intestine. A bowel movement that looks like currant jelly (red and mucus-filled) is a possible symptom.

Any time your child has an illness with severe stomach pain as a complaint, call your doctor. Your doctor will examine your child's abdomen to get clues about the cause of the abdominal pain. A high white blood cell count may indicate appendicitis. X-rays of the abdomen may identify the source of abdominal pain. A barium enema (p. 628) often corrects intussusception by pushing the dislocated portion of the intestine back into place.

Surgical removal of the appendix is needed for appendicitis. Surgery may be needed to treat intussusception if it isn't corrected by the barium enema.

## Sudden Infant Death Syndrome

In the United States, one out of every 500 babies dies of *sudden infant death syndrome,* or SIDS. Most of the victims are between the ages of one month and six months, and die suddenly during sleep.

The cause of SIDS is unknown. The original and most persistent theory to explain these mysterious deaths suggests a defect in the area of the brain that controls breathing. It's thought this defect leads to a sudden stop in normal breathing during sleep.

Newer research suggests that the baby's position during sleep may contribute to SIDS. Infants lying on their stomachs may be at increased risk of SIDS. Some experts recommend putting babies to sleep on their side or back to help prevent SIDS.

It may be possible to prevent some cases of SIDS. Babies at greatest risk of SIDS are those who have stopped breathing previously, who were premature, had a low birth weight, had low *Apgar scores* (a test done right after birth to determine the baby's physical health) and had mothers who were drug users. For these high-risk babies, home monitoring with a special device may be tried to make sure the infant continues to breathe. Training in CPR (p. 596) for parents or caregivers is suggested when the parents are trained to use this special monitoring equipment.

# CHAPTER 3

ADOLESCENTS

Adolescence begins with the physical and emotional changes of *puberty.* Puberty may begin as early as age nine in some girls or as late as age 18 in some boys.

Changing levels of *hormones,* chemical messengers that affect organ growth and function, stimulate the physical and emotional changes of adolescence. During adolescence, the sex hormones—testosterone, estrogen and progesterone—signal the body to begin to mature. Growth hormones continue to be secreted during adolescence, helping the teen become an adult.

Changes during adolescence are normal, but the typical awkwardness, skin problems and the new feelings of sexual desire all seem to come on so quickly that they sometimes *feel* abnormal to the teenager.

**Changes in the maturing male.** When a young man matures physically, his voice deepens and he begins to grow facial, chest and pubic hair. His testicles, the main sexual organs, begin to secrete *androgens,* the male hormones responsible for many of these physical changes. The penis, testicles and *scrotum* (the sac holding the testicles) grow.

Sperm are produced in the testicles under the influence of *testosterone,* the primary male hormone. Without testosterone, the production of sperm would be shut down. For sperm to mature, they need to live in an environment with a cooler temperature than the usual body temperature. This is the reason the testicles are suspended away from the body—so a slightly

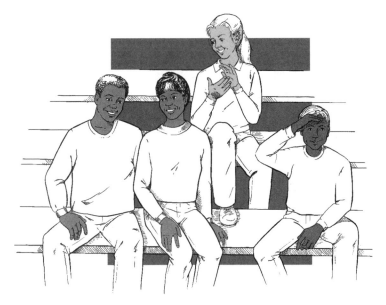

lower temperature can be maintained. Wearing very tight underwear or pants or sitting in a hot tub for a long time can increase the temperature in the scrotum and reduce the number of sperm.

The sperm are stored in the *epididymis* and *vas deferens,* the tubes that the sperm pass through to reach the urethra. Near the place where the vas deferens meets the urethra, the *seminal vesicles* and the *prostate* add nutrients and fluid to the mature sperm. This mixture is called *semen.* Semen is ejaculated through the penis. Almost all young men, before they become sexually active, have one or more "wet dreams," or episodes during the night when semen is ejaculated. Although a wet dream may be embarrassing for the young man, it's completely normal.

**Changes in the maturing female.** The female reproductive system is much more complex than the male's. And it develops earlier than in males.

## Growth and Development in Boys

- Growth spurts in boys typically occur between ages 13 and 15½.
- Sexual changes in boys include the growth of the scrotum and testicles, lengthening of the penis, growth of pubic hair and growth of the seminal vesicles and prostate.
- Growth spurt in height usually begins about one year after the testicles start growing.
- Facial hair and hair under the arms appears about two years after pubic hair.
- First nocturnal ejaculation ("wet dream") occurs between ages 12½ and 14—about one year after accelerated penis growth.
- Production of mature sperm begins between ages 14 and 16. Peak fertility is reached in the late teens or early 20s.

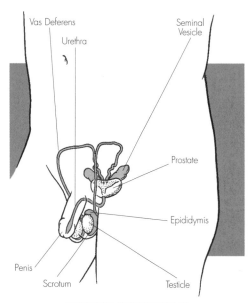

**MALE REPRODUCTIVE TRACT**

The *ovaries*, the main female glands that contain eggs, begin to secrete female hormones. The breasts begin to develop and pubic hair begins to grow. The hormones also stimulate ovulation and *menstruation*, or "periods." This usually occurs a couple of years after the breasts begin to form.

The age at which a young woman begins menstruating, or having periods, varies from as early as age nine to as late as age 16 or so. Girls are born with all the eggs in their ovaries that they'll ever have. These eggs are stored in the ovaries until the girl reaches puberty.

When menstruation begins, an egg develops to maturity about once a month. After it has matured, it's released, a process called *ovulation*. The egg travels down one of the pair of *fallopian tubes* to the *uterus*, or womb. The egg can be fertilized by sperm if the girl has sexual intercourse. If pregnancy doesn't occur, the egg and the buildup of blood and tissue in the uterus are expelled about two weeks following ovulation. Menstruation usually lasts from two to five days and generally occurs every 28 to 32 days.

For more information about menstruation and some of the changes or problems that may be associated with it, see page 382.

**Precocious puberty.** Sometimes puberty occurs at an early age, around eight or nine. This is called *precocious puberty*. This early puberty may be a family trait, or a result of a problem, such as a tumor, that affects the pituitary gland and hypothalamus. These glands are located in the brain. Precocious puberty may also be a result of a tumor or problem in other glands, such as the adrenal glands, ovaries or testicles.

If you think your child is beginning puberty early, take him or her to your doctor for an exam. Your doctor will probably order blood tests to check sex hormone levels. If a tumor or other problem is suspected, your doctor may order a CT scan (p. 632), ultrasound (p. 643) or MRI scan (p. 637) to check for any problems in the brain, adrenal glands, ovaries or testicles.

Treatment for precocious puberty depends on what's causing it. Medicine to regulate hormone production may be needed. Surgery may also be needed if a tumor is present.

Children who go through puberty early need special attention. They're often teased by other children, who make fun of them. Adults may expect them to act more mature than they are because they look older.

Talk to your child about the physical changes and reassure him or her that the changes are normal and just occurring ahead of the usual time. Parents or guardians may also want to explain the situation to the child's teachers and other adults who play a role in the child's life.

**Delayed puberty.** Development can also be delayed in some adolescents. Girls whose development is delayed

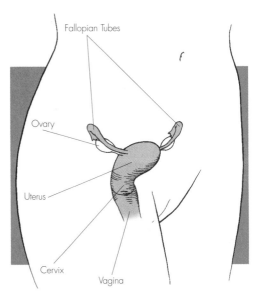

**FEMALE REPRODUCTIVE TRACT**

may not begin to show the physical changes of puberty until age 15 or 16. For a few girls, puberty may be delayed until age 17 or 18. In some boys, puberty may not begin until age 18.

Many times, a parent of an adolescent with delayed growth and sexual maturation also experienced delayed development as a teen. While delayed development may make the adolescent feel different and cause stress and low self-esteem, no serious physical consequences are likely. A medical problem is rarely the cause of the delayed development. Talk to your doctor if you're worried about a problem. But testing may not be called for unless the adolescent has other symptoms of a disease or hormone disturbance.

## Acne

Acne occurs in almost every teen. In most cases, the acne is mild, with only a few pimples. Some teenagers, though, get many pimples. See page 274 for further information about acne.

Although proper skin care is important in managing acne, dirt isn't the reason it occurs. Eating chocolate or greasy foods doesn't cause acne either. The development of acne is actually related to increased levels of sex hormones, called *androgens*. These hormones cause skin glands to produce increased amounts of *sebum.* Sebum is an oily substance. It can mix with skin cells and form a plug that blocks the hair follicles. These blocked follicles can become infected with bacteria that live on the skin. This can lead to pimples, usually on the face, chest or back. Emotional stress or menstruation may provoke an outbreak. Heavy oil-based makeup can also make acne worse.

Good skin care includes washing the skin twice a day with an over-the-counter acne soap and, if needed, applying an over-the-counter acne medicine (p. 614) that contains a drying agent such as benzoyl peroxide or salicylic acid. Scrubbing and squeezing pimples can make the acne worse.

If acne continues or worsens, talk to your doctor. He or she can prescribe medicines, such as oral antibiotics (p. 618), which usually slow serious acne outbreaks and help reduce scarring. Other prescription medicines include tretinoin (p. 617) and isotretinoin (p. 617).

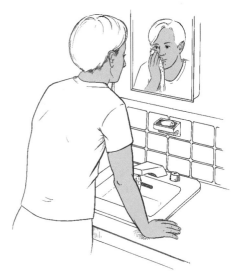

## Alcohol, Tobacco and Drug Use

Drugs, including alcohol and tobacco, are psychologically and physically

## Signs of Drug Use

- Signs of alcohol or other depressant use: clumsiness, laziness, depression or memory loss
- Signs of amphetamine, cocaine or crack use: jumpiness, loss of appetite, nausea or vomiting, irritability, insomnia, increased or irregular heart rate, chest pain, runny nose, "bursts" of energy followed by fatigue and laziness
- Signs of hallucinogenic drug use: uncontrollable laughter or crying, hallucinations, loss of appetite, extreme change in behavior
- Signs of inhalant use: dizziness, drowsiness, slurred speech, stumbling, excitability, irritability, empty spray cans and chemical smell
- Signs of intravenous drug use: unexplained bruises, sores or needle marks
- Signs of marijuana use: red eyes, confused behavior, laziness, increased appetite and dry mouth
- Signs of tobacco use: frequent upper respiratory infections, "smoker's cough," stained teeth and smell of tobacco on clothing, hair and breath

*Extreme chest pain, heart rate irregularities, chronic vomiting, difficulty breathing, unconsciousness and life-threatening behavior require emergency room care.*

addictive. Compared with illegal drugs, tobacco may seem harmless. But tobacco use accounts for more premature deaths than all illegal drugs combined. See page 559 for more information on addictions.

Your doctor can help your adolescent with drug-related problems or refer you to an expert in substance abuse or to an inpatient or outpatient treatment program. Organizations that can help include local chapters of Alcoholics Anonymous or Narcotics Anonymous and local drug hot lines. Check your phone book for telephone numbers. The National Council on Alcoholism and Drug Dependence Helpline (800-475-HOPE) may also be useful. Al-Anon may help provide support for parents of teens with an alcohol problem. For more information about Al-Anon, call 800-356-9996 (or 800-245-3151 in New York).

## Depression

Although depression can occur in childhood, it isn't commonly seen until adolescence. Weight loss or gain, a drop in grades, listlessness, trouble sleeping and trouble concentrating are common symptoms of depression in adolescents. Professional help is urgently needed, especially if your child has talked about suicide or has shown suicidal behavior.

See page 587 for more information about depression and the risk of suicide. Counseling alone helps many episodes of depression, but antidepressant medicine is often an effective addition to counseling. Family therapy is sometimes more effective than individual counseling, especially when depression is related to family problems.

## Eating Disorders

Eating disorders are most common in adolescents, especially teenage girls. Adolescents are bombarded with ads on TV, in magazines, on billboards—nearly everywhere they look—that equate a slender body with happiness and popularity. At a time when they're so eager to please, many adolescent girls become obsessed with weight control. Eating disorders, such as anorexia nervosa (p. 583) or bulimia (p. 584), may be the result.

Eating disorders don't just result from the desire to be thin, they also reflect intense emotional issues. These problems often revolve around a need to be "in control" and to achieve perfection. They may also be rooted in family problems, such as alcoholism, abuse or parents' marriage problems.

Early treatment and a supportive family seem to help people with anorexia recover. In addition to treatment of the physical problems caused by the eating disorder, individual and family psychotherapy, nutritional counseling and, in some cases, antidepressant medicine can be helpful. People with bulimia seem to respond better to treatment than those with anorexia. Relapses are common, especially when stressful situations occur. With professional help, these triggers may be identified before they cause problems.

## Gynecomastia

More than 60% of boys going through puberty have some harmless breast swelling, called *gynecomastia.* It's only rarely connected to a disease. Most often it lasts less than a year and requires no treatment. The cause isn't known, but is probably related to the fact that boys (as well as girls) produce both male and female hormones. As the body determines the proper proportion of these hormones for each sex, the boy may experience some short-term feminine characteristics such as gynecomastia.

## Pregnancy in Teens

The United States has the highest rate of teenage pregnancy of all the developed nations. Four out of 10 girls become pregnant before they reach age 19. Information on pregnancy, child-rearing, adoption and abortion are available for teens.

Teens who face pregnancy may feel guilty, insecure and bad about themselves. Individual counseling may be

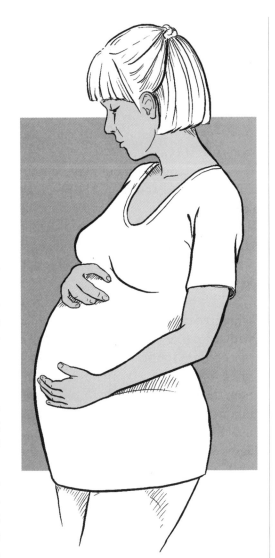

needed for the pregnant teen and the father. Group therapy also provides a supportive and healing environment.

Most teens who give birth keep their babies. Many teen mothers continue to live with their parents during the pregnancy and after the birth of their babies. Supportive parents can help the teen learn necessary parenting, job and social skills.

Illness and death rates for girls ages 12 to 14 who carry their babies to term are higher than for women over 20 years of age. Pregnant teens are at greater risk for health problems, such as poor or excessive weight gain, pregnancy-induced high blood pressure (p. 395), toxemia (p. 662), anemia (p. 391),

### The Importance of Prenatal Medical Care

Studies have shown that the most important factor for avoiding complications in teen pregnancy is to have regular medical care during pregnancy. See page 387 for more information on prenatal health care. Other key factors for avoiding problems are good nutrition and avoidance of tobacco, alcohol and drugs.

prolonged labor and arrest of labor. Many of these health problems may be related to social factors, such as poverty and poor education. The most common contributors to health problems in mother and child are inadequate prenatal health care and poor nutrition.

Continuing in school may be difficult for the pregnant teen. The pregnant teen may need financial and emotional support. Medical care, food and shelter, counseling and education for pregnant teenagers are often available through local social service agencies.

Each year, about 4% of teenagers who give birth choose to place a child with adoptive parents. Babies may be placed for adoption through public or private channels. With public adoption, the birth parents don't have visitation rights. With private adoption, usually arranged through adoption agencies, physicians or lawyers, the birth parents may be able to play a role in the baby's life and meet or choose the baby's adoptive parents. Teens who give up their babies for adoption may require counseling to deal with feelings of loss, depression and grief.

About 400,000 of the 1 million teens who get pregnant each year choose to have an abortion. Abortion has emotional, physical and moral implications for many people. If it's considered, counseling with a doctor, minister or professional trained in abortion counseling is recommended.

## Rebellion and Risk-Taking

Some rebellion and testing of the boundaries in teens is normal. Risk-taking is a common, but often dangerous, part of being a teenager. The rebelliousness often arises from a conflict between feelings of dependence on parents and a desire to be independent.

Your teen's experiments with new values, ideas, hairstyles and clothing may be uncomfortable for you if you try to maintain tight control over your child's behavior. The tighter the control, the more conflict there will be. This, in turn, can push the teen to search out even more outrageous behavior.

Sexual experimentation is a common risk-taking behavior. Drug use, driving recklessly, driving under the influence of alcohol and "overdoing" sports such as biking or skateboarding are common examples of potentially harmful risk-taking behaviors. Education and supportive parenting can help teenagers learn boundaries that match their level of maturity.

Insisting on basic principles such as honesty, self-control and respect for others, while allowing some experimentation, may preserve your sanity and your teenager's. As a general rule, the more responsibility and emotional growth your teen shows, the more freedom he or she should be allowed.

## School Problems

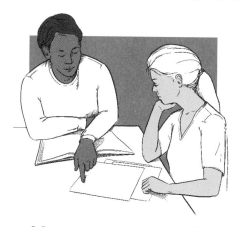

Many teens have problems in school, such as poor study habits, bad grades, skipping classes, trouble reading or other problems. Both physical and behavioral problems may be a source of problems in school. Stress at home and peer pressure can compound these problems.

Attention deficit disorder (p. 369), a learning disorder such as dyslexia (p. 369), depression (p. 376), hyperactivity (p. 367), and such illnesses as asthma (p. 142), diabetes (p. 211), mononucleosis (p. 328) and sickle cell anemia (p. 133) can all affect performance in school.

Behavioral problems include rebellion and risk-taking (p. 378), and alcohol and drug use (p. 375).

How you approach working with your teen to help him or her with school problems will depend greatly on what is contributing to the problems. Talk with your teen to help discover the source of the problem. Try to always remain open-minded and willing to try to communicate with your teen. Your doctor, your teen's teachers or a school or private counselor may also be able to help.

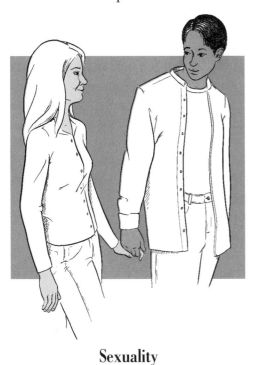

## Sexuality

Sexuality is a normal part of maturing and developing. It's normal for adolescents to be curious about sexuality, their own bodies and the bodies of others. It's important for parents and guardians to provide accurate information about sexuality. Talk to your teen about the changes that occur in both sexes at puberty. This will help the adolescent feel that he or she is normal. Knowledge about sexuality will help adolescents make wise decisions as they face choices in the future.

One of the hallmarks of male puberty is the "wet dream" (p. 373). Wet dreams are an early signal of the beginning of sexual function. They usually begin around age 12 to 14 and may occur occasionally throughout adulthood.

It's also helpful for the adolescent to know that masturbation is normal. It's a normal way of achieving sexual gratification. It's not harmful unless it becomes an obsession, harms interpersonal relationships or is done in unacceptable situations or places. Both boys and girls masturbate, although boys usually begin at an earlier age than girls.

It's not unusual for adolescents to form "crushes" on teachers, other adults and friends of both the opposite and the same sex. It's normal for adolescents to wonder if they're homosexual, regardless of their actual sexual orientation. A small percentage of adolescents may truly have a homosexual or bisexual orientation. If an adolescent is concerned about this, he or she should be encouraged to talk about it with his or her doctor or a counselor to help sort out these feelings.

By age 15, about half of all girls and boys have had sexual intercourse. Although abstinence is the safest choice, prevention of pregnancy (p. 386) and prevention of sexually transmitted diseases (STDs, p. 316) is a responsibility for both boys and girls. Because of the potentially serious consequences of sex, education about sex is essential. See page 556 for more information about how to talk to your teen about sexual issues.

# CHAPTER 4

# WOMEN

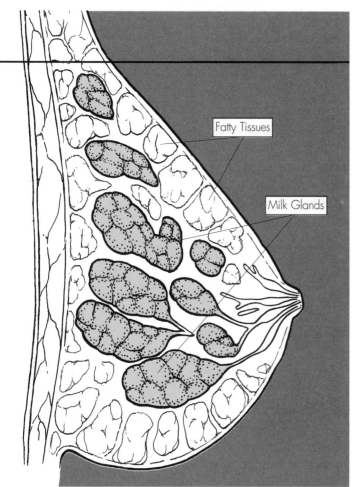

**SIDE VIEW: BREAST**

*Fatty Tissues*

*Milk Glands*

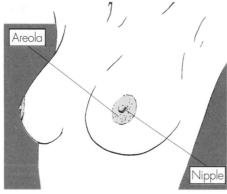

*Areola*

*Nipple*

**FRONT VIEW: BREAST**

The female reproductive system includes many parts. The function of the *breasts* is to produce milk for a baby. The breasts develop during puberty when fat and other tissue deposit on connective tissue that's attached to major chest muscles. Breast size is determined by fat content.

Within the breasts are 17 to 20 milk-producing glands, or *mammary glands.* These glands are connected to pores in the nipples, which are the outlets for breast milk. The dark area of skin around the nipple is called the *areola.*

The main function of the *uterus,* also called the womb, is to provide a safe environment for a baby during the nine months of development before birth. The uterus has two parts, the *fundus,* or main part of the uterus, and the *cervix,* which opens into the vagina. When a woman isn't pregnant, the fundus is about the size and shape of a small pear and usually is collapsed. During pregnancy, the uterus expands, sometimes to more than 500 times its size before pregnancy.

Each month, the uterus gets ready for pregnancy. The uterine lining, called the *endometrium,* thickens, and new blood vessels develop. If a fertilized egg reaches the uterus, it implants in this lush network of nutrient-providing vessels. If pregnancy doesn't occur, the new growth is shed as menstrual fluid, and the menstrual period begins again.

The uterine cavity is narrow at the bottom, forming the hard, muscular cervix. In the center of the cervix is a small opening that allows the flow of sperm in and menstrual fluid out. During childbirth, the cervix opens, or *dilates*, so the baby can move through into the birth canal.

The *ovaries* are two almond-shaped organs that lie on either side of the uterus. When a girl is born, her ovaries already hold all of the eggs, or *ova*, she will ever produce (about 400,000 immature eggs). Starting at puberty, one, or possibly two, mature eggs are produced each month. In the middle of the monthly cycle, the mature egg leaves the ovary. This process is called *ovulation*. The ovaries also manufacture sex hormones that regulate the monthly cycle.

The *fallopian tubes* connect the ovaries to the uterus. They are four to five inches long. The fallopian tubes aren't directly attached to the ovaries—they have funnel-like openings that lie near the ovaries.

After ovulation, one of the fallopian tubes "catches" the egg that has been released from the ovary and propels it toward the uterus with the help of *cilia*, which are tiny, hair-like projections. It takes four to six days for the egg to reach the womb. In the first 24 hours after ovulation, the egg can be fertilized by sperm. In some cases, the fertilized egg becomes implanted in the fallopian tube or elsewhere outside the womb. This is called *ectopic pregnancy* (p. 393) and must be treated surgically.

Pubic hair covers the top part of the vulva, and the bottom part splits into two skin-covered flaps called the *labia majora*. Inside these protective outer lips are the *labia minora*, another set of folds that surrounds the opening to the vagina and the *urethra*, the outlet for urine.

The *clitoris* lies at the top of the labia minora. Only its small, round tip is visible. Its larger part is hidden beneath the skin. The clitoris is the main organ of sexual response in women. It's dense with nerves, blood vessels and the same type of erectile tissue that makes up the

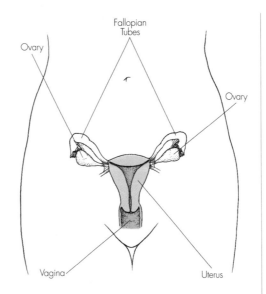

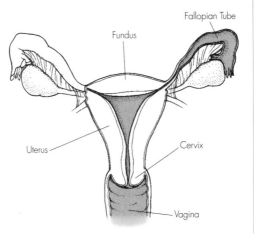

**FEMALE REPRODUCTIVE SYSTEM**

penis. The clitoris is extremely sensitive to touch and, when stimulated, fills with blood and becomes firm.

The *vagina* is about four to six inches long and runs from outside the body to the uterus. The muscular vagina is located between the bladder and the rectum. Its many purposes include providing a passageway for menstrual flow and sperm and serving as the birth canal.

On either side of the vaginal opening lie the *Bartholin's glands*, which secrete fluid. This fluid helps keep the vagina clean, lubricates the vagina during sexual intercourse, provides assistance to swimming sperm when fertilization is possible and protects the

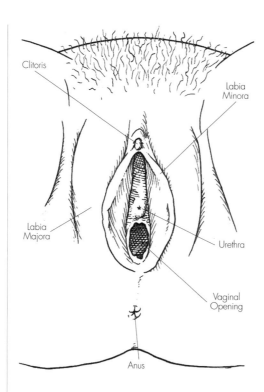

**FEMALE REPRODUCTIVE SYSTEM: VULVAR AREA**

vagina against infection. During childhood, the vaginal entrance is covered by a thin membrane called the *hymen*. This membrane is broken during a female's first sexual intercourse if it hasn't already been broken. It can be easily broken, especially in a child who is physically active, such as in sports.

## Special Issues for Women

### Menstruation

*Menstruation* signals that a girl is physically capable of becoming pregnant. American girls begin menstruation at the average age of 12.7 years, but it's normal for the age of onset to range from nine to 16 years. In other countries, the average age varies from younger to older.

The *menstrual cycle*, also called the period, regularly prepares a female's uterus for the implantation of a fertilized egg. The cycle is controlled by *hormones*, which are chemical messengers that travel through the bloodstream to influence the body's functions. Usually

the cycle lasts 28 to 32 days. Each menstrual cycle begins with the first day of bleeding and lasts until the next menstrual cycle begins.

Each month, the hormones *estrogen* and *progesterone* trigger the uterine lining to build up, mature and then slough off. Estrogen is produced in the first weeks of the cycle, and progesterone and estrogen are produced in the last half of the cycle, after ovulation. Ovulation occurs around the middle of the cycle, usually day 14 of a 28-day cycle, when the uterine lining is most prepared for implantation of the fertilized egg.

The development of a mature egg, the estrogen and progesterone levels, and the course of the menstrual cycle are influenced by hormones called *luteinizing hormone* (LH) and *follicle-stimulating hormone* (FSH). The pituitary gland, a pea-sized structure in the brain, is the main producer of these female hormones. Most women experience some irregularity in their menstrual periods.

Eventually, menopause causes the periods to cease, signaling the end of reproductive function. Usually this occurs between age 45 and 60 years, but in some women, it can occur as early as age 35 or 40. See page 407 for more information on menopause.

**Amenorrhea.** This term describes the absence of the menstrual period. Amenorrhea is classified as either primary or secondary. *Primary amenorrhea* means that the period or cycle never starts. If the onset of puberty is delayed past age 16 to 18 years and the period hasn't started, other hormonal abnormalities may be the cause of amenorrhea. *Secondary amenorrhea* occurs when a women has had normal cyclic periods but suddenly stops having them. Changes in the woman's normal hormone cycle due to stress, illness, rapid and significant loss of body mass, such as that caused by anorexia nervosa (p. 583) or heavy exercise patterns, can disrupt the normal timing of the cycle and delay or stop it. Many women who take birth control pills (p. 550) miss a period or two when they start taking the pill because of the change in hormone stimulation of the uterus.

**Dysmenorrhea.** Painful periods, a condition called *dysmenorrhea*, are common. The cramps may be caused by contractions of the uterus. Dysmenorrhea may also be related to other problems of the uterus, such as infections, tumors and endometriosis (p. 418). Your doctor will probably perform a pelvic exam. An ultrasound (p. 643), cultures of vaginal and uterine fluids, and an exam to look at the inside of the uterus (hysteroscopy, p. 636) may also be needed.

Menstrual cramps may be relieved with analgesic medicines (p. 614). In some women, birth control pills lessen the symptoms of painful menstruation. If an infection is the cause of dysmenorrhea, your doctor may prescribe antibiotics (p. 618). If a problem such as endometriosis is detected, treatment with hormones may be needed.

**Heavy bleeding.** Heavy bleeding may be normal for some women but can be caused by problems in other women. Uterine infections, tumors and endometriosis (p. 418) can cause heavy menstrual flow. Disruption of the hormonal balance can also cause heavy bleeding. Heavy bleeding is a common problem in women who use an intrauterine device (IUD) for birth control. If you have an IUD and the excessive flow is something you don't like, you may need to have the device removed and use another form of birth control.

Persistent heavy periods may reduce your body's supply of iron, causing you to become anemic (p. 133). You may need to take iron supplements. Hormone therapy, such as with birth control pills (p. 550), may reduce the heavy flow and regulate your periods. If these medicines don't work, a surgical procedure called dilatation and curettage (D & C, p. 420) may be done to clean out the uterine lining, allowing the cycle to return to normal in most cases.

**Oligomenorrhea.** Infrequent and irregular periods, called *oligomenorrhea*, are common and usually not a problem. Some women have cycles that normally last as long as 35 to 60 days. The primary difficulty arises in predicting when this long cycle—and the accompanying bleeding—will start. Infrequent periods don't lead to a more serious problem and generally no treatment is needed. If desired, birth control pills can be used to regulate the cycle and make it more predictable.

**Premenstrual syndrome (PMS).** For many women, the body's cyclic hormonal fluctuations seldom cause any problems. But some women are more sensitive to these hormonal and cyclic changes. This response is called *premenstrual syndrome* (PMS). Women affected by PMS experience emotional and physical changes. They may become depressed, moody and anxious during the week or so before menstruation. Their bodies become bloated and tender. The breasts may become very tender. Some women stay in bed for two or three days because of the swelling and abdominal pain.

Wearing a supportive bra and taking oral analgesic medicine (p. 614), and over-the-counter or prescribed diuretics (p. 623) can help reduce discomfort, bloating and water retention. For many women, birth control pills help reduce painful periods, fluid

---

*Symptoms That Need to Be Checked by Your Doctor*

- Periods that never start or suddenly stop
- Periods that are infrequent and irregular
- Painful periods with heavy bleeding
- Mood swings, depression and anxiety along with bloating, breast tenderness and abdominal pain

## Home Remedies for PMS

- Use an over-the-counter analgesic medicine, such as aspirin (p. 615), ibuprofen (p. 617), acetaminophen (p. 614) or naproxen (p. 617) for cramps.
- Minimize your intake of alcohol, caffeine and salt.
- Use diuretics only as prescribed.
- Use a heating pad to ease the pain of cramps.
- Exercise regularly.

retention and the emotional upheavals. Reducing your intake of salt, alcohol and caffeine may improve the condition, too. Various vitamin regimens have been tried with limited success. Antidepressants (p. 619) or antianxiety medicines (p. 618) can control the emotional changes if hormonal therapies don't help.

No specific tests are available to verify that your symptoms are caused by PMS. A physical exam and blood tests may be needed to identify other health problems and to confirm that the symptoms are caused by PMS.

# Sex

The pleasure you derive from your sexual relationship depends greatly on your body, how you feel about your body, how you feel about your partner, the health of your relationship with your partner and many other factors. Sexual intercourse should be a pleasurable experience. It shouldn't be painful. And it should be satisfying. If sex is painful or unsatisfying, you may want to examine the situation to find out the cause so you can address the problem and improve the health of your sexual relationship.

## Orgasm

A wide range of sexual responses is normal. Some women never reach a sexual climax, or *orgasm,* with intercourse, others reach orgasm occasionally, and some women have multiple orgasms. When an orgasm occurs, the muscles in the lower part of the vagina contract. The sensation is pleasurable and creates a feeling of release. But the way orgasms feel or how often they occur is different for everyone. What's normal for one woman may not be normal for another.

Relationships have many variables, and the sexual relationship is only one of them. Work and sleep habits, conflicts, children, financial problems and other circumstances complicate sexual relationships. Sexual arousal requires psychological excitement that's created through visual stimuli and romantic desires. When the psychological excitement is combined with touching, caressing and foreplay, sexual excitement increases and climax is more likely.

If you have a persistent problem reaching sexual climax, talk to your doctor. He or she will go over your sexual history to identify psychological and physical factors that may contribute to diminished sexual response. In addition, your doctor may be able to recommend specific activities to improve your chances of reaching climax or may refer you to another health care professional who can help.

Some of the most common problems that can interfere with sexual response include:

**Fear of pregnancy or disease.** If you don't wish to become pregnant or if you're unsure of your risk of contracting a sexually transmitted disease (STD) your sexual response may be inhibited. Use reliable birth control (p. 550) and follow guidelines to protect yourself against STDs (p. 316). Protection against STDs can be a matter of life and death, and it will no doubt increase your chances of sexual pleasure.

**Hormonal changes.** It's normal to have hormonally triggered times when you're less interested in sex and less likely to reach climax. Many women experience this response during or just after their menstrual period, during or in the months following pregnancy and at various times during or after menopause. Some women experience an increase in sexual desire during these times. No single response is "normal" in any of these situations.

If you experience a lack of interest in sex unrelated to the quality of your relationship, discuss this with your partner. If the lack of desire remains for a long period of time, discuss it with your doctor to determine if a medical treatment, such as hormone therapy, may help.

**Lack of stimulation of the clitoris.** Intercourse may not directly stimulate your clitoris, the part of your genital area that has maximum sensitivity. You may not have an orgasm if your clitoris isn't stimulated. Direct stimulation of your clitoris by you or your partner may be needed to help you reach sexual climax.

**Past sexual abuse.** Women who have been raped or sexually or physically abused may have a diminished sexual response. Seek counseling from a qualified professional as soon after the experience as possible.

**Physical abnormalities.** Physical factors can also add to a diminished sexual response. Several specific physical problems often lead to diminished or unattainable orgasms. Atherosclerosis (p. 111) may result in blockage of the arteries that supply blood to the genitals. Damage to the genital nerves, such as that caused by trauma or diabetes (p. 211), may interfere with sexual response. Local irritation or infection of the vagina, cervix, fallopian tube or bladder can all interfere with orgasm.

**Poor communication.** It's important to communicate clearly and honestly with your partner about which activities or positions help your sexual response and which ones make you uncomfortable. Improve communication with your partner about sex to help him or her become more aware of your needs and desires.

**Poor vaginal lubrication.** Problems with vaginal lubrication can lead to uncomfortable intercourse. Poor vaginal lubrication is perhaps the most correctable difficulty. A vaginal lubricant usually enhances sexual pleasure. If you use condoms, it's important to avoid using oil-based lubricants, such as petroleum jelly (p. 617). These compounds can damage the condom and decrease its usefulness as a birth control or disease prevention device. Instead, use water-based vaginal lubricants (p. 617).

**Relationship problems.** You may have trouble enjoying a sexual relationship with your partner if your relationship is threatened by fights over personal problems, money, children or other issues.

**Uncaring partner.** If your partner is only worried about his or her own sexual enjoyment, you may not be adequately stimulated. As a result, your desire is likely to fade.

**Unrealistic expectations about the sexual response.** A woman who has repeatedly heard that sex is pleasant only for men may have an unhealthy dread of sex that will prevent her from attempting to enjoy a sexual relationship.

The opposite type of expectation may also occur. With all the conflicting information about sexual activity, many people have a preconceived notion of what their sexual response should be. They may expect more from sex than what's realistic. Honesty about one's own feelings and actual response is essential to developing a healthy—and realistic—sexual relationship.

### Painful Sex

Sexual intercourse may be uncomfortable for a woman who is psychologically unprepared for it, whose relationship with her partner is troubled or who has a physical problem that makes intercourse painful. Some of the physical problems that lead to sexual problems include infections, urinary tract problems, abnormalities of the uterus or ovaries, and a condition called *vaginismus* (see below).

Infection of the vagina, the external genitals or the uterus and fallopian tubes often leads to pain during intercourse. Vaginal yeast infections are the most common infections, producing swelling, redness and pain in the vagina during sexual activity. Other infections can cause discharge, tenderness and bleeding during intercourse. Painful intercourse may be the first symptom of a pelvic infection. See your doctor whenever a pattern of pain during sex develops.

Bladder infections (p. 162) or irritation, inflammation of the urethra, and laxity or looseness in the front of the vagina, called *cystocele*, can all produce pain during sexual intercourse. Ovarian cysts (p. 417), tumors of the ovaries (p. 416) or uterus (p. 417), and endometriosis (p. 418) may also cause pain during intercourse.

*Vaginismus* is a condition that leads to painful sex. It has both psychological and physical factors. Poor vaginal lubrication in combination with an excessive constriction of the *pelvic floor muscles* (the muscles around the vaginal opening) make penetration and intercourse difficult or even impossible. The more times you're unable to relax, the more fearful you may become about any sexual activity. This fear, in turn, may make it difficult for you to relax, and the cycle continues.

Treatment for painful intercourse depends on the cause. The treatment for vaginismus includes individual counseling or marital therapy, the use of vaginal dilators during sexual arousal and patience and understanding by the partner. Your doctor can talk with you about dilators and exercises of the pelvic muscles to help reduce the discomfort caused by sexual intercourse. Counseling may be beneficial if severe psychological issues related to past incidents, such as incest, sexual abuse or rape, are playing a role.

## Pregnancy

After an egg is fertilized, it begins to divide into cells and travel down the fallopian tube to the uterus. This journey lasts from five to seven days. When the egg reaches the uterus, it implants itself in the *endometrium,* or the lining of the uterus. Implantation allows the egg to get nourishment for growth from the mother.

The implanted egg sends signals to the ovaries, telling them to continue producing progesterone. This prevents the drop in hormone levels that leads to menstrual bleeding. If the regular monthly bleeding weren't prevented, the egg would be shed with the lining of the uterus during the monthly menstrual period.

One or two weeks after implantation of the fertilized egg, a menstrual period usually is missed. But a few women may have a period, possibly with a lighter and shorter flow, for up to a few months after becoming pregnant. A few weeks after the egg is implanted, changes in the hormones produce tenderness and swelling of the breasts and a full feeling in the abdomen. Many women have episodes of nausea and vomiting (morning sickness) related to these hormone changes.

Women who normally have symptoms of PMS (p. 383) may notice a prolonging of those symptoms at about the same time they miss their period. The emotional and physical symptoms of PMS may continue into the pregnancy for some women, while for others pregnancy provides relief from their monthly symptoms.

A home pregnancy test (p. 636) will allow you to check a urine sample to see if you're pregnant. A hormone called *human chorionic gonadotropin* (HCG) is produced only when a woman is pregnant. This hormone is excreted in the urine. Home pregnancy tests are designed to detect HCG in the urine. A positive test almost always means you're pregnant. But a negative test doesn't always mean you're not pregnant. If you've missed a period but the test is negative, you may not have waited long enough for the test to be positive. If you wait another two weeks to take the test, and your results are still negative, make an appointment to be checked by your doctor.

If your pregnancy test is positive, call your doctor to start prenatal care. Even if your primary care doctor isn't going to provide your prenatal care, he or she can handle other illnesses during your pregnancy.

Always tell a medical caregiver that you're pregnant before any treatment. Avoid alcohol and smoking, even second-hand smoke, for your own health as well as your baby's. Consult your doctor if you need to take any medicine, even over-the-counter drugs, during your pregnancy.

## Prenatal Care

You can start making lifestyle changes even before you're pregnant to help you have a healthy pregnancy. Because you won't know you're pregnant until you miss a period, it's best to make healthy changes while you're trying to conceive. You'll probably hear lots of advice about what to do. Eating right and getting plenty of rest and exercise are keys to feeling your best

and staying your healthiest while you're pregnant.

**Diet.** Start by eating right. Avoid junk foods such as potato chips, soda and pastries. Eat a variety of foods that are high in nutrients, such as fruits, vegetables, grains and lean meats.

Your doctor may prescribe a prenatal vitamin supplement designed specifically for the nutritional demands of pregnancy. Prenatal vitamins contain proper amounts of folic acid, vitamin $B_{12}$ and iron. Folic acid is particularly important before and during pregnancy to help prevent brain or spinal cord problems in the baby.

A weight gain of 25 to 30 pounds is normal and healthy during pregnancy. Attempts to diet during pregnancy or to gain less than 20 pounds may injure the growing baby. On the other hand, excessive weight gain during pregnancy may be difficult to lose after your baby is born, and it also increases your risk of pregnancy-related diabetes (p. 393) and having a large baby.

**Exercise.** In the past, many doctors discouraged any exercise or heavy activity during pregnancy, hoping to reduce the chance for premature labor. More recent evidence suggests just the opposite. A physically fit woman does better during pregnancy, labor and delivery than a woman who isn't in good physical condition.

Early on, most exercise activities can be continued, but as the pregnancy progresses, the changes in your body make strenuous, exhausting or jarring activities unhealthy for you. Walking, using an exercise machine or swimming can be continued safely far into the pregnancy, especially if no complications arise. Sitting in very hot water, such as a hot tub, isn't recommended. Always check with your doctor about any activities you plan to begin or continue during your pregnancy.

### What's an Obstetrician?

*Obstetricians* are doctors who are trained in the specialty of surgery and prevention and treatment of health problems related to pregnancy. These skills overlap into the specialty of gynecology, which addresses women's reproductive health at times other than pregnancy. Many family doctors also deliver babies and take care of women's health problems.

**Genetic counseling.** If any genetic diseases run in your family, talk to your doctor before you get pregnant. He or she can help you assess your risk for having a baby with a genetic disease.

**Sex.** Normal sexual relations during pregnancy cause no problems, although intercourse during the last month of the pregnancy may lead to premature labor. However, many couples who have an overdue pregnancy have tried to induce labor through sexual intercourse with no success. Generally, if you aren't at risk of premature delivery, you can probably continue having sex throughout your entire pregnancy. Once again, your doctor can give you advice about sexual intercourse.

**Things to avoid.** Quit smoking if you smoke. Smoking when you're pregnant can cause miscarriage, bleeding, premature birth and low birth weight. It's also linked to sudden infant death syndrome (SIDS, p. 372). Children of smokers may not do as well on IQ tests, and their physical growth may be slower than other children's.

Avoid drinking alcohol. Drinking when you're pregnant can cause fetal alcohol syndrome (FAS, p. 342).

Illegal drugs, like marijuana and cocaine, raise your risk of miscarriage, premature birth and birth defects. With some drugs, the baby will be born addicted to the drug that the mother used and will go through withdrawal after birth. If you're addicted to alcohol or drugs, ask your doctor to help you get involved in a program that will help you stop, preferably before you become pregnant.

Avoid exposure to materials that could be hazardous to a growing fetus. These materials include radiation, anesthetic gases, carbon disulfide, acids and heavy metals like lead, copper and mercury.

**Other issues.** Before you're pregnant, talk to your doctor if you're not sure if you've had or been vaccinated against rubella (p. 330). Getting the German measles while you're pregnant can be bad for your baby. A blood test can show if you've had it or if you've already been vaccinated. If you haven't had this vaccination, you can get it before you're pregnant to prevent getting German measles while you're pregnant.

Also talk to your doctor about any sexually transmitted diseases (STDs, p. 316) you may have, such as herpes. Many STDs can be passed to the baby during birth. Measures can often be taken to help prevent this.

Ask your doctor before taking any prescription and over-the-counter medicines.

### Stages of pregnancy

The total length of pregnancy is 40 weeks, which includes the two

---

## Toxoplasmosis

*Toxoplasmosis* is a type of parasitic infection. It can be contracted by a pregnant woman and passed to her unborn child. It can lead to birth defects, including blindness and brain damage. This parasite may be present in cat feces. The disease may be transmitted after a pregnant woman handles cat feces, such as when changing the litter box. Raw meat and unpasteurized milk can also carry the parasite. To prevent the infection, ask someone else to clean out your cat's litter box. Don't eat undercooked meat or drink unpasteurized milk.

weeks between your last period and the time of fertilization of the egg. Pregnancy is divided into three parts, or *trimesters*, which each last approximately three months. The changes in both baby and mother are quite different during each of these three periods.

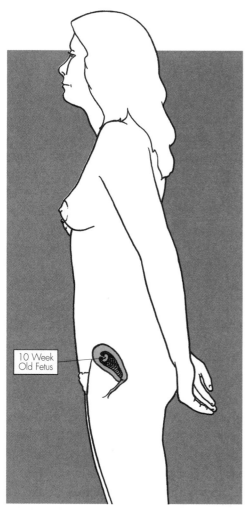

10 Week Old Fetus

**FIRST TRIMESTER**

**First trimester.** Many of the first signs of pregnancy, including nausea and vomiting, tenderness or swelling of the breasts, a sense of fullness in the abdomen and unexplainable fatigue, continue through the first trimester. Other first-trimester symptoms include frequent urination, increasing abdominal size and difficulty sleeping. The nausea, vomiting and breast tenderness often fade by the second trimester.

The first trimester is the riskiest time for the developing fetus. The tissues and organs are forming, and some medicines or exposure to x-rays or other harmful agents can damage these delicate tissues. Birth defects are most likely to develop during the first trimester, and the risk of miscarriage is highest in the first three months of pregnancy. Women can have a spontaneous abortion without even knowing they were pregnant. About 20% of all confirmed pregnancies end with a miscarriage. While repeated miscarriages are usually the result of problems in the uterus, two-thirds of miscarriages are the result of abnormalities in the fetus.

At fertilization, the single cell divides to form a hollow ball of cells as the egg travels down the fallopian tube. Once the egg has implanted in the soft, fertile lining of the uterus, further development takes place as the placenta and covering (the *amniotic sac*) form around the egg. At this stage, the baby is called an *embryo*. Initially, the embryo looks like the embryos of many other animals in their early stages. But within a few weeks, many of the internal organs are formed in the human embryo, and the arms, legs, hands and feet have begun to form. By the end of the first trimester, the baby's heart can be heard with Doppler ultrasound (p. 644). The organs are formed but aren't mature. Tiny fingers and toes are on the hands and feet—quite a change from the one-celled egg fertilized just 11 or so weeks before.

**Second trimester.** The middle three months, or second trimester, usually is the calmest portion of the pregnancy. Many of the early discomforts, such as nausea, vomiting and fatigue, have diminished or disappeared. Although the uterus has greatly increased in size,

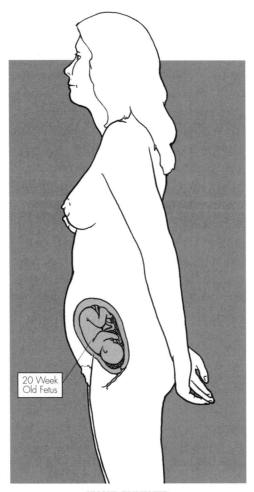

20 Week
Old Fetus

**SECOND TRIMESTER**

you can comfortably continue many of your normal activities.

Sometime between the 15th and 20th weeks of pregnancy, most women feel the baby move or kick for the first time, an event called *quickening*. As the baby continues to grow and mature, the organs expand, the baby's length and weight increase, and more of the organs begin to function, helping with digestion and sending oxygen and nutrients to the tissues. Babies born during this trimester usually aren't able to survive, even with intensive measures and life support. They're just too small and too immature.

A more rapid weight gain begins in the second trimester. Weight gain continues until late in the pregnancy. Follow your doctor's advice and try to stay within the recommendations for weight gain. Call your doctor for instructions if you have any bleeding or pain.

**Third trimester.** In the last trimester, your abdomen grows quite large and feels tight. There's minimal space left in your abdomen for food. The baby presses on your bladder, causing you to urinate often. Reddish marks may appear on your abdomen and breasts as the skin becomes tighter. Tiredness may return, sometimes because it's difficult to find a comfortable position to sleep in. The baby's activity comes in bursts, often when you're trying to sleep. Your joints begin to loosen and creak because of the secretion of a hormone called *relaxin*. Loosening of the hip joints allows delivery through a "relaxed" birth canal. Your feet, hands and face may swell from fluid retention.

While you may be less comfortable during the third trimester, your baby may seem to be having a grand time. Although the baby may be quiet at times, his or her activity can increase until it's uncomfortable for you. Actually, the baby begins to run out of room after the seventh month of pregnancy, so he or she may be trying to stretch out a bit.

Sometime between the 22nd and 25th weeks of pregnancy, the baby reaches a point at which he or she can survive if born prematurely. With the advanced supportive medical techniques available in neonatal intensive care units, younger and younger babies are surviving. The closer the child is born to the end of the pregnancy (36 to 44 weeks), the more mature the baby will be and the less likely to have complications. More mature, or "full-term," babies have more hair and longer fingernails than those born prematurely.

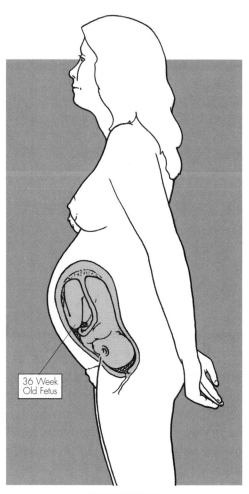

**THIRD TRIMESTER**

## Possible Health Problems of Pregnancy

The changes you experience during pregnancy can produce many uncomfortable symptoms. The majority of these symptoms are mild. But some are more dangerous for you and your baby and should be managed by your doctor.

Sometimes pregnancy doesn't proceed normally. Problems can occur that affect the placenta, the fluid around the baby, the uterus, the baby or the mother. Even problems that seem simple may indicate that a serious complication has developed that needs immediate treatment.

Check with your doctor right away if you have bleeding or a gush of fluid from your vagina, severe pain in your abdomen, headache or rapid swelling of your face, hands or legs during pregnancy.

**Abruptio placentae.** Normally, the placenta is connected to the uterus during pregnancy. If the placenta becomes separated from the uterus before the baby's birth, the condition is called *abruptio placentae.* It occurs about once in every 200 births. It's a serious problem because it can cause severe bleeding. If you're near the end of your pregnancy and abruptio placentae occurs, your doctor will probably choose to do a cesarean section (also called a C-section, p. 403). If the problem occurs before the time when the baby can survive outside the womb, your doctor may prescribe complete bed rest.

**Anemia.** Anemia (p. 133) is a common and often undetected problem. It affects 10% of women in the United States. Low levels of iron in the blood or a lack of vitamins can cause you to have a pale complexion, weakness and a tendency to tire easily. Severe anemia can lead to chest pain, heart palpitations and even heart failure.

During pregnancy, a woman may become anemic, or more anemic, because she doesn't get enough iron in her diet or her body isn't able to absorb the iron. The iron requirements of your baby also deplete your iron supply.

Most women take a prenatal vitamin that includes a small amount of iron, folic acid and vitamin $B_{12}$, nutrients needed for the production of red blood cells.

A low iron content in your blood increases your chances for an infection during pregnancy as well as a miscarriage. Blood loss at the time of delivery can make the anemia worse. Routine blood tests usually identify anemia so it can be treated.

Iron-containing foods, such as meats, whole-grain breads and eggs,

## Medical Tests During Pregnancy

*Your doctor may suggest that you have a number of tests during your pregnancy. The tests can help keep track of how your body is handling the pregnancy and can help find any potential problems early.*

- Amniocentesis (p. 628) to detect abnormalities in the fetus
- Rh-factor test (p. 640) of the mother's blood to see if she has antibodies that may damage the baby's blood cells
- Alpha-fetoprotein (AFP) test (p. 627) to check for increased levels of AFP in the mother's blood, which may indicate that the baby has a serious neural tube defect such as spina bifida (p. 355) or anencephaly (p. 346). Low levels of AFP may indicate a genetic defect such as Down syndrome (p. 348).
- Chorionic villus sampling (p. 631) to detect genetic abnormalities
- Doppler scanning (p. 644) to check the blood flow through the baby's circulatory system, to measure fetal movement and uterine contractions, and to check the baby's response to changes in his or her environment
- Glucose tolerance test (p. 636) to measure the level of sugar in the mother's blood to check for signs of diabetes during pregnancy (p. 393).
- Ultrasound testing or sonogram (p. 643) to estimate the age of the baby, to check for growth problems and to check the health and location of the placenta.

should be eaten in combination with sources of vitamin C, such as citrus fruits, to help increase the amount of iron you absorb from your food. A vitamin/mineral supplement is usually prescribed by your doctor. He or she can also prescribe extra iron in pills if your blood tests show anemia due to low iron.

**Antepartum hemorrhage.** Bleeding before delivery, called *antepartum hemorrhage,* can be caused by conditions that aren't serious, such as a varicose vein of the uterus, or by more serious problems, such as placenta previa (p. 396). The first sign of problems in the pregnancy may be vaginal bleeding without pain. Because this bleeding may be serious for both you and your baby, always report any bleeding during pregnancy to your doctor.

**Backache.** Look at the posture of a woman in the eighth month of pregnancy, and it's easy to understand why her back hurts. The weight of the baby requires a greater curvature in the lower spine, shifting the weight of the upper body further backward. This posture stresses the muscles and ligaments next to the spine and allows them to move more freely.

To compound this stress is the effect caused by the hormone *relaxin.* The hormonal change caused by relaxin loosens the hip joints so the baby can go through the birth canal more easily, but it also produces laxity in the other joints.

Along with the hormonal effects and the change in posture, the uterus and the stressed muscles put pressure on the sciatic nerve, the large nerve that runs from the lower spine to the leg. Extra fluid in the woman's system also irritates the nerves, including the sciatic nerve. The result may be sciatica (p. 247). In addition, the ligament that attaches the uterus to the pelvis also pulls on the back, sometimes causing sharp abdominal and back pains.

Depending on the source of the pain, some posture changes may help. Lying on the side where the pain is occurring may reduce or stop the pain. Lying in the fetal position on your left side often takes the stress off the sciatic nerve. When lying on your back, place pillows under your head and knees. However, lying on your back isn't recommended as your pregnancy progresses, because the increasing weight of the baby may reduce blood return from the lower part of your body, including your uterus. Heating pads, muscle relaxants and pain medicines aren't recommended for back pain during pregnancy.

**Constipation and hemorrhoids.** The entire gastrointestinal tract seems to become lax during pregnancy. Softening of the valve at the top of the stomach allows stomach acids to escape into the esophagus, producing heartburn. The intestine also becomes lax and doesn't push the food through as quickly, causing constipation (p. 177). Straining to have a bowel movement may cause hemorrhoids (p. 189). The other factor that tends to cause hemorrhoids during pregnancy is the way the uterus pushes on the large veins in the pelvis, causing blood to back up into the veins around the rectum.

Over-the-counter laxatives may not be safe to use during pregnancy. Eat a diet high in fiber, including fresh fruits and vegetables, and drink lots of fluids to prevent or reduce the severity of hemorrhoids and constipation.

**Diabetes.** When diabetes (p. 211) develops during pregnancy (*gestational diabetes*), it's a serious complication of pregnancy, yet it may not produce any symptoms until it has already caused damage. This is why your doctor frequently tests your urine and blood and does other tests, such as a glucose tolerance test (p. 636), to check for diabetes.

Diabetes, or elevated blood sugar, is dangerous during pregnancy because the growing baby can't tolerate the extra sugar. A number of these babies are stillborn, and others have deformities or problems with their blood sugar when they're born. Careful control of the blood sugar with diet and insulin prevents serious complications in the baby.

Although few symptoms of diabetes are apparent during pregnancy, there are some warning signs and predictors. If you're overweight, if there's a history of diabetes in your family or if you've previously had a baby weighing more than 9½ to 10 pounds at birth, you're at risk for diabetes during pregnancy. Make sure you see your doctor for scheduled appointments, and contact him or her immediately if you have a problem during your pregnancy.

A very high level of blood sugar indicates that you have diabetes during pregnancy. Some pregnant women have a very mild form of sugar intolerance but don't need insulin. In these women, close monitoring and avoiding sugar are sufficient to control their blood sugar level. In more severe cases, diet changes and insulin are used to keep the blood sugar level down. In all instances of diabetes in the pregnant woman, the baby will be monitored closely to detect any potential problems.

**Ectopic pregnancy.** When an egg is fertilized, it usually travels down the

---

### Diabetes and Pregnancy

If you have diabetes, pregnancy poses a risk for you and an even greater risk for your baby. Newer methods of monitoring have improved the chances of a safe and successful pregnancy in women with diabetes. But a woman who has diabetes must control her blood sugar carefully through diet, exercise and use of insulin.

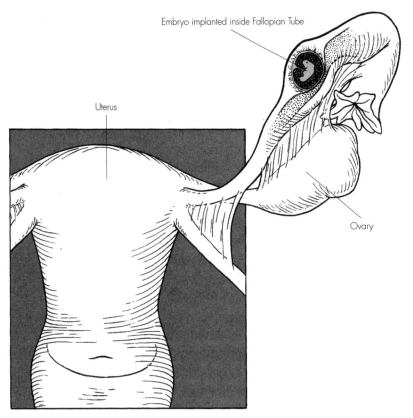

Embryo implanted inside Fallopian Tube

Uterus

Ovary

**ECTOPIC PREGNANCY**

fallopian tube into the uterus. Rarely, the egg will lodge in the fallopian tube, implant there and begin to grow. This condition is called a *tubal pregnancy*. Sometimes the fertilized egg can be pushed out of the tube and inside the abdominal cavity. This is called an *abdominal pregnancy*. When a fertilized egg grows outside the womb, such as in a tubal or abdominal pregnancy, the condition is called an *ectopic pregnancy*. An egg that's growing in a fallopian tube will cause the tube to stretch, resulting in pain. If the problem isn't treated, the tube can rupture and cause internal bleeding. Pain resulting from an ectopic pregnancy usually appears by the sixth week.

Any pain in your abdomen that lasts for more than an hour or two should be checked by your doctor. An ultrasound exam will locate the baby in its amniotic sac and determine its location, whether it's within the uterus or outside the uterus. A ruptured ectopic pregnancy is life-threatening and may require immediate treatment with surgery, blood transfusions and intensive supportive care. An ectopic pregnancy should be removed as soon as possible to prevent severe complications. Surgery to remove the ectopic egg will save the mother's life and protect her reproductive system so she can retain her fertility.

**Genetic defects.** Although they're rare, genetic defects can affect a child even if the parents don't have the disorder. The parents may be carriers of a disease, although they don't have it themselves. Some genetic diseases in babies and young children include cystic fibrosis (p. 348), muscular dystrophy (p. 354), sickle cell anemia (p. 134), Down syndrome (p. 348) and hemophilia (p. 136). Many genetic diseases affect a child only when both parents contribute a faulty gene.

Severe genetic abnormalities often cause miscarriages or stillbirths. Some of these problems can be discovered by testing the fetus. If the parents have already had a child with a serious disorder, a genetic counselor can be helpful in evaluating the possibility of the genetic problem showing up in future children. Specialized testing for genetic problems, such as amniocentesis (p. 628) or chorionic villus sampling (p. 631), before birth may give your doctor important information about certain health problems.

**Growth retardation.** Several factors, including diabetes, drug abuse, genetic abnormalities, heart disease and high blood pressure (p. 123), can slow the growth of the baby. Regular examinations and measurements of the uterus will detect slow growth as soon as possible, so your doctor can

> ## When should I call my doctor?
>
> *If you're pregnant, call your doctor*
> *if you have any of these symptoms:*
> - Severe headaches
> - Painful or increasingly frequent urination
> - Fever or signs of infection
> - Rapid increase in swelling
> - Increase in nausea and vomiting
> - Pain in the abdomen
> - Sudden vaginal bleeding or fluid gush
> - Absence of fetal movement for more than 24 hours
>
> *Any of these signs could mean a serious health problem for mother or baby. Call your doctor immediately for further instructions.*

## Reducing Problems During Pregnancy

- Abstain from alcohol, drugs and smoking.
- Eat a balanced, healthy diet and take your vitamins as prescribed.
- Exercise.
- See your doctor for regular appointments and follow his or her recommendations.
- Watch for any hazardous conditions in your workplace.

order tests to identify the cause of slow growth. Once the problem is identified, various treatments may improve your baby's growth rate and reduce the possibility of premature delivery or fetal respiratory distress syndrome (p. 344).

**Heartburn.** Many gastrointestinal problems are common during pregnancy. Heartburn (p. 187), caused by a backward flow of stomach juices into the esophagus, is common during pregnancy because of the lax valve at the top of the stomach, where the stomach meets the esophagus. As the uterus becomes larger, more pressure is exerted on the stomach, causing stomach fluids to back up into the esophagus. Severe heartburn should be checked by your doctor.

Eating small, bland, low-fat meals greatly reduces the tendency for heartburn. An over-the-counter antacid will relieve symptoms, but check with your doctor before using it on a regular basis. Most of the other medicines for heartburn haven't yet been cleared for use during pregnancy.

**High blood pressure.** Another dangerous complication of pregnancy occurs when the mother's blood pressure becomes elevated. High blood pressure is one of a group of symptoms associated with *preeclampsia*, a serious complication of pregnancy. Other symptoms include swelling of the feet, legs, hands and face. The kidneys may be injured. If the high blood pressure isn't treated, it can lead to convulsions, unconsciousness and even death of the woman and her baby. Worsening of symptoms is a condition called *eclampsia*, and it's one of the most serious problems in pregnancy. High blood pressure alone can injure the baby by reducing the oxygen and other nutrients the baby receives from the placenta. The poor nutrition leads to growth retardation and a greater chance of birth complications.

Your doctor will check your blood pressure and obtain a urine sample at each visit to his or her office or clinic. A significant elevation in blood pressure causes concern and requires careful monitoring. Initially, your doctor may tell you to limit your salt intake. If your blood pressure continues to rise, protein appears in your urine (a sign of kidney problems) and your feet, legs, hands and face swell, then your doctor may order bed rest, medicines or even hospitalization and early delivery by C-section to prevent serious problems for you and your baby.

**Infections during pregnancy.** Certain infections are very dangerous when contracted early in pregnancy. The most dangerous viral infections during pregnancy include AIDS

## Am I having a miscarriage?

- Are you bleeding or having lower abdominal cramps?
- Do you have continuous pain in the lower abdomen?
- Have you passed anything pink or gray in color from your vagina?

*If you're pregnant and answer yes to any of these questions, call your doctor or the local hospital right away for instructions.*

## Possible Causes of Miscarriage

- A genetic problem in the baby
- A problem with the placenta
- A uterine problem, which may be suspected if a woman has more than one miscarriage
- An accident or fall
- Drug or alcohol use

(p. 325), chickenpox (p. 321) cytomegalovirus, rubella (p. 330), hepatitis (p. 204) and herpes (p. 325). Bacterial infections that may harm the mother or the baby include urinary tract infections (p. 162), chlamydia (p. 317), gonorrhea (p. 318), certain streptococcal infections (p. 306) and syphilis (p. 319).

Infections can cause direct damage to the unborn child. Some will cause deformities or retardation. Bladder infections are associated with premature labor. If you become ill with a fever, rash or other symptoms indicating infection, see your doctor right away to rule out these damaging infections.

**Miscarriage and stillbirth.** A pregnancy that ends during the first 20 weeks is called a *miscarriage,* or *spontaneous abortion.* After the 20th week, the death of the baby is called a *stillbirth,* or *intrauterine death.*

Medical problems in the mother, such as bleeding, Rh incompatibility, diabetes and high blood pressure or severe physical deformities in the fetus can lead to miscarriage or stillbirth.

A small amount of bleeding without cramping or pain may signal a *threatened abortion,* the premature separation of the placenta from the uterus. With rest, the placenta often stops separating, and the pregnancy continues normally. If bleeding continues and cramping begins, a miscarriage is likely.

An ultrasound (p. 643) can reveal the status of the baby and placenta and help determine if further bleeding or placental separation is likely. When fetal death occurs later in the pregnancy, the mother may notice that the baby's movement has ceased, and further testing confirms that the baby is no longer alive. Labor will be induced if it doesn't start within a few weeks to prevent loss of blood clotting function in the mother. If the blood's ability to clot is impaired, the mother may begin bleeding severely. This could lead to death.

If you have a miscarriage, your doctor will examine you for signs of infection or excessive blood loss.

A dilatation and curettage (D & C, p. 420) may be recommended to remove any remains of the pregnancy.

Almost all miscarriages are related to a defect in the baby or the placenta, or to a health condition affecting the mother. Miscarriages aren't related to anything the mother did or didn't do. Grief is normal after a miscarriage. Grief may be more pronounced when a child is lost late in pregnancy. Counseling can help you and your partner deal with the loss.

**Nausea and vomiting (morning sickness).** The hormonal changes of pregnancy and their effect on the stomach and intestines can cause nausea and vomiting, especially during the first few months of pregnancy. The more familiar term, *morning sickness,* describes the nausea that hits many women when they first wake up. For some women, nausea and vomiting continue throughout the day or occur in the evening. Most women don't require treatment. For women who have severe symptoms, treatment may be necessary and may include vitamin $B_6$. Admission to the hospital and intravenous fluids may be needed if the vomiting becomes severe and continuous. This condition is called *hyperemesis gravidarum.*

Many of the medicines once used for nausea and vomiting during pregnancy have been taken off the market and are no longer recommended because of their potential to harm the baby. Try to eat a bland, reduced-fat diet and small, frequent meals

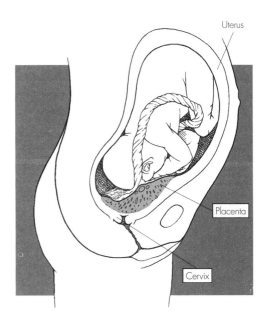

**PLACENTA PREVIA**

instead of a three large meals a day. Keeping something in the stomach all the time seems to help most women. Check with your doctor if your vomiting is severe, causes you to be light-headed or weak, or makes you feel as if you're going to pass out.

**Placenta previa.** Bleeding from the vagina is often the first symptom of *placenta previa,* a condition that occurs when the placenta is close to or covering the lower portion of the uterus. The placenta is normally in the upper part of the uterus. When placenta previa occurs and the *cervix* (the opening of the uterus into the vagina) is completely covered by the placenta, the baby can bleed to death if delivery is forced through the placenta. When placenta previa is present, a C-section is usually done as soon as the baby is mature enough to survive outside the womb. Placenta previa is usually discovered in a routine ultrasound exam. An ultrasound exam may be specially ordered to locate the placenta if your doctor suspects a problem.

**Polyhydramnios.** Excessive amniotic fluid may build up inside the uterus for no apparent reason or because of diabetes, high blood pressure or a pregnancy with twins. This excessive fluid, called *polyhydramnios,* is usually harmless but may lead to premature labor. Your doctor may suggest that you rest or take medicine to prevent uterine contractions and premature labor.

**Postmaturity.** Why does your doctor watch the growth of your uterus and take such care to calculate your estimated date of delivery? Serious damage may occur to a baby who is *postmature,* or not delivered within a few weeks after the expected due date. Problems occur because the placenta begins to degenerate later in the pregnancy, and the baby won't have enough oxygen or nutrients if the pregnancy continues after the placenta begins degenerating. Stillbirths are twice as common in postmature pregnancies as in those delivered on or before the due date. When pregnancy continues for two weeks beyond the due date, labor may be induced by giving the woman medicine to start uterine contractions.

**Premature membrane rupture.** The membranes surrounding the baby are filled with amniotic fluid. As the uterus begins contracting regularly during labor, these membranes break and the fluid gushes out. In some women, the membranes rupture before labor starts. Within a few hours, the regular contractions of labor begin.

When the membranes rupture but labor doesn't start, infection can result. Careful monitoring of the pregnancy, often in the hospital, is required if this happens.

**Rh-factor incompatibility.** A mother who has Rh-negative blood whose baby has Rh-positive blood can develop antibodies to the baby's Rh factor during pregnancy and shortly after labor and delivery. During delivery, the mother is exposed to the Rh-positive

---

## Coping with Stillbirth

- Hold your baby and give him or her a name.
- Take time to cry for the loss of your baby. Include your partner in your grief process.
- Don't immediately destroy or undo the preparations you made at home for the baby.
- Discuss with your doctor any tests that were performed on your baby.
- Seek professional counseling, especially if the effects of the depression last more than a few months, or if the depression becomes so severe that you think about suicide or are unable to perform your normal daily functions.

### If You Want to Breast Feed Your Baby

- Know your hospital's policies for breast feeding in the delivery room and, later, in your hospital room.
- Make sure your doctor knows you want to breast feed as soon as possible, including in the delivery room.
- You may be able to have your baby stay in your room with you part of the time (partial rooming-in), all of the time (full rooming-in) or just when your baby is hungry (demand feeding).
- See page 404 for information about how to prepare for breast feeding and how to get off to a good start.

blood as the baby's blood enters her bloodstream when the placenta separates from the uterus. Later, if the mother carries another Rh-positive child, her antibodies get into the baby's bloodstream during the pregnancy and destroy the baby's red blood cells.

An injection given to the mother late in the pregnancy and after delivery, or after a miscarriage, destroys the circulating Rh factor and prevents antibody formation in the mother. But if the problem is missed and the baby becomes sick because of the mother's antibodies against the baby's Rh-positive blood, a blood transfusion can be given to the baby shortly after birth. A transfusion can even be given before the baby is born if the baby is too small to be delivered. Before these transfusions were possible, most Rh infants died of blood incompatibility.

**Swelling.** You may notice that you tend to retain water during your pregnancy. This can result in swelling, or *edema,* of your extremities, particularly your legs. Rest with your feet up. When you sleep, lie on your left side so your blood will flow better from your legs back to your heart. Cut back on the amount of salt you eat if salty foods seem to make the edema worse. Don't take diuretics (p. 623).

**Trophoblastic tumors.** Tumors may grow from placental tissue during pregnancy. These rare tumors are called *trophoblastic* tumors. A fertilized

egg may not be able to develop because of the rapid growth of the tumor.

A *hydatidiform mole* is usually noncancerous. It grows rapidly in the uterus during pregnancy and destroys the growing fetus. Placental tissue left from a previous pregnancy can result in a hydatidiform mole months or even years later.

A small percentage of hydatidiform moles become cancerous, damaging the uterus and causing bleeding. The tumor may also invade other tissues and spread to distant sites.

An ultrasound and blood tests can help in diagnosis. Treatment involves removing the tumor, usually through a procedure called dilatation and curettage (D & C, p. 420). The uterus is left intact for future pregnancies. If the tumor is cancerous, however, the uterus will be removed and a course of chemotherapy medicines (p. 621) will probably be given to prevent recurrence and spread of the disease.

## Giving Birth

As you get close to your due date, the uterus tones itself with occasional contractions. Some women feel these contractions earlier in the pregnancy, while others don't feel them until quite late. These normal preparatory contractions are called *Braxton Hicks* contractions. For some women, the contractions become strong and regular, mimicking the early stages of labor. "False labor" can

### Skin Color Changes During Pregnancy

During pregnancy, different areas of skin can take in more or less pigment, producing darker or lighter areas. These changes commonly include darker spots on the face (*chloasma*), darkening of the nipples, darkening of the line between the bellybutton and the pubic bone (*linea nigra*) and darkening in areas where the skin is rubbed.

## Why should I take a childbirth class?

*Consider these reasons for deciding to take a childbirth class:*

- It will teach you more about pregnancy and delivery.
- A trained nurse or other health care professional will be able to answer your questions.
- You will meet and share information with other expectant parents.
- It helps the father of the baby or other family members become more involved in the pregnancy.
- Training improves your chances of a less strenuous, shorter and more comfortable labor, with a reduced need for anesthesia or pain medicine.

be identified as irregular contractions that fade with time or with walking.

One sign that labor may begin soon is the loss of the *mucus plug* from the cervix, also called a "bloody show." This mucus may come out at the beginning of labor or a few days before labor actually starts. Another sign is any fluid leak or gush from the vagina. This gush usually means that your "water has broken"—the amniotic sac has ruptured, and labor has started or will soon begin. The amniotic sac can rupture at the beginning of labor or before labor (*premature rupture*), or your doctor may break it during active labor.

Strong regular contractions, leakage of fluid or a gush of fluid let you know that you're beginning labor. When these signs occur, call your doctor or go directly to the hospital, according to the plan you and your doctor have discussed.

**Stages of labor.** When you go into labor, you'll experience three distinct stages outlined below.

*First stage.* During delivery of a baby, a number of changes must occur in the uterus. First, the thick walls of the cervix become thin because the baby's head is pushing on them. The stronger the contractions, the more quickly the baby's head can help to thin the cervix. Cervical thinning is a change that can be felt and

assessed by your nurse or doctor during an exam.

Next, the cervix must dilate, or open, so the baby's head can squeeze through. Your nurse or doctor will tell you how wide the dilation is in centimeters. Full dilation is about 10 centimeters. The baby's head can then push through this opening and enter the vaginal canal. For first-time mothers, the first stage of labor lasts an average of about 12 hours, although it can last for 24 hours or longer for some women. After you've had one child, it's easier for the cervix to thin and dilate, so subsequent first stages of labor tend to be shorter. The average time for the first stage

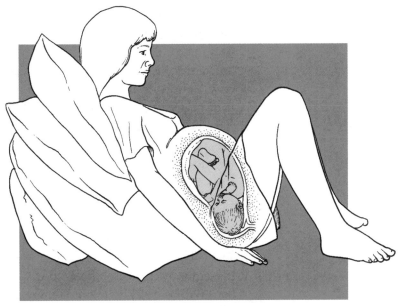

**BABY'S HEAD PUSHING INTO BIRTH CANAL**

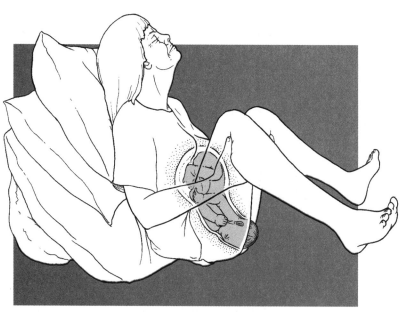

**HEAD EMERGING FROM BIRTH CANAL**

of labor for a second, third or fourth child is only six hours. Generally, the more children a woman has, the shorter her labors become.

*Second stage.* A short pause, or transition, sometimes occurs between the first stage of labor, when the cervix is completely dilated, and the second stage, when the baby begins to move through the birth canal. The second stage of labor is marked by two changes. First, you suddenly feel the strong urge to push to expel the baby. Second, your contractions become stronger than those in the first stage. The desire to push comes as the baby's head moves through the cervix and into the vagina. A full rectum gives you the desire to push to have a bowel movement, and so does the pressure on the rectum caused by the baby's head as it moves into the vagina.

The second stage is completed when the baby moves completely through the birth canal and is born. The baby will still be connected to the placenta by the umbilical cord. The cord will be quickly tied or clamped in two places and cut between the ties.

A woman having her first baby may spend an hour or more pushing the baby through the birth canal. Women giving birth to their second, third or fourth child usually have a much shorter second stage, seldom more than 30 minutes. Their babies are often born with five to 10 pushes.

*Third stage.* The final stage of labor may last only a few minutes. At the most, it usually lasts no more than 20 minutes. In the third stage, the placenta, also called the *afterbirth,* is pushed out as your uterus continues to contract. Your doctor may help the placenta to separate by pulling gently on the umbilical cord while pressing on the contracting uterus. Some bleeding will occur. But the more the uterus contracts, the more the blood vessels of the blood-rich lining of the uterus constrict. This constriction helps the uterus stop bleeding as much. A medicine can also be given to further contract the uterus and prevent postpartum bleeding, a potentially serious complication after childbirth.

**Anesthesia during labor.** Medicine can be used during labor to help reduce the discomfort of the contractions and pain when the baby moves through the birth canal. Oral or intravenous medicine to reduce pain can be given early in the first stage of labor, but this medicine sedates your baby along with you, making it more difficult for your baby to wake up and breathe after delivery. General anesthesia, an older and seldom-used method for vaginal deliveries, can still be used for C-sections (p. 403) if the mother or doctor desires. Today, the most commonly used methods of anesthesia are injections of local anesthetic or epidural anesthesia for vaginal deliveries. Epidural, or spinal, anesthetic is most commonly used during a cesarean section. Talk to your doctor about the types of anesthesia he or she usually recommends. Some methods aren't available at all hospitals.

As the baby's head comes through the vaginal canal, your doctor may make a small incision in your *perineum* (the area between the vagina and the rectum) to prevent the tissue from tearing. This incision is called an *episiotomy.* A small injection of lidocaine or other anesthetic is given to numb the skin before the cut is made. Sutures are usually needed after the birth to close the cut and prevent infection. A deeper injection, called a *pudendal block,* can also be used to numb the other tissues of the vaginal canal, if necessary.

When *spinal anesthesia* is needed, an injection of anesthetic medicine is placed next to the spinal cord with a long needle pushed through a space between the vertebrae. This anesthetic numbs everything from the level of the injection down, preventing both pain and motion. If spinal anesthesia is given before the baby has moved through the birth canal, forceps may be needed to help the baby move through the birth canal. The forceps are placed around the baby's head like a helmet, and the baby is gently pulled through the vagina. *Epidural anesthesia* is similar to spinal anesthesia, but relieves the pain of contractions without restricting all movement. Women who desire a "natural" childbirth may not want oral or spinal medicines, although some women change their minds if delivery pain is unexpectedly severe.

**Monitoring during labor.** You'll be closely monitored during labor and birth. This helps your doctor prevent or correct problems that can occur. Monitoring begins with a general exam, blood tests and checking the cervix when you're admitted. An electronic monitor may be attached to your

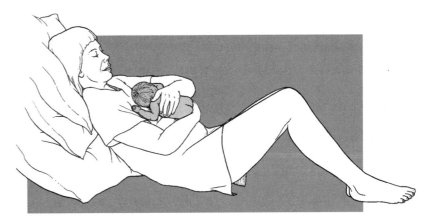

**WOMAN HOLDING NEWBORN**

abdomen to "watch" your contractions and the response of your baby's heart rate to the contractions.

If your baby's heart rate responds normally to the contractions, it means your baby is probably healthy and the cord or placenta isn't being squeezed, or threatened, during contractions. An abnormal response in your baby's heart rate could mean your baby is in trouble, and a C-section may be needed right away. Other samples of blood may be taken or an electrode may be placed on the scalp of the baby to better monitor his or her progress through labor and delivery.

Your doctor will also monitor the length of your labor. If it continues far beyond the normal time, your doctor may order tests or exams to look for problems. It may be that your birth canal or pelvis is too small for the baby's head or that your cervix isn't able to dilate properly. A C-section may be needed.

**Problems of labor.** During labor and delivery, problems can develop that affect the mother or baby. Most problems can be successfully treated by your doctor in a hospital.

*Malpresentation.* During labor, the baby's head becomes a wedge that's used to open the cervix so the baby can squeeze through the vaginal canal. In most births, the baby emerges from the vagina with the back of his or her head toward the ceiling (a position called *occiput anterior*). If the face is toward the ceiling (*occiput posterior*), the baby travels more slowly through the birth canal, and forceps may be needed to guide the baby through the vagina. A C-section is needed when the baby becomes stuck in the birth canal.

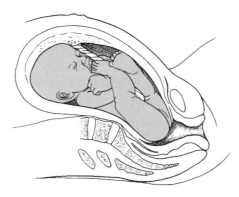

**BREECH PRESENTATION**

The most common malpresentation is the *breech position*, when the baby emerges from the vagina with his or her bottom first. Because the infant may not move into the normal, head-down position until shortly before labor, some babies get caught in the breech position when labor is premature, pushing the baby through the birth canal before he or she has had time to turn around. In the breech position, the baby's head can push down on the umbilical cord, cutting off the baby's oxygen supply. Because of this, most breech babies are delivered by C-section. Sometimes an attempt is made to turn the baby around into a head-down position. Often, this isn't possible.

Another potentially dangerous malpresentation is a *transverse,* or *sideways,* position. Smaller babies, especially premature ones, can end up with one shoulder lodged across the birth canal. The umbilical cord can be compressed, causing severe damage

to the baby. C-section is usually chosen to deliver a baby in this position.

*Premature labor.* When labor begins at least three weeks before the estimated due date, it's said to be premature. Less than 5% of pregnancies end in premature labor and, in many cases, there are no lasting problems in the baby. However, the earlier the birth, the less the baby's organs are able to function on their own.

One of the most common complications of premature labor is respiratory distress syndrome (p. 344), caused by immaturity of the baby's lungs. Sometimes premature labor is caused by maternal problems such as bleeding, high blood pressure (p. 123) or placenta previa (p. 396).

Premature labor can sometimes be stopped by a medicine administered by your doctor. If labor can't be stopped, the premature baby will be kept in a neonatal intensive care unit that provides special life support and intensive monitoring. If a premature delivery seems imminent, medicine can be given to help the baby's lungs mature more quickly before birth. This measure can make premature birth less risky for the baby.

*Prolonged labor.* Prolonged labor (more than 24 hours) is uncommon. Prolonged labor usually occurs because the baby's head is too big to fit through the mother's pelvis or because the uterine contractions are too weak or uncoordinated to push the baby through the birth canal. A special x-ray of the pelvis may be used to check for a disproportion between the size of the baby's skull and the space in your pelvis.

If pelvic size isn't the problem, medicine will probably be given to help your uterus contract more forcefully. Vacuum extraction (p. 403) or, less commonly, forceps (p. 403) may be used when second-stage labor seems to be progressing slowly. Your baby will be delivered by C-section if the head is too big to fit through your pelvis, or if forceps or stimulation of the uterus doesn't work.

*Postpartum hemorrhage.* Uterine contractions continue naturally after delivery of the baby and the placenta. The contractions put pressure on the enlarged blood vessels and help prevent excessive bleeding, or *postpartum hemorrhage.* Hemorrhage is more likely when the uterus has been stretched by the presence of twins or a large number of pregnancies. Excessive bleeding may also occur when labor has been long and hard.

If the contractions stop after delivery, they can sometimes be stimulated by pressing or massaging the uterus. They can also be restarted with medicine. Tears in the vaginal tissues, which may sometimes go through to the rectum, can bleed profusely and require repair. Rarely, surgery will be needed to stop the bleeding and save the mother's life. During surgery, the bleeding blood vessels are tied and the uterus is repaired. If the bleeding can't be stopped by tying the vessels, the uterus may have to be removed.

*Retained placenta.* The third stage of labor usually produces an intact placenta, but in some women, small pieces of the placenta remain inside the uterus. Left there, they could lead to bleeding, infection and uterine scarring. In other women, the contractions trap the entire placenta. Your doctor may need to remove the placenta, using his or her hand to wipe or peel the retained pieces off the walls of the uterus. Anesthetic can be given.

### Postpartum Care

Some bleeding is normal after giving birth. This bleeding gradually changes to a bloody discharge called *lochia* that gradually turns clear. You may have lochia for up to six weeks. The bleeding varies, but usually isn't an extremely heavy flow. At first, the

## Difficult Labor and Delivery

**Cesarean section.** In a C-section, the baby is taken out of the uterus during surgery. A C-section is done when labor isn't progressing the way it should, or if the baby or mother is at risk for any reason. During a C-section, anesthetic is given so you don't feel anything from your waist down. If the C-section is an emergency, a general anesthetic may be used. The doctor makes an incision that opens the uterus, and the baby is removed.

A C-section usually requires more recovery time than a vaginal delivery. Sometimes, women who have had a C-section will need to have another one if they give birth again. Whether or not a woman can have a vaginal delivery after a C-section depends on why the first C-section was done, what type of incision was made, how her current pregnancy and labor have gone, and other factors.

**Forceps.** Forceps may be used if your baby is showing signs of distress or you can't push the baby out. Forceps are two metal tongs that are placed on either side of the baby's head. The baby can then be gently pulled from the birth canal. Sometimes, the baby will be bruised on the sides of the head and have some minor nerve damage.

**Vacuum extraction.** This method is a replacement for forceps and is now used much more often than forceps. A device is attached to the baby's head and is held there with suction. Your doctor can then turn the baby into a better position and gently pull him or her out of the birth canal. There usually are no ill effects, other than some slight bruising on the baby's head that goes away on its own.

## Colostrum

The first milk your breasts produce is called *colostrum*. It may be yellow or clear and is full of antibodies that help fight infection. Colostrum in breast milk may also reduce your baby's risk of jaundice (p. 205).

Your milk will probably come in on the second or third day after your baby is born. Sometimes it doesn't come in until the fifth day. The milk will probably look like skim milk. Your breasts will feel full and tender, and may feel lumpy.

bleeding may be average to quite heavy with clots. If you begin to flow very heavily, call your doctor right away.

After you have a baby, you may go through some changes that can make you feel depressed. Your hormones will go through a drastic change. You'll have a new role as a mother to adjust to. You'll probably be very tired and perhaps feel fat and unattractive. While some mood swings are normal after giving birth, depression can be serious. If you have signs of depression (p. 404), talk to your doctor about it. Depression can be treated.

You may also notice that your desire for sex has declined. This is also normal. You may not become interested in sex again for several months. Your doctor may recommend that you wait several weeks or longer before starting to have sex again. If you have any pain with sex, be sure to let your doctor know. And be sure to use birth control if you don't wish to become pregnant again right away. Having just given birth and breast feeding don't prevent pregnancy. See page 550 for information about birth control and talk to your doctor about choosing the best method for you while you're breast feeding.

You'll also need to keep the area around your vagina—called the *perineum*—clean to help prevent an infection. This is particularly important if you had an episiotomy. Your doctor may recommend that you take a sitz bath every day, or may give you a spray or ointment to use on the area.

### Breast Feeding

Breast milk is better for babies than formula. It's easier to digest than formula, it contains antibodies that help your baby fight infections and it doesn't cost anything. Babies who are breast-fed have fewer ear infections and urinary tract infections than babies who are bottle-fed. Studies have shown that breast feeding may prevent or delay certain conditions, such as allergies, celiac disease and diabetes. Women who breast feed are less likely to develop osteoporosis (p. 244), breast cancer (p. 408) and ovarian cancer (p. 416).

Because breast milk is digested more easily than formula, your baby may get hungrier more often. Breast-fed babies may need to nurse every two or three hours. Try to alternate the breast your baby feeds on. A small safety pin attached to your bra can help you remember.

Your baby may nurse on one or both breasts at each feeding. You should nurse your newborn at least eight times every 24 hours. How much milk your body makes depends on how much your baby nurses—milk production is based on supply and demand. That's why it's best to let your baby, and not a schedule or clock, decide when and how long to nurse. Also, babies differ in how fast they nurse. Some can take as long as 40 minutes.

Even though babies are constantly growing, there are times in which they grow a lot in a short period of time. These are called growth spurts. Your baby may want to nurse more often at these times. For example, growth spurts might occur at two to three weeks, six weeks, three months and between 4 1/2 and six months of age. These times are only averages. Don't be concerned if your baby's growth spurts are at different times. During growth spurts, you can increase the amount of milk your body makes by nursing your baby more frequently.

Because mothers who breast feed don't know exactly how much milk their babies are getting, they often worry whether their babies are getting enough. If your baby is gaining weight and has two or more bowel movements and six to eight wet diapers every 24 hours, then he or she is probably getting enough milk. Don't worry if your baby's stool is soft or if your baby has frequent bowel movements. These things are normal in breast-fed babies because breast milk is digested more easily than formula.

Remember that any medicine you take may be passed to your baby through your milk. Check with your baby's doctor before taking any kind of medicine, even an over-the-counter drug. If you smoke, try to quit before you start breast feeding. See page 31 for tips on quitting. Using illicit drugs while breast feeding is very dangerous for your baby and can cause brain damage and many physical, emotional and mental problems for your baby. An occasional glass of wine or other alcohol may be okay, but if you notice that your baby doesn't seem to want to nurse after you've had alcohol, avoid drinking until you've stopped breast feeding your baby. Also, large amounts of caffeine can overstimulate your baby, so if you usually drink coffee or cola, try to drink caffeine-free drinks.

Your nipples may be tender at first. Let the milk air dry on your nipples. Don't use soap when washing your breasts.

Good breast-feeding technique isn't necessarily second nature. At first, your baby may be sleepy and appear uninterested in eating, or you may worry whether you're producing enough milk. If you have questions about breast feeding, ask your doctor or check your telephone book for the number of your local La Leche League leader or a lactation consultant. Some hospitals offer classes on breast feeding.

Positioning your baby correctly will help prevent sore nipples and can help your baby get the milk more easily. Make sure your baby's gums

## Breast Care During Breast Feeding

- Wear a well-fitting nursing bra.
- Let your baby feed often from both breasts.
- Air dry the nipples after breast feeding.
- Apply heat, such as with a warm wet towel, if your breast is engorged. Express milk from any areas that aren't drained after breast feeding.
- See your doctor if redness, swelling or tenderness persists.

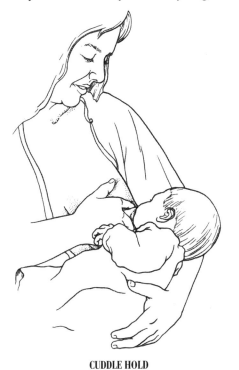

**CUDDLE HOLD**

are on the areola (the dark area around the nipple) and not just around the nipple. There are three popular positions for breast feeding:

**Cuddle hold.** Sit up straight (put pillows behind you for support) and cradle your baby in one arm so that your baby's stomach is facing yours. Hold your breast with the other hand and place your nipple in the baby's mouth. Once your baby begins to nurse, you can let go of your breast. If your baby has trouble keeping your nipple on top of his or her tongue, you can continue to hold your breast in the proper position. You may need to press your breast away from your baby's nostrils so they aren't blocked off. Young babies breathe almost exclusively through their noses.

**Football hold.** Sit up straight and position your baby so that the baby's head is in the palm of your hand and the baby's feet are touching your upper arm. You'll need support, such as the arm of a chair or a pillow, under your arm. This position is good if you've had a C- section or if you have twins.

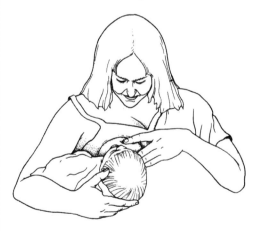

**FOOTBALL HOLD**

**Side-lying position.** Lie down on your side with your baby. Place your baby on his or her side facing you. If you're lying on your right side, your baby will nurse on the right breast. Raise your breast with one hand and

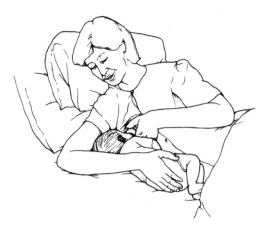

**SIDE-LYING POSITION**

place your nipple in the baby's mouth. In this position, you may need to hold your breast until the baby stops nursing. This position is especially good during the night or if you're recovering from a C-section.

If you breast-feed your infant, practice regular breast care and learn proper techniques. Improper breast-feeding techniques can lead to infections of the breast or nipple.

When the baby suckles, the skin may become irritated. If the skin of the nipple cracks, bacteria may enter. Bacteria also can enter the milk ducts. Keeping the nipples clean and dry reduces this risk. Don't let the baby "chew" on your nipple. This damages the skin and ducts, making infection more likely.

After breast feeding, let your nipples air dry. Wash your nipples daily with warm water. Tell your doctor about any redness or swelling that develops in or around the nipple. Your doctor may prescribe medicine to prevent a more serious infection.

If a woman decides not to breast feed her infant, her breasts may become very swollen, tender and filled with milk. This may also happen if a nursing baby isn't removing enough milk. This is called *engorgement*.

Regular feeding by the baby drains most of the milk produced and usually prevents engorgement. If not, a breast pump can be used to remove some of the milk and relieve the pressure, swelling and tenderness. This can also make it easier for the baby to nurse. After a week or two, your body will produce milk more evenly, reducing the number of engorgement episodes. Use warm compresses and feed the baby more often until the engorgement problems taper off. Also, wear a supportive bra.

It's important to treat engorgement. If the breasts aren't drained on a regular basis, the body may interpret this as the end of the nursing process. As a result, the hormones that stimulate milk production dwindle, and milk production may cease after a few weeks.

## Menopause

*Menopause,* the end of menstrual cycles and fertility, is a normal part of a woman's life. Some women worry about the changes they'll face during menopause. They may have heard stories from friends and relatives about symptoms.

Many women say that with age comes a certain wisdom that helps them deal better with adversity than they might have earlier in life. Some women enjoy improved sexual relationships and freedom from birth control after menopause.

For about half of women who enter menopause, the menstrual cycle becomes irregular and then stops, and they don't have any other symptoms. But the major hormonal changes of menopause can cause distress—both physical and emotional—in some women. Symptoms may last from a few months to 10 years. Symptoms of menopause may include depression, anxiety, irritability, hot flashes, sweating, racing of the heart (palpitations) and headaches.

Decreasing estrogen levels during menopause cause thinning, or *atrophy,* in vaginal tissue. This may result in soreness and dryness during sexual intercourse. Low estrogen levels, especially in thin, white females, may also lead to thinning of the bone, or osteoporosis (p. 244).

Estrogen levels can be checked with a blood test to determine if menopause is the reason your periods have stopped. Otherwise, the absence of your period, along with typical symptoms, may be enough of an indication to start medical treatment if you feel discomfort.

---

### Warning: Bleeding After Menopause

If you have vaginal bleeding after you have ceased to menstruate, check with your doctor immediately. The cause may be noncancerous and easily treated, or it can be a sign of cancer. Because a serious cause is also possible, you should have your doctor find the cause.

---

### Symptoms of Menopause

- Irregular periods or cessation of menstruation
- Hot flashes and sweating
- Emotional changes
- Vaginal dryness and soreness
- Headaches

---

### Advantages and Disadvantages of Hormone Replacement Therapy

**Advantages**
- Protects against heart disease
- Helps maintain good cholesterol levels
- Prevents excessive bone loss that can lead to osteoporosis
- Relieves symptoms of menopause, including dry vaginal tissues
- Limits the frequency of urinary tract infections (p. 162) and urinary incontinence (p. 434) associated with menopause

**Disadvantages**
- May cause bleeding that resembles menstruation
- Increases the risk of endometrial cancer, especially if progesterone isn't used
- May increase the risk of breast cancer, although evidence for this is conflicting

## Possible Signs of Breast Cancer

- A hard, painless lump or mass within the breast that seems to be fixed and doesn't move
- Any new lump, which may not be painful or tender
- Unusual thickening of your breasts
- An indentation or flattening of the contour of the breast
- An area of the breast or nipple that retracts (dimples in)
- A discharge from the nipple, sometimes containing blood

Therapy with estrogen and progesterone, called *hormone replacement therapy,* is now commonly prescribed to reduce the effects of menopause and help prevent osteoporosis. Vaginally delivered estrogen can be used to reduce dryness and pain that may occur during intercourse. Other symptoms may be treated with other medicines if you can't take hormones, if the hormone therapy doesn't help or if you decide you'd rather not use hormones.

The use of oral estrogen also offers two other significant benefits. Estrogen reduces bone loss caused by osteoporosis and provides protection against heart disease. Thus, even if you don't have menopausal symptoms, hormone replacement therapy provides definite benefits after menopause. Consult your doctor to talk about the pros and cons of hormone replacement therapy.

## Taking Care of Your Body

The reproductive system is complex, and most of it is hidden from view. So problems in this area may not be readily noticeable. Good common sense may be your most effective tool for maintaining good health. Eat a well-balanced diet, exercise regularly, get proper rest and avoid undue stress to prevent many health problems. Pay attention to your body and its signals, and seek medical care for any problems. Below are simple steps you can take to help maintain your reproductive health.

## Breasts

Proper breast care throughout a woman's life can prevent some problems and help detect others before they cause harm. Some of the measures you can take are outlined.

### Breast Cancer

Breast cancer is one of the most feared diseases among women. The statistics are alarming—one in nine women will have breast cancer before age 85. It can also occur in men but is 10 times more likely in women. Rather than ignore the possibility of the disease, try to realize that breast cancer is a treatable disease. With early detection, it's often curable.

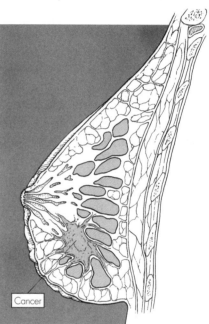

**BREAST CANCER**

One of the ways you can make your own health a priority is to have regular check-ups. A combination of breast self-exams, familiarity with your family's history of breast cancer, regular exams by your doctor and regular mammography can help detect breast cancer early.

**Perform a self-exam of your breasts each month.** This is extremely important. Start early, around age 20, so you can get familiar with what's normal for you. The main thing you're looking for when you do a monthly breast self-exam is a change from what's normal for you.

Do the exam each month a few days after your menstrual period ends.

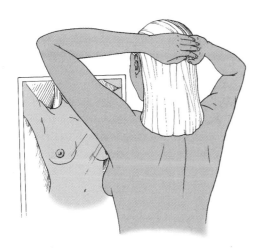

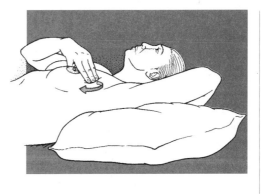

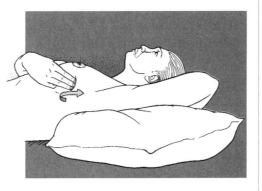

**BREAST SELF-EXAM USING CIRCULAR HAND MOVEMENT**

Your breasts will be less lumpy then. If you don't have a period, do the exam at the same time every month.

Begin by standing in front of a mirror. First put your arms at your sides, then raise them behind your head and then put your hands on your hips and flex your chest muscles. Look at your breasts. Look for any changes in the skin, such as changes in color or texture.

Now lie down. Put a pillow under your left shoulder. Put your left hand behind your head and feel your left breast with the pads of the three middle fingers on your right hand. Start at the outside and work around your breast in circles, moving closer to your nipple with each circle. You can use hand lotion to help your finger pads glide more smoothly over your skin.

Squeeze your nipple gently and look for fluid coming out of the nipple.

Do the same steps with your other breast. You can also check your breasts in the same circular way while standing in the shower. The soap makes your hands glide more easily over your skin.

When you're doing the exam, include the areas up to your collarbone and out to your armpit. Lymph nodes are located in these areas. Cancer can spread to lymph node tissue.

**See your doctor for regular breast exams.** Have your doctor check your breasts every year or two. Go every year when you reach age 40 or older. Your doctor will check your breasts for any lumps or signs of cancer.

**Have a mammogram at proper intervals.** *Mammography* is an x-ray of the breasts. A mammogram often can

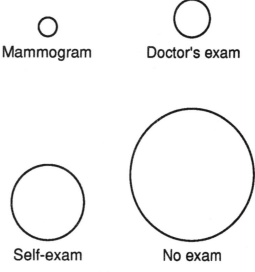

Mammogram          Doctor's exam

Self-exam          No exam

**TYPICAL SIZES OF LUMPS FOUND DURING EXAMS**

show very small lumps that you and your doctor may be unable to feel during a physical exam. Women over age 50 should have a mammogram each year.

If you're between age 40 and 50 and have a family history of breast cancer, have been diagnosed with or treated for breast cancer, or have a precancerous condition, your doctor may suggest you have a mammogram every year or two.

Your doctor may also suggest you have a *baseline mammogram.* This is a mammogram done when you're younger and it can be used to compare with mammograms done later on.

See page 638 for information about mammography.

If you've had breast cancer in one breast or if you have a history of breast cancer in one or more female family members (sister, aunt, mother or grandmother), you have an increased chance of getting breast cancer in the other breast. This is especially true if breast cancer occurred in these relatives before they went through menopause.

Women who started menstruating early (before age 12) or who enter menopause late are at increased risk of breast cancer. Also at increased risk are women who have given birth to a first child after age 30 or who have never had children.

Other possible risk factors include obesity, overuse of alcohol, a diet high in calories and fat, and a high body-fat percent. Whether these characteristics actually increase the risk of breast cancer isn't clear. But losing weight (if you're overweight), moderating your use of alcohol and eating a low-fat diet are lifestyle changes that promote better health.

If you notice any of the changes in the box on page 408, see your doctor right away. Performing a breast exam and knowing about the history of breast cancer in your family will help your doctor determine possible reasons for a lump or discharge. This information also guides your doctor in suggesting the best course for further diagnosis. This may include a mammogram, removing fluid from the lump to test or removing a small part of the area for testing.

If the lump is cancer, many treatments are available. The treatment depends on the type of tumor, how early it's found, how much it has spread and if the tumor is sensitive to hormones.

In most cases, the cancer is removed by surgery. For small tumors, a *lumpectomy* can be done. Larger tumors may need to be removed by removing the whole breast in a surgical procedure called a *modified* or *complete mastectomy.* Lymph nodes under the arm will also be removed to search for spread of the cancer. Radiation therapy (p. 225) or chemotherapy (p. 225) usually follows the surgery to reduce the chances of the cancer's return. In many cases, breast cancer is curable with early detection and a combination of surgery, radiation and chemotherapy.

*Breast reconstruction* following mastectomy can produce remarkable results. There are a wide variety of

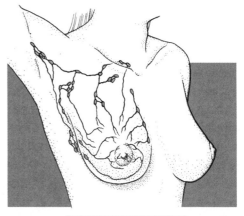

**LOCATION OF LYMPH NODES**

options. You may have a breast implant inserted or undergo one of a number of reconstruction techniques using tissue from other parts of your body. Usually, these procedures are begun at the same time as the mastectomy. Reconstruction of the nipple takes place about three months after the mastectomy. You should discuss the options with your doctor before your mastectomy. You also have the option of deciding on reconstruction later or wearing removable implants (prosthesis) that are part of specially designed bras or other clothing.

## Breast Infections

The dark area around the nipple, called the *areola,* contains several oil-secreting, or *sebaceous,* glands with pores that allow secretions to leave the body. This substance helps keep the nipples from drying out. If one of the pores becomes blocked, the oil is trapped and turns into a waxy substance. This can lead to a nipple infection if the gland is blocked. Infection may cause a small, red, tender, pimple-like sore. Most of these infections heal by themselves. But larger infections may need to be drained by opening the area through surgery.

Breast infections are more common if you're breast feeding. Signs of infection include redness, tenderness and swelling of the breast, sometimes accompanied by fever and swollen lymph nodes in the armpit. When your infant suckles, bacteria can enter the swollen milk ducts during the process of milk production, which is called *lactation.* The bacteria can spread to the glandular or fatty tissue of the breast, as well as to the lymph glands in the armpit on the same side as the infected breast. These glands then become swollen and tender, too. While breast infections are most common during

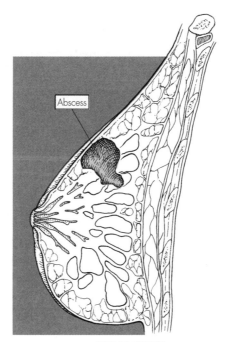

**BREAST ABSCESS**

lactation, they can occur at other times as well.

**Breast abscess.** Once the bacteria spread into the fatty tissue or into the gland itself, they may form a pocket of infection, or *abscess.* The body produces a layer of tissue around these collections to wall them off and prevent spread to surrounding tissues. Sometimes a needle can be used to drain a breast abscess. Your doctor may cut the area open and drain it, especially if it's a large abscess. An abscess must be completely drained or it will come back.

**Mastitis.** When infection spreads into the mammary gland tissue, it causes swelling and redness. This infection is called *mastitis.* Mastitis is usually confined to one segment of the gland. If you are breast feeding, you may see some blood in your milk. When compared with the opposite breast, you may notice that the infected breast feels warmer, has some redness and often is swollen and tender. You can tell the difference between mastitis and an abscess. Mastitis is characterized by hardened, localized areas within the glandular tissue. An abscess has a softer, cyst-like, fluid feeling.

Recognizing an infection early, seeing your doctor to find out if antibiotics may help and applying heat to the infected area may prevent an infection from turning into an abscess. Admission to the hospital for intravenous antibiotics and surgical drainage may be required to treat a severe infection of the breast.

If you are breast feeding, your doctor may advise you to feed your baby only from the noninfected breast until the infection is resolved. Massaging the infected breast to express milk reduces the pain of milk engorgement (p. 406).

### Cosmetic Breast Surgery

For a variety of reasons, many women choose to have their breasts enlarged (*augmented*) or reduced surgically.

During breast enlargement, a breast implant is inserted through an incision in your breast or armpit. Implants are round shells made of rubbery silicone and filled with a saltwater solution called *saline*. They're available in many sizes.

Breast reduction is an option for women who don't like their large breasts or who experience backaches and other problems related to large breasts. During this procedure, the surgeon removes breast tissue, reshapes the remaining tissue and may reduce the size of the areola so it's proportional to the breast size. The breast is also "lifted" and the nipple is placed at a higher position.

Breast enlargement and reduction are usually elective procedures. Even though these procedures generally are free of major complications, they do have the same risks as any surgery and use of anesthesia. They also involve

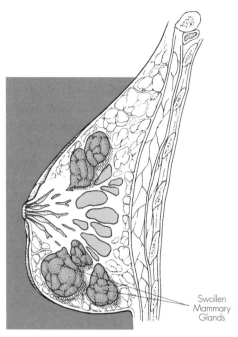

**MASTITIS**

some pain and some temporary activity restriction. The sensitivity of the nipple and ability to breast-feed a baby are often affected by cosmetic surgery. Check with your doctor about this issue.

### Fibrocystic Breast Disease and Other Lumps

The breast consists of two sections: the overlying fatty tissues and the glandular tissue and milk ducts that end at the pores in the nipple. The fatty tissues are smooth and soft, compared with the slightly lumpy and firmer glandular tissue that rests against the rib cage. It's important to know the consistency of your breasts—the smoother fatty tissues, the glandular tissue and any disparities—so you can perform skillful self-exams (p. 408). Until you learn the anatomy of your breasts, it's normal to be unsure about the feeling of the structures, tissues and lumps.

Normally, breasts swell with menstruation and return to normal a few days after the flow. Many women have benign cysts in their breasts that change with menstruation, enlarging, shrinking, becoming tender and then returning to normal. This is called *fibrocystic breast disease.* As the body gains water during the monthly cycle, these cysts gain fluid, too. Many breast cysts are quite small, about the size of a marble, while others may swell to the size of a golf ball.

Many other noncancerous conditions may affect the breast. *Lipomas* are benign fatty tumors that can grow very large. *Fibroadenomas* are benign tumors of the glandular tissue. They're usually round and movable, and are often removed to make sure cancer isn't present. Infection or injury of the breast can also result in a lump.

Most tumors felt in the breast aren't cancer. They are usually cysts that swell with the monthly cycle, are tender and soft, and move within the breast when they're pushed from side to side. Only a small percentage of breast tumors are cancer. Cancerous tumors usually are painless, feel very firm and tend not to move when pushed. The overlying skin or nipple may retract as the mass grows.

The lumps of fibrocystic disease can cause false alarms because they are hard to differentiate from cancerous lumps. While fibrous breasts don't appear to be at higher risk of cancer than other breasts, the unusual cysts and lumps can obscure or hide potentially cancerous lumps.

If you feel a lump in your breast, see your doctor right away. Your doctor will feel the lump, looking for characteristics that indicate whether the lump is cancerous. If the lump appears to be a fluid-filled cyst, your doctor may attempt to draw fluid from it. If the lump is small, repeated exams and a mammogram (p. 638) may be needed. If questions remain about the kind of tumor it is, the lump can be surgically removed or some of its tissue removed and tested to make sure it isn't cancer.

Many women who drink lots of caffeinated beverages report that breast tenderness, small cysts and swelling subside when they stop or reduce their caffeine intake. Women who smoke and have breast discomfort may benefit from stopping smoking.

## Galactorrhea

*Galactorrhea* is a milky discharge from the breast at a time other than pregnancy or after childbirth. It may sometimes be associated with abnormal menstrual periods or weight gain, but most cases of galactorrhea have no known cause. Some cases can be attributed to medicines such as amphetamines (p. 618), antidepressants (p. 619), medicines used to lower blood pressure (p. 619) and tranquilizers (p. 626). If a medicine is the cause, stopping the medicine will take care of the problem. Galactorrhea can also be caused by overproduction of a hormone called *prolactin.* Overproduction of prolactin may occur when a hormone-producing tumor forms in the pituitary gland.

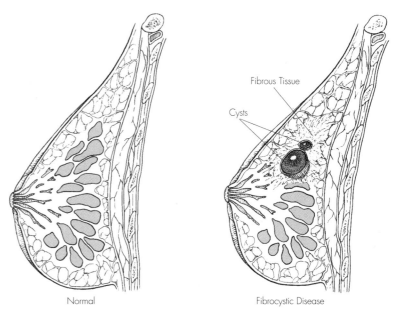

Fibrous Tissue

Cysts

Normal                          Fibrocystic Disease

**NORMAL BREAST VS. FIBROCYSTIC BREAST DISEASE**

## Signs of Cervix Problems

Usually, abnormalities of the cervix aren't obvious. Sometimes, a feeling of irritation during intercourse and spotting between periods occur. Cervical tumors usually don't cause symptoms. At times, there may be mucus or a bloody discharge from the vagina. Symptoms of advanced cancer include weight loss and back pain.

If you notice any abnormal discharge from your breasts, you need to see your doctor for an evaluation. One means of diagnosing the problem is through blood tests that measure various hormone levels. If your prolactin level is high, your doctor will perform a careful examination of your vision and visual fields to look for signs of a pituitary tumor. Other tests may be done. An MRI scan (p. 637) or CT scan (p. 632) of the brain can identify very small swellings in or near the pituitary that may represent a tumor.

If your doctor finds a tumor, he or she will probably prescribe the medicine bromocriptine to lower your body's level of prolactin. Bromocriptine will shrink the tumor and, in most cases, prevent the need for surgery or radiation. Larger tumors may need to be removed surgically. In addition, radiation therapy (p. 225) can be used in combination with surgery or by itself to shrink a pituitary tumor.

In a small percentage of patients, galactorrhea is caused by low levels of thyroid hormone, a condition that can be remedied by taking thyroid medicine (p. 626).

## Cervix

The *cervix* is the lower end of the uterus that opens into the vagina. The cervix is exposed to bacteria, viruses, yeast and chemicals within the vagina. These infectious agents and chemical irritants can react with the cervical tissues to change the cells within the cervix.

**Cervical cancer.** Cancer of the cervix strikes most often after the age of 40 but can be cured if detected early by regular exams. Having regular Pap smears (p. 639) is the first line of defense against cervical cancer. The purpose of a Pap smear is to detect changes in the cervical cells that may indicate a precancerous condition.

Begin having Pap smears when you start having sex or by the time you're 18 years old. Have them at least annually until you've had at least three normal Pap smears. After that, have one at least every three years unless your doctor thinks you need them more often. If you're more than 65 years old and your Pap smears have been negative, you may not need to keep having them. Talk to your doctor about this.

If you have an abnormal Pap smear and undergo treatment for it, you'll probably need to have Pap smears at least every six months for some time, until your doctor tells you it's okay for you to have Pap smears annually or less often. If the Pap smear shows abnormal changes, your doctor may recommend colposcopy (p. 632).

Treatment depends on the severity of the changes seen in the cervical cells. If an area of the cervix appears precancerous, it can be taken out during a procedure called a cone biopsy (p. 633). It may also be destroyed with heat, chemicals or freezing.

If the changes in the cells, called *cervical dysplasia*, are left untreated, the cells may keep changing. Over five to 10 years, the cells can progress to cancerous tumors. Once the cancer has developed, but before it has invaded deeper tissue or spread outside the uterus, it's called *carcinoma in situ*, or CIS. If not treated at this stage, cancer cells further invade the cervix, then may move to the uterus, the vagina and the bladder, and even spread to distant locations in the body.

Extensive surgery may be needed for large areas of abnormal changes. A hysterectomy (p. 418) is usually reserved for cases in which the cellular changes are advanced, when cancer is strongly suspected or when other menstrual abnormalities or large fibroids (p. 419) are present.

If cervical cancer is found in a later stage, removal of the cervix, uterus and fallopian tubes, and radiation therapy (p. 225) will probably be needed. As long as the tumor hasn't spread past the uterus, the prognosis is good.

An increased risk of cervical cancer has been found in women who become sexually active at an early age (before about age 20) and who have many sexual partners. Some viral sexually transmitted diseases (STDs) have been implicated. Human papillomavirus is one of the main STDs associated with cervical problems. If you're sexually active, following guidelines to prevent STDs (p. 32) can help reduce your risk of catching an STD.

Women who have had a hysterectomy (p. 418) don't have to worry about cervical cancer.

**Cervical cysts.** *Nabothian cysts* are fluid-filled knots on the cervix that usually are detected during a pelvic exam. These cysts form when a mucous gland within the cervical tissue is blocked. Cauterization or freezing destroys the abnormal area.

**Cervical dysplasia.** Long-term irritation of the cervical cells caused by chronic infections of the vagina or cervix can lead to abnormal cellular changes. This condition is called *dysplasia*, which means "abnormal cell development." The abnormal pattern of cell growth may or may not be an indication of a precancerous condition. In any case, if it's caught early and treated appropriately, cancer usually doesn't occur.

Hormone therapy, such as the use of birth control pills, may also be a cause of cervical dysplasia. If a Pap smear shows dysplasia, your doctor

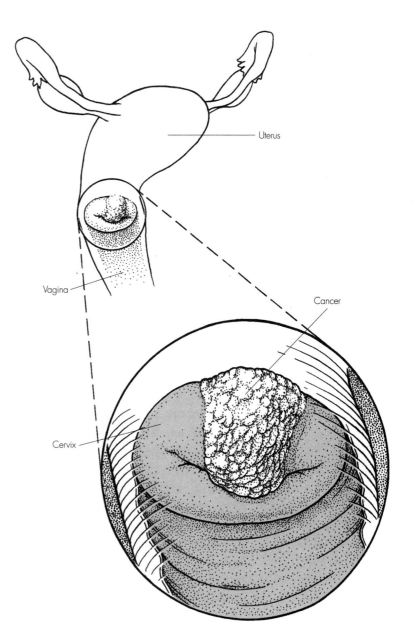

**CERVICAL CANCER**

may recommend that you stop taking the hormones.

**Cervical erosion.** Small sores may form on the cervix as a result of irritation caused by an infection, hormone use or pregnancy. Abnormal bleeding or discharge from the vagina suggests this abnormality. By using heat, freezing techniques or chemicals, the abnormal area can be destroyed. Mucus-like discharge may occur for 15 to 20 days after these treatments.

## Pelvic Exams

A *pelvic exam* involves inspection of the outer genitals and some of the inner structures as well. Your doctor will use a device called a *speculum* to expand the vaginal canal. During this exam, he or she will perform a Pap smear (p. 639). Your doctor may also palpate your reproductive organs to feel for any problems with your uterus and ovaries. Your rectum and lower abdomen also are checked. This palpation may be a little uncomfortable, but it's a quick procedure. A breast exam is usually done when you have your pelvic exam.

**Cervical polyps.** Any time a mucus-producing cell becomes inflamed, it can produce a polyp. These mucus-filled sacs aren't cancerous but may cause bleeding or discharge. The cervical polyp can be easily removed.

## Ovaries

Your *ovaries* are responsible for holding all of your eggs from the day you are born. An egg is released about once a month. This release is called *ovulation*. The ovaries also manufacture sex hormones that regulate your monthly cycle.

**Ovarian cancer.** Because of the location of the ovaries deep within the abdomen, ovarian cancer is virtually impossible to detect in its early stages. During a pelvic exam, your doctor can feel the ovaries. Further studies will be done if enlargement is found. Many women with ovarian cancer don't have symptoms until the cancer is advanced. They may see their doctor because of weight loss, abdominal swelling, fatigue and general ill health. The swelling comes from fluid buildup in the abdomen, a condition called *ascites*. When discovered at this later stage, the cancer usually isn't curable.

See your doctor regularly for pelvic exams that assess the size and shape of your reproductive organs. Enlargement of an ovary may be caused by an ovarian cyst, scar tissue or, rarely, cancer.

An ultrasound (p. 643) can be done to assess the size and shape of the ovaries. Your doctor may want to perform a laparoscopy (p. 637) to obtain a tissue sample.

If ovarian enlargement is suspected to be related to cancer, the ovary should be surgically removed as soon as possible. In some cases, your doctor may recommend a complete hysterectomy (p. 418).

Along with surgery, chemotherapy (p. 225) or radiation therapy (p. 225) may be needed. These treatments destroy cancerous cells that may have spread to near or distant tissues.

Ovarian cancer is uncommon. No specific risk factors are known, although if someone in your immediate family has had ovarian cancer, you may be at increased risk.

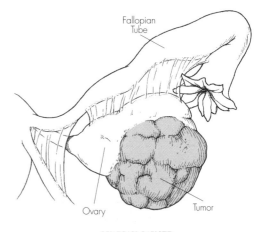

Fallopian Tube

Ovary                    Tumor

**OVARIAN CANCER**

## Pelvic Inflammatory Disease

*Pelvic inflammatory disease,* or PID, occurs when bacteria grow in and around the fallopian tubes, ovaries and uterus. Often the bacteria are sexually transmitted organisms, such as the bacteria that cause gonorrhea (p. 318) or chlamydia (p. 317). Infections of the female organs may not always be a sexually transmitted disease. A miscarriage, an abortion or use of a contraceptive intrauterine device (IUD) can also result in infection.

A long-standing pelvic infection may cause occasional pain, some vaginal discharge, pain with intercourse or infertility. The severe symptoms of a fast-developing, or acute, pelvic infection usually force the woman to seek medical care.

A pelvic exam may be done to obtain cultures of the secretions. Any bacterial cause of infection usually can be identified in a culture. An ultrasound (p. 643) or x-ray of the abdomen may help your doctor diagnose the source of the infection.

Oral or intravenous antibiotics (p. 618) and analgesics (p. 618) are used to treat the infection. Surgery can repair damage that results from the infection. This repair may improve a woman's chances of conceiving.

**Ovarian cysts.** Eggs, or *ova,* develop in the ovary. As they reach maturity, a small sac of fluid forms around the egg as it moves toward the surface. This sac, called a *follicular cyst,* usually bursts, shedding the mature egg into the abdomen to be swept into the fallopian tube and uterus.

Follicular cysts are a normal part of a woman's menstrual cycle. But sometimes they don't burst when they are small. Instead, they continue to fill with fluid and grow. Some become the size of a golf ball or larger. Pain and abdominal discomfort or a change in menstrual activity can occur when these cysts become the size of a marble or larger.

Most enlarged follicular cysts burst by themselves and require no further treatment. Pain or abdominal swelling may send you to your doctor for relief. He or she may detect an ovarian cyst during a pelvic exam, but some cysts aren't easily discovered. An ultrasound may reveal the location and size of the cyst, as well as other cysts or abnormalities.

The cyst can be removed during surgery or drained through a laparoscope (p. 637). The fluid will be examined to make sure the cyst is not cancerous. The ovary and fallopian tube may need to be removed if the cyst is large. Fertility is maintained if one ovary and fallopian tube remain on the opposite side. Recurrent cysts can be treated with cyclic hormone medicine to prevent the egg from maturing and the cyst from forming.

### Uterus

**Endometrial cancer.** Cancer of the uterus begins in the lining of the uterus, or *endometrium.* Most women with endometrial cancer are more than 50 years old. Endometrial cancer is difficult to detect because it doesn't produce any changes on a Pap smear (p. 639). Fortunately, endometrial cancer grows very slowly and spreads to other tissues only in the very last stages. So the outlook for cure is usually good.

If you're at increased risk of endometrial cancer, your

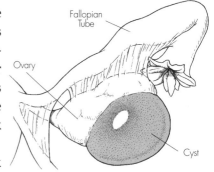

Fallopian Tube

Ovary

Cyst

**OVARIAN CYST**

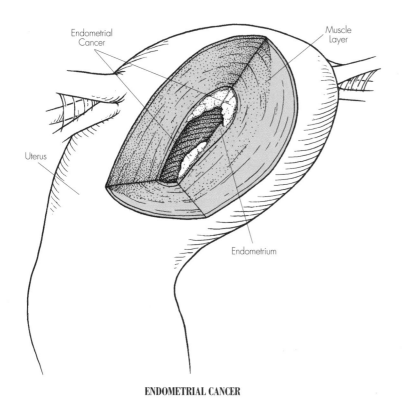

Labels: Endometrial Cancer · Muscle Layer · Uterus · Endometrium

**ENDOMETRIAL CANCER**

### Risk Factors for Endometrial Cancer

- A family history of uterine cancer
- A history of irregular or no ovulation
- Never being pregnant or having a baby
- Being overweight
- Having taken estrogen without progesterone (estrogen causes thickening of the endometrium, and progesterone inhibits this growth)

doctor may recommend regular analysis of samples of endometrial tissue, called an endometrial biopsy or sampling (p. 634).

If cancer cells are found on an endometrial sampling or if the uterus is enlarged and bleeding after menopause, a dilatation and curettage (D & C, p. 420) will be done to obtain more tissue for diagnosis. Treatment for endometrial cancer usually includes a hysterectomy. This procedure ensures removal of the tumor, and the chance of further spread of cancer is reduced. If the cancer has spread, chemotherapy (p. 225) or radiation therapy (p. 225)

can be used to improve the chance of long-term survival.

### Hysterectomy

This surgery is done to remove the uterus. Sometimes, both ovaries, the fallopian tubes and other nearby tissue may also need to be removed. The surgery usually involves removing the organs through an incision low on the abdomen or through the vagina. Hysterectomy is a major surgery. Most women must take six weeks off of work and must avoid lifting heavy objects. After a hysterectomy, you will no longer have periods. You may need to talk to your doctor about taking hormone replacement therapy (p. 407) if your ovaries are also removed.

**Endometriosis.** The lining of the uterus, also called the endometrium, "bulks up" in response to female hormones and is shed at the end of each menstrual cycle if an egg isn't fertilized. When an egg is fertilized, it attaches to the endometrial lining, grows and gets nutrition from the tissue. Sometimes, the endometrium spreads outside the uterus to other female organs, including the fallopian tubes and the ovaries. The term for this abnormal spread of uterine lining is *endometriosis*.

Under the influence of hormones, the areas of extra endometrial tissue may spread and increase in size. As with the endometrial lining of the uterus, the endometrial tissue outside the uterus secretes blood into the abdomen, fallopian tubes or near the ovaries during each menstrual period. These collections of blood irritate the nearby tissues. Severe, untreated endometriosis leads to scarring and infertility.

Women with endometriosis may have few or no apparent symptoms for years. Then they may notice they're having particularly heavy or painful periods. The worsening of heavy bleeding or painful periods may suggest to your doctor the possibility of endometriosis. An ultrasound (p. 643) of the uterus is helpful to look for other problems that may be responsible for the pain. A laparoscopy (p. 637) may be needed to evaluate the uterus, fallopian tubes and ovaries. A biopsy can be taken at the same time, if needed.

The primary treatment for endometriosis is the use of cyclic female hormones to reduce the amount of bleeding into the abdomen. In more severe cases, synthetic male hormones may be prescribed to reduce the swelling and tenderness. Male hormones reduce the level of female hormones that stimulate the endometrium.

Some doctors are using laser therapy to destroy abnormal endometrial cells. Surgery, such as hysterectomy (p. 418), can be done when other methods don't work.

**Fibroids.** The wall of the uterus consists of a tough, fibrous outer layer, an ever-changing soft, inner layer called the endometrium and a thick middle layer of smooth muscle cells. The muscular portion of the uterus stretches during pregnancy but sometimes contracts forcibly during menstrual periods, causing cramps. The smooth muscle layer contracts under the influence of hormones.

A noncancerous tumor of these smooth muscle cells can form in the wall of the uterus. This tumor will produce a lump, or *fibroid.* The medical term for this tumor is *leiomyoma.* Fibroids range from the size of a grape

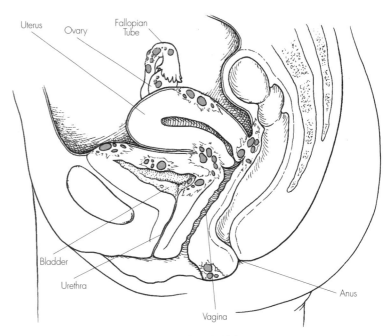

**ENDOMETRIOSIS**

to the size of a softball and even to the size of a watermelon in extreme cases.

Small fibroids cause no pain and no changes in the menstrual cycle or flow. Multiple or larger fibroids may produce heavier, more painful periods. Miscarriages may occur when a large fibroid is present during pregnancy. When hormone levels are reduced during menopause, fibroids often shrink to a very small size.

Most fibroids are found during a regular pelvic exam. If they're large or if your period has become longer,

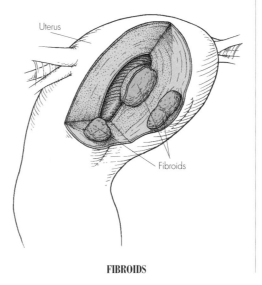

**FIBROIDS**

## Dilatation and Curettage

Dilatation and curettage (D & C) is a procedure done to scrape away the top layer of the uterine lining, or *endometrium*. During the procedure, the cervix, the opening to the uterus, is dilated, or widened. This allows a *curette* to be inserted into the uterus. The procedure may be mildly uncomfortable and some bleeding occurs afterward. Analgesics (p. 618) or anesthesia may be used. A D & C can be used for many purposes, including treating disorders or as a means of obtaining a sample of the endometrium to test.

heavier or more painful, further studies may be done. An ultrasound exam may define the size, number and position of the fibroid tumors. A procedure called dilatation and curettage (D & C, above) may be done to make sure endometrial or uterine cancer isn't present. Fibroids are removed surgically by cutting the tumor from the wall of the uterus or by removing the entire uterus.

**Uterine prolapse.** The muscles and ligaments attached to and holding the uterus in place at the top of the vagina are stretched during pregnancy and childbirth. The more children a woman has, the looser these muscles and ligaments become. Age tends to decrease the strength and elasticity of tissues. The combination of aging and multiple births can weaken the muscles until the uterus falls into the vagina, even pushing the cervix out of the vaginal opening.

Childbirth and aging also allow the tissues of the vaginal wall to stretch. When the bladder is full of urine, it may protrude into the vagina (a condition called *cystocele*). The rectum may protrude into the vagina as well (*rectocele*). Discomfort, burning during urination, incontinence and pain may result from the prolapsed uterus. These symptoms may develop during the middle to later years of a woman's life.

Exercises, including Kegel's exercises (p. 168), to strengthen the muscles are recommended as the first line of response to the problem, especially in its early stages. A special support for the uterus (called a *pessary*) can be placed in the vagina to prevent the discomfort. But the only permanent solution to a prolapsed uterus is surgical correction. With this surgery, the uterus is placed in its normal position, and sutures are used to hold it in place.

## Vagina

The vagina leads from your uterus and cervix to the outside of your body. Glands inside the vagina and cervix produce a fluid that flows out of the vagina and helps keep the vagina clean by carrying out old cells. Usually, this discharge is clear or milky and doesn't have an unpleasant odor. The discharge is slightly thicker when you're ovulating, breast feeding or sexually excited. During your menstrual period, blood mixes with the discharge.

*Vaginitis* is the most common infection of the female reproductive tract. The main symptom is a change in the vaginal discharge. Often, vaginal itching and burning are also present. A number of factors can promote these uncomfortable infections, including the use of personal hygiene products and certain medicines, and even some clothing and underclothing. Sometimes, an infection may be passed from an infected sexual partner.

**Bacterial vaginosis.** A number of bacterial infections can cause a profuse, fishy-smelling vaginal discharge. Swelling of the vagina and vulva may also be noted. The most common cause of these symptoms is the *Gardnerella vaginalis* bacteria. Why some women get this infection isn't certain. The infection doesn't seem to be related to sexual activity. This type of infection responds well to either oral antibiotics or vaginal antibiotic creams.

**Chlamydia.** Chlamydia is an infection of the cervix, but it also causes a vaginal discharge. A chlamydia infection is caused by bacteria that can be passed during sex. It can be treated with antibiotics (p. 618). See page 317 for more information about chlamydia.

**Gonorrhea.** As with chlamydia, gonorrhea is an STD that can cause an increase in vaginal discharge. It can also be treated with antibiotics. See page 318 for more information about gonorrhea.

**Trichomonas vaginitis.** Caused by a tiny, one-celled parasite, this infection produces a foamy, greenish-yellow, foul-smelling discharge. It also causes painful urination. Oral medicines can treat this type of infection.

Both partners should be treated at the same time to prevent reinfection.

**Yeast vaginitis.** Vaginitis caused by yeast is the most common vaginal infection. It's called *vaginal candidiasis,* or a "yeast infection." Bacteria normally live in the vagina in balance with yeast organisms. When this balance is thrown off, the yeast may begin to overgrow and irritate the vaginal lining and outer genitalia. The balance can be thrown off if you're taking antibiotics for another infection, if you're using birth control pills, if you're pregnant or have diabetes, or if you stay hot and sweaty for long periods of time. Sometimes, no reason can be found.

The discharge often resembles small, whitish curds. Itching and swelling of the genitals are common. Treatment with an over-the-counter or prescription medicine for a vaginal yeast infection usually cures the problem.

Treatment usually involves putting a medicine into your vagina. This medicine may be a cream that you put into your vagina with a special plunger or a suppository that you insert into your vagina. Creams can also help relieve the itching on the outside.

## Preventing Vaginitis

- Wear cotton panties during the day and don't wear any at night. This will allow your genital area to "breathe."
- Don't wear anything tight around your genital area.
- If you think your detergent or fabric softener may be irritating, switch brands.
- Avoid hot tubs if you have recurring infections.
- The latex in condoms and diaphragms, and the sperm-killing gels used for birth control can be irritating. Talk to your doctor about other types of birth control if you think any of these things bother you.
- Avoid having sex when you have vaginitis. Sometimes you and your partner can pass infections back and forth. If you choose to have sex while you have vaginitis, use a condom to help prevent the infection from spreading.

## Vulva

The *vulva* encompasses the folds of skin just outside your vagina. Excessive itching of the female genitals, sometimes accompanied by tenderness, redness and swelling, can be a difficult and embarrassing problem. There are many causes for excessive genital itching. Some of the causes are listed below.

**Allergic skin reaction.** Feminine hygiene sprays, deodorants in tampons or pads, detergents used to wash underclothes and even the dyes in certain clothes can produce redness, itching and peeling of the skin on or near the genitals. Identifying and removing the offending chemical irritant may be difficult. If the irritant can be avoided, itching and tenderness resolve within a few days. Over-the-counter medicine is available to reduce itching and discomfort.

**Estrogen deficiency.** Women may have dryness and itching of the vulva or genital region during or after menopause. A lack of estrogen causes these tissues to become dry. An itching sensation may result when the estrogen level drops during menopause. Treatment with topical or oral estrogen reduces the itching and dryness. The itching and dryness can also cause discomfort during intercourse.

**Pruritus vulvae.** *Pruritus vulvae* means "itching of the female genitals." It's used to describe itching when no exact cause can be found. Your doctor may do some tests to check for possible causes before making this diagnosis.

**Vulvar cancer.** *Vulvar cancer* is similar to other types of skin cancer. It may first appear as a shallow ulcer that doesn't heal or as a lump that ulcerates, crusts and doesn't heal. A sexually transmitted disease (STD, p. 316) may be suspected. When treatment doesn't heal the sores, a biopsy is needed to check for cancer.

Complete removal of the cancerous sore, along with some surrounding skin and lymph nodes, usually cures the cancer. Radiation therapy (p. 225) may be needed if the lymph nodes show that the cancer has spread. The slow rate of growth of vulvar cancer, along with easy access and visibility, usually make it relatively easy to catch in its early stages when the cure rate is high.

**Yeast infections.** Some women develop yeast or fungal infections of the skin around the genitals. These infections can cause itching and sometimes swelling or redness of the vulva. See page 421 for more information about vaginal yeast infections.

# CHAPTER 5

# MEN

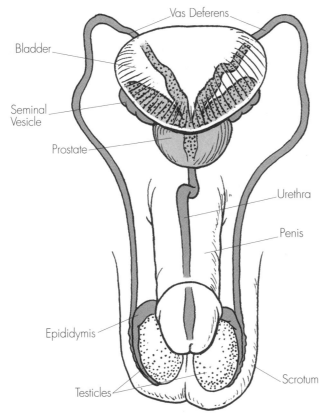

Bladder

Vas Deferens

Seminal Vesicle

Prostate

Urethra

Penis

Epididymis

Testicles

Scrotum

**MALE REPRODUCTIVE SYSTEM: FRONT VIEW**

The male's reproductive system shares a number of organs with the urinary system. The bladder empties through the *urethra*, which is within the penis. *Semen* is ejaculated through the urethra as well. During sexual intercourse, the penis becomes hard, or erect. Nerves close the opening at the base of the bladder, so the semen can flow out the urethra without mixing with urine.

The male reproductive system consists of the *testicles*, which are in the scrotum; the *urethra*, which is connected to the testicles by the *epididymis*, and the *vas deferens*, which is a tube that carries the sperm to the prostate gland.

*Sperm* are produced in the testicles, where the temperature is lower than in the rest of the body. The lower temperature helps keep the sperm alive and healthy. The *scrotum* is made of thin skin. It hangs outside the body so the testicles can remain cooler. Sperm are stored in the epididymis and the ducts inside the testicles.

During intercourse and ejaculation, sperm are rhythmically squeezed into the vas deferens, which carry the sperm through the *seminal vesicles* and *prostate gland* and out through the urethra. The prostate gland and seminal vesicles add fluid to the sperm to make them more mobile.

## Special Issues for Men

### Impotence

It can be extremely distressing for any man who has been having erections and sexual intercourse normally to suddenly have trouble getting or keeping an erection (*impotence*). Most men at some time have problems with getting and keeping erections. The possibility of impotence should be considered when these problems occur about 25% of the time or more.

Male sexual responses (arousal, erection and climax) are fueled by visual and psychological stimuli. Men who are tired, very stressed or having problems in a relationship may have a diminished sexual response or may

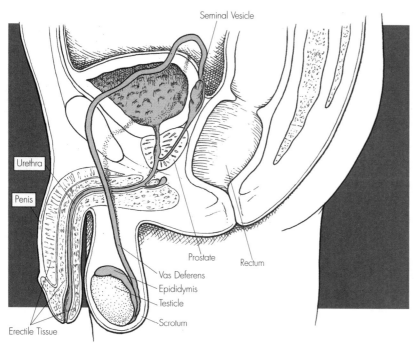

Seminal Vesicle

Urethra

Penis

Prostate

Rectum

Vas Deferens

Epididymis

Testicle

Scrotum

Erectile Tissue

**MALE REPRODUCTIVE SYSTEM: SIDE VIEW**

not be able to maintain an erection. Failure to perform sexually can lead to fears of future failure. Anxiety can make the situation even worse. Sexual failure may be one of the most difficult psychological issues for men to deal with.

The causes of impotence are physical in about half of men who have difficulty getting or keeping an erection. Diabetes (p. 211), atherosclerosis (p. 111), kidney disease, liver disease and male hormone deficiencies can reduce the ability to maintain an erection. Some men who have had prostate surgery may have impotence.

Men whose impotence is caused by stress or psychological problems will still have erections during sleep or in the morning as they awaken. Physical disease reduces these normal sleep-cycle erections. This is the easiest way to tell the difference between a physical cause of impotence and a psychological or stress-related cause.

Various medicines can also interfere with a man's sexual function. For example, some medicines for high blood pressure reduce the function that's essential to stimulate and maintain an erection. Alcohol use also reduces the ability to maintain an erection. Any medicines that cause drowsiness, such as tranquilizers (p. 626) or antihistamines (p. 615), may also contribute to impotence.

Sexual desire is often absent in men who are seriously depressed. Treatment with antidepressants (p. 619) usually restores sexual desire.

A thorough physical exam plus blood tests for diabetes and low testosterone levels will provide some basic information about possible physical causes of impotence. Your doctor may also review what medicines you take and ask you about alcohol use. Your doctor will also ask you about life stresses, relationship problems or conflicts, or sexual fears.

New treatments, such as injections and devices that are surgically placed in the penis, can allow a man to have an erection if he is unable to do so because of physical problems. Also available is a vacuum pump that pulls blood into the erectile tissues of the penis. This artificial erection is held in place with a pressure device at the base of the penis.

**Orgasm**

Most men reach a sexual climax, or *orgasm*, during intercourse. Generally, the man must have a reasonably erect penis for an orgasm to occur.

Right before an orgasm occurs, the man will have the feeling that the orgasm is inevitable, or can't be stopped. The amount of time it takes a man to have an orgasm varies. It may take only a few minutes, several minutes or longer.

When an orgasm occurs, the rhythmic squeezing of the sperm into the vas deferens gives the man an intensely pleasurable sense of release. After an orgasm, the man can't have another orgasm right away. It usually takes about 10 to 20 minutes for enough sperm to gather for another ejaculation.

Sometimes men aren't able to reach an orgasm. Complex psychological issues can be the cause. Not giving your partner your full attention and not concentrating on the sensations of intercourse can contribute to not reaching an orgasm. If you're having problems reaching orgasm, talk to your doctor.

### Painful Intercourse

Most of the time, physical problems are the reason for pain in men during intercourse. Several infections, including jock itch (p. 430), herpes (p. 318) and urethritis (p. 320), along with skin irritation caused by spermicides, can produce pain during intercourse. Infections in the prostate gland, epididymis or urethra can produce an aching or burning discomfort both before and during intercourse. More serious diseases, such as cancer of the penis (p. 426) or testicles (p. 429), also may be the cause of the pain.

An exam by your doctor will likely reveal the problem. The diseases that produce pain with intercourse can usually be treated.

### Premature Ejaculation

Premature ejaculation is described as reaching climax before penetration or very soon after vaginal penetration. After ejaculation, the penis quickly becomes limp, or flaccid. It's normal for premature ejaculation to happen occasionally when you're very excited. Frustration may grow if this happens often.

Although premature ejaculation is categorized as a sexual dysfunction, it's actually common in adolescents and in men who haven't had sex for a long time. For intercourse that's satisfying for both partners, the timing of climax needs to be tested, learned and refined over time.

Try not to feel guilty or worry if you're unable to control your climax. Emotions often strongly influence sexual performance, so the more guilt and frustration you feel, the more difficulty you may have.

The "squeeze" technique has proved to be the most successful method of treating premature ejaculation. When the man nears climax, he or his partner squeezes firmly (but not so hard as to cause bruising) just under the *glans*, or head, of the penis for five to 10 seconds. This decreases the level of excitement so that stimulation can be resumed. Each time the man nears climax, he or his partner can use the squeeze technique so that sexual stimulation can be prolonged. With repeated use of this method, the man can usually achieve better control.

Talking with your partner about sexual problems is an essential part of a healthy relationship. Good communication can help a sexual relationship flourish.

### Sex

Hormonal changes that begin with puberty extend into adulthood as men face relationship issues and concerns or awareness regarding sexual performance. How you feel about your sexuality depends greatly on how you feel about your body, how you feel about your partner and many other factors.

Sexual intercourse should be a pleasurable experience. It shouldn't be painful or stressful. And it should be satisfying. If sex is painful, stressful or unsatisfying, you may want to examine the situation to find out the cause so you can address the problem and improve the health of your sexual relationship. Talk to your doctor openly

---

## Some Reasons For Impotence

### Psychological reasons

- Job/life stress
- Fear of pain, pregnancy or poor sexual performance
- Poor communication between sexual partners
- Problems with your relationship with your partner (anger, guilt)

### Physical reasons

- Drinking too much alcohol
- Atherosclerosis
- Diabetes
- Various medicines, such as high blood pressure medicine
- Use of street drugs such as cocaine and marijuana
- Prostate surgery

about any concerns you have. He or she can help you find solutions.

## Taking Care of Your Body

You can help prevent serious medical problems by paying attention to your body and seeking medical help if you notice changes in how you feel. Some men are reluctant to seek medical advice. This is unfortunate, because most medical conditions can be treated. But, of course, treatment can't begin if you don't ask for help. Stay in tune with your body and talk to your doctor about any concerns you have.

## Penis

The penis has functions for both the urinary and the reproductive systems. The urethra, which is a tube within the penis, expels both urine from the bladder and semen from the testicles and epididymis. The penis is made of tissue that allows it to become erect during sexual excitement.

### Balanitis

An infection of the head of the penis is called *balanitis*. It's usually caused by a fungus, often *Candida albicans.* Balanitis causes swelling, redness and tenderness at the end of the penis. Good hygiene and cleansing of the head of the penis, which is also called the glans, are essential to prevent infection.

In uncircumcised men, the glans is covered by the foreskin, which extends over the end of the penis. The foreskin should be pulled back while bathing so the glans can be cleansed. Cleaning this area prevents buildup of secretions (*smegma*) and thereby reduces the risk of infection. In circumcised men, the foreskin has been removed.

Soaking in a bathtub may help cleanse the area and prevent an infection from getting worse. The more swollen and tender the area becomes, the more it will hurt during urination or erection. When compared with uncircumcised men who don't practice good hygiene, circumcised men seem less likely to get balanitis and less likely to spread this and other infections to their sex partners. Uncircumcised men who practice good penile hygiene have little or no increased rate of infection.

Treatments for balanitis include gentle cleansing, applying antifungal ointment (p. 615), taking an oral antibiotic (p. 618) if a bacterial infection is present and, sometimes, a partial or complete circumcision.

Good hygiene prevents balanitis. Upon reaching puberty, uncircumcised boys should be taught to retract, or pull back, the foreskin and clean the glans several times a week.

### Cancer of the Penis

Uncircumcised men who haven't practiced good hygiene through the years are most at risk for penile cancer. Cancer of the penis begins as a warty-looking growth, a white patch or a shallow sore on the glans or other part of the penis.

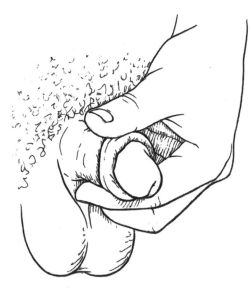

**PULLING BACK THE FORESKIN**

A smear, culture or biopsy of a small sample of tissue taken from the sore will help your doctor decide whether the growth is cancer or a sexually transmitted disease (STD). Some STDs, such as human papillomavirus, have been associated with penile cancer. Follow guidelines to prevent STDs (p. 32) if you choose to be sexually active.

Surgical removal of the tumor can cure the disease if cancer cells haven't spread to the lymph nodes in the groin or the rest of the body. Radiation therapy (p. 225) to the area, including the lymph nodes or areas of possible spread, is another option for treatment. Chemotherapy (p. 225) and laser therapy are also used. Penile cancer is curable if it's discovered and treated early.

### Curvature of the Penis

Curvature of the penis, or *Peyronie's disease,* can become so severe that it causes erections to be painful and interferes with sexual activity. The cause is related to a buildup of fibrous material in the penis. The reason this occurs isn't known. The condition may go away on its own over many months. Treatment may include surgery to remove the fibrous material or injections of corticosteroids (p. 622).

### Priapism

This rare condition affects the erectile tissue in the penis. It results in an erection that lasts for many hours and often becomes painful. The erection may occur without sexual arousal. Once the penis becomes swollen with blood, the veins that drain the blood become clogged. As a result, pressure builds and the penis may throb with pain. Hours of pressure can damage the tissue, leading to permanent impotence. Priapism is a medical emergency. Rapid treatment is essential to preserve sexual function.

Medicines that are usually given to treat blood pressure may relieve priapism. But if medicine doesn't work quickly, your doctor may try to temporarily block the nerves leading to the penis, or try to locate the clog in the veins and correct it. Home remedies such as cool compresses or ice don't usually help relieve a blockage. Delaying treatment may result in greater damage.

## Prostate

The prostate gland is located under the bladder. It surrounds the urethra where the urethra leaves the bladder. The prostate gland's main function is to produce a special fluid that mixes with sperm and seminal fluid before ejaculation. The fluid helps make sperm more able to move once it's ejaculated into the female's reproductive tract. This helps the sperm fertilize an egg.

### Benign Prostatic Hypertrophy

*Benign prostatic hypertrophy* is a common problem in older men. The prostate gland becomes larger and interferes with urination. Men with benign prostatic hypertrophy may notice a decrease in the size of the urine stream and may have frequent urinary tract infections. Repeated infections of the urinary tract caused by an enlarged prostate can damage the kidneys and lead to kidney failure if not treated early or adequately.

Generally, as a man ages, his prostate gland becomes larger and more stiff. Most of this change is caused by the normal aging process, although prostate infections can contribute to the process. As the prostate grows it may pinch the urethra. The urine stream may then become smaller and less forceful. The bladder may not be emptied completely. The urine that's left in the bladder can stagnate and become infected. In some men, the bladder may suddenly become blocked so that urine can't flow out. When this happens, the full bladder causes pain, and the bladder must be drained with a catheter.

Your doctor will probably check your prostate gland if you have signs of an infection or if your urine stream changes. A rectal exam is the easiest way to find out the size and shape of the prostate. Urine testing may also be done to check for infection, and an IVP (p. 636) may be needed to see if the swollen prostate gland is pushing into the bladder.

If you're having trouble urinating, get medical help right away. You may need to have a catheter placed in your bladder to drain it. Don't wait until it's totally impossible to urinate, because then it's become a serious medical emergency.

Your doctor may want to look in your bladder with a *cystoscope*, a thin tube that's passed into the urethra and into the bladder. The cystoscope lets the doctor see the inside of your bladder. If the prostate is causing severe blockage, a *transurethral resection of the prostate* (TURP) can be done. This operation involves removing some of the prostate with a device that's passed through the penile urethra. A possible complication of any prostate surgery is impotence, although it occurs in only 5% of men who have TURP.

Complete removal of the prostate isn't usually needed unless prostate cancer is present. Symptoms of infection are usually checked out with urine tests. Medicines are available to help slow the growth of the prostate. Surgery may be recommended before the prostate becomes so large that it completely blocks urine flow.

### Prostate Cancer

As with benign prostatic hypertrophy, prostate cancer is more common in older men. This tumor tends to grow very slowly. Most men with prostate cancer live with the disease for many years without symptoms until it's found during a routine prostate exam (digital rectal exam, p. 633).

A new blood test called prostate-specific antigen (PSA, p. 640) may sometimes detect prostate cancer before it can be felt in a prostate exam. Further studies of the prostate allow the doctor to confirm the diagnosis. Other tests may be ordered to check for cancer spread if the tumor is large or if other symptoms or tests suggest the cancer has spread.

Treatment of prostate cancer includes surgery, chemotherapy, radiation and hormonal therapy. The type of treatment depends on the tumor—how large it is, how much it has spread, how fast it's growing—and the

Seminal Vesicle

Bladder

Urethra

Enlarged Prostate compressing Urethra

Bladder and Prostate sectioned (side view)

**BENIGN PROSTATIC HYPERTROPHY**

patient's age, overall health and personal feelings about the risks and benefits of the different treatment options.

Because surgical removal of the prostate can cause impotence, some men choose other kinds of treatment. In older men with a slow-growing, small tumor, the tumor may be watched closely at regular exams but not treated. Removing the testicles to reduce hormone levels or giving the man estrogen, a female hormone to block the hormones produced by the testicles, can reduce the prostate cancer's growth. In some men these treatments may prevent the need for surgery and its potential side effects. But these treatments reduce sexual desire and function in many men.

## Prostatitis

The bladder is often the source of an infection that spreads to the prostate. A prostate infection can cause swelling of the prostate, tenderness and, sometimes, symptoms of urinary tract infection. Swelling where the urethra is surrounded by the prostate may slow or change the flow of urine. Difficulty starting to urinate may be the first symptom of this infection. The symptoms may come on slowly and be mild. This is called *chronic prostatitis*. Symptoms of *acute prostatitis* progress quickly and include severe pain in the area between the anus and the scrotum (the perineum), fever, aches and chills. Chronic prostatitis is more common than acute prostatitis.

Chronic infection of the prostate can be hard to verify. Urine tests may not show bacteria. A prostate exam can help confirm a prostate infection.

Most cases of chronic prostatitis can be treated with oral antibiotics. Several long courses of antibiotics may be required to prevent return of the infection. Take sitz baths and avoid alcohol, coffee and tea. These drinks make your body produce more urine, which may cause the bladder to rapidly expand. When the bladder expands with urine, symptoms may worsen.

Antibiotic (p. 618) treatment when the symptoms of prostatitis are first noticed may prevent chronic infection and great discomfort. Taking an antibiotic for a sufficient time will reduce the chance of recurrence. Rarely, prostatitis is contracted through sexual contact. Following recommendations to prevent sexually transmitted diseases (STDs, p. 316) can help decrease the risk of prostatitis.

## Testicles

The testicles are where the sperm are produced. The testicles are enclosed in the scrotum, which hangs outside of the body so that the temperature of the testicles can be kept lower than in the rest of the body. The lower temperature helps keep the sperm healthy.

### Cancer of the Testicle

Cancer of the testicle is more common in men between the ages of 20 and 40 than in older men. Men who have an undescended testicle (p. 355), even if it has been corrected by surgery, have a higher risk for this type of cancer. Cancer of the testicle can spread through the lymph system to the abdomen and lungs.

The primary sign of this cancer is a painless, hard lump on the surface of the testicle or a general, painless

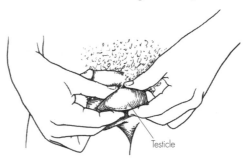

Testicle

**TESTICULAR SELF-EXAM**

*Testicular
Self-Exam*

During a bath or shower, gently feel the surface of your testicles. You're looking for a lump on the surface of the testicles, rather than on your scrotum. Use both hands to examine each testicle one at a time. Put your index and middle fingers underneath the testicle and your thumb on top. Then roll the testicle gently between your thumb and fingers. Don't worry if one testicle is bigger than the other. That's normal. Don't confuse the epididymis on the upper back side of each testicle with a lump. After examining your testicles, check your scrotum for any lumps or varicoceles (p. 432). Any lump should be checked by your doctor to find out what it is and if you need treatment. It's recommended that you check yourself every week.

## Jock Itch

*Jock itch* is the commonly used name for tinea cruris. It's a fungal, or yeast, infection in the groin area. It causes itching and redness. Flare-ups are most common during the summer months. Wearing tight clothes, sweating and being overweight seem to help the organisms grow. You can help prevent jock itch by keeping your genital area dry and clean, and not sharing towels with other people. Your doctor can give you a cream or lotion to use on the area, or may suggest antifungal medicines (p. 615) you can buy without a prescription. Even after treatment, jock itch can come back from time to time.

increase in size of the testicles. Other symptoms include a dull, achy feeling of heaviness in the scrotum, groin or lower abdomen, or a sudden buildup of fluid in the scrotum. Regular self-exam of the testicles (see box) is important to catch this cancer early. A careful exam by your doctor and further studies, including a biopsy, may be needed to confirm the diagnosis. Other swelling around the testicle, such as hydrocele (below), may also appear as painless lumps near the testicles.

Surgical removal of the testicle and local lymph nodes, chemotherapy (p. 225) and radiation therapy (p. 225) can be used to treat cancer of the testicle. When caught early and treated aggressively, this type of cancer is very curable.

### Epididymitis

The *epididymis* is the tube behind each testicle, where the sperm ducts empty. It acts as a storage place for sperm and a place where sperm mature. The epididymis feeds into the vas deferens. During ejaculation, the muscles within these tubes contract rhythmically to push the sperm through the urethra. The epididymis

can become infected by bacteria that enter it from the urethra, prostate gland or bladder. This is called *epididymitis*. Pain and minor swelling behind one of the testicles may be symptoms of this infection.

Epididymitis may be caused by a sexually transmitted disease (STD), such as chlamydia (p. 317) or gonorrhea (p. 318). The swelling, tenderness and pain usually occur quite suddenly. The pain involves the entire scrotum on one side. It's important to see a doctor quickly to make sure of the diagnosis and begin treatment. After repeated episodes of epididymitis, the surrounding tissue can scar. This scarring can result in an enlarged epididymis that may eventually require removal. Chronic epididymitis is treated with antibiotics (p. 618) and anti-inflammatory medicines (p. 619).

In younger men, it's important to make sure that the pain isn't caused by a twisted epididymis *(torsion)*. Most of these infections get better a few days after oral antibiotics are started. Following guidelines to prevent STDs (p. 32) can help reduce the likelihood of epididymitis due to an STD.

### Hydrocele

As the testicle migrates from the abdomen into the scrotum while the fetus is still forming in the womb, a small amount of *peritoneum,* or lining of the abdomen, may descend into the scrotum along with the testicle. This extra membrane can produce a sac that's filled with fluid. The sac is called a *hydrocele.*

If you have a hydrocele, you may notice a soft, painless swelling around one of the testicles. The fluid in the sac doesn't cause cancer, infertility or infection. No treatment is needed unless the hydrocele becomes large or tender. Then the hydrocele can be

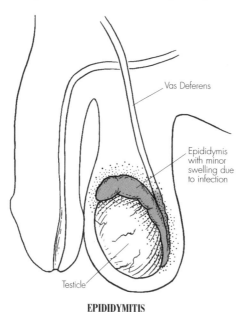

Vas Deferens

Epididymis with minor swelling due to infection

Testicle

**EPIDIDYMITIS**

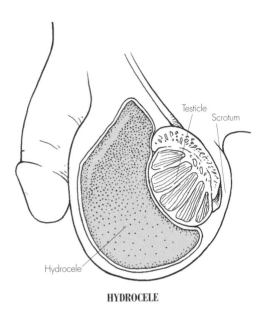

**HYDROCELE**

removed with surgery. Most men with a hydrocele have no problems.

## Spermatocele

Often a lump in the scrotum is an *epididymal cyst*. These cysts are also called *spermatoceles,* because sperm build up in the epididymis. The epididymis is the tube that carries sperm to the seminal vesicles and the prostate gland. Any mass in the testicle should be checked by your doctor. Spermatoceles can slowly grow and become tender.

Treatment isn't usually needed. If the cyst produces symptoms that are bothersome, the cyst may be surgically removed. As long as the other testicle is normal, fertility isn't affected by surgery.

## Testicular Torsion

*Testicular torsion* occurs mostly in adolescents and young men. The testicles are attached to the body by a cord of tissue that includes the vas deferens, the testicular artery and vein, and a nerve. If one of the testicles twists on this cord, the blood supply to that testicle can be cut off. The twisting of the testicle causes pain so severe you may become nauseated or vomit. Swelling of the testicle then develops.

The torsion may reverse itself within a few minutes, relieving the pain and swelling. But if it persists, see your doctor right away or go to an emergency room. The testicle can be damaged within minutes or hours if its blood supply is cut off. Immediate treatment can prevent damage to the testicle.

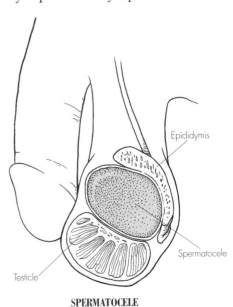

**SPERMATOCELE**

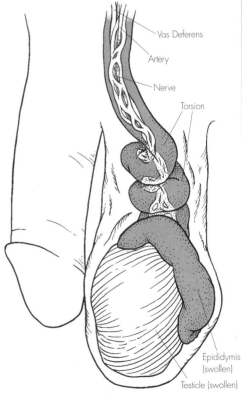

**TESTICULAR TORSION**

If you have testicular torsion, surgery will probably be needed within a few hours to restore the blood supply and prevent loss of the testicle. A testicle that has been without blood supply for more than a few hours may have to be removed. This can be decided by your doctor when he or she examines the testicle during surgery.

### Trauma to a Testicle

Injury to a testicle is one of the most painful injuries for a man. The intense pain can cause fainting, nausea and vomiting, as well as a general feeling of illness. Most of the time, testicular injury produces pain that goes away within minutes or hours. Usually the testicle isn't damaged. If the trauma is more serious or if pain, swelling or bruising in the scrotum doesn't go away, the injury should be checked by a doctor.

Serious injuries to the genital area may require repeated exams to make sure healing is complete. Any cuts in the area will require careful surgical inspection to make sure the spermatic cord and other structures are okay. Surgery may be required to remove excess blood and to stop the bleeding in the scrotum. Very rarely, the testicle or tissues around it are so badly damaged that removal is the only treatment possible.

> ### Preventing Testicular Trauma
>
> If you play contact sports, wear a protective supporter with an athletic cup to prevent damage to the testicles. If you've already lost one testicle, you should consider not playing contact sports so you can be sure your remaining testicle and your fertility are preserved. Athletic supporters and cups can be purchased at most sporting goods stores.

> ### EMERGENCY: Severe Pain in a Testicle
>
> Severe pain in one testicle may mean a serious problem. Even if you haven't had an injury, seek medical attention immediately to avoid possible loss of the testicle. A blow to the testicle can produce bleeding in the scrotum. In such cases, the scrotum may have to be surgically drained. An inguinal hernia (p. 191), when part of the intestine slips into the scrotum, can be serious if the bowel becomes blocked. Testicular torsion, another condition that may cause severe pain in a testicle, may require emergency surgery. See your doctor right away if you have severe pain in a testicle.

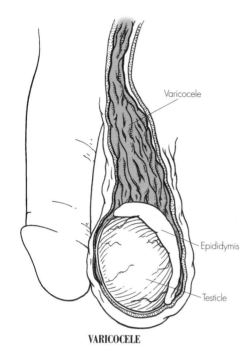

**VARICOCELE**

### Varicocele

Just as veins in the legs can swell, twist and turn bluish, so can veins in the scrotum. The result is *varicocele*. The process is caused by the destruction of the tiny valves that control the flow of blood in the veins. This problem is present in up to 20% of men. The condition may first be discovered by your doctor during a routine exam of the genitals. If a varicocele appears suddenly, an evaluation is necessary.

A varicocele is often described as feeling like "a bag of worms." The area in the scrotum may ache or feel vaguely uncomfortable. More than 95% of varicoceles occur on the left side because of the way veins drain blood on that side.

Varicoceles may reduce fertility in a small number of men. Because of this, they're sometimes surgically removed. Doctors don't usually recommend removal unless a possible decrease in fertility is a great concern, if the varicocele causes discomfort or if you're bothered by its appearance. A well-fitting protective supporter worn during athletic activities may reduce the discomfort of a varicocele.

# CHAPTER 6

# THE ELDERLY

Changes in our bodies occur throughout our lives. From the time we're conceived, our bodies are changing, maturing and growing. As we age, our health care needs change. Problems that are only minor issues for younger adults become more serious in elderly people. New health concerns also arise in the elderly.

The way we live as we grow older also changes. Sometimes we need more help as we become less able to care for ourselves. Our families may want to become more involved in our care, or we may need the care that a nursing home can provide. These are the realities of growing older.

While many tough decisions need to be made as we age, growing older doesn't have to be a negative or frightening experience. With age comes wisdom and perspective. It can be a time of great pleasure, as you have more time to enjoy special hobbies and the people around you.

## Special Issues for the Elderly

While many health problems become more common in older adults, don't blame age for every pain or problem. Although your body will eventually weaken with age, you can do many things to stay healthy as you grow older. Stay as physically active as possible. Get involved with activities and clubs. Keep your mind active and stay informed.

### Accidents and Falls

Many factors make accidents and falls more common in older adults. As we age, our balance becomes less certain. This can interfere with the ability to walk and move. An elderly person's sense of surroundings may also fade. These things combine with joint pain and muscle weakness to increase the risk of accidents and falls.

A number of common diseases can also contribute to falls. Atherosclerosis (p. 111) can cause dizziness or fainting spells. Parkinson's disease (p. 56) affects balance and the ability to walk. Diabetes

---

*Health Problems That Are More Common in Older Adults*

Alzheimer's disease (p. 53)
Arthritis (p. 229)
Atherosclerosis (p. 111)
Benign prostatic hypertrophy (p. 427)
Cancer (p. 224)
Chronic obstructive pulmonary disease (p. 145)
Decreased hearing (p. 77)
Diabetes (p. 211)
Glaucoma (p. 68)
Heart disease (p. 113)
High blood pressure (p. 123)
Osteoporosis (p. 244)
Parkinson's disease (p. 56)
Shingles (p. 331)
Stroke (p. 59)
Trigeminal neuralgia (p. 61)
Urinary incontinence (p. 434)

## Grief

As you age, you're more likely to face situations that can lead to grief. These may include the death of loved ones and friends, the loss of health to illness, and the loss of familiar roles you have played in your life. Grief is a normal reaction to loss. But it can become unhealthy if it doesn't progress through normal stages and lessen over time. See page 568 for more information about the grieving process.

(p. 211) may make the feet and legs numb. Osteoporosis (p. 244) makes bones brittle and more likely to break. Medicines for diseases like high blood pressure (p. 123) may make older people unsteady on their feet. Vision problems also can contribute to falls.

Falls can cause serious problems for older people. Broken bones, especially hip fractures, take a long time to heal and may require surgery. A hip fracture in an older person can even cause death. This is because it can make a person bedridden, which leads to weakness and illnesses. Inactivity may allow the formation of blood clots, which can travel through the veins and block large veins in the lungs (pulmonary embolism, p. 157).

Another complication of falls is head injury (p. 50). Head injury from a fall can cause bleeding next to the brain (subdural hematoma, p. 46). The tissues of the brain bleed more easily in the elderly, and even a relatively minor injury can cause a great deal of bleeding.

The type of tests done after an accident or fall depends on the injury. X-rays of the arms, legs, ribs, spine and skull are often done, since even minor falls can cause serious damage in elderly people.

See the box below for what you can do to reduce your risk of falls. Try

to stay as active as possible. If pain, weakness, weight or breathing problems prevent activity, talk to your doctor about medicines or exercises that may help. Make every effort to stay active.

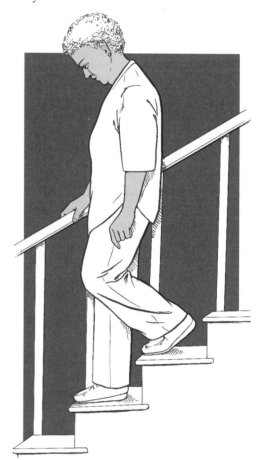

### Incontinence

As the body ages, the tissues near the bladder and the muscular rings (*sphincters*) that control opening and closing of the urethra and rectum may

## How to Prevent Falls

- Cover any loose electrical cords.
- Have strong handrails on each side of a stairway and use the handrails when going up or down the stairs. Make sure the stairs are well lighted. If your stairs are carpeted, be sure the carpeting is tacked down securely.
- Don't have loose throw rugs on the floor. They can slip and make you fall.
- Install supports or handrails near the toilet and around the bathtub.
- Use a cane or walker if you're unsteady.
- Talk to your doctor about any medicines you may be taking that could cause dizziness or unsteadiness.
- Have your vision tested regularly, especially if you wear glasses.

---

### Future Considerations

You may want to consider filling out some extra paperwork. It's a good idea to think about what may happen if you become ill or are in an accident and can't speak for yourself. Patient advance directives for terminal care, a power of attorney and a will are all things to consider. In patient advance directives for terminal care, you can direct how you want your health care managed in the event you can't speak for yourself. In a power of attorney, you can assign to someone you trust the responsibility of speaking for you if you can't speak for yourself. Another option is the health care proxy. In a will, you can outline where you want all of your belongings to go in the event you die. Talk to your doctor about these options. You may want to talk to a lawyer for help with a power of attorney and a will.

---

weaken and stretch. This can lead to *incontinence* (involuntary loss of control) of the bladder and the rectum.

Bladder infections (p. 162) or prostate infections (p. 429) can also lead to incontinence. Some injuries to the brain or nerves, such as in a stroke (p. 59) or in damage to the spine or the nerves around the bladder, can also lead to incontinence.

Be sure and talk to your doctor if you begin having incontinence. It can often be treated. Antibiotics (p. 618) may help if you have an infection of your bladder or prostate. In women who have gone through menopause, hormone replacement therapy (p. 407) or estrogen vaginal cream may decrease dryness and irritation in the vagina and urethra, and improve tissue strength. Sometimes, bladder retraining may be helpful if you have urinary incontinence. See page 167 for more information about bladder retraining.

No one should "just live" with incontinence. Various incontinence aids, such as pads, help you to remain active. Many treatments are available. In women, bladder incontinence may be corrected with surgery.

### Medicine Use

The average older adult takes 4.5 prescription medicines and 3.5 over-the-counter medicines. The more medicines you take, the more likely you are to have side effects or interactions between two medicines. The more medicines you take, the harder it is to remember when to take what medicine.

Be sure your doctor knows about all the medicines you take, both prescription and over-the-counter. This is especially important if you see different doctors for different problems. The doctors may not know what medicines your other doctors have prescribed. It may be helpful to take your medicines with you when you visit your doctor.

It's important to take your medicines correctly. Some medicine must be

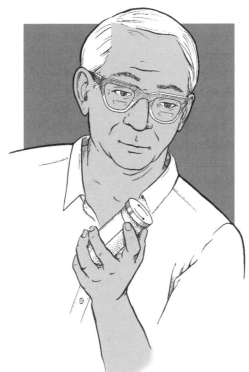

taken with food so that it won't upset your stomach. Other medicine is best taken on an empty stomach so that your body can absorb it better.

Ask your doctor for written instructions about taking your medicine so that you won't have to memorize them. The instructions can provide you with answers to such questions as: Should the medicine be taken at the same time every day? At meals or with food? What should I do if I forget to take a dose?

Ask about possible side effects of your medicine. Tell your doctor if you notice changes in how you're feeling after you start taking a medicine. Don't just stop taking the medicine on your own. Talk to your doctor first. Sometimes you can take another medicine or the dosage can be changed so that you won't have side effects.

Older people are often more sensitive to the effects and side effects of a medicine. Their livers and kidneys don't process medicine as quickly as in younger adults. If you have side effects from a medicine, smaller doses may be needed. Work with your doctor to minimize both the number of medicines you take and how often you take the medicines.

### Memory Problems

As we age, the brain loses cells. The body also makes a lower amount of the chemical the brain cells need to work properly. The older you are, the more likely that these changes will affect your memory.

*Short-term memory* (the last few seconds and minutes) and *remote memory* (last few hours through most recent years) aren't usually affected by aging. But *recent memory* may be affected. You may need a little more time to make decisions. You may forget names of people you've met recently. These are normal changes.

Help yourself remember things by keeping lists and sticking to a routine. Put important items, such as your keys or medicine, in the same place every time. Repeat and write down names when you meet new people. Use landmarks to help you remember how to get somewhere. If you're having trouble remembering a word or name, run through the ABCs in your mind. This can help "tweak" your memory when you "hear" the first letter of a word.

While many people become a little forgetful as they get older, a rapid loss of memory usually indicates a serious problem. One type of serious memory problem is dementia (p. 53). It's a progressive, permanent decline in all mental ability, including memory. Causes can include stroke (p. 59), brain tumor (p. 47) or Alzheimer's disease (p. 53).

### Skin Changes

The skin changes with aging, gradually becoming thinner and less elastic, until the outer layers become thin and fragile. These changes are caused by the gradual breakdown of the connective tissue in the skin.

**Age spots.** Sometimes these are called "liver spots." These spots are dark patches caused by a local increase in the skin's pigment. Use sunscreen to help prevent age spots or to keep them from getting darker. Bleaching creams can sometimes make them fade.

**Bruises.** As your skin becomes more fragile, you may bruise (p. 138) more often and more easily. A bruise occurs when you bleed underneath your skin.

**Dry skin.** Especially in the winter, dry and itchy skin can be a constant irritant. Try over-the-counter moisturizing creams or lotions for relief. Petroleum jelly is the cheapest and most effective moisturizer, but it may feel too

---

*Memory Problems That Aren't Typical of Aging*

- Not remembering how to do something you've done frequently
- Problems learning new things
- Repeating phrases or stories in the same conversation
- Not being able to keep track of what happens each day
- Marked changes in personality
- Losing interest in daily activities and how you look
- Depression
- Confusion
- Feeling restless and anxious
- Loss of social manners
- Trouble handling money

greasy for you. If over-the-counter products don't work, talk to your doctor. Prescription creams may help.

**Skin cancer.** Cancer of the skin (p. 290) is more common in elderly people, simply because your skin has been exposed to the sun for many years. Any sore or spot that doesn't heal or that grows should be checked by your doctor.

**Wrinkles.** The skin breaks down with age, which results in wrinkles. Your genes and the amount of time you've spent in the sun over the years will determine how wrinkled your skin becomes. There is no magic remedy for wrinkles. If you're concerned about your appearance, you can talk to your doctor about treatment or plastic surgery.

## Special Issues for Caregivers

With more people surviving into their 80s and 90s, the issue of "eldercare" is becoming increasingly important. Nearly one-third of all working adults provide some care for an older family member.

Health problems, memory loss, difficulties with the senses and a general loss of function make it natural for elderly persons to feel depressed and hopeless. These feelings may explain the increased rate of suicide among the elderly.

Whatever we can do to give the lives of the elderly more meaning is well worth the effort. Wherever the elderly person lives, display plenty of pictures of the family, including the elderly person's parents, children, grandchildren and great-grandchildren.

Encourage family members and friends to visit or write often. Letters and visits help the elderly to feel remembered and loved. Help the elderly person stay as active as possible and maintain self-worth by asking for help

with chores and duties if he or she lives with you. Listen to important memories. Encourage your parent to record memories on an audiotape or videotape or to write them down so they can be shared from generation to generation. This record not only gives the elderly person a sense of value, it preserves family traditions.

When determining the best environment and caregiver for an elderly parent, the thoughts and feelings of the parent and the family must be considered. Consider the amount of care that's needed as well as the limitations of the elderly person and the potential caregivers. If possible, arrange a "trial run" before a more lasting decision is made. Be aware that decisions about caring for an elderly loved one are often influenced more by a sense of duty or guilt than by an objective evaluation of the situation. The ideal arrangement is a mutual agreement between the elderly parent and the family.

Before making a life-changing decision about your elderly parent's living arrangements, discuss his or her medical condition, prognosis and physical limitations with your parent's doctor so you understand the extent of care that's needed. Medical professionals use the term "levels of care" to identify the amount of help and care the elderly parent needs. These levels of care range from general independence, with minimal help, to skilled nursing care in a nursing home.

### The Elderly Person Living at Home

Older adults who are able to live in their own home may be able to handle most or all of their own care. They may need only some help with finances, meal preparation, yard work and housecleaning. They may just need someone to talk to. If memory problems exist, someone may

### Elder Abuse and Neglect

Elderly persons, both men and women, are sometimes mistreated by their spouses, adult children or other caretakers. The typical victims of this type of abuse are physically and financially unable to leave the situation. Often, abuse isn't intentional but results when caregivers are too busy to take proper care of an elderly parent, for example. In other situations, abuse is intentional. Alternatives are available to reduce stress on caregivers or to take the elderly person out of the abusive situation. See page 577 for more information about elder abuse.

need to stay with them to keep them from wandering off and to make sure medicines are taken correctly. Hired help or an adult day care center may be needed for people who can't take care of themselves. In many areas, a home nursing program is available for medical needs. A home aide can be assigned to help with duties around the house.

Investigate the community-based services and resources in your area. Elderly people often know something about nursing homes in their areas, but they may know little about available community services such as in-home nursing programs. Even doctors and other health care professionals may not be aware of the community services available for the elderly. Although these services aren't available in all areas, many can be found by calling your local hospital or your community services office.

One invaluable support service is adult day care, which can provide support to the elderly parent and the family in many ways. There are about 1,500 of these facilities in the U.S. More than 60,000 people receive such care each day in the U.S. The elderly parent continues to live in his or her own home but spends the day in the day care center, which provides supervision, protection and activities. The adult day care center can free the caregiver to work or meet other demands during the day. Almost half of all caregivers work outside the home either full or part time, and many caregivers have children of their own. Adult day care offers resources, counseling and education to help family members deal with the stresses of caring for an elderly parent.

### Caring for the Elderly in Your Home

Three-fourths of caregivers are women. Since women generally have a

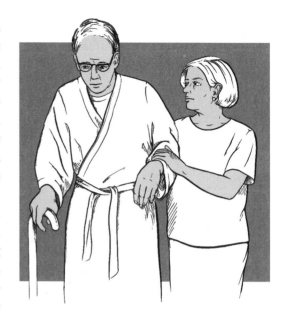

longer life expectancy than men, more wives than husbands eventually must care for a sick or disabled spouse. When there is no spouse, adult children usually assume responsibility for the elderly parent. Daughters outnumber sons as caregivers four to one, and unmarried daughters take on this role more often than those who are married. Only about 10% of elderly people live with their adult children, but that figure is expected to rise as the number of elderly adults increases.

Adult children also may hire a caregiver to stay with the elderly parent at home part or all the time. These caregivers can be found through local agencies, churches or want ads in the newspaper.

Caring for an elderly parent is stressful. Caregivers may have depression and anxiety, and their family and social life may be disrupted. The burden felt by the adult child depends greatly on his or her ability to care for the elderly parent while continuing to meet other responsibilities.

Another problem is the adult child's concern about the decline or death of an aging parent. When the parent is ill or health begins to decline, the adult child may try to "save" the parent from death and to preserve the bond between parent and child. Anxiety stems from the adult child's awareness that these efforts won't prevent the parent's decline and eventual death. Anxiety can motivate the adult child to care for the parent. High levels of anxiety may have a reverse effect, however, reducing the adult child's ability or willingness to give care.

Other factors may also affect a person's ability to care for a parent. Many people have disabilities or other chronic illnesses and are physically unable to care for another person. Some people live far away from their older relatives and are unable to move nearby. Some are limited by job and financial restrictions.

The amount of stress felt by the adult child is related to the amount of social support provided by family or friends. This may be why some studies show that women are less likely than men to experience severe stress and strain in a caregiving situation. Women are more likely than men to have a network of friends, neighbors and church groups. But studies also reveal that daughters seem to be at risk for depression more than sons. Adult daughters report more illness and more negative emotional effects related to their parents' living situation than adult sons do, perhaps because the daughters are typically more involved with meeting the everyday needs of their elderly parents. Time pressures associated with parent care and the parent's tendency to be demanding are also factors that may lead to depression.

Finding and encouraging others to help care for your elderly parent will allow you to feel more relaxed if you are the caregiver. Knowing that others can be called on in an emergency helps reduce the feeling of, "If I don't do it, who will?" Recognize your limits and try to function within them. Seek help if you need counseling. Keep yourself physically and emotionally fit with proper diet and exercise, and build a network of friends and helpers who can help you on a regular basis.

Adult children who choose to care for an elderly parent in their home should evaluate the situation before taking on this responsibility. Moving your parent into your home may represent a cost savings when compared to the cost of a nursing home or other residential facility. But before making this move you should also assess the effect of this arrangement on your own health, time and energy. Also consider realistically whether the arrangement will cause conflicting demands by other family members or by your employer. Discuss every aspect of the proposed change with all members of the family.

Studies have shown that caregivers who join support groups are

## Questions to Ask Before You Choose to Care for an Elderly Person at Home

- Will I need to lift the person frequently? Am I physically able to do this?
- Will meeting the person's daily needs be too much for me physically and emotionally?
- How will the additional stress affect my physical health?
- Is my home large enough for an extra person?
- How will the stress of taking care of the person affect my other family members?
- Are there other people to provide care when I need a break?

## Families That May Have the Most Trouble Taking Care of an Elderly Person in the Home

- Those in which only one caregiver is available without any other help
- Homes that are already overcrowded—this situation could lead to neglect or abuse of the elderly parent
- Families in which a great deal of marital or relationship conflict is already causing stress
- Families in which other problems, such as alcohol or drug dependence, trouble with adolescents or financial problems, keep emotions near the boiling point

less likely to use nursing homes or other facilities than those who don't participate in these groups. In these groups, caregivers share experiences and express their feelings. Participation in such a group helps relieve feelings of isolation that are common among caregivers.

Such groups also may provide training in moving, lifting and bathing elderly persons, information about giving medicines, and on the aging process.

### Nursing Home Care

For many adult children, placing a parent in a nursing home is a last resort. When this decision is made, other alternatives may have been exhausted. The family may have already experienced a great deal of stress in caring for the elderly parent and in making the decision.

Making this decision doesn't necessarily relieve the stress. Sometimes family stress continues, or even increases, after the elderly parent goes to the nursing home. The sources of stress may include the quality of care the parent is receiving, the adequacy of staffing in the nursing home and the staff members' attitudes toward both the parent and adult child. One of the best ways for the caregiver to reduce his or her anxiety is to continue to help the parent with some tasks after the move to the nursing home.

It's a great help when the nursing home staff is sensitive to a family's feelings and problems. The nursing home should provide a calm, warm, quiet and comfortable place for visits by family members. Support groups and educational groups for the family members are also an important resource that the nursing home may offer. These groups can help ease tensions as well as give practical help, such as financial counseling, and provide information about additional resources for the family.

Placing a parent in an institution should never be viewed as neglect, but as one option in the continuum of care for the elderly person. In some cases, this arrangement may be the only appropriate option, and it may be a better alternative than home care.

# PART 5

# A Child's Guide to Health

442 Keeping Your Body Clean

444 Eating Right

446 Exercising

448 Avoiding Illness

450 Taking Care of Your Teeth

452 Your Body and Stress

454 Going to the Doctor

456 Going to the Hospital

458 Medicines: How to Use Them

460 Responding to an Accident

462 Alcohol, Cigarettes & Illegal Drugs

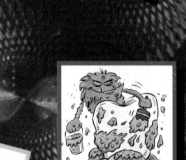

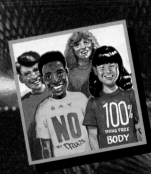

# KEEPING Your Body CLEAN

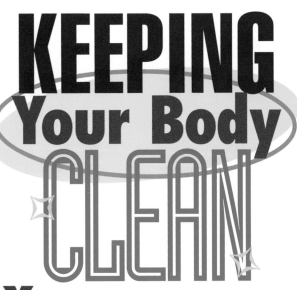

**Y**ou may not always like taking a bath or shower. But staying clean helps you stay healthy.

Your skin is your body's largest organ. It covers every square inch of you. It helps your body temperature stay the same in all kinds of weather. And it protects the organs inside you.

Every day your skin sheds a layer of cells. Every day oil and water come to the surface of your skin. Together, the oil and water make sweat, or *perspiration*. Dry, dead skin cells mix with dirt and sweat. The mixture of skin cells, sweat and dirt make a good place for *bacteria* to grow. Bacteria are germs. They can cause infections, such as in cuts and scrapes.

Bathing daily washes away the dirt, sweat and dead skin cells.

Because your skin is clean, bacteria will not grow there. You stay healthier because you are clean.

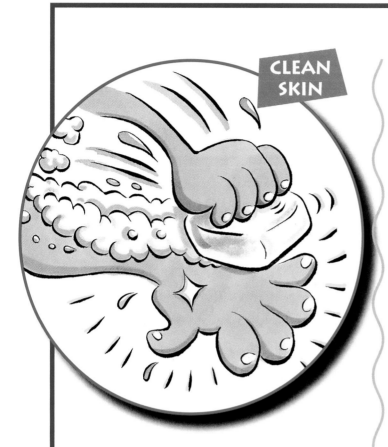

CLEAN SKIN

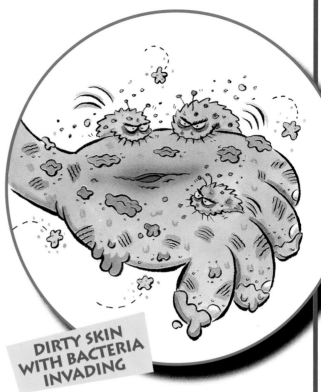

DIRTY SKIN WITH BACTERIA INVADING

Remember when you take a bath to wash behind your ears. Clean your elbows, fingers, knees, toes and private parts—and remember to wash your face. Wash your hair, too. Be sure to rinse away all the soap.

Clean your fingernails when you take a bath. If there is still some dirt under your fingernails after your bath and you cannot get it out yourself, ask someone to help you remove it. A good nail file will probably do the job.

Staying clean takes more than just a bath or shower every day. Staying clean means washing your hands before and after you eat. It means washing your hands after you go to the bathroom and before you handle any type of food. So when you help in the kitchen, wash your hands before you touch the food. Any time your hands get dirty, wash them.

Staying clean is important. If you stay clean, you have a much better chance of staying well.

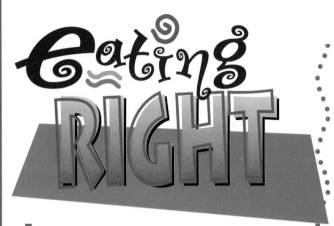

# Eating RIGHT

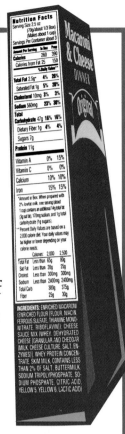

Jill loves macaroni and cheese. She often wishes she could have it for lunch *and* dinner.

She asks her dad if macaroni is good for her.

He says yes, as long as she eats other healthy foods with it. If she eats only macaroni, she would not be eating a balanced diet. She would not be getting all of the vitamins and minerals she needs to help her grow and stay healthy.

Her dad pulls a box of macaroni and cheese from the shelf. They look on the side of the box and find the list of nutrition facts and ingredients. They see that the macaroni is made from enriched flour and has added vitamins. The cheese sauce mix is made from cheese and milk in a dried form. Jill learned about

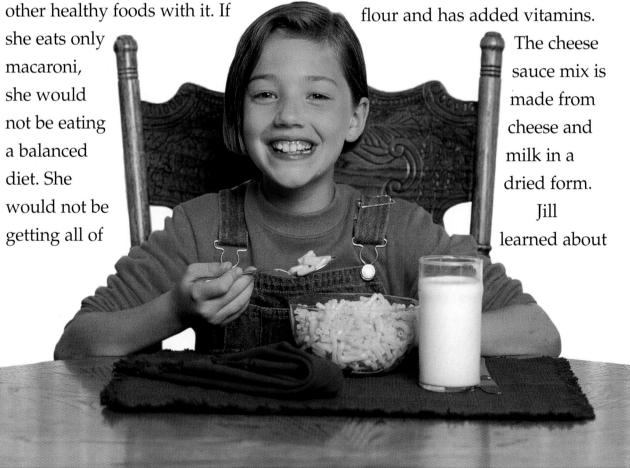

a balanced diet in school. She knows she needs to eat foods that have different vitamins and minerals. She has seen a picture of the food pyramid. It shows how much she should eat from each food group every day.

"Which group is macaroni and cheese in?" she wondered.

Look at the picture of the food pyramid. Can you figure out which food group macaroni and cheese is in? (Hint: It is in two groups. Find the answer below.)

Next, can you plan a nutritious meal that includes macaroni and cheese *and* something from each of the other food groups?

You need one or two servings from the *Fruit and Vegetable Groups* and one or two servings from the *Meat, Egg, Nut, Bean Group.*

FRUIT AND VEGETABLE
   GROUPS:_____

   FRUIT AND VEGETABLE
      GROUPS:_____

      MEAT, EGG, NUT, BEAN
         GROUP:_____

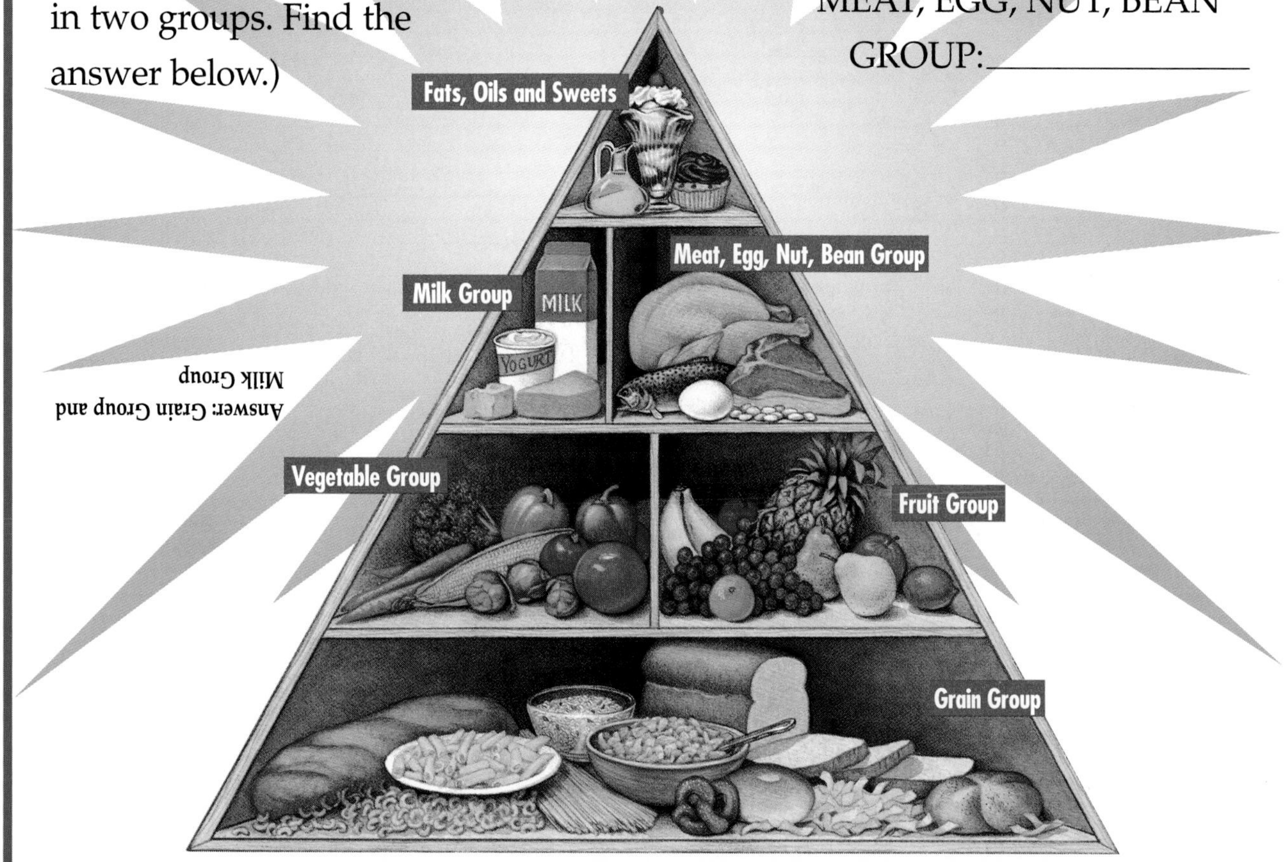

Answer: Grain Group and Milk Group

**Fats, Oils and Sweets**

**Milk Group** MILK

YOGURT

**Meat, Egg, Nut, Bean Group**

**Vegetable Group**

**Fruit Group**

**Grain Group**

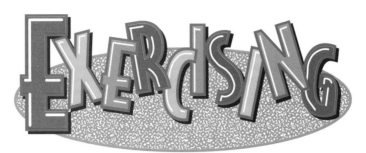

# EXERCISING

**G**rant has a long hill to climb on his bicycle. But he has a problem. He is already tired because he has been playing hard all afternoon. He wonders if he can make it up the hill.

What Grant needs to help him climb the hill on his bike is *strength* and *endurance*. How strong he is and how long he will be able to keep going depend on the amount of exercise he has had in the past weeks. If he has been exercising regularly, he will probably make it to the top of the hill.

If you want to have strong muscles and be physically fit, you need to exercise every day. Exercise makes you breathe faster and more deeply. When you do so, oxygen and nutrients in your blood move faster through your body. This helps you feel better.

Exercises that cause your heart to beat quickly are called *aerobic exercises*.

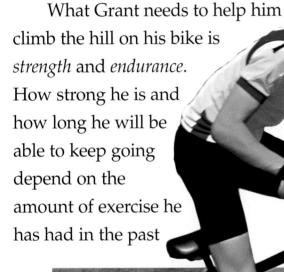

This kind of exercise makes your heart and lungs stronger.

If you want to run or swim or play ball or dance longer than you can now, here is what you can do:

(1) Set a goal for how much exercise, like running or jumping rope or bike riding, you want to be able to do.

(2) Time yourself to see how long you can do it today. Write this time down.

(3) Tomorrow, do the same activity, but do it a little longer.

(4) Keep gradually increasing the length of time you do the exercise until you reach your goal.

Over several weeks you will find you have much more endurance and strength.

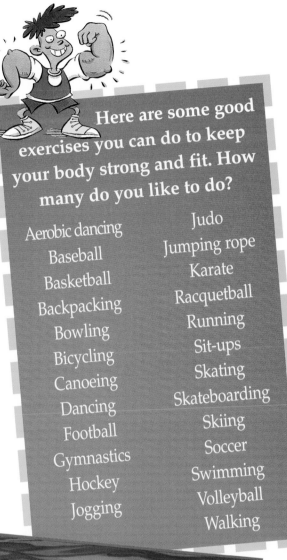

Here are some good exercises you can do to keep your body strong and fit. How many do you like to do?

Aerobic dancing
Baseball
Basketball
Backpacking
Bowling
Bicycling
Canoeing
Dancing
Football
Gymnastics
Hockey
Jogging

Judo
Jumping rope
Karate
Racquetball
Running
Sit-ups
Skating
Skateboarding
Skiing
Soccer
Swimming
Volleyball
Walking

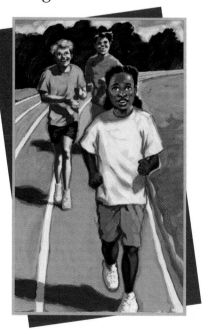

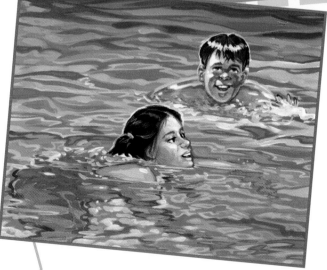

# AVOIDING ILLNESS

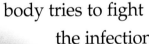

**P**am has a cold. Her throat is sore and her nose is stuffy. She feels rotten. "How did I catch this awful cold?" Pam wonders. "It is not even winter."

Pam has a cold because she was exposed to a *virus*. A virus is a type of germ that can make you sick. It is a tiny organism that gets into your body and can attach itself to your throat and nose. The virus *grows* and irritates the linings of your throat and nose. Your body tries to fight the infection

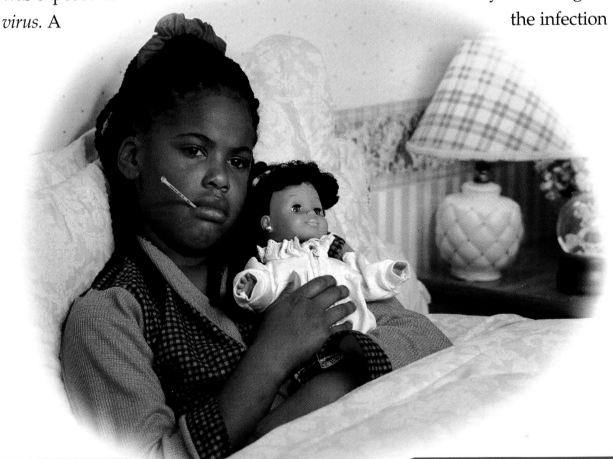

by releasing chemicals into the tissues of your nose and throat. This process produces redness and pain.

Pam's mother takes her to their family doctor. Pam asks her doctor

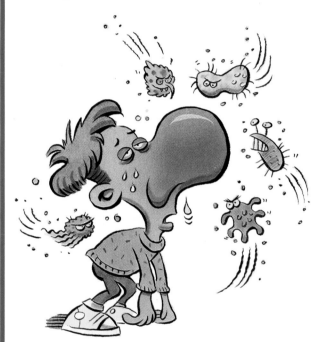

how she can stop catching colds. Her doctor tells her that most viruses are passed around when you touch the hands of someone who has the infection and then touch your nose or mouth with your hands or eat with your hands.

The best way to keep someone else's virus from infecting you is to wash your hands. You should do this after touching the

hands of someone who has a cold or the flu. You can even avoid diseases like chickenpox and strep throat by washing your hands often during the day.

Some viruses are passed through the air when a person coughs or sneezes. But what can you do to keep from catching every virus that comes through the air? You can keep your body healthy by eating three nutritious meals a day, getting plenty of sleep and exercising regularly. If your doctor recommends it, you can also take vitamins. And do not forget: Wash your hands often.

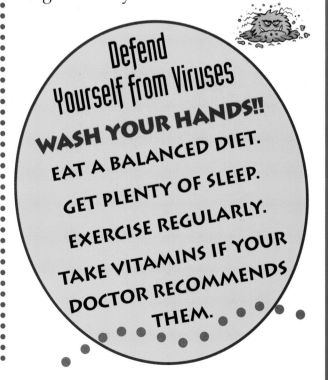

Defend Yourself from Viruses

WASH YOUR HANDS!!

EAT A BALANCED DIET.

GET PLENTY OF SLEEP.

EXERCISE REGULARLY.

TAKE VITAMINS IF YOUR DOCTOR RECOMMENDS THEM.

# Taking Care of your Teeth

Angela and Heather both have healthy teeth because they take good care of them. Angela still has her first set of teeth, which are called *primary* teeth. Some people call them baby teeth. Heather, who is older, has already lost her primary teeth. She now has her *permanent* teeth.

"Why do I have to brush my teeth if I am going to lose them anyway?" Angela asks.

"Because if you don't, they can rot," says Heather. "Rotten teeth look bad."

Their mother comes into the bathroom and gives Angela another reason to brush her teeth. She says that if her primary teeth decay, her permanent teeth might grow in crooked.

Heather takes care of her teeth because she does not want them to decay. She also knows she cannot grow another set to take their place. If she loses her teeth, she would not be able to eat foods that need chewing.

Tooth decay is caused by bits of food left on and between your teeth.

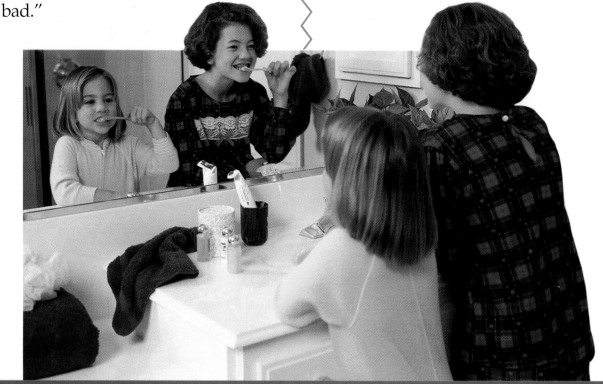

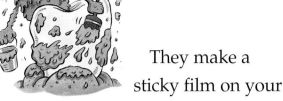

They make a sticky film on your teeth called *plaque.* The germs that live in the plaque make an acid that can slowly eat a hole in your tooth. This hole is called a *cavity.*

You probably already know one kind of food that harms your teeth. *Sugar.* Sugar is one reason you should not eat too much candy or drink a lot of sodas. But other foods can be just as bad for your teeth as sugar. All kinds of food can leave a sticky film, or plaque, on your teeth. That's why it is important to brush your teeth after eating.

You can reduce your chances of having cavities by brushing your teeth after you eat, in the morning and before you go to sleep. Brush with a toothbrush and use toothpaste that has a special ingredient called fluoride. Be sure to brush every tooth. Take your time. Be gentle. Move the brush in small circles across all the tooth surfaces. Also, gently brush your gums. This helps keep them healthy, too.

Before you go to bed, use dental floss to clean between your teeth. Dental floss is a strong, thread-like material that helps you remove the plaque and food stuck between your teeth. Have your mom or dad or another adult show you how to floss.

You may also need to have your teeth *sealed* and treated with fluoride every year. With sealing, your dentist brushes a special coating on the teeth to help protect them from cavities.

## Preventing Tooth Decay

- Brush with a fluoride toothpaste after eating, in the morning and before you go to sleep.
- Floss daily to remove plaque from between teeth.
- Limit snacking between meals, unless you brush afterward.
- Use a fluoride rinse to help your teeth resist decay.
- Have regular dental checkups.
- Have your parents ask your dentist about having your teeth sealed.

# YOUR BODY and STRESS

**K**evin lies awake in bed listening to his parents arguing. It seems to him that they fight a lot. Kevin is beginning to fear that his parents might get a divorce. His best friend's parents got a divorce last year. Kevin feels sad and afraid. What would happen to him if *his* parents divorced? He feels tears come to his eyes. Finally, when the argument is over, he falls asleep.

The next morning he has a very bad stomachache.

Kevin is feeling *stress*. Stress sometimes affects your body. It can make your stomach feel as if it is tied in a knot. It can make you feel like you are going to throw up. It can cause sickness in many different ways. It can even make you dizzy. Kevin's stomach hurts because he is worried. Worry is one way we feel stress.

We can even feel stress when *good* things happen. Enjoying a vacation, winning a sports event or being in a school play can be stressful. Stress can come from both happy and unhappy situations.

One good way to handle stress is to *think* about what has caused it. Then you can *try to change* what is causing it. Also, you can let someone know how you feel. *Talking about your feelings* often reduces your stress and helps you feel better. Another great way to keep stress from making you sick is to *exercise.*

Kevin talks with his parents at breakfast. He tells them that when they argue, he is afraid they might get a divorce. They are surprised,

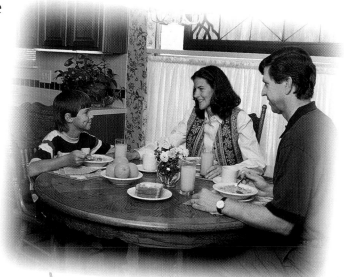

but they understand what Kevin is feeling. They tell Kevin they are sorry they have upset him. Then they tell him they still love each other and they love him and they are not going to divorce each other. This makes Kevin feel much better.

As he walks to the school bus he realizes . . . *his stomachache is gone!*

## When You Feel Stress

Think about what is causing it.

Try to change what is causing it.

Talk to someone about your feelings.

Exercise.

**A**llison and her mother walk into the doctor's office. Allison looks around the waiting room. It is very quiet except for some music playing softly. She feels afraid.

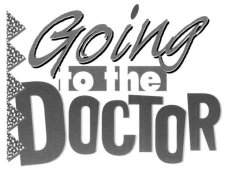

Going to the DOCToR

Do you ever feel afraid when you have to go to the doctor? Maybe it will help to know what to expect when you get there.

After you check in with the receptionist, a nurse will come to the waiting room and call your name. The nurse will take you to the area where the doctor examines patients. You will stand on a scale to see how much you weigh. You may also be measured to find out how tall you are. Then you and your parent or guardian will be led into an *exam room*. There the nurse will hold your wrist and feel your *pulse*. Your pulse tells the nurse how fast your heart is beating.

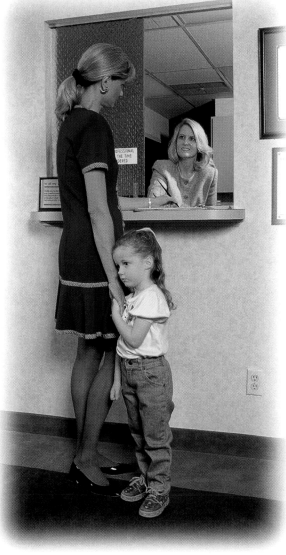

Your *temperature* will be taken and your *blood pressure* checked. Your doctor will be able to tell if you are running a fever. Your blood pressure tells your doctor the pressure of your blood as it flows through your blood vessels. None of these exams hurt.

When your doctor comes into the room, he or she will visit with you and ask you how you are doing.

Your doctor might first look into your ears with a tiny light. Then you will probably be asked to open your mouth and stick out your tongue so the doctor can see your throat. Your doctor will press on the glands of your neck to make sure they are not swollen, which can be a sign of an infection. Then your doctor will probably use an instrument, called a *stethoscope*, to listen to your lungs and heart. None of these exams hurt.

One reason to go to the doctor is to get your *immunization shots*. These shots are needed to keep you from getting certain diseases, such as measles, mumps and polio. You probably already have received several shots. They sting a little, but only for a second.

If you are feeling bad, your doctor will ask you questions about how and where you hurt. If your stomach aches, your doctor will gently push on your stomach and ask questions about the pain. If you hurt somewhere else, your doctor will examine that part of your body to find out what is causing the pain.

When your doctor decides what your illness is, this is called a *diagnosis*. Then he or she will tell you and your parent or guardian what kind of treatment you need. You may get a *prescription*, which is a paper telling the pharmacist what medicine you need. The prescription also says how much medicine you need to take and how often.

Fortunately, Allison is very healthy, so she does not need a prescription. She just needs an immunization shot. The doctor gives her a shot that doesn't hurt much at all.

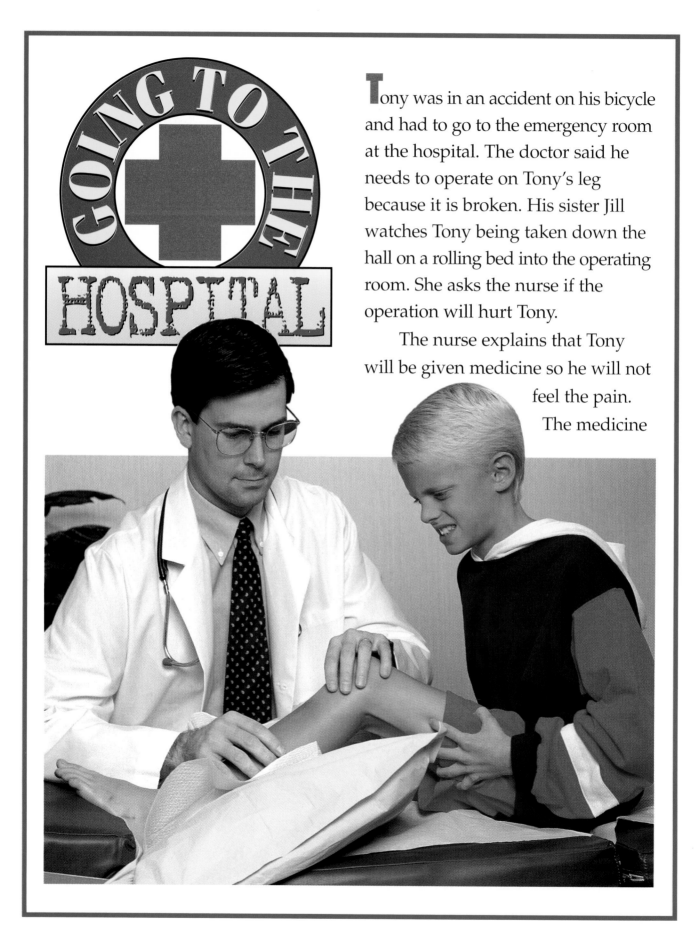

## GOING TO THE HOSPITAL

Tony was in an accident on his bicycle and had to go to the emergency room at the hospital. The doctor said he needs to operate on Tony's leg because it is broken. His sister Jill watches Tony being taken down the hall on a rolling bed into the operating room. She asks the nurse if the operation will hurt Tony.

The nurse explains that Tony will be given medicine so he will not feel the pain.

The medicine

will make him fall asleep. He will not wake up until the surgery is over.

When Tony wakes up, he will feel a little confused and sleepy at first. The nurses will be there to talk to him. When he is completely awake, he will be rolled to his hospital room. There, another nurse will make sure he is comfortable. This nurse will give Tony more medicine, if he needs it. And best of all, this nurse will bring him meals and things to drink.

The doctor taking care of Tony is an *orthopedic surgeon*. That is a doctor who works with bones.

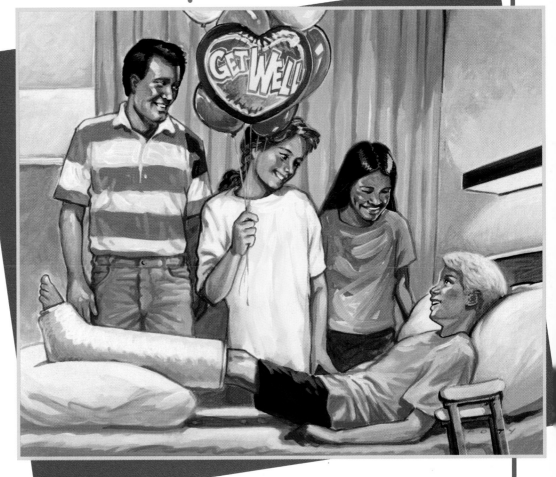

The doctor will put a long cast on Tony's leg, but he will be able to walk with crutches. While Tony is in the hospital, he can have visitors in his room. Some visitors will bring him flowers, balloons and cards.

No one really wants to get hurt or be sick. But if you *are* hurt or sick, going to the hospital can help you get well again.

# MEDICINES:
# HOW TO *use* THEM

**W**hen you get sick, you may need to take medicine. Because there are many kinds of illnesses, there are many kinds of medicines. Medicines may help you feel better or cure your illness.

Some medicines are prescribed for you by your family doctor. This type of medicine is called *prescription* medicine, and you must go to a *pharmacy* to get it. A pharmacy is run by a man or woman called a *pharmacist*, who knows how to read the prescription from your doctor and give you the right medicine.

Some medicines can be bought at a store without a prescription. These are called *nonprescription*, or *over-the-counter*, medicines.

Take medicine *only* when an adult you know tells you to. Taking the wrong medicine or the wrong amount can be dangerous. Medicine can make you sicker if it is not the right medicine for you. Both prescription and nonprescription medicines can be dangerous if they are not taken correctly.

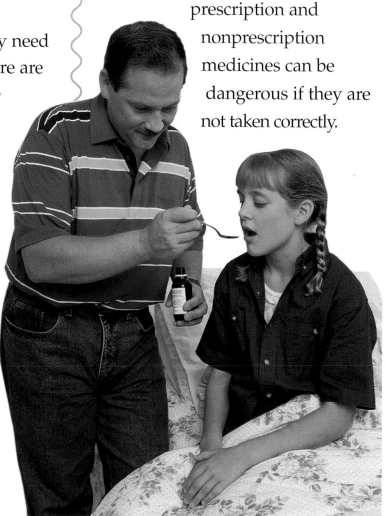

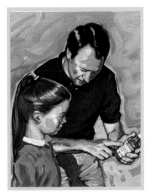

The directions for using medicines are on the label. Be sure you read them carefully or get someone you trust to read them for you, and then follow them carefully.

*Antibiotics* are one type of medicine that your doctor may prescribe. Antibiotics can help you get well when you have an illness caused by *bacteria*, a kind of germ. An example of an illness caused by bacteria is strep throat. It is very important to finish all of your antibiotic prescription, even if you start feeling better before you finish taking all of the pills.

Remember that antibiotics cannot cure all illnesses. Colds and flu are caused by *viruses*, another type of germ, and antibiotics do not work against viruses.

## How to Be Safe With Medicines

✓ Check with an adult you know you can trust before taking any medicine.

✓ Read the directions on the label before using a medicine or have someone you know you can trust read them for you.

✓ Use medicines *exactly* the way the directions tell you to use them.

✓ Tell your parent or someone who takes care of you if you feel weak while you are taking medicine. Also, tell someone if your stomach is upset or you get a rash on your skin while you are taking any medicine. Upset stomach, a rash and feeling weak are examples of *side effects* of medicine and can be early signs of more serious problems.

✓ Do not take two or more medicines at the same time, unless your doctor tells you to.

✓ Do not take a medicine if you are not sure what it is for.

✓ Throw the medicine away if the expiration date—the date marked on the bottle label to show when it is no longer good to take—has passed.

# Responding to an ACCIDENT

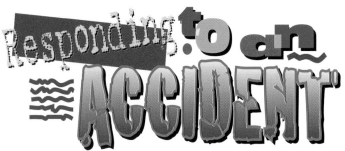

You probably have seen stories on TV about a child who has saved someone's life. These stories are about children who have made the right decision in an accident. What should you do in case there is an accident?

When an accident has hurt someone badly, it is an *emergency*. In an emergency, it is very important for you to stay calm. This will help you think more clearly. Then try to find an adult to help. If you cannot find an adult,

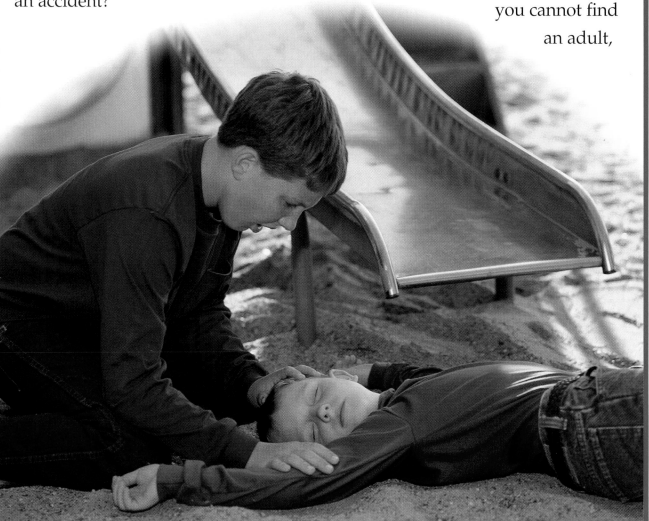

you may need to find a telephone and call *911* or *0*. These are emergency numbers you can use to get help.

If you call 911, tell the operator:

▶ Where you are. (The address, if you know it, or the nearest street corner or building.)

▶ The kind of accident you have seen.

▶ Your name and the telephone number you are calling from.

Do not hang up until the operator tells you to.

Some accidents are not serious. But you may be the only one who can help until an adult arrives. For a

cut on the skin, or a wound, you can give first aid. Here is what to do:

✚ Do not touch the wound or the blood with your hands.

✚ Wash the wound with soap and cool, running water. Use a clean cloth.

✚ Cover the wound with a bandage. You can make a bandage with a clean cloth if a bandage is not available.

✚ Push down gently on the bandage if the wound is bleeding. This slows down the flow of blood.

✚ Stay calm until help comes. Try to help calm the injured person. Keep pushing down gently on the bandage if the wound is bleeding.

# Alcohol, cigarettes & Illegal Drugs

Even though alcohol and cigarettes are legal for adults, using them is not healthy. Alcohol and cigarettes are not legal for young people.

Drinking too much alcohol can cause health problems and can also cause problems with your relationships with other people. Alcohol is also a major cause of car wrecks. Alcohol makes you respond slower to things that happen.

Drinking problems tend to run in families. So if you have a parent, sister or brother who drinks too much, you may need to be extra careful not to fall into the same pattern.

If someone in your house drinks too much, you may find it helpful to talk to a school counselor, another adult or a friend about it. It can be hard to live around someone who drinks.

Just say NO!

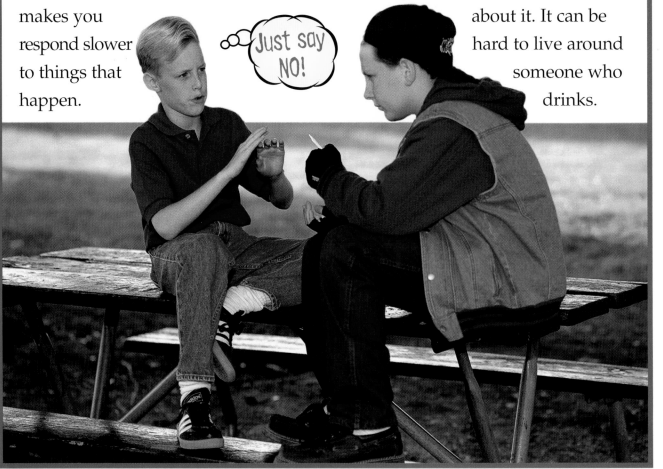

You probably have already heard how bad cigarettes are for your health. They can cause all sorts of problems, including cancer in your lungs and throat. They also smell bad and cause bad breath. Even just being around people who smoke can lead to health problems. These problems can be caused by *secondary*, or *passive*, smoke.

You may find it hard not to smoke or drink if one of your friends wants you to try it. But it is much easier to never start than it is to stop after you get addicted! If your friends do not understand that you do not want to try smoking or drinking, find new friends who respect what you want to do.

Illegal drugs are not just against the law. They are also very dangerous. Your brain is the part of your body that is harmed the most by illegal drugs. If you take an illegal drug, your brain will become confused. Some drugs can even destroy brain cells. Other parts of your body, such as your heart, can also be harmed. Some of the more common illegal drugs are marijuana, cocaine and crack, and LSD.

Marijuana is an illegal drug that is smoked. It has a lot of other names, like "pot," "mary jane," "weed," "smoke" or "grass." People who smoke marijuana forget things. They feel mixed up. Using marijuana for a long time can cause long-lasting damage to your brain. You should never use marijuana if you want to stay healthy.

Cocaine comes as a white powder, or as a lump, called *crack* or *rock*. Crack is a form of cocaine that is smoked. Cocaine speeds up some of the body's systems. It makes the heart beat very fast. Cocaine can kill a person if the heart beats way too fast. It makes people feel like they have a lot of

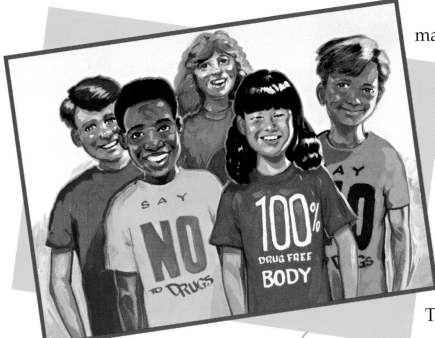

may feel like he or she can do anything. Some people inhale fumes from paint thinners, glue, hair sprays and other common sprays kept around the home. They get a "high" feeling by doing this. They also risk serious problems. These fumes go into the lungs and blood very quickly. They can cause stomachaches, throwing up, passing out, heart problems and brain damage. They can even kill you—even the first time you use them.

energy. But it keeps them from sleeping well, so they cannot work or play very well, either.

Crack causes quick changes in the way people feel. One minute they feel happy. The next minute, they feel awful. They often do not know whether something is real or not.

LSD, or "acid," causes what is called "tripping." Tripping means that the person sees things that are not really there. Acid may seem harmless. It often comes on little slips of paper that are put on the tongue. But acid can be very harmful because it makes it hard for a person to tell what is real. A person on acid

If someone offers you an illegal drug, do not accept! You may be told that the drug will make you feel better. It is not true!

You may be told that trying an illegal drug is a grown-up thing to do. It is not! It is against the law to use illegal drugs. It also hurts your body and mind.

Stay alive and stay healthy. Say no to drugs.

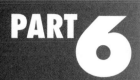

# PART 6

# SELF-CARE FLOWCHARTS

| | TOPIC | PAGE | | TOPIC | PAGE |
|---|---|---|---|---|---|
| 1 | Hair Loss | 466 | 24 | Chest Pain, Chronic | 501 |
| 2 | Headaches | 467 | 25 | Chest Pain in Infants and Children | 503 |
| 3 | Fever | 469 | 26 | Hand/Wrist/Arm Problems | 504 |
| 4 | Fever in Infants and Children | 472 | 27 | Abdominal Pain, Acute | 505 |
| 5 | Eye Problems | 474 | 28 | Abdominal Pain, Chronic | 507 |
| 6 | Facial Swelling | 476 | 29 | Nausea and Vomiting | 509 |
| 7 | Ear Problems | 477 | 30 | Nausea and Vomiting in Infants and Children | 511 |
| 8 | Hearing Problems | 479 | 31 | Lower Back Pain | 512 |
| 9 | Mouth Problems | 480 | 32 | Elimination Problems | 514 |
| 10 | Mouth Problems in Infants and Children | 482 | 33 | Elimination Problems in Infants and Children | 515 |
| 11 | Tooth Problems | 483 | 34 | Diarrhea | 516 |
| 12 | Feeding Problems in Infants and Children | 484 | 35 | Urination Problems | 518 |
| 13 | Neck Pain | 485 | 36 | Genital Problems in Infants | 520 |
| 14 | Neck Swelling | 486 | 37 | Genital Problems in Women | 521 |
| 15 | Throat Problems | 487 | 38 | Menstrual Cycle Problems | 523 |
| 16 | Cough | 488 | 39 | Genital Problems in Men | 525 |
| 17 | Cold and Flu | 490 | 40 | Hip Problems | 527 |
| 18 | Shoulder Problems | 491 | 41 | Leg Problems | 528 |
| 19 | Breast Problems in Women | 493 | 42 | Knee Problems | 530 |
| 20 | Breast Problems in Men | 494 | 43 | Ankle Problems | 532 |
| 21 | Shortness of Breath | 495 | 44 | Foot Problems | 533 |
| 22 | Shortness of Breath in a Child or Infant | 498 | 45 | Skin Rashes and Other Changes | 535 |
| 23 | Chest Pain, Acute | 499 | | | |

# TOPIC 1 Hair Loss

Many reasons can be found for temporary or permanent hair loss. Some causes are reversible, as shown in this chart.

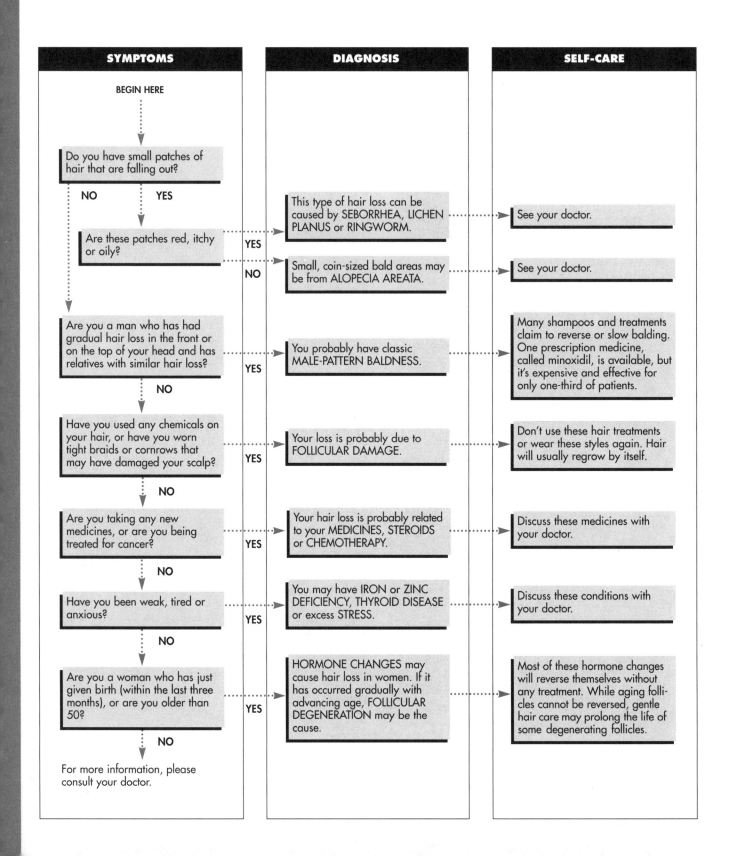

| SYMPTOMS | DIAGNOSIS | SELF-CARE |
|---|---|---|
| **BEGIN HERE** | | |
| Do you have small patches of hair that are falling out? | | |
| NO          YES | | |
| Are these patches red, itchy or oily? → **YES** | This type of hair loss can be caused by SEBORRHEA, LICHEN PLANUS or RINGWORM. | See your doctor. |
| **NO** | Small, coin-sized bald areas may be from ALOPECIA AREATA. | See your doctor. |
| Are you a man who has had gradual hair loss in the front or on the top of your head and has relatives with similar hair loss? **YES** | You probably have classic MALE-PATTERN BALDNESS. | Many shampoos and treatments claim to reverse or slow balding. One prescription medicine, called minoxidil, is available, but it's expensive and effective for only one-third of patients. |
| **NO** | | |
| Have you used any chemicals on your hair, or have you worn tight braids or cornrows that may have damaged your scalp? **YES** | Your loss is probably due to FOLLICULAR DAMAGE. | Don't use these hair treatments or wear these styles again. Hair will usually regrow by itself. |
| **NO** | | |
| Are you taking any new medicines, or are you being treated for cancer? **YES** | Your hair loss is probably related to your MEDICINES, STEROIDS or CHEMOTHERAPY. | Discuss these medicines with your doctor. |
| **NO** | | |
| Have you been weak, tired or anxious? **YES** | You may have IRON or ZINC DEFICIENCY, THYROID DISEASE or excess STRESS. | Discuss these conditions with your doctor. |
| **NO** | | |
| Are you a woman who has just given birth (within the last three months), or are you older than 50? **YES** | HORMONE CHANGES may cause hair loss in women. If it has occurred gradually with advancing age, FOLLICULAR DEGENERATION may be the cause. | Most of these hormone changes will reverse themselves without any treatment. While aging follicles cannot be reversed, gentle hair care may prolong the life of some degenerating follicles. |
| **NO** | | |
| For more information, please consult your doctor. | | |

# TOPIC 2 Headaches

Pain in one area or multiple areas of the head sometimes is accompanied by other symptoms. There are many causes for headaches.

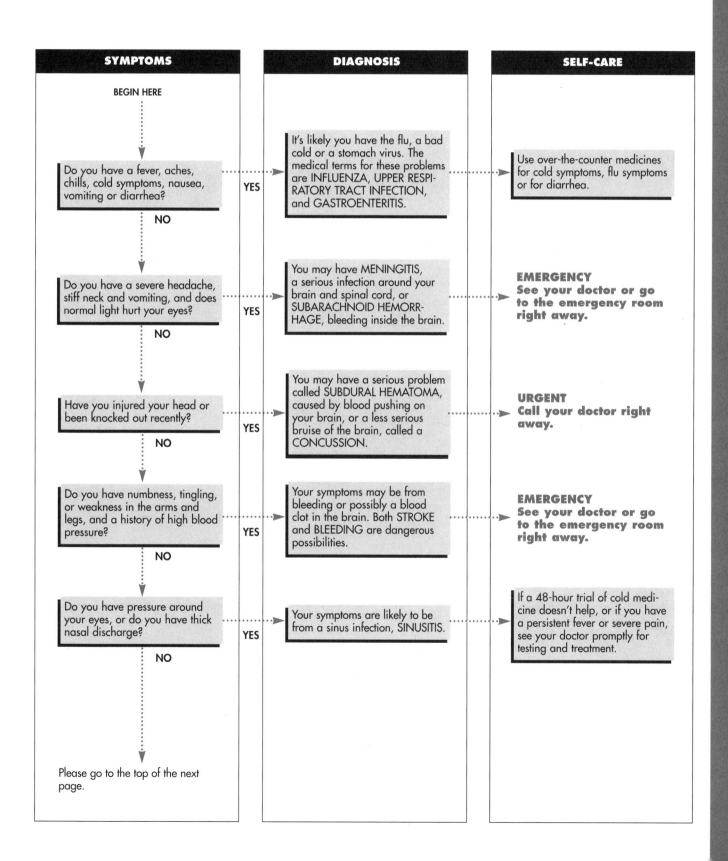

| SYMPTOMS | DIAGNOSIS | SELF-CARE |
|---|---|---|

**BEGIN HERE**

Do you have a fever, aches, chills, cold symptoms, nausea, vomiting or diarrhea? — **YES** → It's likely you have the flu, a bad cold or a stomach virus. The medical terms for these problems are INFLUENZA, UPPER RESPIRATORY TRACT INFECTION, and GASTROENTERITIS. → Use over-the-counter medicines for cold symptoms, flu symptoms or for diarrhea.

**NO**

Do you have a severe headache, stiff neck and vomiting, and does normal light hurt your eyes? — **YES** → You may have MENINGITIS, a serious infection around your brain and spinal cord, or SUBARACHNOID HEMORRHAGE, bleeding inside the brain. → **EMERGENCY** **See your doctor or go to the emergency room right away.**

**NO**

Have you injured your head or been knocked out recently? — **YES** → You may have a serious problem called SUBDURAL HEMATOMA, caused by blood pushing on your brain, or a less serious bruise of the brain, called a CONCUSSION. → **URGENT** **Call your doctor right away.**

**NO**

Do you have numbness, tingling, or weakness in the arms and legs, and a history of high blood pressure? — **YES** → Your symptoms may be from bleeding or possibly a blood clot in the brain. Both STROKE and BLEEDING are dangerous possibilities. → **EMERGENCY** **See your doctor or go to the emergency room right away.**

**NO**

Do you have pressure around your eyes, or do you have thick nasal discharge? — **YES** → Your symptoms are likely to be from a sinus infection, SINUSITIS. → If a 48-hour trial of cold medicine doesn't help, or if you have a persistent fever or severe pain, see your doctor promptly for testing and treatment.

**NO**

Please go to the top of the next page.

## TOPIC 2 Headaches

continued.

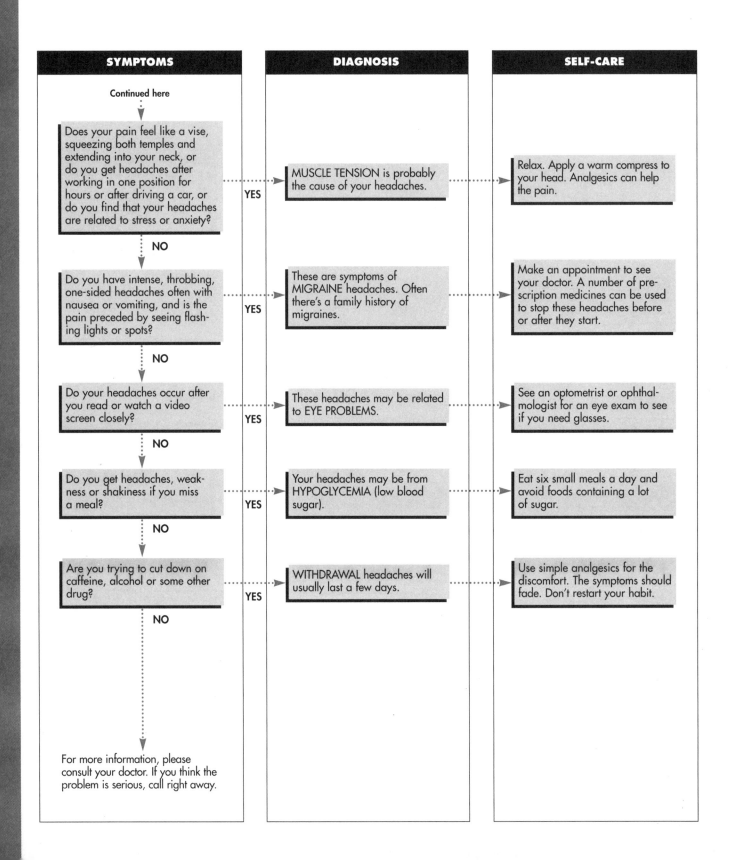

| SYMPTOMS | DIAGNOSIS | SELF-CARE |
|---|---|---|
| **Continued here** | | |
| Does your pain feel like a vise, squeezing both temples and extending into your neck, or do you get headaches after working in one position for hours or after driving a car, or do you find that your headaches are related to stress or anxiety? **YES** | MUSCLE TENSION is probably the cause of your headaches. | Relax. Apply a warm compress to your head. Analgesics can help the pain. |
| **NO** | | |
| Do you have intense, throbbing, one-sided headaches often with nausea or vomiting, and is the pain preceded by seeing flashing lights or spots? **YES** | These are symptoms of MIGRAINE headaches. Often there's a family history of migraines. | Make an appointment to see your doctor. A number of prescription medicines can be used to stop these headaches before or after they start. |
| **NO** | | |
| Do your headaches occur after you read or watch a video screen closely? **YES** | These headaches may be related to EYE PROBLEMS. | See an optometrist or ophthalmologist for an eye exam to see if you need glasses. |
| **NO** | | |
| Do you get headaches, weakness or shakiness if you miss a meal? **YES** | Your headaches may be from HYPOGLYCEMIA (low blood sugar). | Eat six small meals a day and avoid foods containing a lot of sugar. |
| **NO** | | |
| Are you trying to cut down on caffeine, alcohol or some other drug? **YES** | WITHDRAWAL headaches will usually last a few days. | Use simple analgesics for the discomfort. The symptoms should fade. Don't restart your habit. |
| **NO** | | |
| For more information, please consult your doctor. If you think the problem is serious, call right away. | | |

## TOPIC 3 Fever

A fever is defined as a temperature 1° or more above the normal 98.6°. Mild or short-term elevations are common with minor infections. High fevers, with temperatures of 103° and above, can signal a potentially dangerous infection. Contact your doctor in case of a high fever or if a lower fever doesn't resolve with simple treatments.

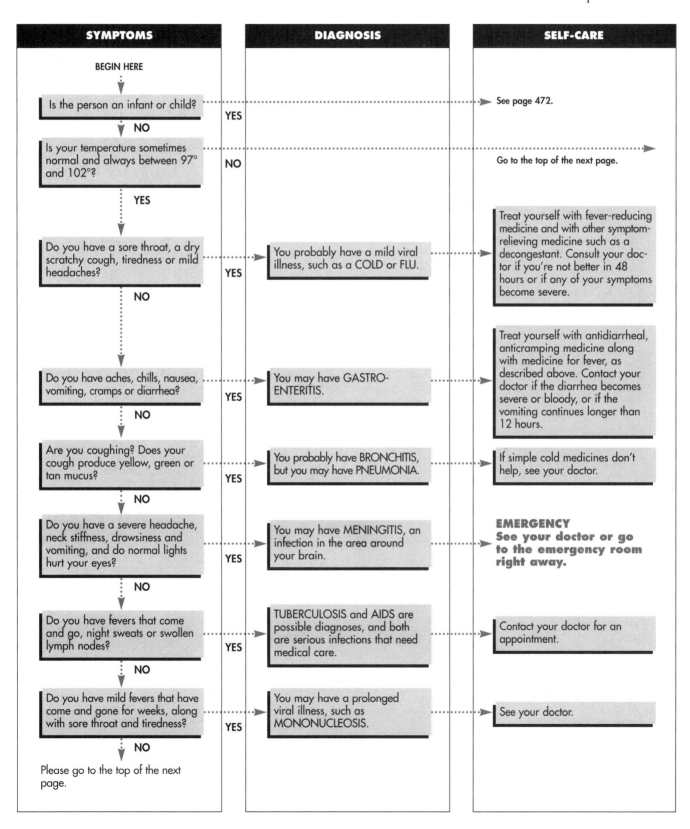

| SYMPTOMS | DIAGNOSIS | SELF-CARE |
|---|---|---|

BEGIN HERE

Is the person an infant or child? — **YES** → See page 472.

↓ **NO**

Is your temperature sometimes normal and always between 97° and 102°? — **NO** → Go to the top of the next page.

↓ **YES**

Do you have a sore throat, a dry scratchy cough, tiredness or mild headaches? — **YES** → You probably have a mild viral illness, such as a COLD or FLU. → Treat yourself with fever-reducing medicine and with other symptom-relieving medicine such as a decongestant. Consult your doctor if you're not better in 48 hours or if any of your symptoms become severe.

↓ **NO**

Do you have aches, chills, nausea, vomiting, cramps or diarrhea? — **YES** → You may have GASTRO-ENTERITIS. → Treat yourself with antidiarrheal, anticramping medicine along with medicine for fever, as described above. Contact your doctor if the diarrhea becomes severe or bloody, or if the vomiting continues longer than 12 hours.

↓ **NO**

Are you coughing? Does your cough produce yellow, green or tan mucus? — **YES** → You probably have BRONCHITIS, but you may have PNEUMONIA. → If simple cold medicines don't help, see your doctor.

↓ **NO**

Do you have a severe headache, neck stiffness, drowsiness and vomiting, and do normal lights hurt your eyes? — **YES** → You may have MENINGITIS, an infection in the area around your brain. → **EMERGENCY See your doctor or go to the emergency room right away.**

↓ **NO**

Do you have fevers that come and go, night sweats or swollen lymph nodes? — **YES** → TUBERCULOSIS and AIDS are possible diagnoses, and both are serious infections that need medical care. → Contact your doctor for an appointment.

↓ **NO**

Do you have mild fevers that have come and gone for weeks, along with sore throat and tiredness? — **YES** → You may have a prolonged viral illness, such as MONONUCLEOSIS. → See your doctor.

↓ **NO**

Please go to the top of the next page.

# TOPIC 3 Fever

continued.

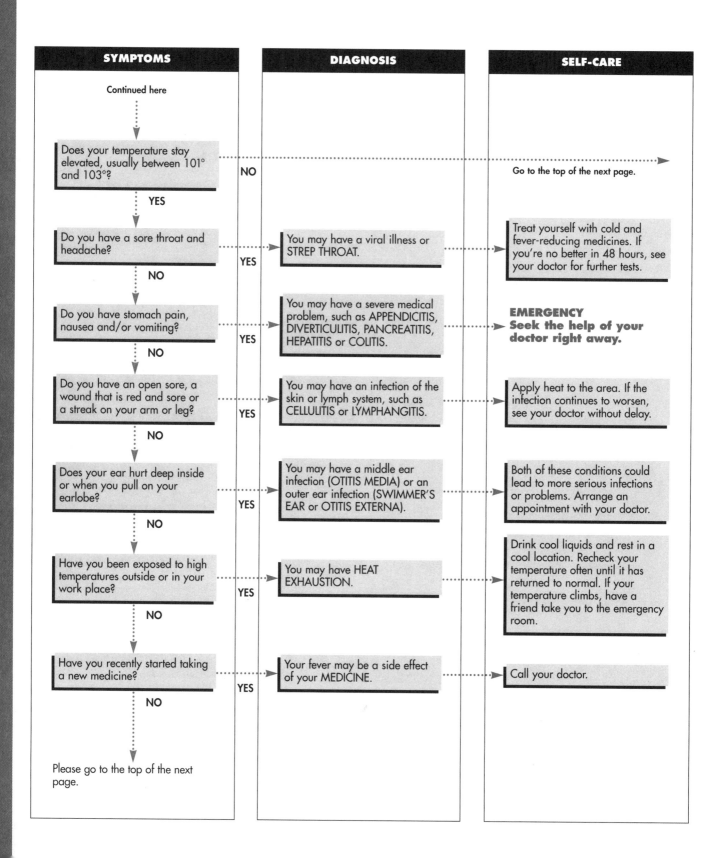

| SYMPTOMS | DIAGNOSIS | SELF-CARE |
|---|---|---|

Continued here

Does your temperature stay elevated, usually between 101° and 103°?

**NO** → Go to the top of the next page.

**YES**

Do you have a sore throat and headache?

**YES** → You may have a viral illness or STREP THROAT. → Treat yourself with cold and fever-reducing medicines. If you're no better in 48 hours, see your doctor for further tests.

**NO**

Do you have stomach pain, nausea and/or vomiting?

**YES** → You may have a severe medical problem, such as APPENDICITIS, DIVERTICULITIS, PANCREATITIS, HEPATITIS or COLITIS. → **EMERGENCY Seek the help of your doctor right away.**

**NO**

Do you have an open sore, a wound that is red and sore or a streak on your arm or leg?

**YES** → You may have an infection of the skin or lymph system, such as CELLULITIS or LYMPHANGITIS. → Apply heat to the area. If the infection continues to worsen, see your doctor without delay.

**NO**

Does your ear hurt deep inside or when you pull on your earlobe?

**YES** → You may have a middle ear infection (OTITIS MEDIA) or an outer ear infection (SWIMMER'S EAR or OTITIS EXTERNA). → Both of these conditions could lead to more serious infections or problems. Arrange an appointment with your doctor.

**NO**

Have you been exposed to high temperatures outside or in your work place?

**YES** → You may have HEAT EXHAUSTION. → Drink cool liquids and rest in a cool location. Recheck your temperature often until it has returned to normal. If your temperature climbs, have a friend take you to the emergency room.

**NO**

Have you recently started taking a new medicine?

**YES** → Your fever may be a side effect of your MEDICINE. → Call your doctor.

**NO**

Please go to the top of the next page.

**TOPIC 3** Fever

continued.

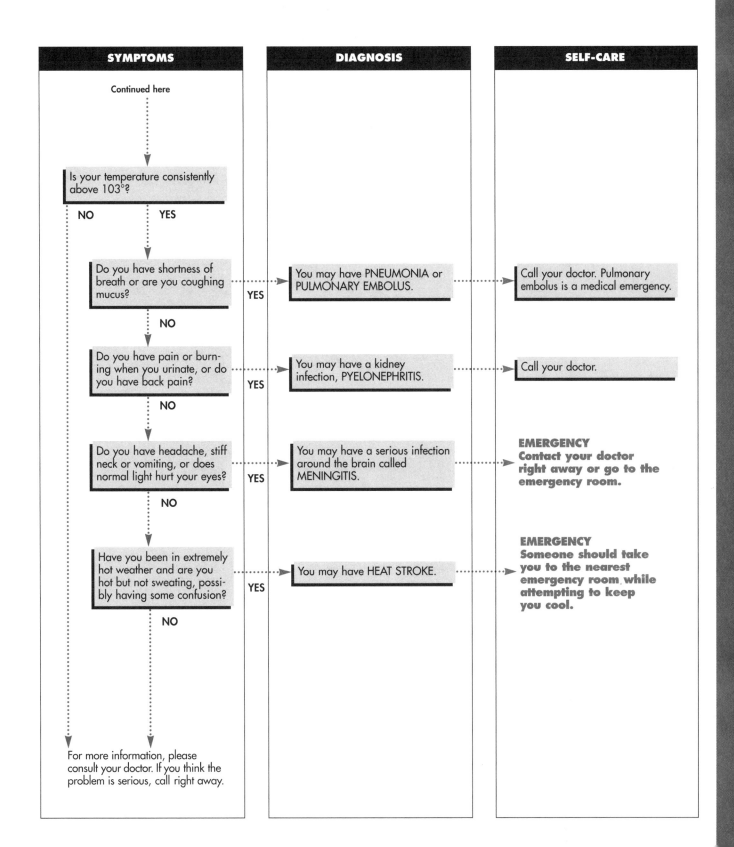

| SYMPTOMS | DIAGNOSIS | SELF-CARE |
|---|---|---|

Continued here

Is your temperature consistently above 103°?

NO     YES

Do you have shortness of breath or are you coughing mucus?

YES → You may have PNEUMONIA or PULMONARY EMBOLUS. → Call your doctor. Pulmonary embolus is a medical emergency.

NO

Do you have pain or burning when you urinate, or do you have back pain?

YES → You may have a kidney infection, PYELONEPHRITIS. → Call your doctor.

NO

Do you have headache, stiff neck or vomiting, or does normal light hurt your eyes?

YES → You may have a serious infection around the brain called MENINGITIS. → **EMERGENCY Contact your doctor right away or go to the emergency room.**

NO

Have you been in extremely hot weather and are you hot but not sweating, possibly having some confusion?

YES → You may have HEAT STROKE. → **EMERGENCY Someone should take you to the nearest emergency room, while attempting to keep you cool.**

NO

For more information, please consult your doctor. If you think the problem is serious, call right away.

# TOPIC 4 Fever in Infants and Children

Checking temperatures rectally or axillarily (under the arm) is necessary in small children because they're not able to hold a thermometer in their mouth. Axillary temperatures are generally 1° lower than rectal temperatures. Temperatures above 105° (oral) can be dangerous, and immediate action must be taken.

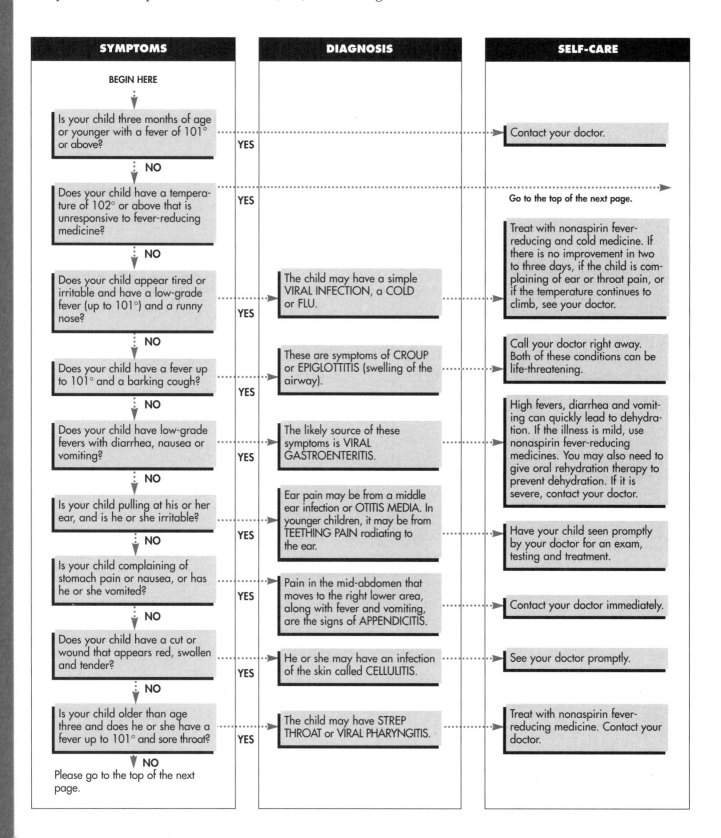

**SYMPTOMS**

BEGIN HERE

Is your child three months of age or younger with a fever of 101° or above? — **YES**

NO

Does your child have a temperature of 102° or above that is unresponsive to fever-reducing medicine? — **YES**

NO

Does your child appear tired or irritable and have a low-grade fever (up to 101°) and a runny nose? — **YES**

NO

Does your child have a fever up to 101° and a barking cough? — **YES**

NO

Does your child have low-grade fevers with diarrhea, nausea or vomiting? — **YES**

NO

Is your child pulling at his or her ear, and is he or she irritable? — **YES**

NO

Is your child complaining of stomach pain or nausea, or has he or she vomited? — **YES**

NO

Does your child have a cut or wound that appears red, swollen and tender? — **YES**

NO

Is your child older than age three and does he or she have a fever up to 101° and sore throat? — **YES**

NO

Please go to the top of the next page.

**DIAGNOSIS**

The child may have a simple VIRAL INFECTION, a COLD or FLU.

These are symptoms of CROUP or EPIGLOTTITIS (swelling of the airway).

The likely source of these symptoms is VIRAL GASTROENTERITIS.

Ear pain may be from a middle ear infection or OTITIS MEDIA. In younger children, it may be from TEETHING PAIN radiating to the ear.

Pain in the mid-abdomen that moves to the right lower area, along with fever and vomiting, are the signs of APPENDICITIS.

He or she may have an infection of the skin called CELLULITIS.

The child may have STREP THROAT or VIRAL PHARYNGITIS.

**SELF-CARE**

Contact your doctor.

Go to the top of the next page.

Treat with nonaspirin fever-reducing and cold medicine. If there is no improvement in two to three days, if the child is complaining of ear or throat pain, or if the temperature continues to climb, see your doctor.

Call your doctor right away. Both of these conditions can be life-threatening.

High fevers, diarrhea and vomiting can quickly lead to dehydration. If the illness is mild, use nonaspirin fever-reducing medicines. You may also need to give oral rehydration therapy to prevent dehydration. If it is severe, contact your doctor.

Have your child seen promptly by your doctor for an exam, testing and treatment.

Contact your doctor immediately.

See your doctor promptly.

Treat with nonaspirin fever-reducing medicine. Contact your doctor.

## TOPIC 4 Fever in Infants and Children

continued.

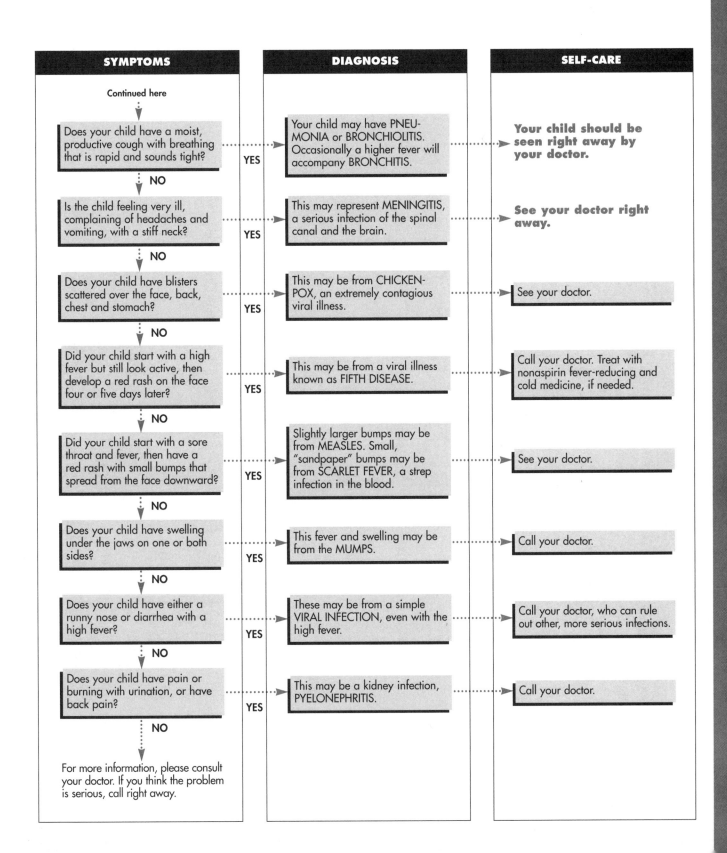

| SYMPTOMS | DIAGNOSIS | SELF-CARE |
|---|---|---|
| Continued here | | |
| Does your child have a moist, productive cough with breathing that is rapid and sounds tight? **YES** | Your child may have PNEUMONIA or BRONCHIOLITIS. Occasionally a higher fever will accompany BRONCHITIS. | **Your child should be seen right away by your doctor.** |
| **NO** | | |
| Is the child feeling very ill, complaining of headaches and vomiting, with a stiff neck? **YES** | This may represent MENINGITIS, a serious infection of the spinal canal and the brain. | **See your doctor right away.** |
| **NO** | | |
| Does your child have blisters scattered over the face, back, chest and stomach? **YES** | This may be from CHICKENPOX, an extremely contagious viral illness. | See your doctor. |
| **NO** | | |
| Did your child start with a high fever but still look active, then develop a red rash on the face four or five days later? **YES** | This may be from a viral illness known as FIFTH DISEASE. | Call your doctor. Treat with nonaspirin fever-reducing and cold medicine, if needed. |
| **NO** | | |
| Did your child start with a sore throat and fever, then have a red rash with small bumps that spread from the face downward? **YES** | Slightly larger bumps may be from MEASLES. Small, "sandpaper" bumps may be from SCARLET FEVER, a strep infection in the blood. | See your doctor. |
| **NO** | | |
| Does your child have swelling under the jaws on one or both sides? **YES** | This fever and swelling may be from the MUMPS. | Call your doctor. |
| **NO** | | |
| Does your child have either a runny nose or diarrhea with a high fever? **YES** | These may be from a simple VIRAL INFECTION, even with the high fever. | Call your doctor, who can rule out other, more serious infections. |
| **NO** | | |
| Does your child have pain or burning with urination, or have back pain? **YES** | This may be a kidney infection, PYELONEPHRITIS. | Call your doctor. |
| **NO** | | |
| For more information, please consult your doctor. If you think the problem is serious, call right away. | | |

# TOPIC 5 Eye Problems

Pain, redness and loss of vision are important problems that require medical attention.
Eye problems can warn us of other health problems as well.

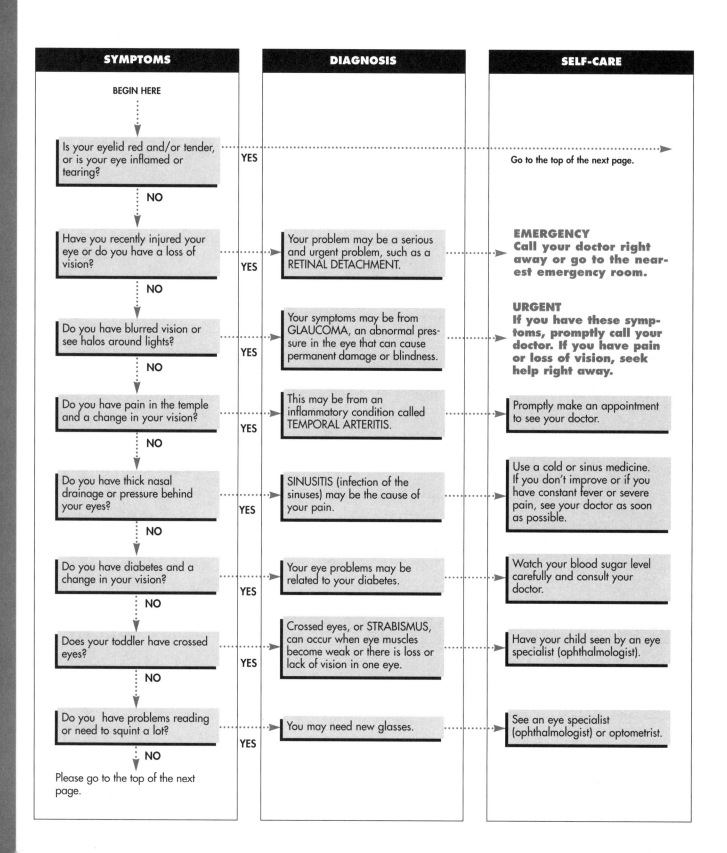

| SYMPTOMS | DIAGNOSIS | SELF-CARE |
|---|---|---|
| **BEGIN HERE** | | |
| Is your eyelid red and/or tender, or is your eye inflamed or tearing? — **YES** | | Go to the top of the next page. |
| **NO** | | |
| Have you recently injured your eye or do you have a loss of vision? — **YES** | Your problem may be a serious and urgent problem, such as a RETINAL DETACHMENT. | **EMERGENCY** Call your doctor right away or go to the nearest emergency room. |
| **NO** | | |
| Do you have blurred vision or see halos around lights? — **YES** | Your symptoms may be from GLAUCOMA, an abnormal pressure in the eye that can cause permanent damage or blindness. | **URGENT** If you have these symptoms, promptly call your doctor. If you have pain or loss of vision, seek help right away. |
| **NO** | | |
| Do you have pain in the temple and a change in your vision? — **YES** | This may be from an inflammatory condition called TEMPORAL ARTERITIS. | Promptly make an appointment to see your doctor. |
| **NO** | | |
| Do you have thick nasal drainage or pressure behind your eyes? — **YES** | SINUSITIS (infection of the sinuses) may be the cause of your pain. | Use a cold or sinus medicine. If you don't improve or if you have constant fever or severe pain, see your doctor as soon as possible. |
| **NO** | | |
| Do you have diabetes and a change in your vision? — **YES** | Your eye problems may be related to your diabetes. | Watch your blood sugar level carefully and consult your doctor. |
| **NO** | | |
| Does your toddler have crossed eyes? — **YES** | Crossed eyes, or STRABISMUS, can occur when eye muscles become weak or there is loss or lack of vision in one eye. | Have your child seen by an eye specialist (ophthalmologist). |
| **NO** | | |
| Do you have problems reading or need to squint a lot? — **YES** | You may need new glasses. | See an eye specialist (ophthalmologist) or optometrist. |
| **NO** | | |
| Please go to the top of the next page. | | |

## TOPIC 5 Eye Problems

continued.

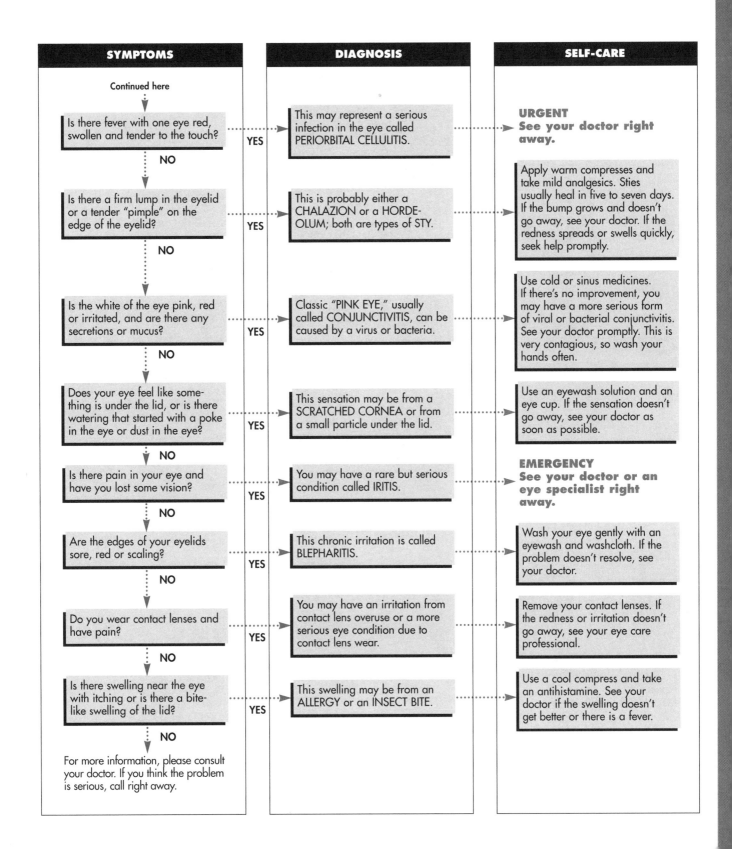

| SYMPTOMS | DIAGNOSIS | SELF-CARE |
|---|---|---|
| Continued here | | |
| Is there fever with one eye red, swollen and tender to the touch? **YES** | This may represent a serious infection in the eye called PERIORBITAL CELLULITIS. | **URGENT** **See your doctor right away.** |
| **NO** | | |
| Is there a firm lump in the eyelid or a tender "pimple" on the edge of the eyelid? **YES** | This is probably either a CHALAZION or a HORDE-OLUM; both are types of STY. | Apply warm compresses and take mild analgesics. Sties usually heal in five to seven days. If the bump grows and doesn't go away, see your doctor. If the redness spreads or swells quickly, seek help promptly. |
| **NO** | | |
| Is the white of the eye pink, red or irritated, and are there any secretions or mucus? **YES** | Classic "PINK EYE," usually called CONJUNCTIVITIS, can be caused by a virus or bacteria. | Use cold or sinus medicines. If there's no improvement, you may have a more serious form of viral or bacterial conjunctivitis. See your doctor promptly. This is very contagious, so wash your hands often. |
| **NO** | | |
| Does your eye feel like something is under the lid, or is there watering that started with a poke in the eye or dust in the eye? **YES** | This sensation may be from a SCRATCHED CORNEA or from a small particle under the lid. | Use an eyewash solution and an eye cup. If the sensation doesn't go away, see your doctor as soon as possible. |
| **NO** | | |
| Is there pain in your eye and have you lost some vision? **YES** | You may have a rare but serious condition called IRITIS. | **EMERGENCY** **See your doctor or an eye specialist right away.** |
| **NO** | | |
| Are the edges of your eyelids sore, red or scaling? **YES** | This chronic irritation is called BLEPHARITIS. | Wash your eye gently with an eyewash and washcloth. If the problem doesn't resolve, see your doctor. |
| **NO** | | |
| Do you wear contact lenses and have pain? **YES** | You may have an irritation from contact lens overuse or a more serious eye condition due to contact lens wear. | Remove your contact lenses. If the redness or irritation doesn't go away, see your eye care professional. |
| **NO** | | |
| Is there swelling near the eye with itching or is there a bite-like swelling of the lid? **YES** | This swelling may be from an ALLERGY or an INSECT BITE. | Use a cool compress and take an antihistamine. See your doctor if the swelling doesn't get better or there is a fever. |
| **NO** | | |
| For more information, please consult your doctor. If you think the problem is serious, call right away. | | |

# TOPIC 6 Facial Swelling

This chart helps distinguish various types of swelling on the face.

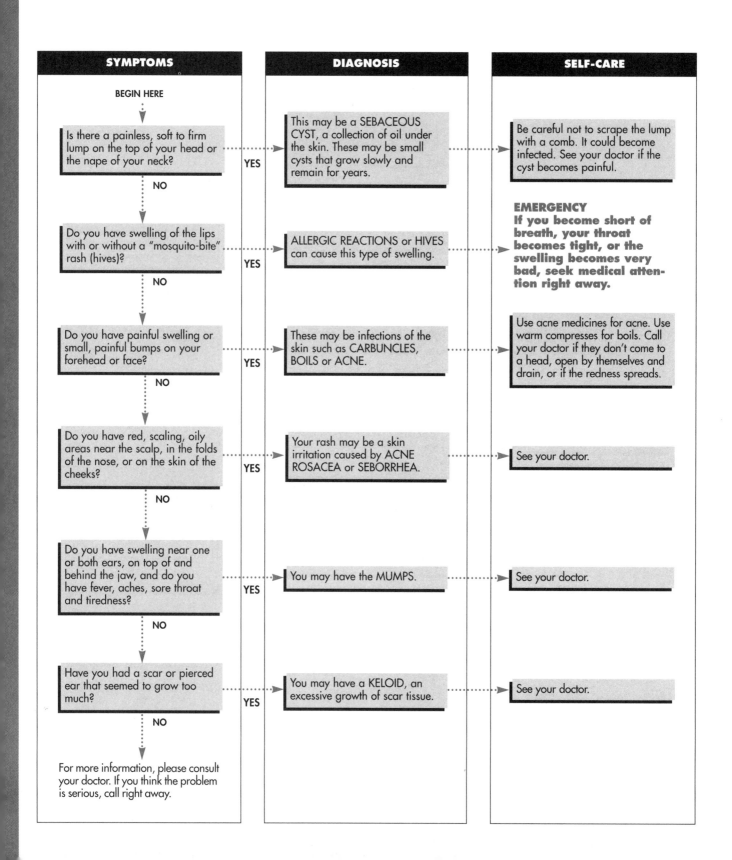

| SYMPTOMS | DIAGNOSIS | SELF-CARE |
|---|---|---|
| **BEGIN HERE** | | |
| Is there a painless, soft to firm lump on the top of your head or the nape of your neck? — **YES** | This may be a SEBACEOUS CYST, a collection of oil under the skin. These may be small cysts that grow slowly and remain for years. | Be careful not to scrape the lump with a comb. It could become infected. See your doctor if the cyst becomes painful. |
| **NO** | | **EMERGENCY** |
| Do you have swelling of the lips with or without a "mosquito-bite" rash (hives)? — **YES** | ALLERGIC REACTIONS or HIVES can cause this type of swelling. | **If you become short of breath, your throat becomes tight, or the swelling becomes very bad, seek medical attention right away.** |
| **NO** | | |
| Do you have painful swelling or small, painful bumps on your forehead or face? — **YES** | These may be infections of the skin such as CARBUNCLES, BOILS or ACNE. | Use acne medicines for acne. Use warm compresses for boils. Call your doctor if they don't come to a head, open by themselves and drain, or if the redness spreads. |
| **NO** | | |
| Do you have red, scaling, oily areas near the scalp, in the folds of the nose, or on the skin of the cheeks? — **YES** | Your rash may be a skin irritation caused by ACNE ROSACEA or SEBORRHEA. | See your doctor. |
| **NO** | | |
| Do you have swelling near one or both ears, on top of and behind the jaw, and do you have fever, aches, sore throat and tiredness? — **YES** | You may have the MUMPS. | See your doctor. |
| **NO** | | |
| Have you had a scar or pierced ear that seemed to grow too much? — **YES** | You may have a KELOID, an excessive growth of scar tissue. | See your doctor. |
| **NO** | | |
| For more information, please consult your doctor. If you think the problem is serious, call right away. | | |

## TOPIC 7 Ear Problems

Pain or drainage from the ear may mean an infection. But pain in or around the ear isn't always an infection of the middle ear.

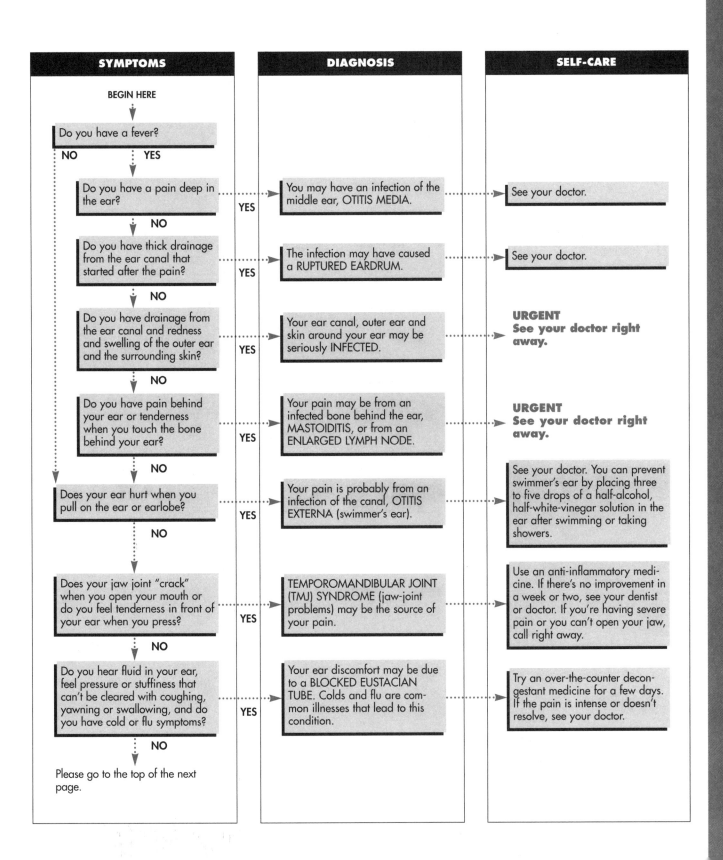

| SYMPTOMS | DIAGNOSIS | SELF-CARE |
|---|---|---|
| BEGIN HERE | | |
| Do you have a fever? | | |
| NO / YES | | |
| Do you have a pain deep in the ear? — YES | You may have an infection of the middle ear, OTITIS MEDIA. | See your doctor. |
| NO | | |
| Do you have thick drainage from the ear canal that started after the pain? — YES | The infection may have caused a RUPTURED EARDRUM. | See your doctor. |
| NO | | |
| Do you have drainage from the ear canal and redness and swelling of the outer ear and the surrounding skin? — YES | Your ear canal, outer ear and skin around your ear may be seriously INFECTED. | URGENT See your doctor right away. |
| NO | | |
| Do you have pain behind your ear or tenderness when you touch the bone behind your ear? — YES | Your pain may be from an infected bone behind the ear, MASTOIDITIS, or from an ENLARGED LYMPH NODE. | URGENT See your doctor right away. |
| NO | | |
| Does your ear hurt when you pull on the ear or earlobe? — YES | Your pain is probably from an infection of the canal, OTITIS EXTERNA (swimmer's ear). | See your doctor. You can prevent swimmer's ear by placing three to five drops of a half-alcohol, half-white-vinegar solution in the ear after swimming or taking showers. |
| NO | | |
| Does your jaw joint "crack" when you open your mouth or do you feel tenderness in front of your ear when you press? — YES | TEMPOROMANDIBULAR JOINT (TMJ) SYNDROME (jaw-joint problems) may be the source of your pain. | Use an anti-inflammatory medicine. If there's no improvement in a week or two, see your dentist or doctor. If you're having severe pain or you can't open your jaw, call right away. |
| NO | | |
| Do you hear fluid in your ear, feel pressure or stuffiness that can't be cleared with coughing, yawning or swallowing, and do you have cold or flu symptoms? — YES | Your ear discomfort may be due to a BLOCKED EUSTACIAN TUBE. Colds and flu are common illnesses that lead to this condition. | Try an over-the-counter decongestant medicine for a few days. If the pain is intense or doesn't resolve, see your doctor. |
| NO | | |
| Please go to the top of the next page. | | |

# TOPIC 7  Ear Problems

continued.

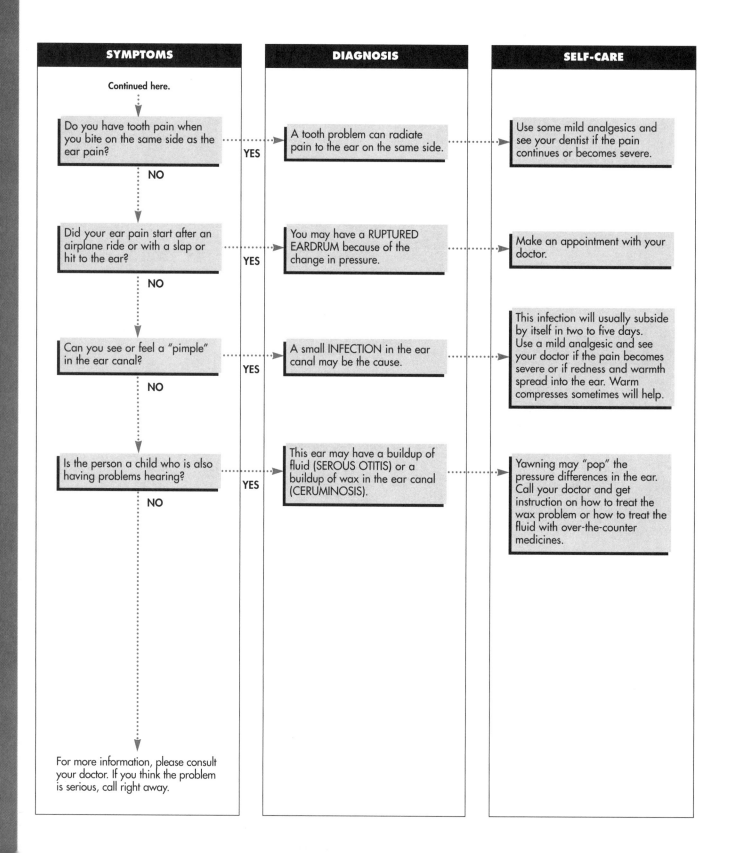

| SYMPTOMS | DIAGNOSIS | SELF-CARE |
|---|---|---|

**Continued here.**

Do you have tooth pain when you bite on the same side as the ear pain?

**YES** → A tooth problem can radiate pain to the ear on the same side. → Use some mild analgesics and see your dentist if the pain continues or becomes severe.

**NO**

Did your ear pain start after an airplane ride or with a slap or hit to the ear?

**YES** → You may have a RUPTURED EARDRUM because of the change in pressure. → Make an appointment with your doctor.

**NO**

Can you see or feel a "pimple" in the ear canal?

**YES** → A small INFECTION in the ear canal may be the cause. → This infection will usually subside by itself in two to five days. Use a mild analgesic and see your doctor if the pain becomes severe or if redness and warmth spread into the ear. Warm compresses sometimes will help.

**NO**

Is the person a child who is also having problems hearing?

**YES** → This ear may have a buildup of fluid (SEROUS OTITIS) or a buildup of wax in the ear canal (CERUMINOSIS). → Yawning may "pop" the pressure differences in the ear. Call your doctor and get instruction on how to treat the wax problem or how to treat the fluid with over-the-counter medicines.

**NO**

For more information, please consult your doctor. If you think the problem is serious, call right away.

# TOPIC 8 Hearing Problems

Losses in the ability to hear or discriminate sounds is a common disability.
This flow chart will help direct you if hearing loss is a problem for you or a family member.

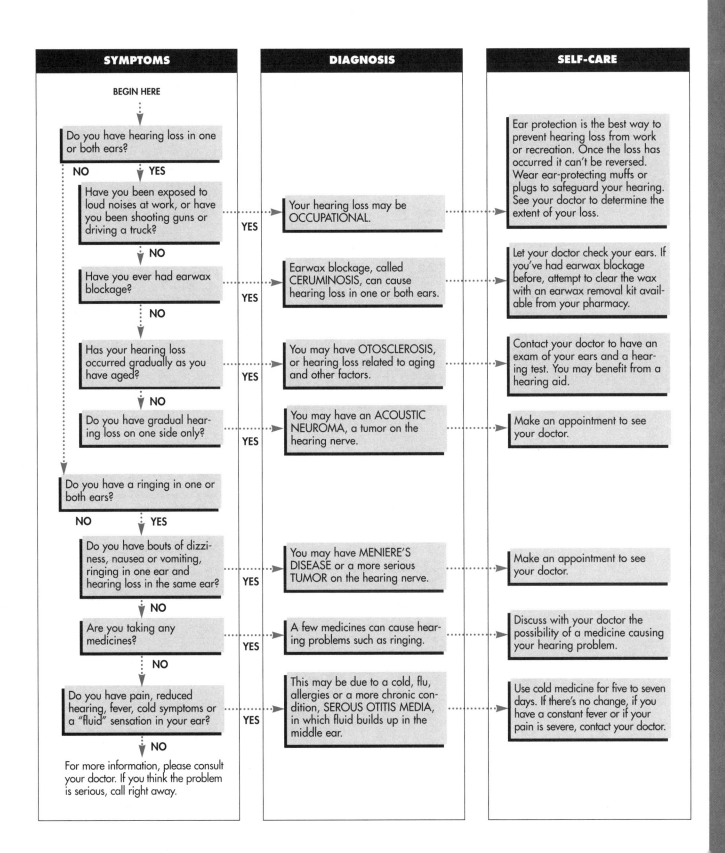

| SYMPTOMS | DIAGNOSIS | SELF-CARE |
|---|---|---|

**BEGIN HERE**

Do you have hearing loss in one or both ears?

NO     YES

Have you been exposed to loud noises at work, or have you been shooting guns or driving a truck? — YES → Your hearing loss may be OCCUPATIONAL. → Ear protection is the best way to prevent hearing loss from work or recreation. Once the loss has occurred it can't be reversed. Wear ear-protecting muffs or plugs to safeguard your hearing. See your doctor to determine the extent of your loss.

NO

Have you ever had earwax blockage? — YES → Earwax blockage, called CERUMINOSIS, can cause hearing loss in one or both ears. → Let your doctor check your ears. If you've had earwax blockage before, attempt to clear the wax with an earwax removal kit available from your pharmacy.

NO

Has your hearing loss occurred gradually as you have aged? — YES → You may have OTOSCLEROSIS, or hearing loss related to aging and other factors. → Contact your doctor to have an exam of your ears and a hearing test. You may benefit from a hearing aid.

NO

Do you have gradual hearing loss on one side only? — YES → You may have an ACOUSTIC NEUROMA, a tumor on the hearing nerve. → Make an appointment to see your doctor.

Do you have a ringing in one or both ears?

NO     YES

Do you have bouts of dizziness, nausea or vomiting, ringing in one ear and hearing loss in the same ear? — YES → You may have MENIERE'S DISEASE or a more serious TUMOR on the hearing nerve. → Make an appointment to see your doctor.

NO

Are you taking any medicines? — YES → A few medicines can cause hearing problems such as ringing. → Discuss with your doctor the possibility of a medicine causing your hearing problem.

NO

Do you have pain, reduced hearing, fever, cold symptoms or a "fluid" sensation in your ear? — YES → This may be due to a cold, flu, allergies or a more chronic condition, SEROUS OTITIS MEDIA, in which fluid builds up in the middle ear. → Use cold medicine for five to seven days. If there's no change, if you have a constant fever or if your pain is severe, contact your doctor.

NO

For more information, please consult your doctor. If you think the problem is serious, call right away.

# TOPIC 9 Mouth Problems

Mouth problems are very common. For more information, check Topic 15.

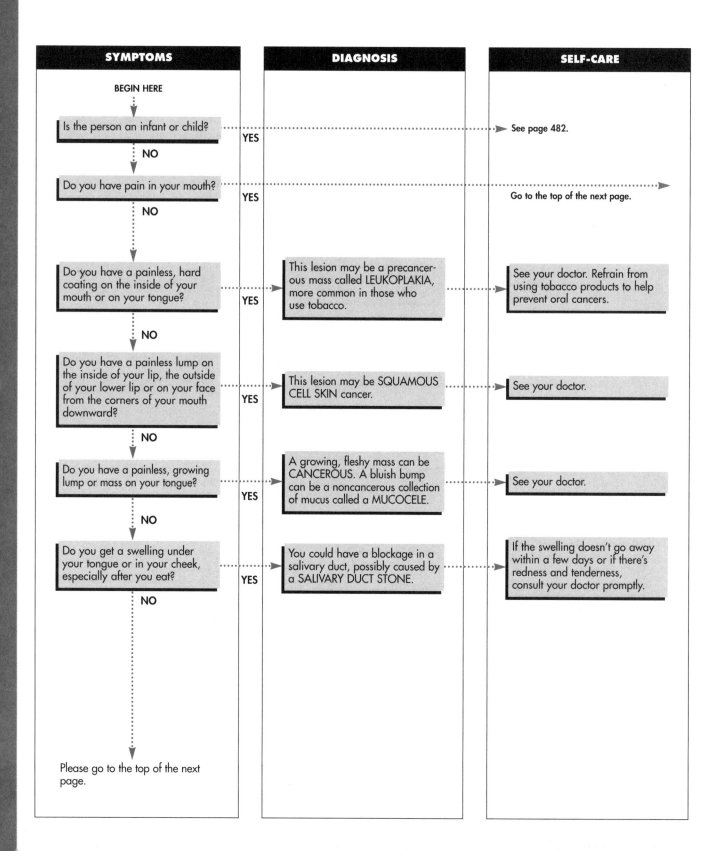

| SYMPTOMS | DIAGNOSIS | SELF-CARE |
|---|---|---|

**BEGIN HERE**

Is the person an infant or child? — **YES** ⟶ See page 482.

**NO**

Do you have pain in your mouth? — **YES** ⟶ Go to the top of the next page.

**NO**

Do you have a painless, hard coating on the inside of your mouth or on your tongue? — **YES** ⟶ This lesion may be a precancerous mass called LEUKOPLAKIA, more common in those who use tobacco. ⟶ See your doctor. Refrain from using tobacco products to help prevent oral cancers.

**NO**

Do you have a painless lump on the inside of your lip, the outside of your lower lip or on your face from the corners of your mouth downward? — **YES** ⟶ This lesion may be SQUAMOUS CELL SKIN cancer. ⟶ See your doctor.

**NO**

Do you have a painless, growing lump or mass on your tongue? — **YES** ⟶ A growing, fleshy mass can be CANCEROUS. A bluish bump can be a noncancerous collection of mucus called a MUCOCELE. ⟶ See your doctor.

**NO**

Do you get a swelling under your tongue or in your cheek, especially after you eat? — **YES** ⟶ You could have a blockage in a salivary duct, possibly caused by a SALIVARY DUCT STONE. ⟶ If the swelling doesn't go away within a few days or if there's redness and tenderness, consult your doctor promptly.

**NO**

Please go to the top of the next page.

**TOPIC 9** Mouth Problems

continued.

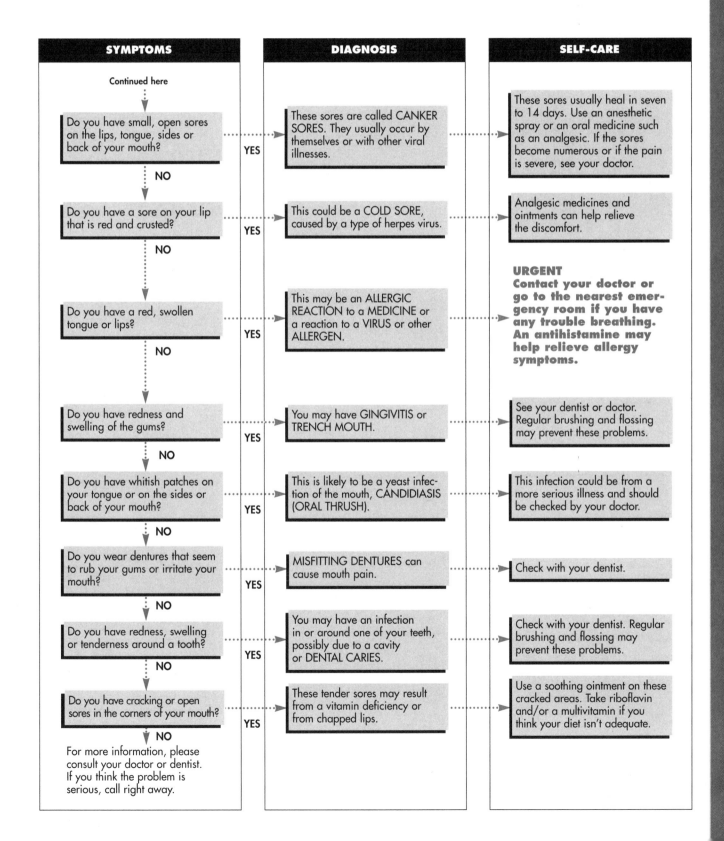

| SYMPTOMS | DIAGNOSIS | SELF-CARE |
|---|---|---|

Continued here

Do you have small, open sores on the lips, tongue, sides or back of your mouth?
**YES** → These sores are called CANKER SORES. They usually occur by themselves or with other viral illnesses. → These sores usually heal in seven to 14 days. Use an anesthetic spray or an oral medicine such as an analgesic. If the sores become numerous or if the pain is severe, see your doctor.

**NO**

Do you have a sore on your lip that is red and crusted?
**YES** → This could be a COLD SORE, caused by a type of herpes virus. → Analgesic medicines and ointments can help relieve the discomfort.

**NO**

Do you have a red, swollen tongue or lips?
**YES** → This may be an ALLERGIC REACTION to a MEDICINE or a reaction to a VIRUS or other ALLERGEN. → **URGENT Contact your doctor or go to the nearest emergency room if you have any trouble breathing. An antihistamine may help relieve allergy symptoms.**

**NO**

Do you have redness and swelling of the gums?
**YES** → You may have GINGIVITIS or TRENCH MOUTH. → See your dentist or doctor. Regular brushing and flossing may prevent these problems.

**NO**

Do you have whitish patches on your tongue or on the sides or back of your mouth?
**YES** → This is likely to be a yeast infection of the mouth, CANDIDIASIS (ORAL THRUSH). → This infection could be from a more serious illness and should be checked by your doctor.

**NO**

Do you wear dentures that seem to rub your gums or irritate your mouth?
**YES** → MISFITTING DENTURES can cause mouth pain. → Check with your dentist.

**NO**

Do you have redness, swelling or tenderness around a tooth?
**YES** → You may have an infection in or around one of your teeth, possibly due to a cavity or DENTAL CARIES. → Check with your dentist. Regular brushing and flossing may prevent these problems.

**NO**

Do you have cracking or open sores in the corners of your mouth?
**YES** → These tender sores may result from a vitamin deficiency or from chapped lips. → Use a soothing ointment on these cracked areas. Take riboflavin and/or a multivitamin if you think your diet isn't adequate.

**NO**

For more information, please consult your doctor or dentist. If you think the problem is serious, call right away.

# TOPIC 10 Mouth Problems in Infants and Children

Many different causes exist for a child's sore mouth. This chart will help you to decide how to best care for this problem.

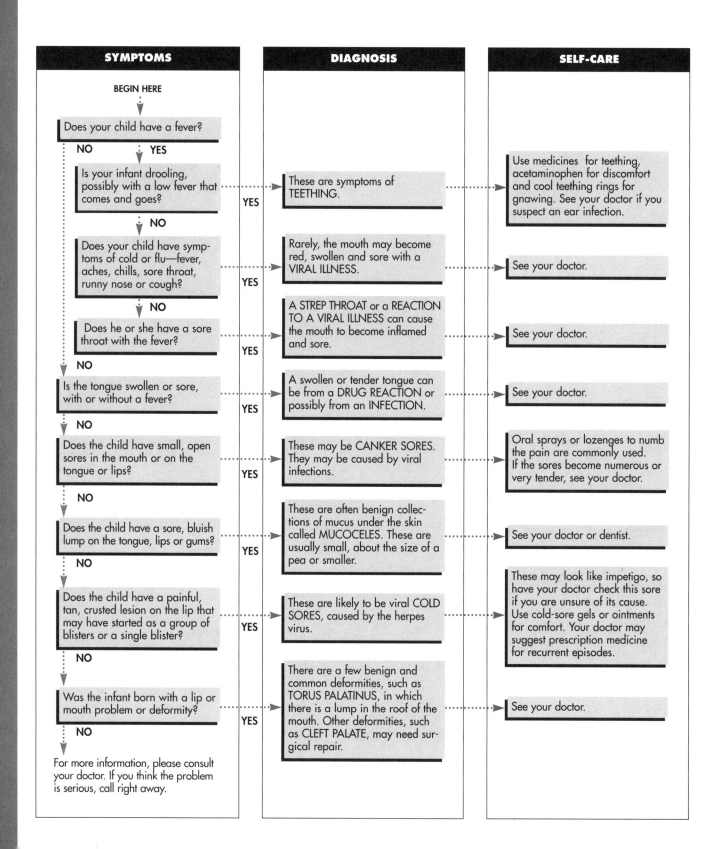

| SYMPTOMS | DIAGNOSIS | SELF-CARE |
|---|---|---|
| **BEGIN HERE** | | |
| Does your child have a fever? | | |
| NO / YES | | |
| Is your infant drooling, possibly with a low fever that comes and goes? — **YES** | These are symptoms of TEETHING. | Use medicines for teething, acetaminophen for discomfort and cool teething rings for gnawing. See your doctor if you suspect an ear infection. |
| NO | | |
| Does your child have symptoms of cold or flu—fever, aches, chills, sore throat, runny nose or cough? **YES** | Rarely, the mouth may become red, swollen and sore with a VIRAL ILLNESS. | See your doctor. |
| NO | | |
| Does he or she have a sore throat with the fever? **YES** | A STREP THROAT or a REACTION TO A VIRAL ILLNESS can cause the mouth to become inflamed and sore. | See your doctor. |
| NO | | |
| Is the tongue swollen or sore, with or without a fever? **YES** | A swollen or tender tongue can be from a DRUG REACTION or possibly from an INFECTION. | See your doctor. |
| NO | | |
| Does the child have small, open sores in the mouth or on the tongue or lips? **YES** | These may be CANKER SORES. They may be caused by viral infections. | Oral sprays or lozenges to numb the pain are commonly used. If the sores become numerous or very tender, see your doctor. |
| NO | | |
| Does the child have a sore, bluish lump on the tongue, lips or gums? **YES** | These are often benign collections of mucus under the skin called MUCOCELES. These are usually small, about the size of a pea or smaller. | See your doctor or dentist. |
| NO | | |
| Does the child have a painful, tan, crusted lesion on the lip that may have started as a group of blisters or a single blister? **YES** | These are likely to be viral COLD SORES, caused by the herpes virus. | These may look like impetigo, so have your doctor check this sore if you are unsure of its cause. Use cold-sore gels or ointments for comfort. Your doctor may suggest prescription medicine for recurrent episodes. |
| NO | | |
| Was the infant born with a lip or mouth problem or deformity? **YES** | There are a few benign and common deformities, such as TORUS PALATINUS, in which there is a lump in the roof of the mouth. Other deformities, such as CLEFT PALATE, may need surgical repair. | See your doctor. |
| NO | | |
| For more information, please consult your doctor. If you think the problem is serious, call right away. | | |

## TOPIC 11 Tooth Problems

A tooth that causes ongoing pain can be due to a serious problem.
Use this chart to determine if an immediate exam is needed.

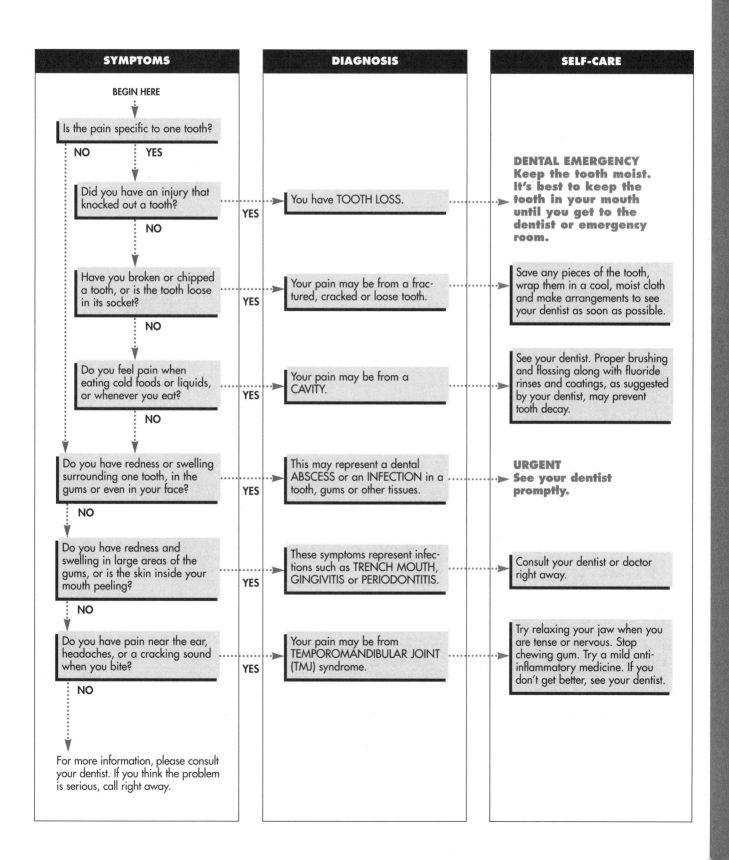

| SYMPTOMS | DIAGNOSIS | SELF-CARE |
|---|---|---|

BEGIN HERE

Is the pain specific to one tooth? — NO / YES

Did you have an injury that knocked out a tooth? — YES → You have TOOTH LOSS. → **DENTAL EMERGENCY Keep the tooth moist. It's best to keep the tooth in your mouth until you get to the dentist or emergency room.**

NO

Have you broken or chipped a tooth, or is the tooth loose in its socket? — YES → Your pain may be from a fractured, cracked or loose tooth. → Save any pieces of the tooth, wrap them in a cool, moist cloth and make arrangements to see your dentist as soon as possible.

NO

Do you feel pain when eating cold foods or liquids, or whenever you eat? — YES → Your pain may be from a CAVITY. → See your dentist. Proper brushing and flossing along with fluoride rinses and coatings, as suggested by your dentist, may prevent tooth decay.

NO

Do you have redness or swelling surrounding one tooth, in the gums or even in your face? — YES → This may represent a dental ABSCESS or an INFECTION in a tooth, gums or other tissues. → **URGENT See your dentist promptly.**

NO

Do you have redness and swelling in large areas of the gums, or is the skin inside your mouth peeling? — YES → These symptoms represent infections such as TRENCH MOUTH, GINGIVITIS or PERIODONTITIS. → Consult your dentist or doctor right away.

NO

Do you have pain near the ear, headaches, or a cracking sound when you bite? — YES → Your pain may be from TEMPOROMANDIBULAR JOINT (TMJ) syndrome. → Try relaxing your jaw when you are tense or nervous. Stop chewing gum. Try a mild anti-inflammatory medicine. If you don't get better, see your dentist.

NO

For more information, please consult your dentist. If you think the problem is serious, call right away.

# TOPIC 12 Feeding Problems in Infants and Children

Parents are often frustrated when a child has problems with feedings, especially if he or she wakes often or cries during the night. Follow this chart for information and care suggestions for infant feeding problems.

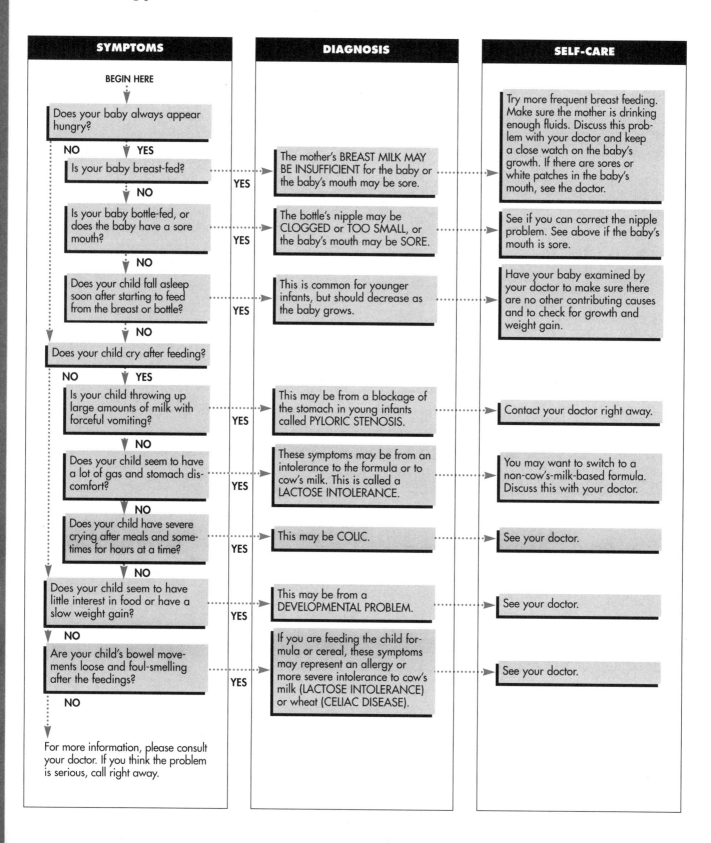

**SYMPTOMS**

BEGIN HERE

Does your baby always appear hungry?

NO — YES

Is your baby breast-fed?

NO

Is your baby bottle-fed, or does the baby have a sore mouth?

NO

Does your child fall asleep soon after starting to feed from the breast or bottle?

NO

Does your child cry after feeding?

NO — YES

Is your child throwing up large amounts of milk with forceful vomiting?

NO

Does your child seem to have a lot of gas and stomach discomfort?

NO

Does your child have severe crying after meals and sometimes for hours at a time?

NO

Does your child seem to have little interest in food or have a slow weight gain?

NO

Are your child's bowel movements loose and foul-smelling after the feedings?

NO

For more information, please consult your doctor. If you think the problem is serious, call right away.

**DIAGNOSIS**

YES — The mother's BREAST MILK MAY BE INSUFFICIENT for the baby or the baby's mouth may be sore.

YES — The bottle's nipple may be CLOGGED or TOO SMALL, or the baby's mouth may be SORE.

YES — This is common for younger infants, but should decrease as the baby grows.

YES — This may be from a blockage of the stomach in young infants called PYLORIC STENOSIS.

YES — These symptoms may be from an intolerance to the formula or to cow's milk. This is called a LACTOSE INTOLERANCE.

YES — This may be COLIC.

YES — This may be from a DEVELOPMENTAL PROBLEM.

YES — If you are feeding the child formula or cereal, these symptoms may represent an allergy or more severe intolerance to cow's milk (LACTOSE INTOLERANCE) or wheat (CELIAC DISEASE).

**SELF-CARE**

Try more frequent breast feeding. Make sure the mother is drinking enough fluids. Discuss this problem with your doctor and keep a close watch on the baby's growth. If there are sores or white patches in the baby's mouth, see the doctor.

See if you can correct the nipple problem. See above if the baby's mouth is sore.

Have your baby examined by your doctor to make sure there are no other contributing causes and to check for growth and weight gain.

Contact your doctor right away.

You may want to switch to a non-cow's-milk-based formula. Discuss this with your doctor.

See your doctor.

See your doctor.

See your doctor.

# TOPIC 13 Neck Pain

The proverbial "pain in the neck" can be caused by stress or by a number of health problems, including some that may have serious consequences. Follow this chart for suggestions if you have been suffering from stiffness, soreness or cramps in the neck.

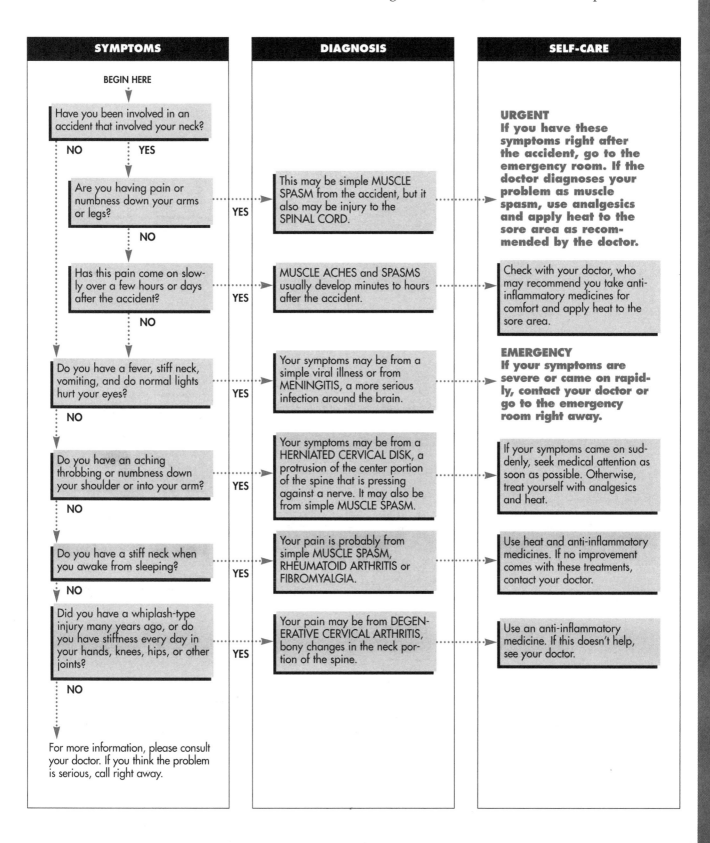

**SYMPTOMS**

BEGIN HERE

Have you been involved in an accident that involved your neck?

NO          YES

Are you having pain or numbness down your arms or legs?

NO

Has this pain come on slowly over a few hours or days after the accident?

NO

Do you have a fever, stiff neck, vomiting, and do normal lights hurt your eyes?

NO

Do you have an aching throbbing or numbness down your shoulder or into your arm?

NO

Do you have a stiff neck when you awake from sleeping?

NO

Did you have a whiplash-type injury many years ago, or do you have stiffness every day in your hands, knees, hips, or other joints?

NO

For more information, please consult your doctor. If you think the problem is serious, call right away.

**DIAGNOSIS**

YES → This may be simple MUSCLE SPASM from the accident, but it also may be injury to the SPINAL CORD.

YES → MUSCLE ACHES and SPASMS usually develop minutes to hours after the accident.

YES → Your symptoms may be from a simple viral illness or from MENINGITIS, a more serious infection around the brain.

YES → Your symptoms may be from a HERNIATED CERVICAL DISK, a protrusion of the center portion of the spine that is pressing against a nerve. It may also be from simple MUSCLE SPASM.

YES → Your pain is probably from simple MUSCLE SPASM, RHEUMATOID ARTHRITIS or FIBROMYALGIA.

YES → Your pain may be from DEGENERATIVE CERVICAL ARTHRITIS, bony changes in the neck portion of the spine.

**SELF-CARE**

**URGENT**
**If you have these symptoms right after the accident, go to the emergency room. If the doctor diagnoses your problem as muscle spasm, use analgesics and apply heat to the sore area as recommended by the doctor.**

Check with your doctor, who may recommend you take anti-inflammatory medicines for comfort and apply heat to the sore area.

**EMERGENCY**
**If your symptoms are severe or came on rapidly, contact your doctor or go to the emergency room right away.**

If your symptoms came on suddenly, seek medical attention as soon as possible. Otherwise, treat yourself with analgesics and heat.

Use heat and anti-inflammatory medicines. If no improvement comes with these treatments, contact your doctor.

Use an anti-inflammatory medicine. If this doesn't help, see your doctor.

# TOPIC 14 Neck Swelling

Any swelling on the neck causes concern. Yet most such swellings aren't cancerous. Check this chart if you have any swelling or lumps on your neck.

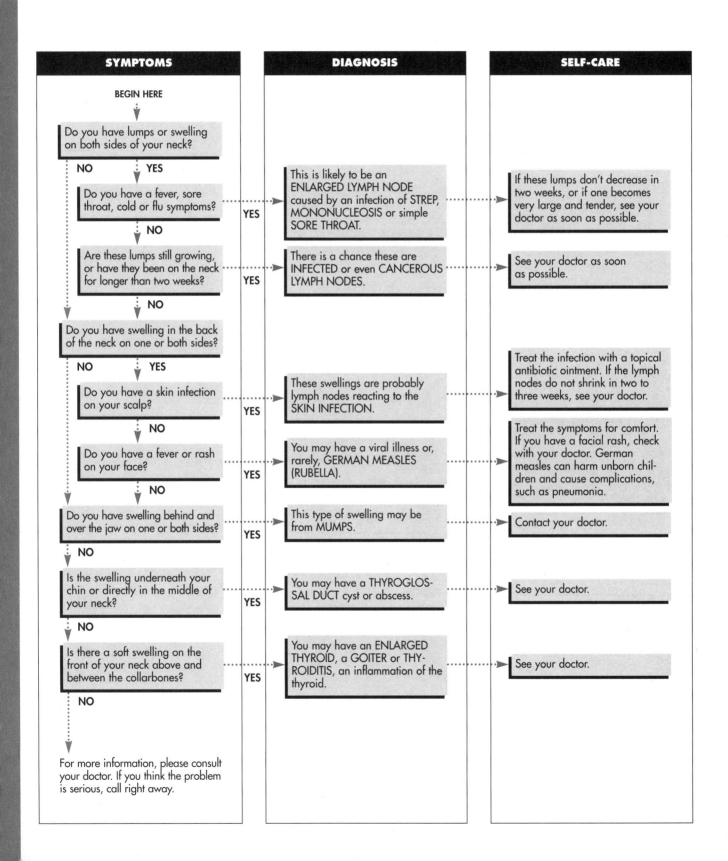

| SYMPTOMS | DIAGNOSIS | SELF-CARE |
|---|---|---|
| **BEGIN HERE** | | |
| Do you have lumps or swelling on both sides of your neck? | | |
| NO    YES | | |
| Do you have a fever, sore throat, cold or flu symptoms? — **YES** | This is likely to be an ENLARGED LYMPH NODE caused by an infection of STREP, MONONUCLEOSIS or simple SORE THROAT. | If these lumps don't decrease in two weeks, or if one becomes very large and tender, see your doctor as soon as possible. |
| NO | | |
| Are these lumps still growing, or have they been on the neck for longer than two weeks? — **YES** | There is a chance these are INFECTED or even CANCEROUS LYMPH NODES. | See your doctor as soon as possible. |
| NO | | |
| Do you have swelling in the back of the neck on one or both sides? | | |
| NO    YES | | |
| Do you have a skin infection on your scalp? — **YES** | These swellings are probably lymph nodes reacting to the SKIN INFECTION. | Treat the infection with a topical antibiotic ointment. If the lymph nodes do not shrink in two to three weeks, see your doctor. |
| NO | | |
| Do you have a fever or rash on your face? — **YES** | You may have a viral illness or, rarely, GERMAN MEASLES (RUBELLA). | Treat the symptoms for comfort. If you have a facial rash, check with your doctor. German measles can harm unborn children and cause complications, such as pneumonia. |
| NO | | |
| Do you have swelling behind and over the jaw on one or both sides? — **YES** | This type of swelling may be from MUMPS. | Contact your doctor. |
| NO | | |
| Is the swelling underneath your chin or directly in the middle of your neck? — **YES** | You may have a THYROGLOSSAL DUCT cyst or abscess. | See your doctor. |
| NO | | |
| Is there a soft swelling on the front of your neck above and between the collarbones? — **YES** | You may have an ENLARGED THYROID, a GOITER or THYROIDITIS, an inflammation of the thyroid. | See your doctor. |
| NO | | |
| For more information, please consult your doctor. If you think the problem is serious, call right away. | | |

# TOPIC 15 Throat Problems

Tenderness with swallowing or pain in the back of the throat, along with other cold and flu symptoms, is common. This chart will direct you in the appropriate care for this common problem.

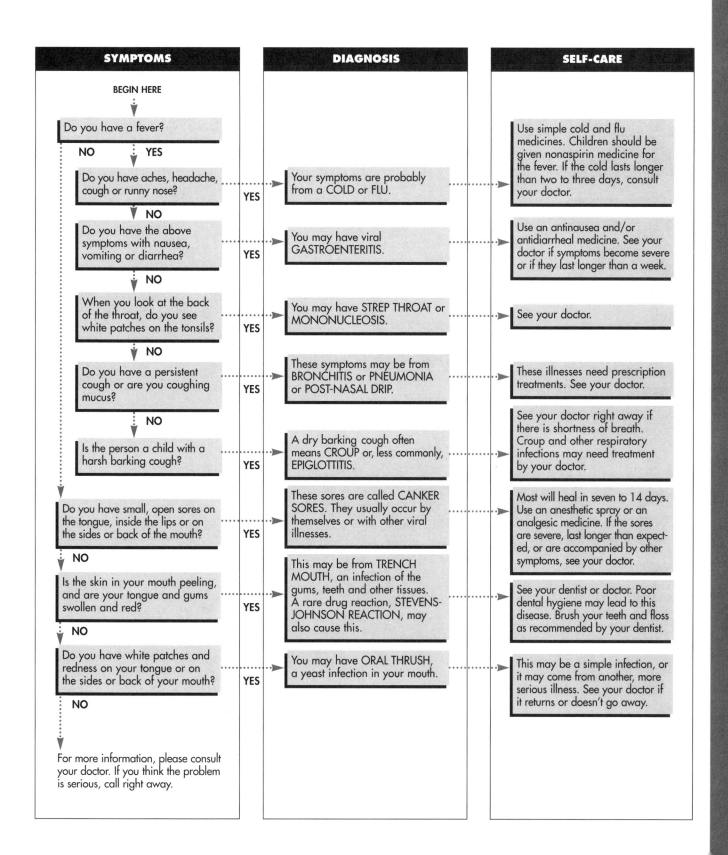

**SYMPTOMS**

BEGIN HERE

Do you have a fever?

NO → YES

Do you have aches, headache, cough or runny nose?
YES →

NO

Do you have the above symptoms with nausea, vomiting or diarrhea?
YES →

NO

When you look at the back of the throat, do you see white patches on the tonsils?
YES →

NO

Do you have a persistent cough or are you coughing mucus?
YES →

NO

Is the person a child with a harsh barking cough?
YES →

Do you have small, open sores on the tongue, inside the lips or on the sides or back of the mouth?
YES →

NO

Is the skin in your mouth peeling, and are your tongue and gums swollen and red?
YES →

NO

Do you have white patches and redness on your tongue or on the sides or back of your mouth?
YES →

NO

For more information, please consult your doctor. If you think the problem is serious, call right away.

**DIAGNOSIS**

Your symptoms are probably from a COLD or FLU.

You may have viral GASTROENTERITIS.

You may have STREP THROAT or MONONUCLEOSIS.

These symptoms may be from BRONCHITIS or PNEUMONIA or POST-NASAL DRIP.

A dry barking cough often means CROUP or, less commonly, EPIGLOTTITIS.

These sores are called CANKER SORES. They usually occur by themselves or with other viral illnesses.

This may be from TRENCH MOUTH, an infection of the gums, teeth and other tissues. A rare drug reaction, STEVENS-JOHNSON REACTION, may also cause this.

You may have ORAL THRUSH, a yeast infection in your mouth.

**SELF-CARE**

Use simple cold and flu medicines. Children should be given nonaspirin medicine for the fever. If the cold lasts longer than two to three days, consult your doctor.

Use an antinausea and/or antidiarrheal medicine. See your doctor if symptoms become severe or if they last longer than a week.

See your doctor.

These illnesses need prescription treatments. See your doctor.

See your doctor right away if there is shortness of breath. Croup and other respiratory infections may need treatment by your doctor.

Most will heal in seven to 14 days. Use an anesthetic spray or an analgesic medicine. If the sores are severe, last longer than expected, or are accompanied by other symptoms, see your doctor.

See your dentist or doctor. Poor dental hygiene may lead to this disease. Brush your teeth and floss as recommended by your dentist.

This may be a simple infection, or it may come from another, more serious illness. See your doctor if it returns or doesn't go away.

# TOPIC 16 Cough

This annoying symptom has many causes. Follow this chart to help identify your problem and find suggestions for self-care.

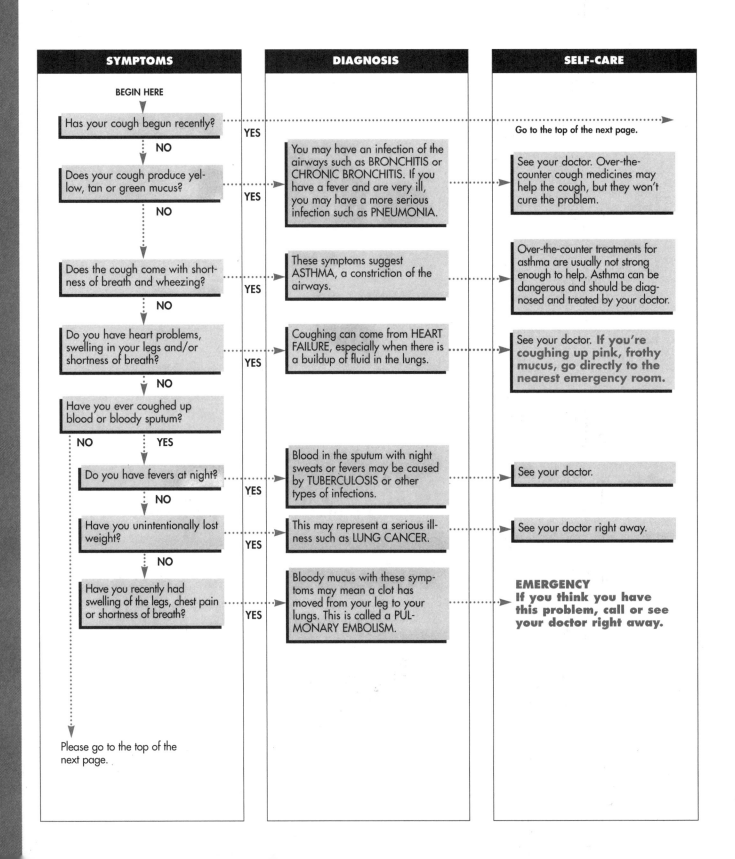

| SYMPTOMS | DIAGNOSIS | SELF-CARE |
|---|---|---|

**BEGIN HERE**

Has your cough begun recently? — **YES** → Go to the top of the next page.

**NO**

Does your cough produce yellow, tan or green mucus? — **YES** → You may have an infection of the airways such as BRONCHITIS or CHRONIC BRONCHITIS. If you have a fever and are very ill, you may have a more serious infection such as PNEUMONIA. → See your doctor. Over-the-counter cough medicines may help the cough, but they won't cure the problem.

**NO**

Does the cough come with shortness of breath and wheezing? — **YES** → These symptoms suggest ASTHMA, a constriction of the airways. → Over-the-counter treatments for asthma are usually not strong enough to help. Asthma can be dangerous and should be diagnosed and treated by your doctor.

**NO**

Do you have heart problems, swelling in your legs and/or shortness of breath? — **YES** → Coughing can come from HEART FAILURE, especially when there is a buildup of fluid in the lungs. → See your doctor. **If you're coughing up pink, frothy mucus, go directly to the nearest emergency room.**

**NO**

Have you ever coughed up blood or bloody sputum?

**NO** | **YES**

Do you have fevers at night? — **YES** → Blood in the sputum with night sweats or fevers may be caused by TUBERCULOSIS or other types of infections. → See your doctor.

**NO**

Have you unintentionally lost weight? — **YES** → This may represent a serious illness such as LUNG CANCER. → See your doctor right away.

**NO**

Have you recently had swelling of the legs, chest pain or shortness of breath? — **YES** → Bloody mucus with these symptoms may mean a clot has moved from your leg to your lungs. This is called a PULMONARY EMBOLISM. → **EMERGENCY** If you think you have this problem, call or see your doctor right away.

Please go to the top of the next page.

# TOPIC 16 Cough

continued.

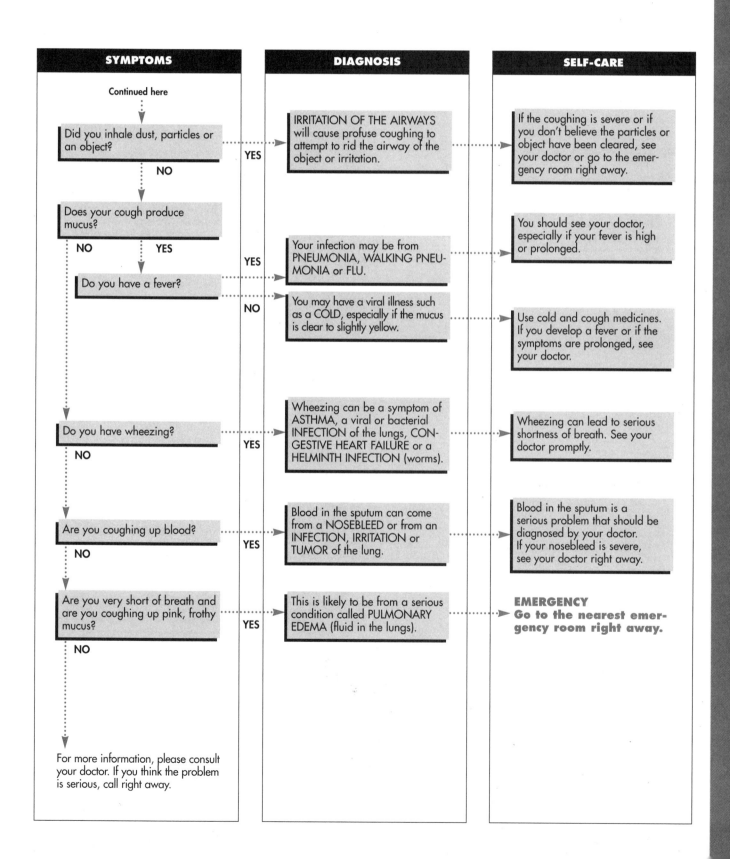

| SYMPTOMS | DIAGNOSIS | SELF-CARE |
|---|---|---|

Continued here

Did you inhale dust, particles or an object?   **YES** → IRRITATION OF THE AIRWAYS will cause profuse coughing to attempt to rid the airway of the object or irritation. → If the coughing is severe or if you don't believe the particles or object have been cleared, see your doctor or go to the emergency room right away.

**NO**

Does your cough produce mucus?

**NO**     **YES**

Do you have a fever?   **YES** → Your infection may be from PNEUMONIA, WALKING PNEUMONIA or FLU. → You should see your doctor, especially if your fever is high or prolonged.

**NO** → You may have a viral illness such as a COLD, especially if the mucus is clear to slightly yellow. → Use cold and cough medicines. If you develop a fever or if the symptoms are prolonged, see your doctor.

Do you have wheezing?   **YES** → Wheezing can be a symptom of ASTHMA, a viral or bacterial INFECTION of the lungs, CONGESTIVE HEART FAILURE or a HELMINTH INFECTION (worms). → Wheezing can lead to serious shortness of breath. See your doctor promptly.

**NO**

Are you coughing up blood?   **YES** → Blood in the sputum can come from a NOSEBLEED or from an INFECTION, IRRITATION or TUMOR of the lung. → Blood in the sputum is a serious problem that should be diagnosed by your doctor. If your nosebleed is severe, see your doctor right away.

**NO**

Are you very short of breath and are you coughing up pink, frothy mucus?   **YES** → This is likely to be from a serious condition called PULMONARY EDEMA (fluid in the lungs). → **EMERGENCY** Go to the nearest emergency room right away.

**NO**

For more information, please consult your doctor. If you think the problem is serious, call right away.

# TOPIC 17 Cold and Flu

Many people need some direction in how to treat the symptoms of a cold or flu and in knowing when to see a doctor. Other illnesses may also begin with flu- or cold-like symptoms. Self-care is often all that is needed to treat these common viral illnesses.

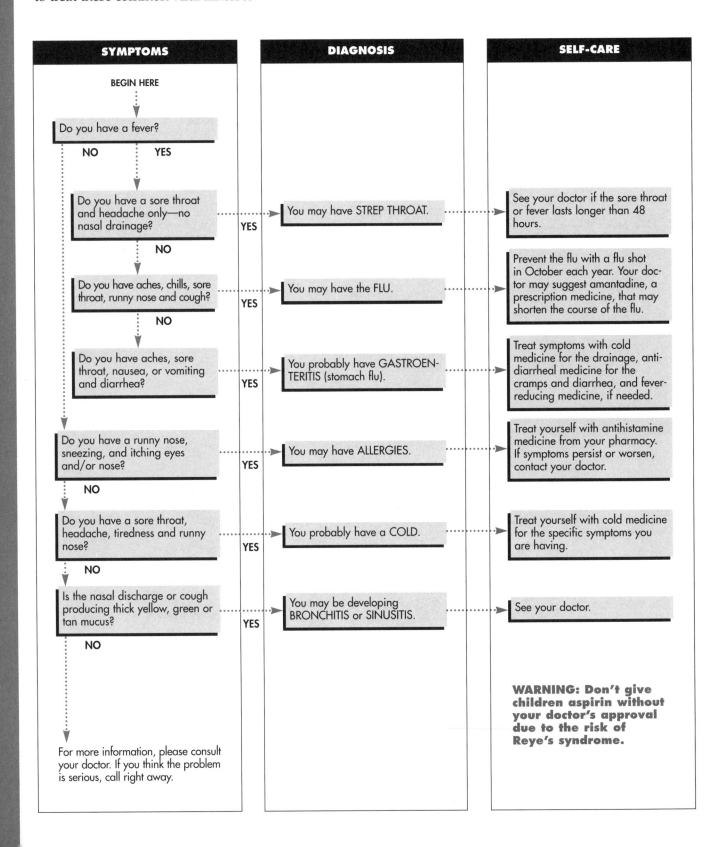

| SYMPTOMS | DIAGNOSIS | SELF-CARE |
|---|---|---|

**BEGIN HERE**

Do you have a fever?
NO / YES

Do you have a sore throat and headache only—no nasal drainage? → **YES** → You may have STREP THROAT. → See your doctor if the sore throat or fever lasts longer than 48 hours.

NO

Do you have aches, chills, sore throat, runny nose and cough? → **YES** → You may have the FLU. → Prevent the flu with a flu shot in October each year. Your doctor may suggest amantadine, a prescription medicine, that may shorten the course of the flu.

NO

Do you have aches, sore throat, nausea, or vomiting and diarrhea? → **YES** → You probably have GASTROEN-TERITIS (stomach flu). → Treat symptoms with cold medicine for the drainage, anti-diarrheal medicine for the cramps and diarrhea, and fever-reducing medicine, if needed.

Do you have a runny nose, sneezing, and itching eyes and/or nose? → **YES** → You may have ALLERGIES. → Treat yourself with antihistamine medicine from your pharmacy. If symptoms persist or worsen, contact your doctor.

NO

Do you have a sore throat, headache, tiredness and runny nose? → **YES** → You probably have a COLD. → Treat yourself with cold medicine for the specific symptoms you are having.

NO

Is the nasal discharge or cough producing thick yellow, green or tan mucus? → **YES** → You may be developing BRONCHITIS or SINUSITIS. → See your doctor.

NO

For more information, please consult your doctor. If you think the problem is serious, call right away.

**WARNING: Don't give children aspirin without your doctor's approval due to the risk of Reye's syndrome.**

# TOPIC 18 Shoulder Problems

Shoulder injures, arthritis and bursitis are common problems in adults, each causing severe pain, discomfort and immobility. Look on this chart to help define your shoulder problem.

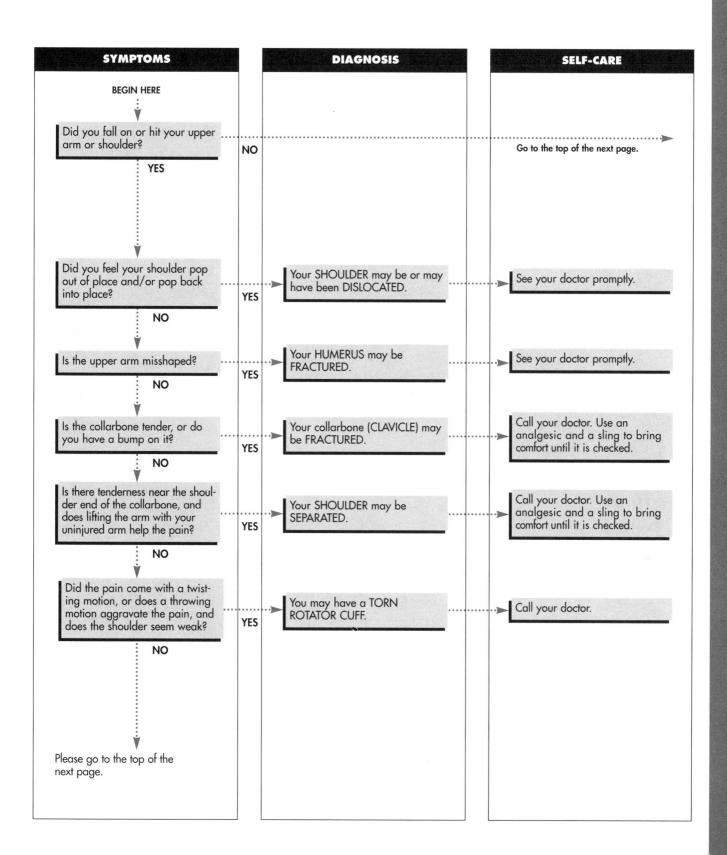

| SYMPTOMS | DIAGNOSIS | SELF-CARE |
|---|---|---|
| **BEGIN HERE** | | |
| Did you fall on or hit your upper arm or shoulder? **NO** | | Go to the top of the next page. |
| **YES** | | |
| Did you feel your shoulder pop out of place and/or pop back into place? **YES** | Your SHOULDER may be or may have been DISLOCATED. | See your doctor promptly. |
| **NO** | | |
| Is the upper arm misshaped? **YES** | Your HUMERUS may be FRACTURED. | See your doctor promptly. |
| **NO** | | |
| Is the collarbone tender, or do you have a bump on it? **YES** | Your collarbone (CLAVICLE) may be FRACTURED. | Call your doctor. Use an analgesic and a sling to bring comfort until it is checked. |
| **NO** | | |
| Is there tenderness near the shoulder end of the collarbone, and does lifting the arm with your uninjured arm help the pain? **YES** | Your SHOULDER may be SEPARATED. | Call your doctor. Use an analgesic and a sling to bring comfort until it is checked. |
| **NO** | | |
| Did the pain come with a twisting motion, or does a throwing motion aggravate the pain, and does the shoulder seem weak? **YES** | You may have a TORN ROTATOR CUFF. | Call your doctor. |
| **NO** | | |
| Please go to the top of the next page. | | |

# TOPIC 18 Shoulder Problems

continued.

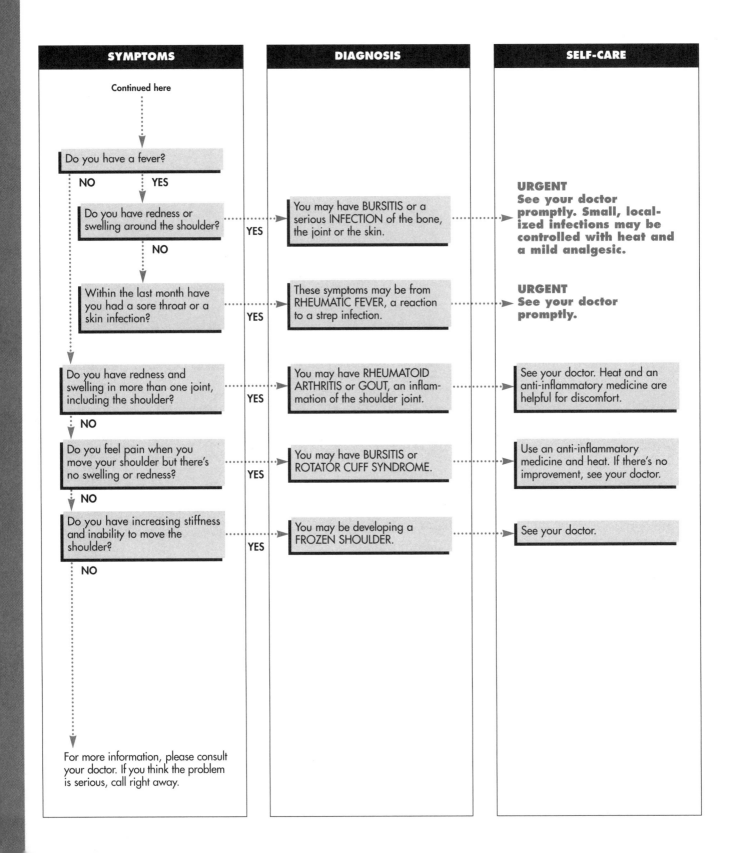

| SYMPTOMS | DIAGNOSIS | SELF-CARE |
|---|---|---|

**Continued here**

Do you have a fever?
NO    YES

Do you have redness or swelling around the shoulder?
NO

You may have BURSITIS or a serious INFECTION of the bone, the joint or the skin.
YES

**URGENT**
**See your doctor promptly. Small, localized infections may be controlled with heat and a mild analgesic.**

Within the last month have you had a sore throat or a skin infection?
YES

These symptoms may be from RHEUMATIC FEVER, a reaction to a strep infection.

**URGENT**
**See your doctor promptly.**

Do you have redness and swelling in more than one joint, including the shoulder?
YES
NO

You may have RHEUMATOID ARTHRITIS or GOUT, an inflammation of the shoulder joint.

See your doctor. Heat and an anti-inflammatory medicine are helpful for discomfort.

Do you feel pain when you move your shoulder but there's no swelling or redness?
YES
NO

You may have BURSITIS or ROTATOR CUFF SYNDROME.

Use an anti-inflammatory medicine and heat. If there's no improvement, see your doctor.

Do you have increasing stiffness and inability to move the shoulder?
YES
NO

You may be developing a FROZEN SHOULDER.

See your doctor.

For more information, please consult your doctor. If you think the problem is serious, call right away.

# **TOPIC 19** Breast Problems in Women

Both men and women can experience breast problems. Lumps, pain, discharge or skin problems can signal both minor and more serious problems.

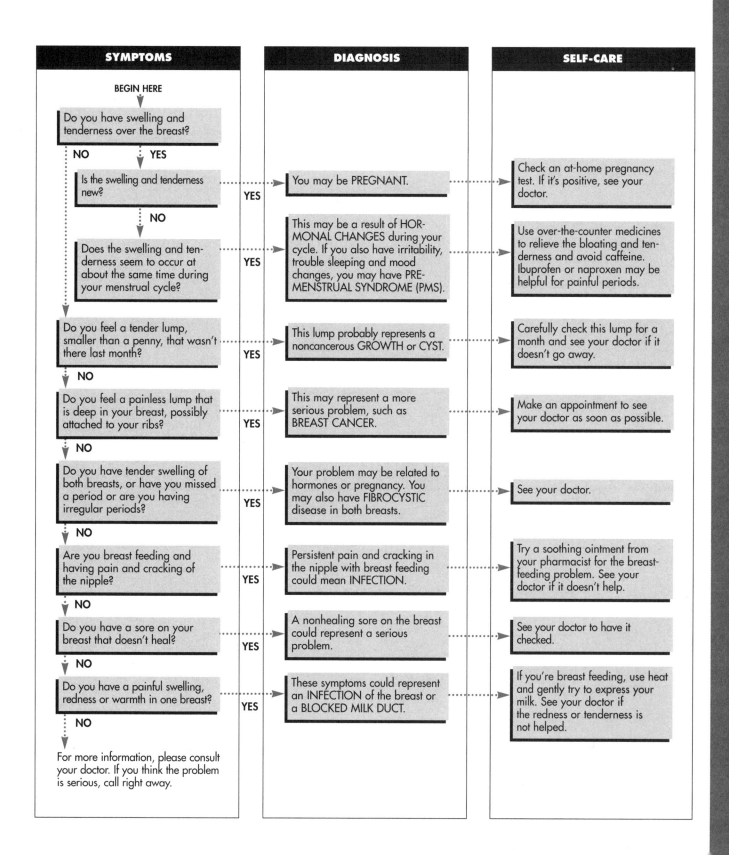

| SYMPTOMS | DIAGNOSIS | SELF-CARE |
|---|---|---|

**BEGIN HERE**

Do you have swelling and tenderness over the breast? — NO / YES

Is the swelling and tenderness new? — YES → You may be PREGNANT. → Check an at-home pregnancy test. If it's positive, see your doctor.

NO

Does the swelling and tenderness seem to occur at about the same time during your menstrual cycle? — YES → This may be a result of HORMONAL CHANGES during your cycle. If you also have irritability, trouble sleeping and mood changes, you may have PREMENSTRUAL SYNDROME (PMS). → Use over-the-counter medicines to relieve the bloating and tenderness and avoid caffeine. Ibuprofen or naproxen may be helpful for painful periods.

Do you feel a tender lump, smaller than a penny, that wasn't there last month? — YES → This lump probably represents a noncancerous GROWTH or CYST. → Carefully check this lump for a month and see your doctor if it doesn't go away.

NO

Do you feel a painless lump that is deep in your breast, possibly attached to your ribs? — YES → This may represent a more serious problem, such as BREAST CANCER. → Make an appointment to see your doctor as soon as possible.

NO

Do you have tender swelling of both breasts, or have you missed a period or are you having irregular periods? — YES → Your problem may be related to hormones or pregnancy. You may also have FIBROCYSTIC disease in both breasts. → See your doctor.

NO

Are you breast feeding and having pain and cracking of the nipple? — YES → Persistent pain and cracking in the nipple with breast feeding could mean INFECTION. → Try a soothing ointment from your pharmacist for the breast-feeding problem. See your doctor if it doesn't help.

NO

Do you have a sore on your breast that doesn't heal? — YES → A nonhealing sore on the breast could represent a serious problem. → See your doctor to have it checked.

NO

Do you have a painful swelling, redness or warmth in one breast? — YES → These symptoms could represent an INFECTION of the breast or a BLOCKED MILK DUCT. → If you're breast feeding, use heat and gently try to express your milk. See your doctor if the redness or tenderness is not helped.

NO

For more information, please consult your doctor. If you think the problem is serious, call right away.

# TOPIC 20 Breast Problems in Men

Men can also experience problems with their breasts.

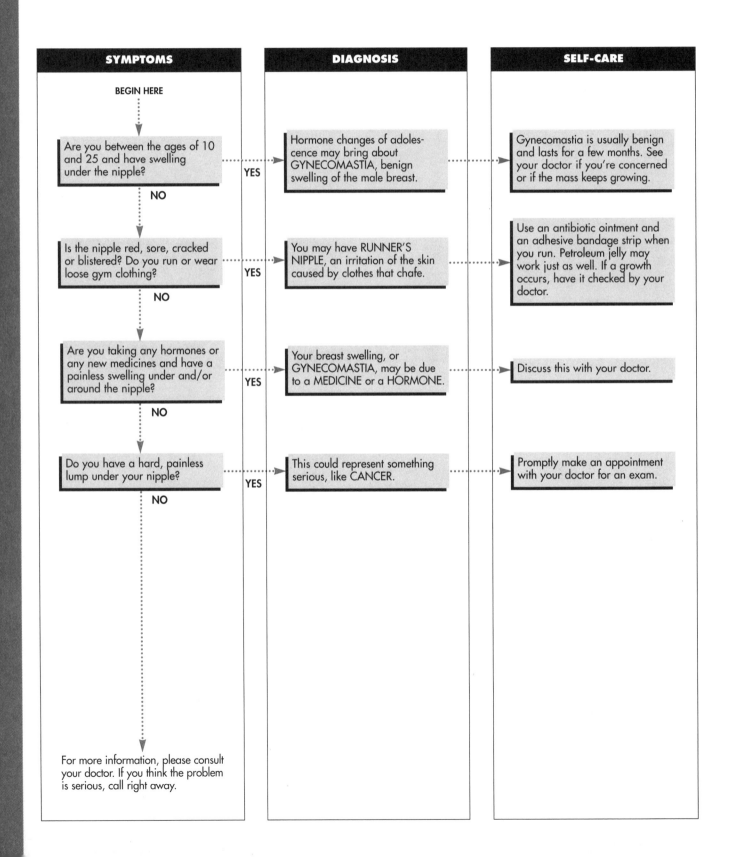

**SYMPTOMS**

BEGIN HERE

Are you between the ages of 10 and 25 and have swelling under the nipple?

YES

NO

Is the nipple red, sore, cracked or blistered? Do you run or wear loose gym clothing?

YES

NO

Are you taking any hormones or any new medicines and have a painless swelling under and/or around the nipple?

YES

NO

Do you have a hard, painless lump under your nipple?

YES

NO

For more information, please consult your doctor. If you think the problem is serious, call right away.

**DIAGNOSIS**

Hormone changes of adolescence may bring about GYNECOMASTIA, benign swelling of the male breast.

You may have RUNNER'S NIPPLE, an irritation of the skin caused by clothes that chafe.

Your breast swelling, or GYNECOMASTIA, may be due to a MEDICINE or a HORMONE.

This could represent something serious, like CANCER.

**SELF-CARE**

Gynecomastia is usually benign and lasts for a few months. See your doctor if you're concerned or if the mass keeps growing.

Use an antibiotic ointment and an adhesive bandage strip when you run. Petroleum jelly may work just as well. If a growth occurs, have it checked by your doctor.

Discuss this with your doctor.

Promptly make an appointment with your doctor for an exam.

# TOPIC 21 Shortness of Breath

This worrisome symptom has many acute and chronic causes. Follow this flowchart for more information about the diseases in which shortness of breath occurs.

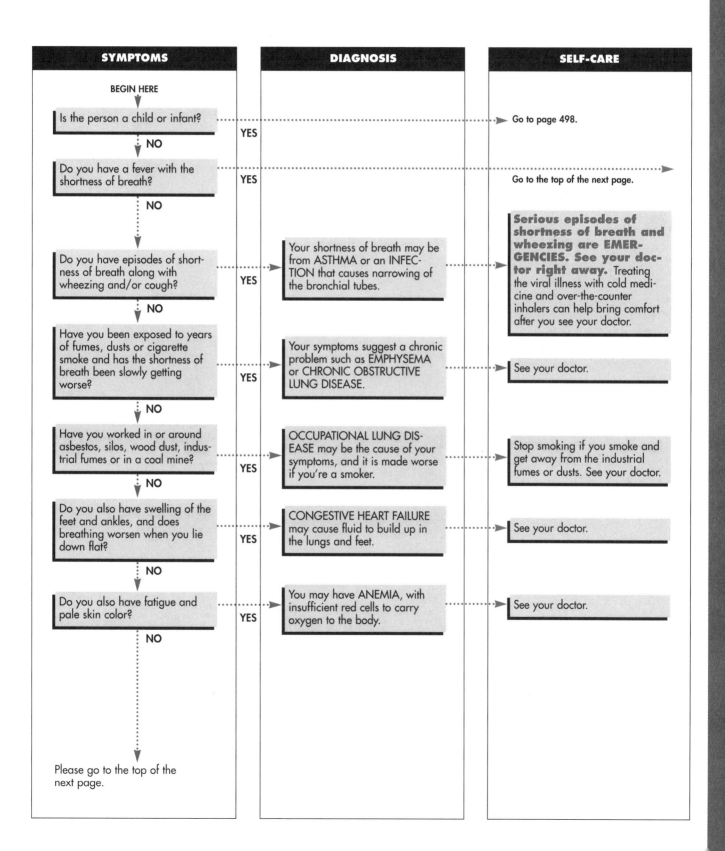

**SYMPTOMS**

BEGIN HERE

Is the person a child or infant? ···· YES ····> Go to page 498.

NO

Do you have a fever with the shortness of breath? ···· YES ····> Go to the top of the next page.

NO

Do you have episodes of shortness of breath along with wheezing and/or cough? ···· YES

NO

Have you been exposed to years of fumes, dusts or cigarette smoke and has the shortness of breath been slowly getting worse? ···· YES

NO

Have you worked in or around asbestos, silos, wood dust, industrial fumes or in a coal mine? ···· YES

NO

Do you also have swelling of the feet and ankles, and does breathing worsen when you lie down flat? ···· YES

NO

Do you also have fatigue and pale skin color? ···· YES

NO

Please go to the top of the next page.

**DIAGNOSIS**

Your shortness of breath may be from ASTHMA or an INFECTION that causes narrowing of the bronchial tubes.

Your symptoms suggest a chronic problem such as EMPHYSEMA or CHRONIC OBSTRUCTIVE LUNG DISEASE.

OCCUPATIONAL LUNG DISEASE may be the cause of your symptoms, and it is made worse if you're a smoker.

CONGESTIVE HEART FAILURE may cause fluid to build up in the lungs and feet.

You may have ANEMIA, with insufficient red cells to carry oxygen to the body.

**SELF-CARE**

**Serious episodes of shortness of breath and wheezing are EMERGENCIES. See your doctor right away.** Treating the viral illness with cold medicine and over-the-counter inhalers can help bring comfort after you see your doctor.

See your doctor.

Stop smoking if you smoke and get away from the industrial fumes or dusts. See your doctor.

See your doctor.

See your doctor.

# TOPIC 21 Shortness of Breath

continued.

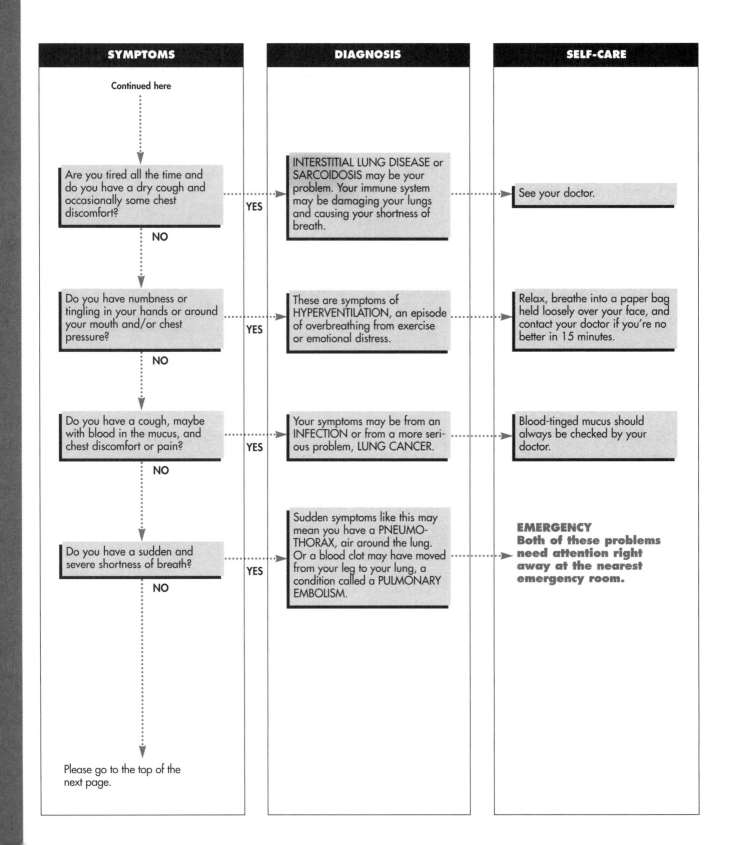

| SYMPTOMS | DIAGNOSIS | SELF-CARE |
|---|---|---|

Continued here

Are you tired all the time and do you have a dry cough and occasionally some chest discomfort? — **YES** → INTERSTITIAL LUNG DISEASE or SARCOIDOSIS may be your problem. Your immune system may be damaging your lungs and causing your shortness of breath. → See your doctor.

**NO**

Do you have numbness or tingling in your hands or around your mouth and/or chest pressure? — **YES** → These are symptoms of HYPERVENTILATION, an episode of overbreathing from exercise or emotional distress. → Relax, breathe into a paper bag held loosely over your face, and contact your doctor if you're no better in 15 minutes.

**NO**

Do you have a cough, maybe with blood in the mucus, and chest discomfort or pain? — **YES** → Your symptoms may be from an INFECTION or from a more serious problem, LUNG CANCER. → Blood-tinged mucus should always be checked by your doctor.

**NO**

Do you have a sudden and severe shortness of breath? — **YES** → Sudden symptoms like this may mean you have a PNEUMO-THORAX, air around the lung. Or a blood clot may have moved from your leg to your lung, a condition called a PULMONARY EMBOLISM. → **EMERGENCY Both of these problems need attention right away at the nearest emergency room.**

**NO**

Please go to the top of the next page.

**TOPIC 21** Shortness of Breath

continued.

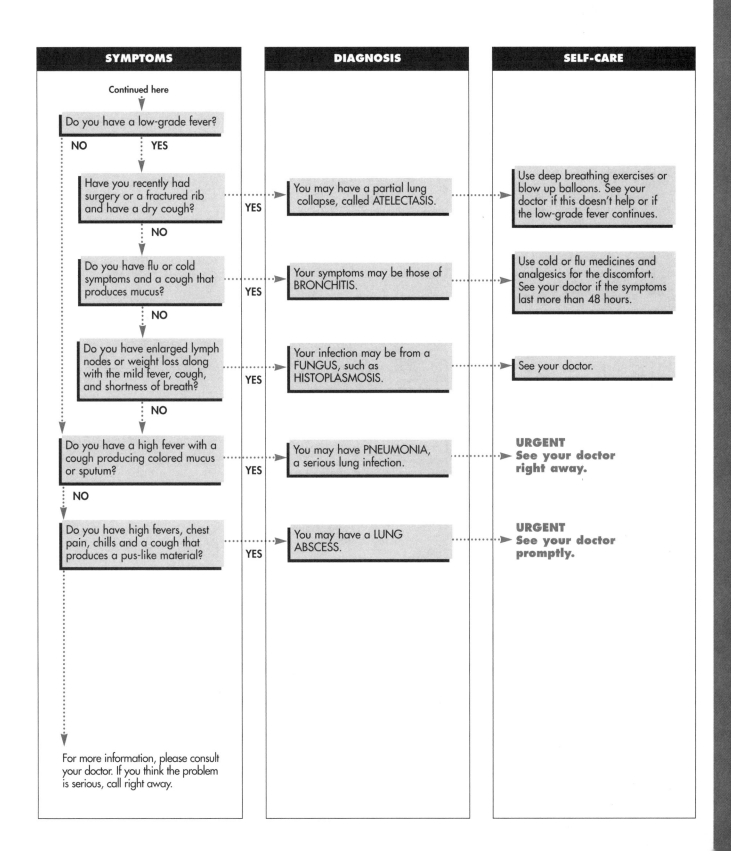

| SYMPTOMS | DIAGNOSIS | SELF-CARE |
|---|---|---|

Continued here

Do you have a low-grade fever?

NO          YES

Have you recently had surgery or a fractured rib and have a dry cough?

YES → You may have a partial lung collapse, called ATELECTASIS. → Use deep breathing exercises or blow up balloons. See your doctor if this doesn't help or if the low-grade fever continues.

NO

Do you have flu or cold symptoms and a cough that produces mucus?

YES → Your symptoms may be those of BRONCHITIS. → Use cold or flu medicines and analgesics for the discomfort. See your doctor if the symptoms last more than 48 hours.

NO

Do you have enlarged lymph nodes or weight loss along with the mild fever, cough, and shortness of breath?

YES → Your infection may be from a FUNGUS, such as HISTOPLASMOSIS. → See your doctor.

NO

Do you have a high fever with a cough producing colored mucus or sputum?

YES → You may have PNEUMONIA, a serious lung infection. → **URGENT See your doctor right away.**

NO

Do you have high fevers, chest pain, chills and a cough that produces a pus-like material?

YES → You may have a LUNG ABSCESS. → **URGENT See your doctor promptly.**

For more information, please consult your doctor. If you think the problem is serious, call right away.

# TOPIC 22 Shortness of Breath in a Child or Infant

This is a very serious symptom in children and should never be ignored. Knowing a doctor has diagnosed and is treating the problem should bring comfort, but if it becomes worse, always call or be seen right away. This chart describes some common causes of shortness of breath.

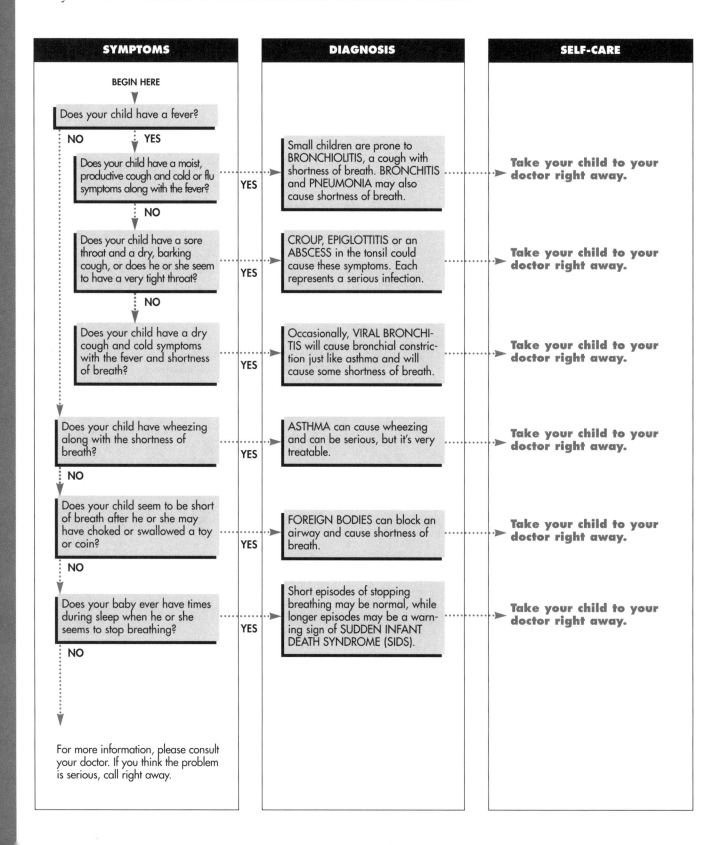

| SYMPTOMS | DIAGNOSIS | SELF-CARE |
|---|---|---|
| **BEGIN HERE** | | |
| Does your child have a fever? | | |
| NO — YES | | |
| Does your child have a moist, productive cough and cold or flu symptoms along with the fever? **YES** | Small children are prone to BRONCHIOLITIS, a cough with shortness of breath. BRONCHITIS and PNEUMONIA may also cause shortness of breath. | Take your child to your doctor right away. |
| NO | | |
| Does your child have a sore throat and a dry, barking cough, or does he or she seem to have a very tight throat? **YES** | CROUP, EPIGLOTTITIS or an ABSCESS in the tonsil could cause these symptoms. Each represents a serious infection. | Take your child to your doctor right away. |
| NO | | |
| Does your child have a dry cough and cold symptoms with the fever and shortness of breath? **YES** | Occasionally, VIRAL BRONCHITIS will cause bronchial constriction just like asthma and will cause some shortness of breath. | Take your child to your doctor right away. |
| Does your child have wheezing along with the shortness of breath? **YES** | ASTHMA can cause wheezing and can be serious, but it's very treatable. | Take your child to your doctor right away. |
| NO | | |
| Does your child seem to be short of breath after he or she may have choked or swallowed a toy or coin? **YES** | FOREIGN BODIES can block an airway and cause shortness of breath. | Take your child to your doctor right away. |
| NO | | |
| Does your baby ever have times during sleep when he or she seems to stop breathing? **YES** | Short episodes of stopping breathing may be normal, while longer episodes may be a warning sign of SUDDEN INFANT DEATH SYNDROME (SIDS). | Take your child to your doctor right away. |
| NO | | |
| For more information, please consult your doctor. If you think the problem is serious, call right away. | | |

# TOPIC 23 Chest Pain, Acute

Severe, sudden chest pain can represent a life-threatening problem.
Follow this chart for more information.

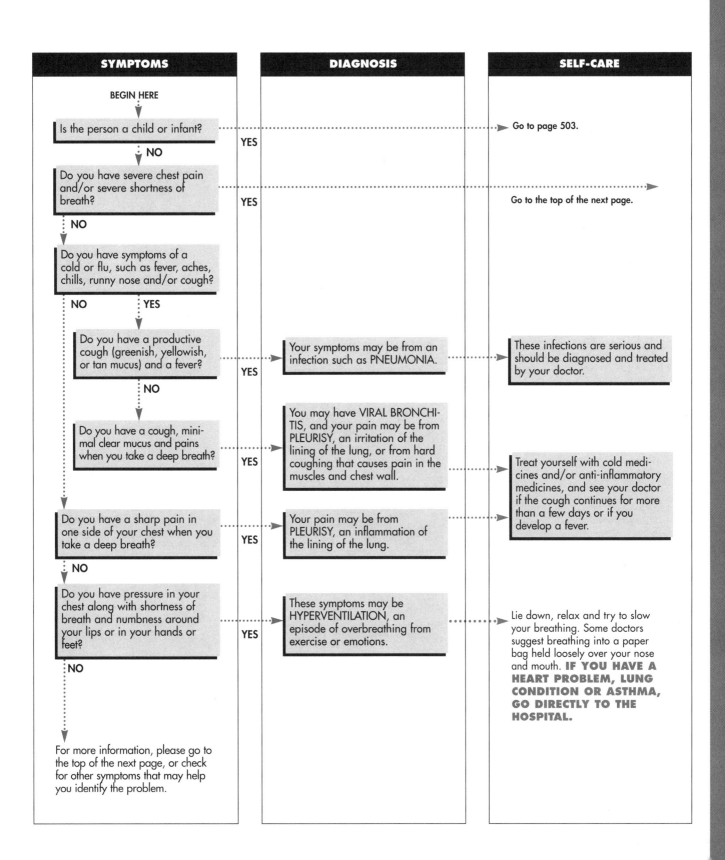

| SYMPTOMS | DIAGNOSIS | SELF-CARE |
|---|---|---|

**BEGIN HERE**

Is the person a child or infant?
— YES → Go to page 503.

NO

Do you have severe chest pain and/or severe shortness of breath?
— YES → Go to the top of the next page.

NO

Do you have symptoms of a cold or flu, such as fever, aches, chills, runny nose and/or cough?

NO       YES

Do you have a productive cough (greenish, yellowish, or tan mucus) and a fever?
— YES → Your symptoms may be from an infection such as PNEUMONIA. ⋯→ These infections are serious and should be diagnosed and treated by your doctor.

NO

Do you have a cough, minimal clear mucus and pains when you take a deep breath?
— YES → You may have VIRAL BRONCHITIS, and your pain may be from PLEURISY, an irritation of the lining of the lung, or from hard coughing that causes pain in the muscles and chest wall. ⋯→ Treat yourself with cold medicines and/or anti-inflammatory medicines, and see your doctor if the cough continues for more than a few days or if you develop a fever.

Do you have a sharp pain in one side of your chest when you take a deep breath?
— YES → Your pain may be from PLEURISY, an inflammation of the lining of the lung. ⋯↗

NO

Do you have pressure in your chest along with shortness of breath and numbness around your lips or in your hands or feet?
— YES → These symptoms may be HYPERVENTILATION, an episode of overbreathing from exercise or emotions. ⋯→ Lie down, relax and try to slow your breathing. Some doctors suggest breathing into a paper bag held loosely over your nose and mouth. **IF YOU HAVE A HEART PROBLEM, LUNG CONDITION OR ASTHMA, GO DIRECTLY TO THE HOSPITAL.**

NO

For more information, please go to the top of the next page, or check for other symptoms that may help you identify the problem.

# TOPIC 23 Chest Pain, Acute

continued.

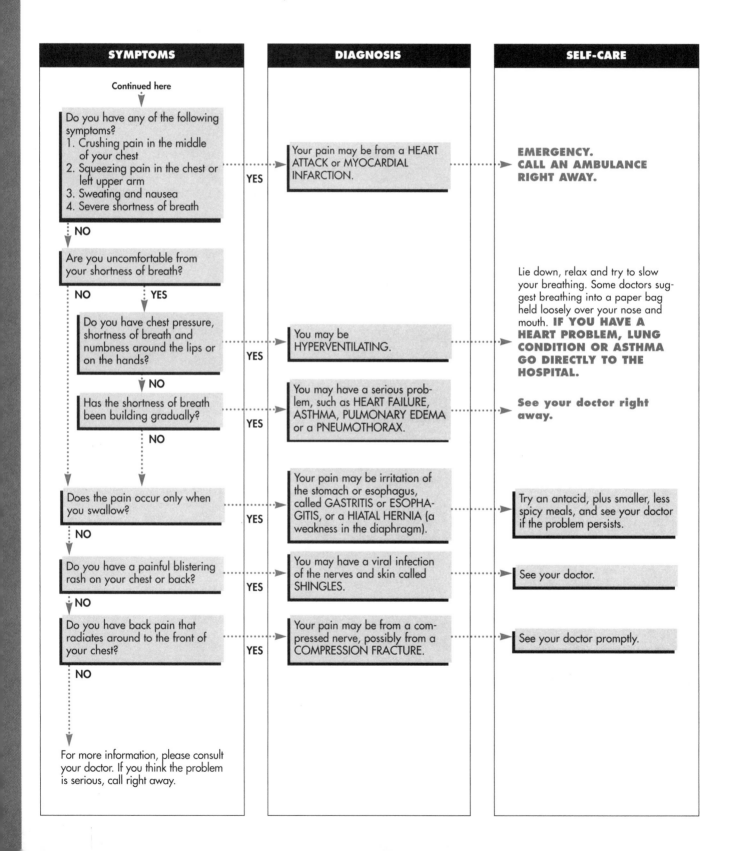

| SYMPTOMS | DIAGNOSIS | SELF-CARE |
|---|---|---|
| **Continued here** | | |
| Do you have any of the following symptoms? 1. Crushing pain in the middle of your chest 2. Squeezing pain in the chest or left upper arm 3. Sweating and nausea 4. Severe shortness of breath    **YES** | Your pain may be from a HEART ATTACK or MYOCARDIAL INFARCTION. | **EMERGENCY. CALL AN AMBULANCE RIGHT AWAY.** |
| **NO** | | |
| Are you uncomfortable from your shortness of breath? **NO**   **YES** | | Lie down, relax and try to slow your breathing. Some doctors suggest breathing into a paper bag held loosely over your nose and mouth. **IF YOU HAVE A HEART PROBLEM, LUNG CONDITION OR ASTHMA GO DIRECTLY TO THE HOSPITAL.** |
| Do you have chest pressure, shortness of breath and numbness around the lips or on the hands?   **YES** | You may be HYPERVENTILATING. | |
| **NO** | | |
| Has the shortness of breath been building gradually?   **YES** | You may have a serious problem, such as HEART FAILURE, ASTHMA, PULMONARY EDEMA or a PNEUMOTHORAX. | **See your doctor right away.** |
| **NO** | | |
| Does the pain occur only when you swallow?   **YES** | Your pain may be irritation of the stomach or esophagus, called GASTRITIS or ESOPHAGITIS, or a HIATAL HERNIA (a weakness in the diaphragm). | Try an antacid, plus smaller, less spicy meals, and see your doctor if the problem persists. |
| **NO** | | |
| Do you have a painful blistering rash on your chest or back?   **YES** | You may have a viral infection of the nerves and skin called SHINGLES. | See your doctor. |
| **NO** | | |
| Do you have back pain that radiates around to the front of your chest?   **YES** | Your pain may be from a compressed nerve, possibly from a COMPRESSION FRACTURE. | See your doctor promptly. |
| **NO** | | |
| For more information, please consult your doctor. If you think the problem is serious, call right away. | | |

# TOPIC 24 Chest Pain, Chronic

Many different types of problems can cause discomfort, shortness of breath, pain with swallowing, and many other symptoms in the chest area. This chart may help you pinpoint your problem as you confirm your symptoms.

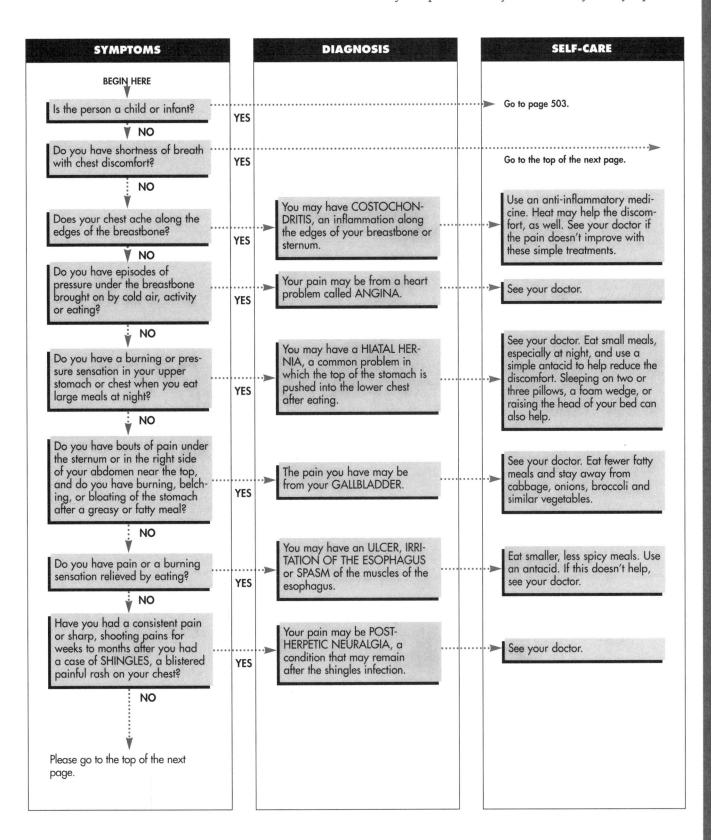

**SYMPTOMS**

BEGIN HERE

Is the person a child or infant? — YES

Do you have shortness of breath with chest discomfort? — YES

Does your chest ache along the edges of the breastbone? — YES

Do you have episodes of pressure under the breastbone brought on by cold air, activity or eating? — YES

Do you have a burning or pressure sensation in your upper stomach or chest when you eat large meals at night? — YES

Do you have bouts of pain under the sternum or in the right side of your abdomen near the top, and do you have burning, belching, or bloating of the stomach after a greasy or fatty meal? — YES

Do you have pain or a burning sensation relieved by eating? — YES

Have you had a consistent pain or sharp, shooting pains for weeks to months after you had a case of SHINGLES, a blistered painful rash on your chest? — YES

Please go to the top of the next page.

**DIAGNOSIS**

You may have COSTOCHONDRITIS, an inflammation along the edges of your breastbone or sternum.

Your pain may be from a heart problem called ANGINA.

You may have a HIATAL HERNIA, a common problem in which the top of the stomach is pushed into the lower chest after eating.

The pain you have may be from your GALLBLADDER.

You may have an ULCER, IRRITATION OF THE ESOPHAGUS or SPASM of the muscles of the esophagus.

Your pain may be POST-HERPETIC NEURALGIA, a condition that may remain after the shingles infection.

**SELF-CARE**

Go to page 503.

Go to the top of the next page.

Use an anti-inflammatory medicine. Heat may help the discomfort, as well. See your doctor if the pain doesn't improve with these simple treatments.

See your doctor.

See your doctor. Eat small meals, especially at night, and use a simple antacid to help reduce the discomfort. Sleeping on two or three pillows, a foam wedge, or raising the head of your bed can also help.

See your doctor. Eat fewer fatty meals and stay away from cabbage, onions, broccoli and similar vegetables.

Eat smaller, less spicy meals. Use an antacid. If this doesn't help, see your doctor.

See your doctor.

# TOPIC 24 Chest Pain, Chronic

continued.

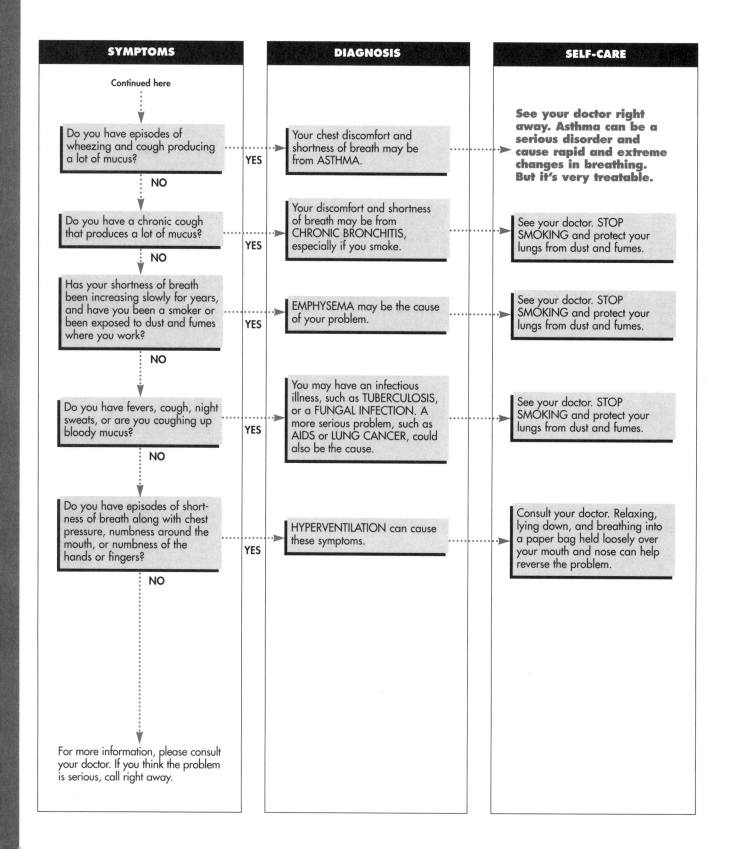

| SYMPTOMS | DIAGNOSIS | SELF-CARE |
|---|---|---|

**Continued here**

Do you have episodes of wheezing and cough producing a lot of mucus?

**YES** → Your chest discomfort and shortness of breath may be from ASTHMA. → **See your doctor right away. Asthma can be a serious disorder and cause rapid and extreme changes in breathing. But it's very treatable.**

**NO**

Do you have a chronic cough that produces a lot of mucus?

**YES** → Your discomfort and shortness of breath may be from CHRONIC BRONCHITIS, especially if you smoke. → See your doctor. STOP SMOKING and protect your lungs from dust and fumes.

**NO**

Has your shortness of breath been increasing slowly for years, and have you been a smoker or been exposed to dust and fumes where you work?

**YES** → EMPHYSEMA may be the cause of your problem. → See your doctor. STOP SMOKING and protect your lungs from dust and fumes.

**NO**

Do you have fevers, cough, night sweats, or are you coughing up bloody mucus?

**YES** → You may have an infectious illness, such as TUBERCULOSIS, or a FUNGAL INFECTION. A more serious problem, such as AIDS or LUNG CANCER, could also be the cause. → See your doctor. STOP SMOKING and protect your lungs from dust and fumes.

**NO**

Do you have episodes of shortness of breath along with chest pressure, numbness around the mouth, or numbness of the hands or fingers?

**YES** → HYPERVENTILATION can cause these symptoms. → Consult your doctor. Relaxing, lying down, and breathing into a paper bag held loosely over your mouth and nose can help reverse the problem.

**NO**

For more information, please consult your doctor. If you think the problem is serious, call right away.

# TOPIC 25 Chest Pain in Infants and Children

This problem isn't reserved for adults only, but may occur in a child as well. Most of the causes aren't serious, but may require a doctor's attention. Follow this chart for more information when your child has chest pain.

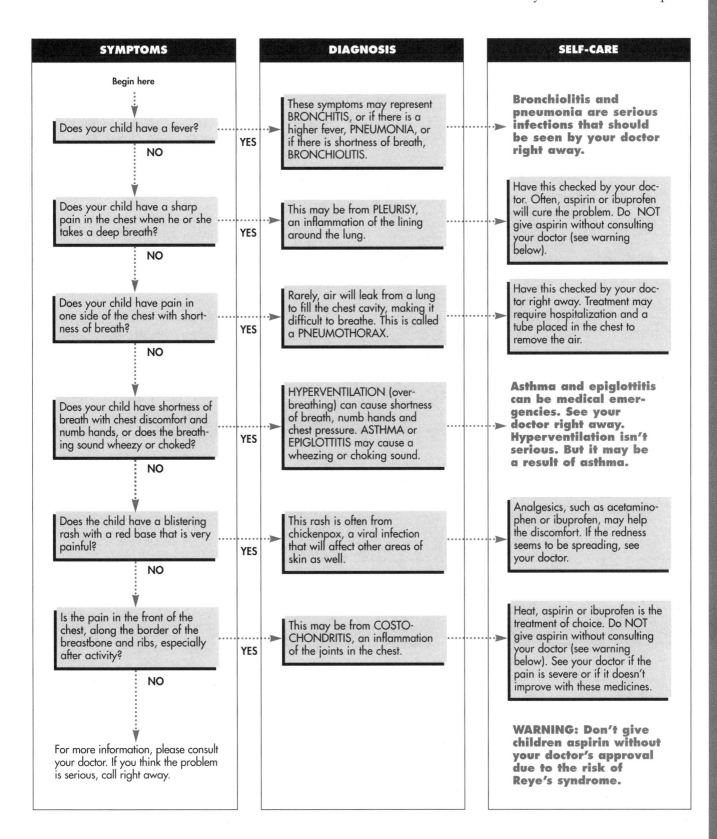

**SYMPTOMS**

Begin here

Does your child have a fever? — **YES**

**NO**

Does your child have a sharp pain in the chest when he or she takes a deep breath? — **YES**

**NO**

Does your child have pain in one side of the chest with shortness of breath? — **YES**

**NO**

Does your child have shortness of breath with chest discomfort and numb hands, or does the breathing sound wheezy or choked? — **YES**

**NO**

Does the child have a blistering rash with a red base that is very painful? — **YES**

**NO**

Is the pain in the front of the chest, along the border of the breastbone and ribs, especially after activity? — **YES**

**NO**

For more information, please consult your doctor. If you think the problem is serious, call right away.

**DIAGNOSIS**

These symptoms may represent BRONCHITIS, or if there is a higher fever, PNEUMONIA, or if there is shortness of breath, BRONCHIOLITIS.

This may be from PLEURISY, an inflammation of the lining around the lung.

Rarely, air will leak from a lung to fill the chest cavity, making it difficult to breathe. This is called a PNEUMOTHORAX.

HYPERVENTILATION (over-breathing) can cause shortness of breath, numb hands and chest pressure. ASTHMA or EPIGLOTTITIS may cause a wheezing or choking sound.

This rash is often from chickenpox, a viral infection that will affect other areas of skin as well.

This may be from COSTO-CHONDRITIS, an inflammation of the joints in the chest.

**SELF-CARE**

**Bronchiolitis and pneumonia are serious infections that should be seen by your doctor right away.**

Have this checked by your doctor. Often, aspirin or ibuprofen will cure the problem. Do NOT give aspirin without consulting your doctor (see warning below).

Have this checked by your doctor right away. Treatment may require hospitalization and a tube placed in the chest to remove the air.

**Asthma and epiglottitis can be medical emergencies. See your doctor right away. Hyperventilation isn't serious. But it may be a result of asthma.**

Analgesics, such as acetaminophen or ibuprofen, may help the discomfort. If the redness seems to be spreading, see your doctor.

Heat, aspirin or ibuprofen is the treatment of choice. Do NOT give aspirin without consulting your doctor (see warning below). See your doctor if the pain is severe or if it doesn't improve with these medicines.

**WARNING: Don't give children aspirin without your doctor's approval due to the risk of Reye's syndrome.**

# TOPIC 26 Hand/Wrist/Arm Problems

A number of common injuries, aches and pain in the hands, wrists and arms occur with sporting activities or work. Follow this flowchart for instructions on self-care and when to see your doctor.

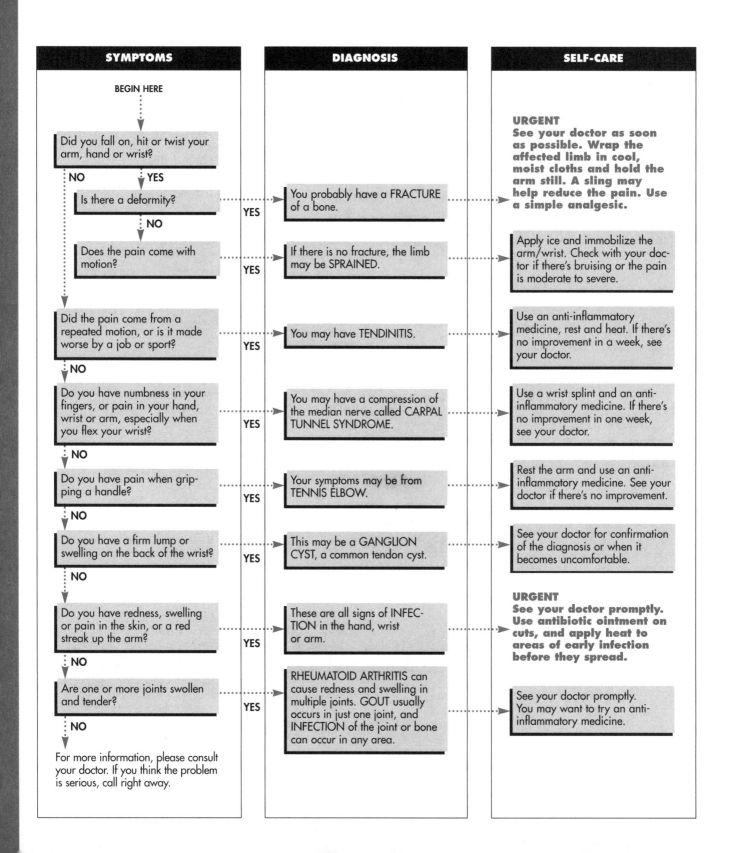

**SYMPTOMS**

BEGIN HERE

Did you fall on, hit or twist your arm, hand or wrist?

NO — YES

Is there a deformity?

NO

Does the pain come with motion?

Did the pain come from a repeated motion, or is it made worse by a job or sport?

NO

Do you have numbness in your fingers, or pain in your hand, wrist or arm, especially when you flex your wrist?

NO

Do you have pain when gripping a handle?

NO

Do you have a firm lump or swelling on the back of the wrist?

NO

Do you have redness, swelling or pain in the skin, or a red streak up the arm?

NO

Are one or more joints swollen and tender?

NO

For more information, please consult your doctor. If you think the problem is serious, call right away.

**DIAGNOSIS**

YES — You probably have a FRACTURE of a bone.

YES — If there is no fracture, the limb may be SPRAINED.

YES — You may have TENDINITIS.

YES — You may have a compression of the median nerve called CARPAL TUNNEL SYNDROME.

YES — Your symptoms may be from TENNIS ELBOW.

YES — This may be a GANGLION CYST, a common tendon cyst.

YES — These are all signs of INFECTION in the hand, wrist or arm.

YES — RHEUMATOID ARTHRITIS can cause redness and swelling in multiple joints. GOUT usually occurs in just one joint, and INFECTION of the joint or bone can occur in any area.

**SELF-CARE**

**URGENT**
**See your doctor as soon as possible. Wrap the affected limb in cool, moist cloths and hold the arm still. A sling may help reduce the pain. Use a simple analgesic.**

Apply ice and immobilize the arm/wrist. Check with your doctor if there's bruising or the pain is moderate to severe.

Use an anti-inflammatory medicine, rest and heat. If there's no improvement in a week, see your doctor.

Use a wrist splint and an anti-inflammatory medicine. If there's no improvement in one week, see your doctor.

Rest the arm and use an anti-inflammatory medicine. See your doctor if there's no improvement.

See your doctor for confirmation of the diagnosis or when it becomes uncomfortable.

**URGENT**
**See your doctor promptly. Use antibiotic ointment on cuts, and apply heat to areas of early infection before they spread.**

See your doctor promptly. You may want to try an anti-inflammatory medicine.

## TOPIC 27 Abdominal Pain, Acute

Just about everyone has had a "stomachache" at one time or another. But severe abdominal pain, also called acute, is nothing to be ignored. It often indicates a serious problem. Follow this chart for more information about abdominal pain that has recently started. See Topic 28 for abdominal pain that has occurred for more than three days.

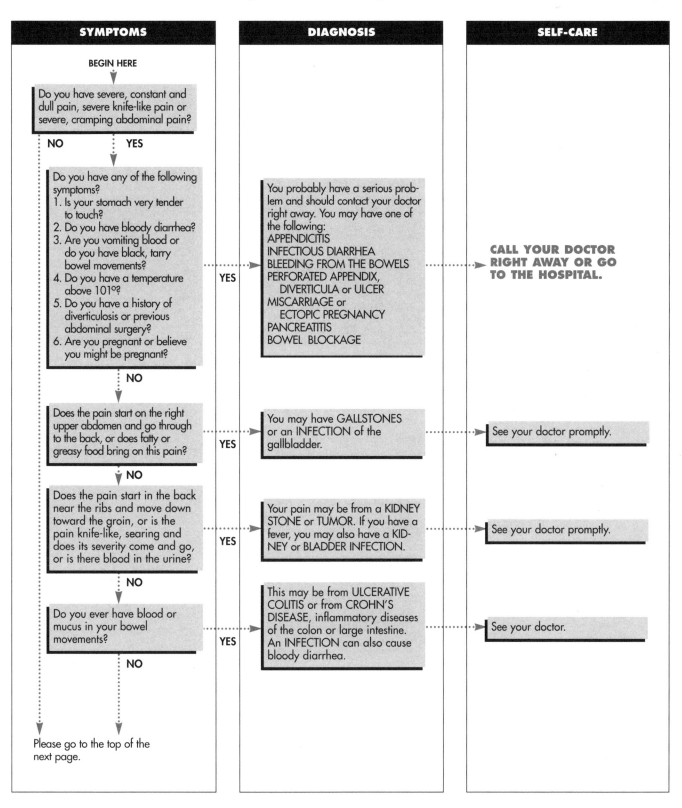

| SYMPTOMS | DIAGNOSIS | SELF-CARE |
|---|---|---|

**BEGIN HERE**

Do you have severe, constant and dull pain, severe knife-like pain or severe, cramping abdominal pain?

NO    YES

Do you have any of the following symptoms?
1. Is your stomach very tender to touch?
2. Do you have bloody diarrhea?
3. Are you vomiting blood or do you have black, tarry bowel movements?
4. Do you have a temperature above 101°?
5. Do you have a history of diverticulosis or previous abdominal surgery?
6. Are you pregnant or believe you might be pregnant?

YES →

You probably have a serious problem and should contact your doctor right away. You may have one of the following:
APPENDICITIS
INFECTIOUS DIARRHEA
BLEEDING FROM THE BOWELS
PERFORATED APPENDIX, DIVERTICULA or ULCER
MISCARRIAGE or ECTOPIC PREGNANCY
PANCREATITIS
BOWEL BLOCKAGE

→ **CALL YOUR DOCTOR RIGHT AWAY OR GO TO THE HOSPITAL.**

NO

Does the pain start on the right upper abdomen and go through to the back, or does fatty or greasy food bring on this pain?

YES →

You may have GALLSTONES or an INFECTION of the gallbladder.

→ See your doctor promptly.

NO

Does the pain start in the back near the ribs and move down toward the groin, or is the pain knife-like, searing and does its severity come and go, or is there blood in the urine?

YES →

Your pain may be from a KIDNEY STONE or TUMOR. If you have a fever, you may also have a KIDNEY or BLADDER INFECTION.

→ See your doctor promptly.

NO

Do you ever have blood or mucus in your bowel movements?

YES →

This may be from ULCERATIVE COLITIS or from CROHN'S DISEASE, inflammatory diseases of the colon or large intestine. An INFECTION can also cause bloody diarrhea.

→ See your doctor.

NO

Please go to the top of the next page.

# TOPIC 27 Abdominal Pain, Acute

continued.

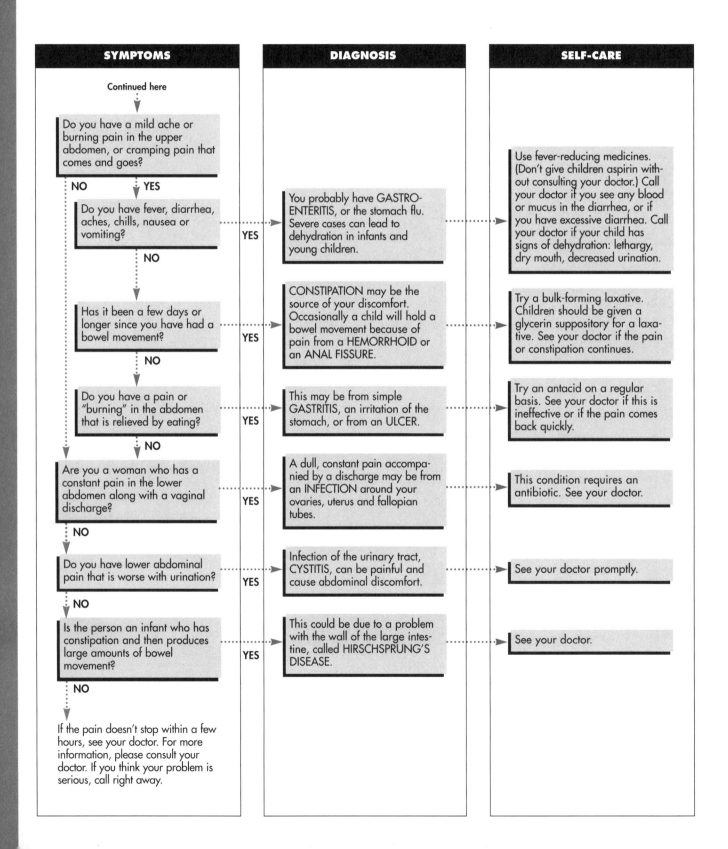

**SYMPTOMS**

Continued here

Do you have a mild ache or burning pain in the upper abdomen, or cramping pain that comes and goes?

NO    YES

Do you have fever, diarrhea, aches, chills, nausea or vomiting?

NO

Has it been a few days or longer since you have had a bowel movement?

NO

Do you have a pain or "burning" in the abdomen that is relieved by eating?

NO

Are you a woman who has a constant pain in the lower abdomen along with a vaginal discharge?

NO

Do you have lower abdominal pain that is worse with urination?

NO

Is the person an infant who has constipation and then produces large amounts of bowel movement?

NO

If the pain doesn't stop within a few hours, see your doctor. For more information, please consult your doctor. If you think your problem is serious, call right away.

**DIAGNOSIS**

YES — You probably have GASTRO-ENTERITIS, or the stomach flu. Severe cases can lead to dehydration in infants and young children.

YES — CONSTIPATION may be the source of your discomfort. Occasionally a child will hold a bowel movement because of pain from a HEMORRHOID or an ANAL FISSURE.

YES — This may be from simple GASTRITIS, an irritation of the stomach, or from an ULCER.

YES — A dull, constant pain accompanied by a discharge may be from an INFECTION around your ovaries, uterus and fallopian tubes.

YES — Infection of the urinary tract, CYSTITIS, can be painful and cause abdominal discomfort.

YES — This could be due to a problem with the wall of the large intestine, called HIRSCHSPRUNG'S DISEASE.

**SELF-CARE**

Use fever-reducing medicines. (Don't give children aspirin without consulting your doctor.) Call your doctor if you see any blood or mucus in the diarrhea, or if you have excessive diarrhea. Call your doctor if your child has signs of dehydration: lethargy, dry mouth, decreased urination.

Try a bulk-forming laxative. Children should be given a glycerin suppository for a laxative. See your doctor if the pain or constipation continues.

Try an antacid on a regular basis. See your doctor if this is ineffective or if the pain comes back quickly.

This condition requires an antibiotic. See your doctor.

See your doctor promptly.

See your doctor.

# TOPIC 28 Abdominal Pain, Chronic

Dull ongoing abdominal pain, called chronic, may be the most difficult to diagnose, causing frustration for both you and your doctor. Do your symptoms fit one of the diagnoses contained in this chart?

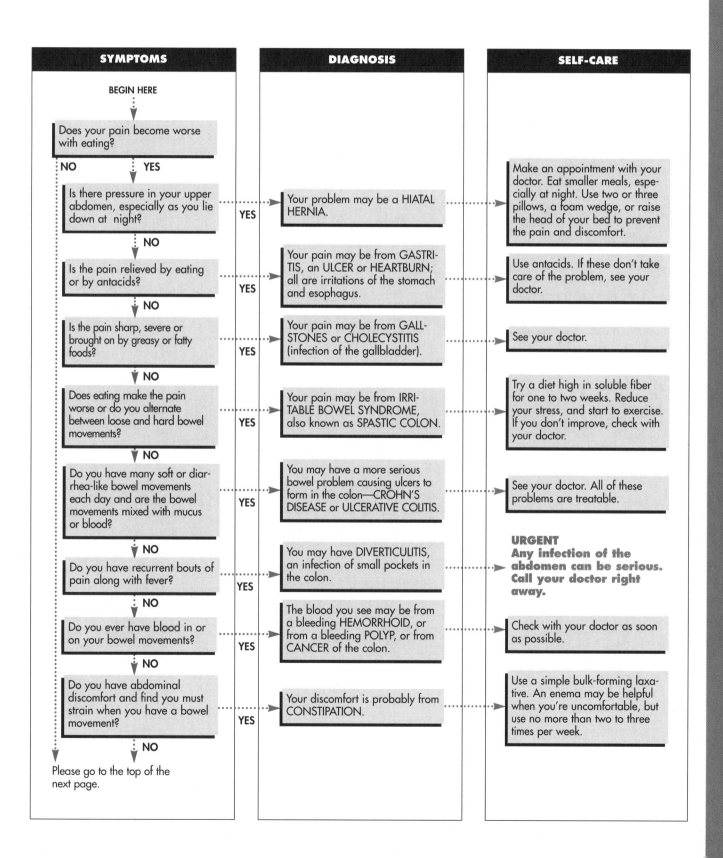

| SYMPTOMS | DIAGNOSIS | SELF-CARE |
|---|---|---|

**BEGIN HERE**

Does your pain become worse with eating?

NO / YES

Is there pressure in your upper abdomen, especially as you lie down at night? — **YES** → Your problem may be a HIATAL HERNIA. → Make an appointment with your doctor. Eat smaller meals, especially at night. Use two or three pillows, a foam wedge, or raise the head of your bed to prevent the pain and discomfort.

NO

Is the pain relieved by eating or by antacids? — **YES** → Your pain may be from GASTRITIS, an ULCER or HEARTBURN; all are irritations of the stomach and esophagus. → Use antacids. If these don't take care of the problem, see your doctor.

NO

Is the pain sharp, severe or brought on by greasy or fatty foods? — **YES** → Your pain may be from GALLSTONES or CHOLECYSTITIS (infection of the gallbladder). → See your doctor.

NO

Does eating make the pain worse or do you alternate between loose and hard bowel movements? — **YES** → Your pain may be from IRRITABLE BOWEL SYNDROME, also known as SPASTIC COLON. → Try a diet high in soluble fiber for one to two weeks. Reduce your stress, and start to exercise. If you don't improve, check with your doctor.

NO

Do you have many soft or diarrhea-like bowel movements each day and are the bowel movements mixed with mucus or blood? — **YES** → You may have a more serious bowel problem causing ulcers to form in the colon—CROHN'S DISEASE or ULCERATIVE COLITIS. → See your doctor. All of these problems are treatable.

NO

Do you have recurrent bouts of pain along with fever? — **YES** → You may have DIVERTICULITIS, an infection of small pockets in the colon. → **URGENT Any infection of the abdomen can be serious. Call your doctor right away.**

NO

Do you ever have blood in or on your bowel movements? — **YES** → The blood you see may be from a bleeding HEMORRHOID, or from a bleeding POLYP, or from CANCER of the colon. → Check with your doctor as soon as possible.

NO

Do you have abdominal discomfort and find you must strain when you have a bowel movement? — **YES** → Your discomfort is probably from CONSTIPATION. → Use a simple bulk-forming laxative. An enema may be helpful when you're uncomfortable, but use no more than two to three times per week.

NO

Please go to the top of the next page.

# TOPIC 28 Abdominal Pain, Chronic

continued.

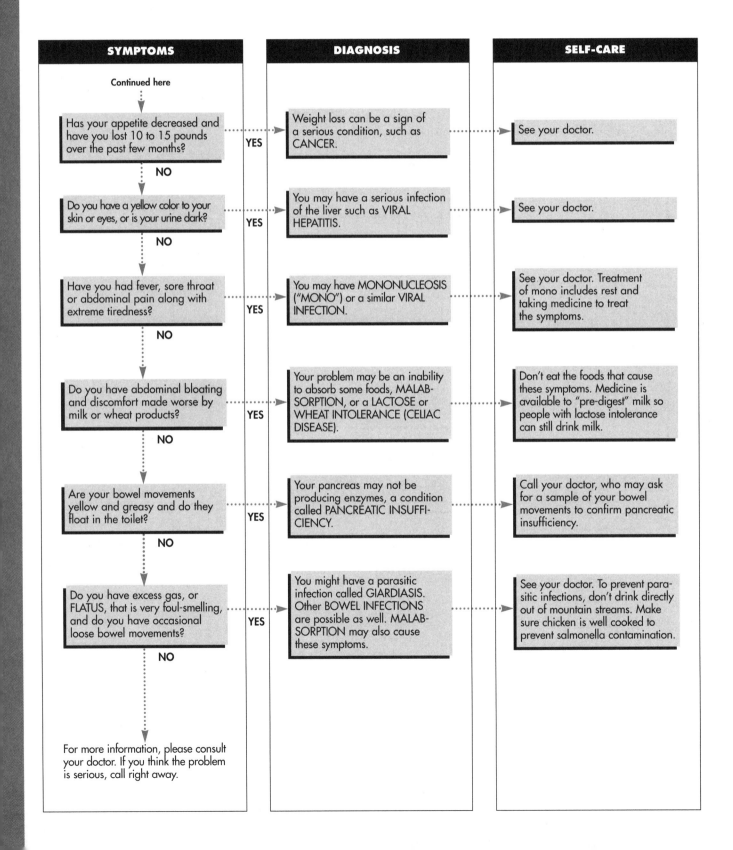

| SYMPTOMS | DIAGNOSIS | SELF-CARE |
|---|---|---|

**Continued here**

Has your appetite decreased and have you lost 10 to 15 pounds over the past few months? — **YES** → Weight loss can be a sign of a serious condition, such as CANCER. → See your doctor.

**NO**

Do you have a yellow color to your skin or eyes, or is your urine dark? — **YES** → You may have a serious infection of the liver such as VIRAL HEPATITIS. → See your doctor.

**NO**

Have you had fever, sore throat or abdominal pain along with extreme tiredness? — **YES** → You may have MONONUCLEOSIS ("MONO") or a similar VIRAL INFECTION. → See your doctor. Treatment of mono includes rest and taking medicine to treat the symptoms.

**NO**

Do you have abdominal bloating and discomfort made worse by milk or wheat products? — **YES** → Your problem may be an inability to absorb some foods, MALABSORPTION, or a LACTOSE or WHEAT INTOLERANCE (CELIAC DISEASE). → Don't eat the foods that cause these symptoms. Medicine is available to "pre-digest" milk so people with lactose intolerance can still drink milk.

**NO**

Are your bowel movements yellow and greasy and do they float in the toilet? — **YES** → Your pancreas may not be producing enzymes, a condition called PANCREATIC INSUFFICIENCY. → Call your doctor, who may ask for a sample of your bowel movements to confirm pancreatic insufficiency.

**NO**

Do you have excess gas, or FLATUS, that is very foul-smelling, and do you have occasional loose bowel movements? — **YES** → You might have a parasitic infection called GIARDIASIS. Other BOWEL INFECTIONS are possible as well. MALABSORPTION may also cause these symptoms. → See your doctor. To prevent parasitic infections, don't drink directly out of mountain streams. Make sure chicken is well cooked to prevent salmonella contamination.

**NO**

For more information, please consult your doctor. If you think the problem is serious, call right away.

# TOPIC 29 Nausea and Vomiting

Many illnesses can cause stomach pain, nausea and vomiting. Some are mild sicknesses that will pass by themselves, but others are serious and need medical attention.

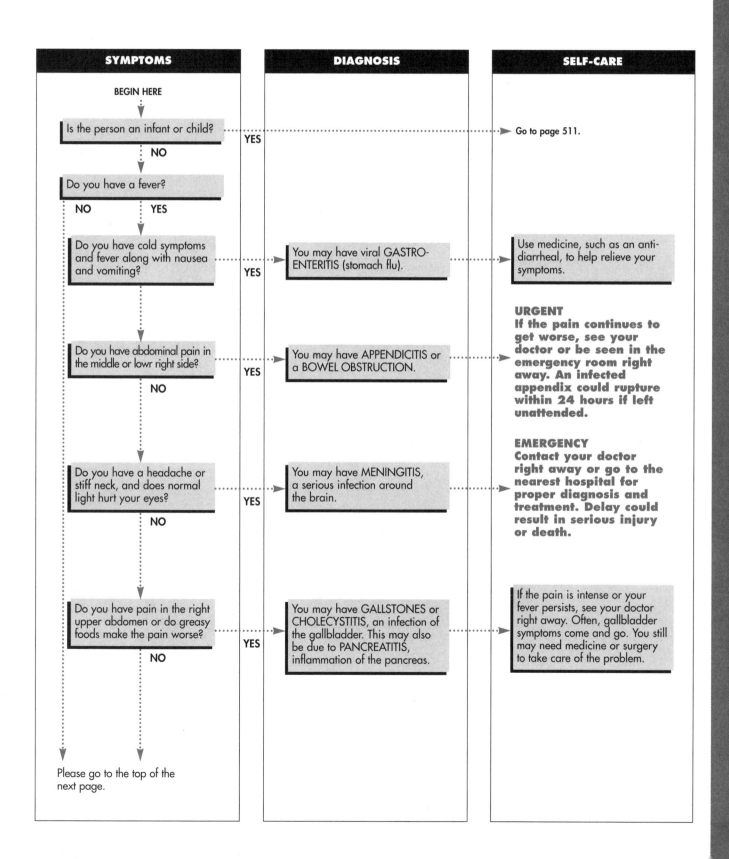

| SYMPTOMS | DIAGNOSIS | SELF-CARE |
|---|---|---|
| **BEGIN HERE** | | |
| Is the person an infant or child? — **YES** | | Go to page 511. |
| **NO** | | |
| Do you have a fever? | | |
| **NO**   **YES** | | |
| Do you have cold symptoms and fever along with nausea and vomiting? — **YES** | You may have viral GASTRO-ENTERITIS (stomach flu). | Use medicine, such as an anti-diarrheal, to help relieve your symptoms. |
| Do you have abdominal pain in the middle or lowr right side? — **YES** | You may have APPENDICITIS or a BOWEL OBSTRUCTION. | **URGENT** **If the pain continues to get worse, see your doctor or be seen in the emergency room right away. An infected appendix could rupture within 24 hours if left unattended.** |
| **NO** | | |
| Do you have a headache or stiff neck, and does normal light hurt your eyes? — **YES** | You may have MENINGITIS, a serious infection around the brain. | **EMERGENCY** **Contact your doctor right away or go to the nearest hospital for proper diagnosis and treatment. Delay could result in serious injury or death.** |
| **NO** | | |
| Do you have pain in the right upper abdomen or do greasy foods make the pain worse? — **YES** | You may have GALLSTONES or CHOLECYSTITIS, an infection of the gallbladder. This may also be due to PANCREATITIS, inflammation of the pancreas. | If the pain is intense or your fever persists, see your doctor right away. Often, gallbladder symptoms come and go. You still may need medicine or surgery to take care of the problem. |
| **NO** | | |

Please go to the top of the next page.

# TOPIC 29 Nausea and Vomiting

continued.

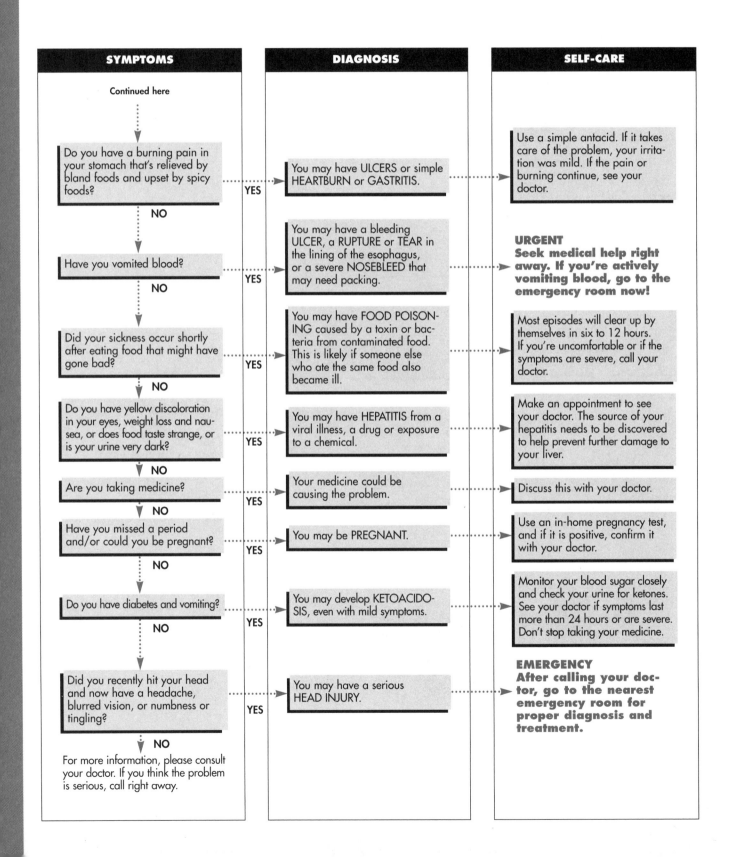

| SYMPTOMS | DIAGNOSIS | SELF-CARE |
|---|---|---|

**Continued here**

Do you have a burning pain in your stomach that's relieved by bland foods and upset by spicy foods? — **YES**

You may have ULCERS or simple HEARTBURN or GASTRITIS.

Use a simple antacid. If it takes care of the problem, your irritation was mild. If the pain or burning continue, see your doctor.

**NO**

Have you vomited blood? — **YES**

You may have a bleeding ULCER, a RUPTURE or TEAR in the lining of the esophagus, or a severe NOSEBLEED that may need packing.

**URGENT**
**Seek medical help right away. If you're actively vomiting blood, go to the emergency room now!**

**NO**

Did your sickness occur shortly after eating food that might have gone bad? — **YES**

You may have FOOD POISONING caused by a toxin or bacteria from contaminated food. This is likely if someone else who ate the same food also became ill.

Most episodes will clear up by themselves in six to 12 hours. If you're uncomfortable or if the symptoms are severe, call your doctor.

**NO**

Do you have yellow discoloration in your eyes, weight loss and nausea, or does food taste strange, or is your urine very dark? — **YES**

You may have HEPATITIS from a viral illness, a drug or exposure to a chemical.

Make an appointment to see your doctor. The source of your hepatitis needs to be discovered to help prevent further damage to your liver.

**NO**

Are you taking medicine? — **YES**

Your medicine could be causing the problem.

Discuss this with your doctor.

**NO**

Have you missed a period and/or could you be pregnant? — **YES**

You may be PREGNANT.

Use an in-home pregnancy test, and if it is positive, confirm it with your doctor.

**NO**

Do you have diabetes and vomiting? — **YES**

You may develop KETOACIDOSIS, even with mild symptoms.

Monitor your blood sugar closely and check your urine for ketones. See your doctor if symptoms last more than 24 hours or are severe. Don't stop taking your medicine.

**NO**

Did you recently hit your head and now have a headache, blurred vision, or numbness or tingling? — **YES**

You may have a serious HEAD INJURY.

**EMERGENCY**
**After calling your doctor, go to the nearest emergency room for proper diagnosis and treatment.**

**NO**

For more information, please consult your doctor. If you think the problem is serious, call right away.

# TOPIC 30 Nausea and Vomiting in Infants and Children

Parents often feel uncomfortable when their children are unable to eat or hold down food or fluids.
Many mild illnesses may lead to a "sour stomach" or an inability to hold down food.
Follow this chart for more information about these problems.

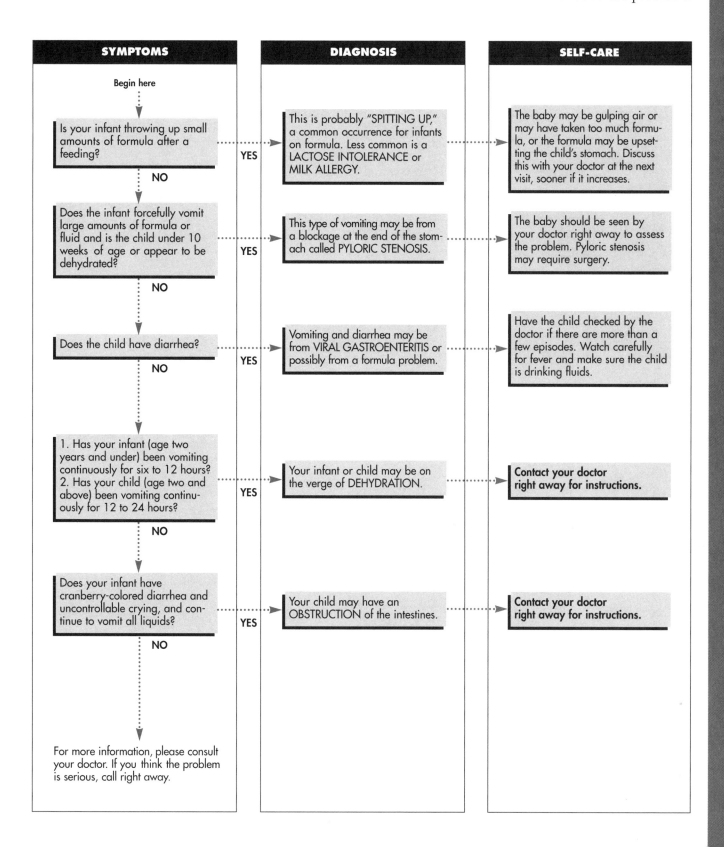

| SYMPTOMS | DIAGNOSIS | SELF-CARE |
|---|---|---|

**Begin here**

Is your infant throwing up small amounts of formula after a feeding?   **YES** → This is probably "SPITTING UP," a common occurrence for infants on formula. Less common is a LACTOSE INTOLERANCE or MILK ALLERGY. → The baby may be gulping air or may have taken too much formula, or the formula may be upsetting the child's stomach. Discuss this with your doctor at the next visit, sooner if it increases.

**NO**

Does the infant forcefully vomit large amounts of formula or fluid and is the child under 10 weeks of age or appear to be dehydrated?   **YES** → This type of vomiting may be from a blockage at the end of the stomach called PYLORIC STENOSIS. → The baby should be seen by your doctor right away to assess the problem. Pyloric stenosis may require surgery.

**NO**

Does the child have diarrhea?   **YES** → Vomiting and diarrhea may be from VIRAL GASTROENTERITIS or possibly from a formula problem. → Have the child checked by the doctor if there are more than a few episodes. Watch carefully for fever and make sure the child is drinking fluids.

**NO**

1. Has your infant (age two years and under) been vomiting continuously for six to 12 hours?
2. Has your child (age two and above) been vomiting continuously for 12 to 24 hours?   **YES** → Your infant or child may be on the verge of DEHYDRATION. → **Contact your doctor right away for instructions.**

**NO**

Does your infant have cranberry-colored diarrhea and uncontrollable crying, and continue to vomit all liquids?   **YES** → Your child may have an OBSTRUCTION of the intestines. → **Contact your doctor right away for instructions.**

**NO**

For more information, please consult your doctor. If you think the problem is serious, call right away.

# TOPIC 31 Lower Back Pain

Back pain and discomfort with movement are common problems, often originating from overuse of the back muscles. Other causes of back pain are also described in this chart.

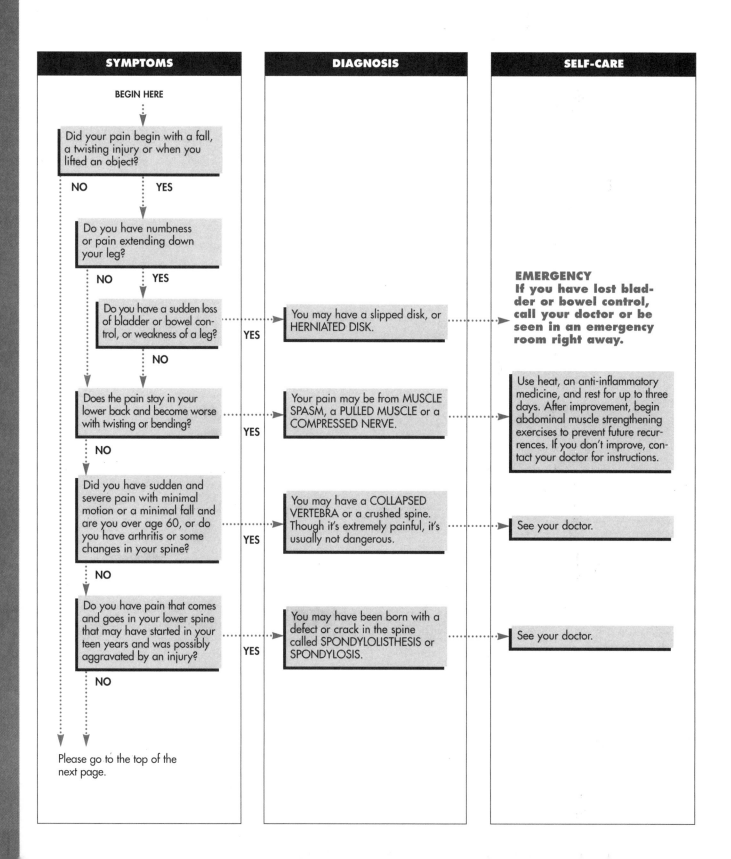

**SYMPTOMS**

BEGIN HERE

Did your pain begin with a fall, a twisting injury or when you lifted an object?

NO     YES

Do you have numbness or pain extending down your leg?

NO     YES

Do you have a sudden loss of bladder or bowel control, or weakness of a leg? — YES

NO

Does the pain stay in your lower back and become worse with twisting or bending? — YES

NO

Did you have sudden and severe pain with minimal motion or a minimal fall and are you over age 60, or do you have arthritis or some changes in your spine? — YES

NO

Do you have pain that comes and goes in your lower spine that may have started in your teen years and was possibly aggravated by an injury? — YES

NO

Please go to the top of the next page.

**DIAGNOSIS**

You may have a slipped disk, or HERNIATED DISK.

Your pain may be from MUSCLE SPASM, a PULLED MUSCLE or a COMPRESSED NERVE.

You may have a COLLAPSED VERTEBRA or a crushed spine. Though it's extremely painful, it's usually not dangerous.

You may have been born with a defect or crack in the spine called SPONDYLOLISTHESIS or SPONDYLOSIS.

**SELF-CARE**

**EMERGENCY**
**If you have lost bladder or bowel control, call your doctor or be seen in an emergency room right away.**

Use heat, an anti-inflammatory medicine, and rest for up to three days. After improvement, begin abdominal muscle strengthening exercises to prevent future recurrences. If you don't improve, contact your doctor for instructions.

See your doctor.

See your doctor.

**TOPIC 31** Lower Back Pain

continued.

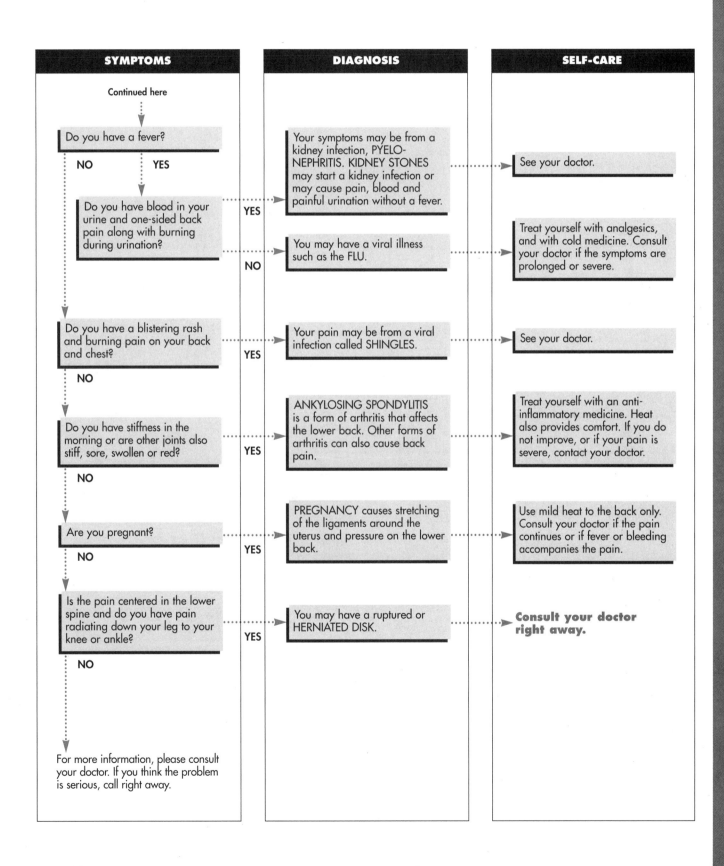

| SYMPTOMS | DIAGNOSIS | SELF-CARE |
|---|---|---|

Continued here

Do you have a fever?

NO          YES

Do you have blood in your urine and one-sided back pain along with burning during urination?

YES → Your symptoms may be from a kidney infection, PYELO-NEPHRITIS. KIDNEY STONES may start a kidney infection or may cause pain, blood and painful urination without a fever. → See your doctor.

NO → You may have a viral illness such as the FLU. → Treat yourself with analgesics, and with cold medicine. Consult your doctor if the symptoms are prolonged or severe.

Do you have a blistering rash and burning pain on your back and chest?

YES → Your pain may be from a viral infection called SHINGLES. → See your doctor.

NO

Do you have stiffness in the morning or are other joints also stiff, sore, swollen or red?

YES → ANKYLOSING SPONDYLITIS is a form of arthritis that affects the lower back. Other forms of arthritis can also cause back pain. → Treat yourself with an anti-inflammatory medicine. Heat also provides comfort. If you do not improve, or if your pain is severe, contact your doctor.

NO

Are you pregnant?

YES → PREGNANCY causes stretching of the ligaments around the uterus and pressure on the lower back. → Use mild heat to the back only. Consult your doctor if the pain continues or if fever or bleeding accompanies the pain.

NO

Is the pain centered in the lower spine and do you have pain radiating down your leg to your knee or ankle?

YES → You may have a ruptured or HERNIATED DISK. → **Consult your doctor right away.**

NO

For more information, please consult your doctor. If you think the problem is serious, call right away.

# TOPIC 32 Elimination Problems

Use this chart when you or a family member has pain, itching or blood with a bowel movement.

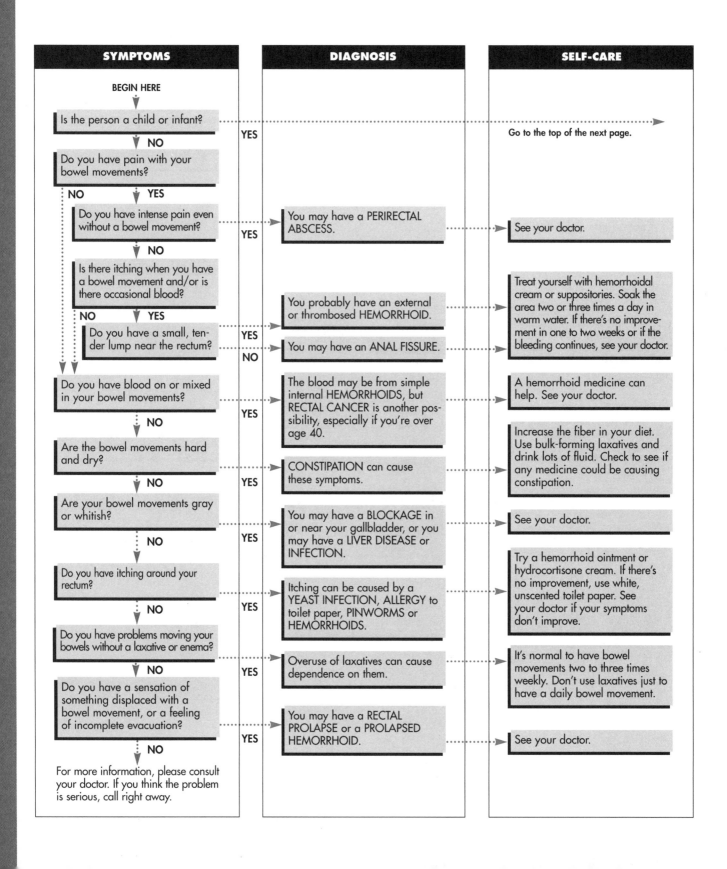

| SYMPTOMS | DIAGNOSIS | SELF-CARE |
|---|---|---|

**BEGIN HERE**

Is the person a child or infant? — **YES** → Go to the top of the next page.

**NO**

Do you have pain with your bowel movements?

**NO** / **YES**

Do you have intense pain even without a bowel movement? — **YES** → You may have a PERIRECTAL ABSCESS. → See your doctor.

**NO**

Is there itching when you have a bowel movement and/or is there occasional blood?

**NO** / **YES**

Do you have a small, tender lump near the rectum? — **YES** → You probably have an external or thrombosed HEMORRHOID. → Treat yourself with hemorrhoidal cream or suppositories. Soak the area two or three times a day in warm water. If there's no improvement in one to two weeks or if the bleeding continues, see your doctor.

**NO** → You may have an ANAL FISSURE.

Do you have blood on or mixed in your bowel movements? — **YES** → The blood may be from simple internal HEMORRHOIDS, but RECTAL CANCER is another possibility, especially if you're over age 40. → A hemorrhoid medicine can help. See your doctor.

**NO**

Are the bowel movements hard and dry? — **YES** → CONSTIPATION can cause these symptoms. → Increase the fiber in your diet. Use bulk-forming laxatives and drink lots of fluid. Check to see if any medicine could be causing constipation.

**NO**

Are your bowel movements gray or whitish? — **YES** → You may have a BLOCKAGE in or near your gallbladder, or you may have a LIVER DISEASE or INFECTION. → See your doctor.

**NO**

Do you have itching around your rectum? — **YES** → Itching can be caused by a YEAST INFECTION, ALLERGY to toilet paper, PINWORMS or HEMORRHOIDS. → Try a hemorrhoid ointment or hydrocortisone cream. If there's no improvement, use white, unscented toilet paper. See your doctor if your symptoms don't improve.

**NO**

Do you have problems moving your bowels without a laxative or enema? — **YES** → Overuse of laxatives can cause dependence on them. → It's normal to have bowel movements two to three times weekly. Don't use laxatives just to have a daily bowel movement.

**NO**

Do you have a sensation of something displaced with a bowel movement, or a feeling of incomplete evacuation? — **YES** → You may have a RECTAL PROLAPSE or a PROLAPSED HEMORRHOID. → See your doctor.

**NO**

For more information, please consult your doctor. If you think the problem is serious, call right away.

# TOPIC 33 Elimination Problems in Infants and Children

Use this chart when an infant or child has changes in bowel movements.

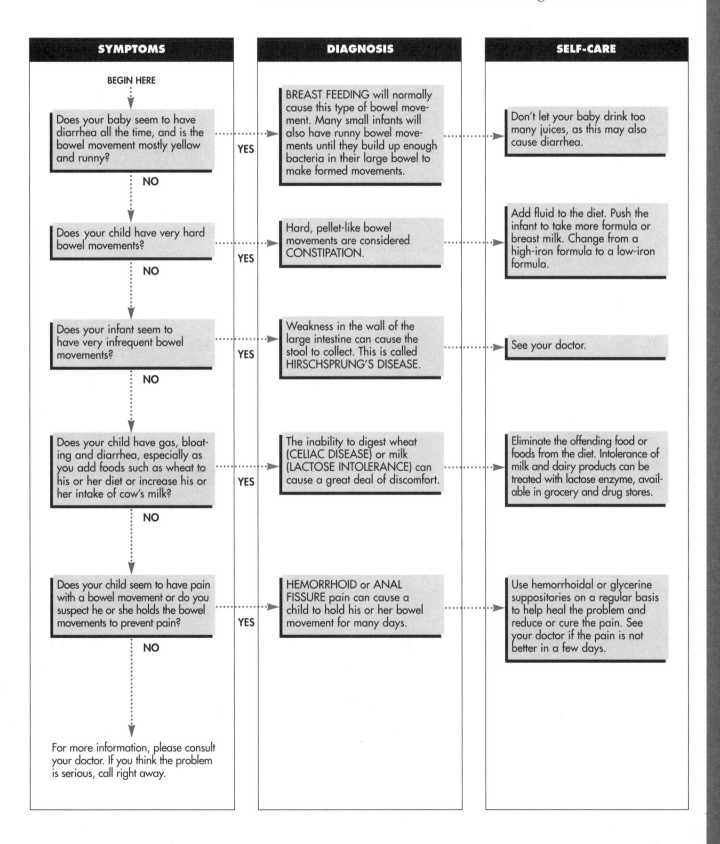

| SYMPTOMS | DIAGNOSIS | SELF-CARE |
|---|---|---|

**BEGIN HERE**

Does your baby seem to have diarrhea all the time, and is the bowel movement mostly yellow and runny? — **YES** → BREAST FEEDING will normally cause this type of bowel movement. Many small infants will also have runny bowel movements until they build up enough bacteria in their large bowel to make formed movements. → Don't let your baby drink too many juices, as this may also cause diarrhea.

**NO**

Does your child have very hard bowel movements? — **YES** → Hard, pellet-like bowel movements are considered CONSTIPATION. → Add fluid to the diet. Push the infant to take more formula or breast milk. Change from a high-iron formula to a low-iron formula.

**NO**

Does your infant seem to have very infrequent bowel movements? — **YES** → Weakness in the wall of the large intestine can cause the stool to collect. This is called HIRSCHSPRUNG'S DISEASE. → See your doctor.

**NO**

Does your child have gas, bloating and diarrhea, especially as you add foods such as wheat to his or her diet or increase his or her intake of cow's milk? — **YES** → The inability to digest wheat (CELIAC DISEASE) or milk (LACTOSE INTOLERANCE) can cause a great deal of discomfort. → Eliminate the offending food or foods from the diet. Intolerance of milk and dairy products can be treated with lactose enzyme, available in grocery and drug stores.

**NO**

Does your child seem to have pain with a bowel movement or do you suspect he or she holds the bowel movements to prevent pain? — **YES** → HEMORRHOID or ANAL FISSURE pain can cause a child to hold his or her bowel movement for many days. → Use hemorrhoidal or glycerine suppositories on a regular basis to help heal the problem and reduce or cure the pain. See your doctor if the pain is not better in a few days.

**NO**

For more information, please consult your doctor. If you think the problem is serious, call right away.

# TOPIC 34 Diarrhea

Loose or watery bowel movements, sometimes with unusual colors or consistencies, create an uncomfortable condition that usually stops by itself. Work through this chart to make sure the diarrhea doesn't need immediate attention.

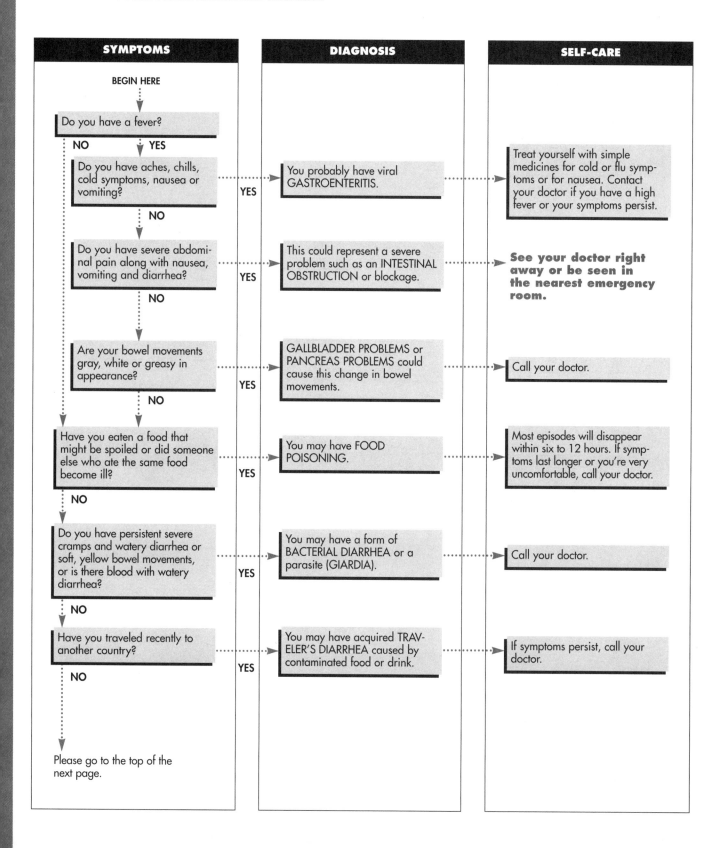

| SYMPTOMS | DIAGNOSIS | SELF-CARE |
|---|---|---|

**BEGIN HERE**

Do you have a fever?

NO — YES

Do you have aches, chills, cold symptoms, nausea or vomiting?

YES → You probably have viral GASTROENTERITIS. → Treat yourself with simple medicines for cold or flu symptoms or for nausea. Contact your doctor if you have a high fever or your symptoms persist.

NO

Do you have severe abdominal pain along with nausea, vomiting and diarrhea?

YES → This could represent a severe problem such as an INTESTINAL OBSTRUCTION or blockage. → **See your doctor right away or be seen in the nearest emergency room.**

NO

Are your bowel movements gray, white or greasy in appearance?

YES → GALLBLADDER PROBLEMS or PANCREAS PROBLEMS could cause this change in bowel movements. → Call your doctor.

NO

Have you eaten a food that might be spoiled or did someone else who ate the same food become ill?

YES → You may have FOOD POISONING. → Most episodes will disappear within six to 12 hours. If symptoms last longer or you're very uncomfortable, call your doctor.

NO

Do you have persistent severe cramps and watery diarrhea or soft, yellow bowel movements, or is there blood with watery diarrhea?

YES → You may have a form of BACTERIAL DIARRHEA or a parasite (GIARDIA). → Call your doctor.

NO

Have you traveled recently to another country?

YES → You may have acquired TRAVELER'S DIARRHEA caused by contaminated food or drink. → If symptoms persist, call your doctor.

NO

Please go to the top of the next page.

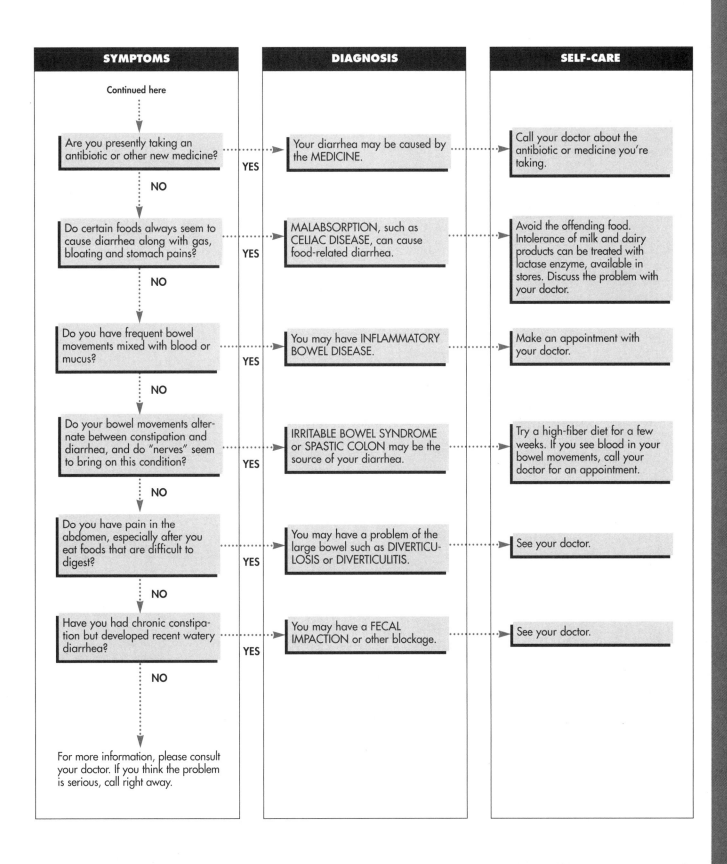

| SYMPTOMS | DIAGNOSIS | SELF-CARE |
|---|---|---|

Continued here

Are you presently taking an antibiotic or other new medicine? — **YES** → Your diarrhea may be caused by the MEDICINE. → Call your doctor about the antibiotic or medicine you're taking.

**NO**

Do certain foods always seem to cause diarrhea along with gas, bloating and stomach pains? — **YES** → MALABSORPTION, such as CELIAC DISEASE, can cause food-related diarrhea. → Avoid the offending food. Intolerance of milk and dairy products can be treated with lactase enzyme, available in stores. Discuss the problem with your doctor.

**NO**

Do you have frequent bowel movements mixed with blood or mucus? — **YES** → You may have INFLAMMATORY BOWEL DISEASE. → Make an appointment with your doctor.

**NO**

Do your bowel movements alternate between constipation and diarrhea, and do "nerves" seem to bring on this condition? — **YES** → IRRITABLE BOWEL SYNDROME or SPASTIC COLON may be the source of your diarrhea. → Try a high-fiber diet for a few weeks. If you see blood in your bowel movements, call your doctor for an appointment.

**NO**

Do you have pain in the abdomen, especially after you eat foods that are difficult to digest? — **YES** → You may have a problem of the large bowel such as DIVERTICULOSIS or DIVERTICULITIS. → See your doctor.

**NO**

Have you had chronic constipation but developed recent watery diarrhea? — **YES** → You may have a FECAL IMPACTION or other blockage. → See your doctor.

**NO**

For more information, please consult your doctor. If you think the problem is serious, call right away.

# TOPIC 35 Urination Problems

Both men and women can experience pain and difficulty with urination caused by common conditions, as well as more serious problems. Follow this chart for more information about these symptoms and their care.

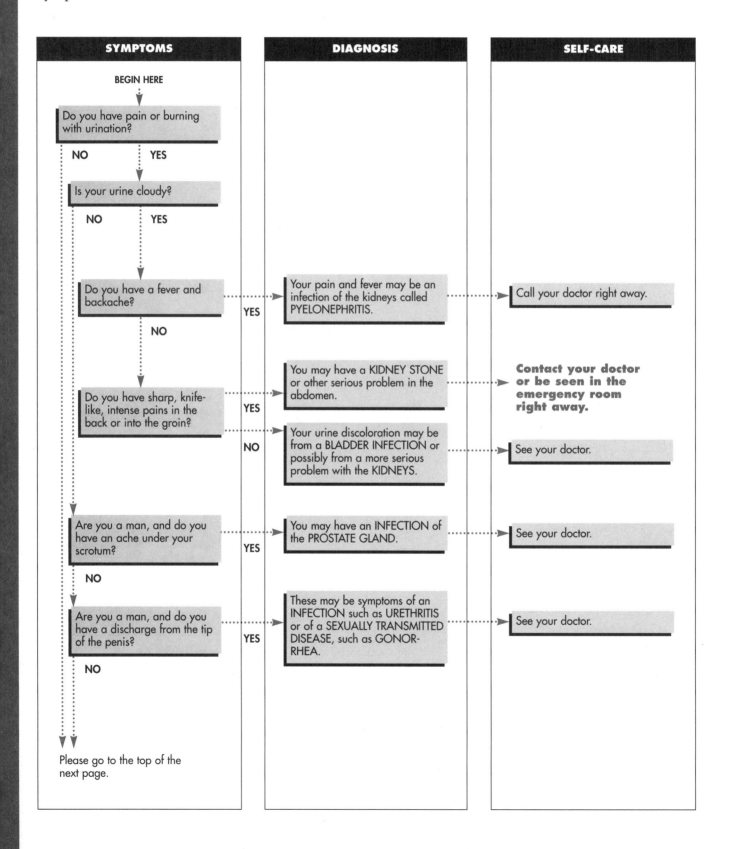

| SYMPTOMS | DIAGNOSIS | SELF-CARE |
|---|---|---|

**BEGIN HERE**

Do you have pain or burning with urination?
NO    YES

Is your urine cloudy?
NO    YES

Do you have a fever and backache?
YES → Your pain and fever may be an infection of the kidneys called PYELONEPHRITIS. → Call your doctor right away.
NO

Do you have sharp, knife-like, intense pains in the back or into the groin?
YES → You may have a KIDNEY STONE or other serious problem in the abdomen. → **Contact your doctor or be seen in the emergency room right away.**
NO → Your urine discoloration may be from a BLADDER INFECTION or possibly from a more serious problem with the KIDNEYS. → See your doctor.

Are you a man, and do you have an ache under your scrotum?
YES → You may have an INFECTION of the PROSTATE GLAND. → See your doctor.
NO

Are you a man, and do you have a discharge from the tip of the penis?
YES → These may be symptoms of an INFECTION such as URETHRITIS or of a SEXUALLY TRANSMITTED DISEASE, such as GONOR-RHEA. → See your doctor.
NO

Please go to the top of the next page.

**TOPIC 35** Urination Problems

continued.

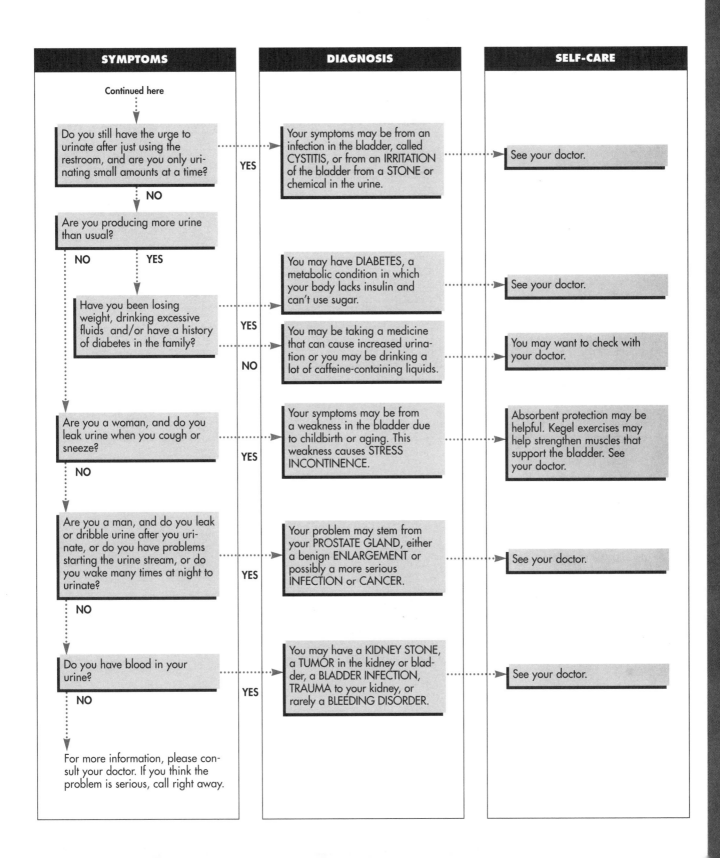

| SYMPTOMS | DIAGNOSIS | SELF-CARE |
|---|---|---|

Continued here

Do you still have the urge to urinate after just using the restroom, and are you only urinating small amounts at a time? — **YES** → Your symptoms may be from an infection in the bladder, called CYSTITIS, or from an IRRITATION of the bladder from a STONE or chemical in the urine. → See your doctor.

**NO**

Are you producing more urine than usual?

**NO**     **YES**

Have you been losing weight, drinking excessive fluids and/or have a history of diabetes in the family? — **YES** → You may have DIABETES, a metabolic condition in which your body lacks insulin and can't use sugar. → See your doctor.

**NO** → You may be taking a medicine that can cause increased urination or you may be drinking a lot of caffeine-containing liquids. → You may want to check with your doctor.

Are you a woman, and do you leak urine when you cough or sneeze? — **YES** → Your symptoms may be from a weakness in the bladder due to childbirth or aging. This weakness causes STRESS INCONTINENCE. → Absorbent protection may be helpful. Kegel exercises may help strengthen muscles that support the bladder. See your doctor.

**NO**

Are you a man, and do you leak or dribble urine after you urinate, or do you have problems starting the urine stream, or do you wake many times at night to urinate? — **YES** → Your problem may stem from your PROSTATE GLAND, either a benign ENLARGEMENT or possibly a more serious INFECTION or CANCER. → See your doctor.

**NO**

Do you have blood in your urine? — **YES** → You may have a KIDNEY STONE, a TUMOR in the kidney or bladder, a BLADDER INFECTION, TRAUMA to your kidney, or rarely a BLEEDING DISORDER. → See your doctor.

**NO**

For more information, please consult your doctor. If you think the problem is serious, call right away.

# TOPIC 36 Genital Problems in Infants

Any deformity or change in the genitals is of obvious concern to parents. Yet many of these changes can be corrected. Follow this chart for more information.

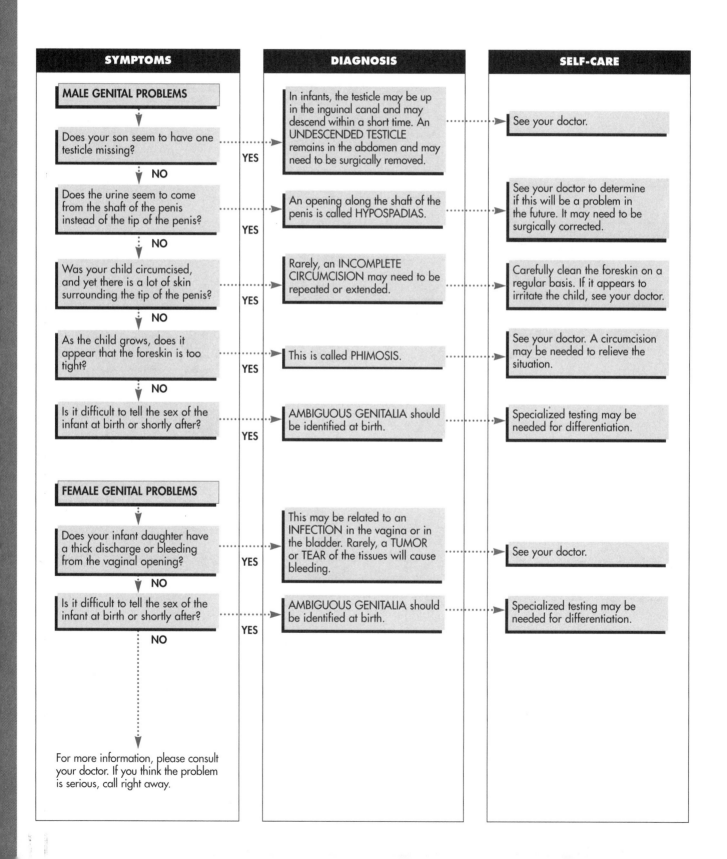

**SYMPTOMS**

**MALE GENITAL PROBLEMS**

Does your son seem to have one testicle missing?

YES

NO

Does the urine seem to come from the shaft of the penis instead of the tip of the penis?

YES

NO

Was your child circumcised, and yet there is a lot of skin surrounding the tip of the penis?

YES

NO

As the child grows, does it appear that the foreskin is too tight?

YES

NO

Is it difficult to tell the sex of the infant at birth or shortly after?

YES

**FEMALE GENITAL PROBLEMS**

Does your infant daughter have a thick discharge or bleeding from the vaginal opening?

YES

NO

Is it difficult to tell the sex of the infant at birth or shortly after?

YES

NO

For more information, please consult your doctor. If you think the problem is serious, call right away.

**DIAGNOSIS**

In infants, the testicle may be up in the inguinal canal and may descend within a short time. An UNDESCENDED TESTICLE remains in the abdomen and may need to be surgically removed.

An opening along the shaft of the penis is called HYPOSPADIAS.

Rarely, an INCOMPLETE CIRCUMCISION may need to be repeated or extended.

This is called PHIMOSIS.

AMBIGUOUS GENITALIA should be identified at birth.

This may be related to an INFECTION in the vagina or in the bladder. Rarely, a TUMOR or TEAR of the tissues will cause bleeding.

AMBIGUOUS GENITALIA should be identified at birth.

**SELF-CARE**

See your doctor.

See your doctor to determine if this will be a problem in the future. It may need to be surgically corrected.

Carefully clean the foreskin on a regular basis. If it appears to irritate the child, see your doctor.

See your doctor. A circumcision may be needed to relieve the situation.

Specialized testing may be needed for differentiation.

See your doctor.

Specialized testing may be needed for differentiation.

# TOPIC 37 Genital Problems in Women

Vaginal irritation and discharge are common problems for many women. Check this chart for help in understanding and self-treating many of these problems.

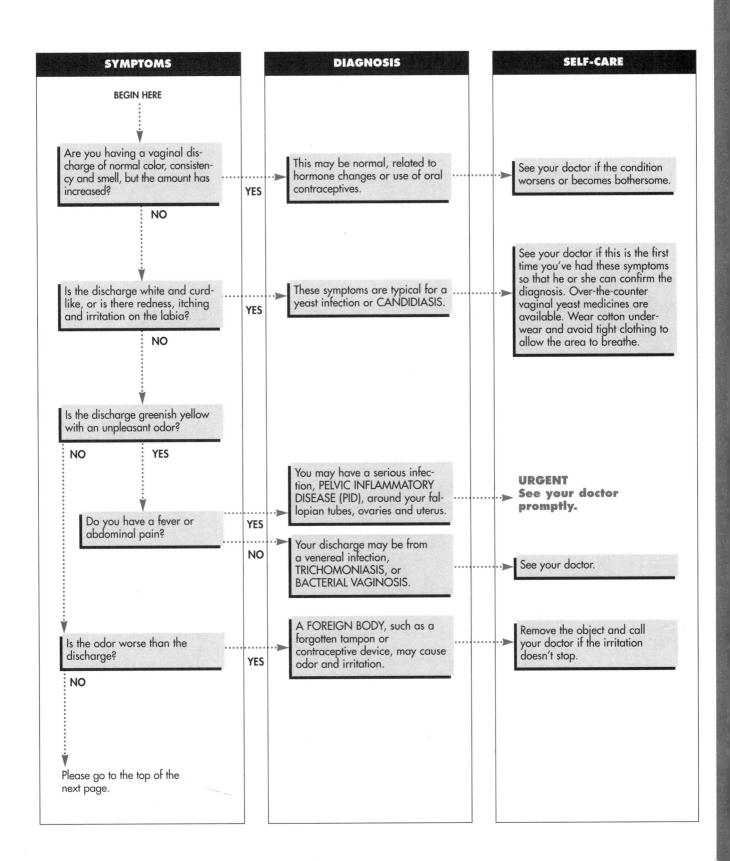

| SYMPTOMS | DIAGNOSIS | SELF-CARE |
|---|---|---|

**BEGIN HERE**

Are you having a vaginal discharge of normal color, consistency and smell, but the amount has increased?

**YES** → This may be normal, related to hormone changes or use of oral contraceptives. → See your doctor if the condition worsens or becomes bothersome.

**NO**

Is the discharge white and curd-like, or is there redness, itching and irritation on the labia?

**YES** → These symptoms are typical for a yeast infection or CANDIDIASIS. → See your doctor if this is the first time you've had these symptoms so that he or she can confirm the diagnosis. Over-the-counter vaginal yeast medicines are available. Wear cotton underwear and avoid tight clothing to allow the area to breathe.

**NO**

Is the discharge greenish yellow with an unpleasant odor?

**NO**          **YES**

Do you have a fever or abdominal pain?

**YES** → You may have a serious infection, PELVIC INFLAMMATORY DISEASE (PID), around your fallopian tubes, ovaries and uterus. → **URGENT See your doctor promptly.**

**NO** → Your discharge may be from a venereal infection, TRICHOMONIASIS, or BACTERIAL VAGINOSIS. → See your doctor.

Is the odor worse than the discharge?

**YES** → A FOREIGN BODY, such as a forgotten tampon or contraceptive device, may cause odor and irritation. → Remove the object and call your doctor if the irritation doesn't stop.

**NO**

Please go to the top of the next page.

# TOPIC 37 Genital Problems in Women

continued.

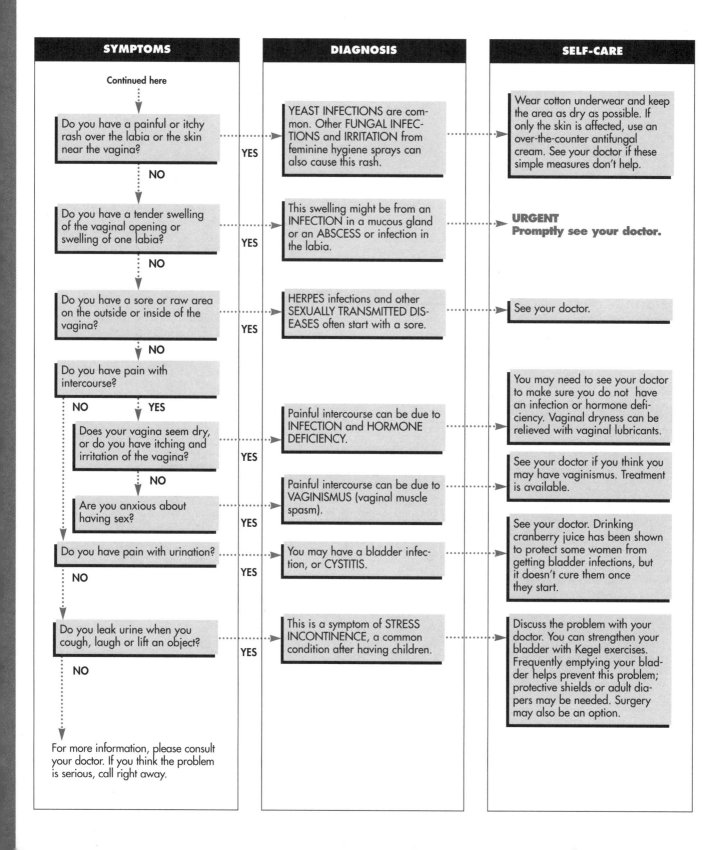

| SYMPTOMS | DIAGNOSIS | SELF-CARE |
|---|---|---|

**Continued here**

Do you have a painful or itchy rash over the labia or the skin near the vagina? — **YES** → YEAST INFECTIONS are common. Other FUNGAL INFECTIONS and IRRITATION from feminine hygiene sprays can also cause this rash. → Wear cotton underwear and keep the area as dry as possible. If only the skin is affected, use an over-the-counter antifungal cream. See your doctor if these simple measures don't help.

**NO**

Do you have a tender swelling of the vaginal opening or swelling of one labia? — **YES** → This swelling might be from an INFECTION in a mucous gland or an ABSCESS or infection in the labia. → **URGENT** **Promptly see your doctor.**

**NO**

Do you have a sore or raw area on the outside or inside of the vagina? — **YES** → HERPES infections and other SEXUALLY TRANSMITTED DISEASES often start with a sore. → See your doctor.

**NO**

Do you have pain with intercourse?

**NO** / **YES**

Does your vagina seem dry, or do you have itching and irritation of the vagina? — **YES** → Painful intercourse can be due to INFECTION and HORMONE DEFICIENCY. → You may need to see your doctor to make sure you do not have an infection or hormone deficiency. Vaginal dryness can be relieved with vaginal lubricants.

**NO**

Are you anxious about having sex? — **YES** → Painful intercourse can be due to VAGINISMUS (vaginal muscle spasm). → See your doctor if you think you may have vaginismus. Treatment is available.

Do you have pain with urination? — **YES** → You may have a bladder infection, or CYSTITIS. → See your doctor. Drinking cranberry juice has been shown to protect some women from getting bladder infections, but it doesn't cure them once they start.

**NO**

Do you leak urine when you cough, laugh or lift an object? — **YES** → This is a symptom of STRESS INCONTINENCE, a common condition after having children. → Discuss the problem with your doctor. You can strengthen your bladder with Kegel exercises. Frequently emptying your bladder helps prevent this problem; protective shields or adult diapers may be needed. Surgery may also be an option.

**NO**

For more information, please consult your doctor. If you think the problem is serious, call right away.

# TOPIC 38  Menstrual Cycle Problems

From missed periods to painful periods, menstrual cycle problems are common and often benign. Follow this chart for information regarding a change in your cycle.

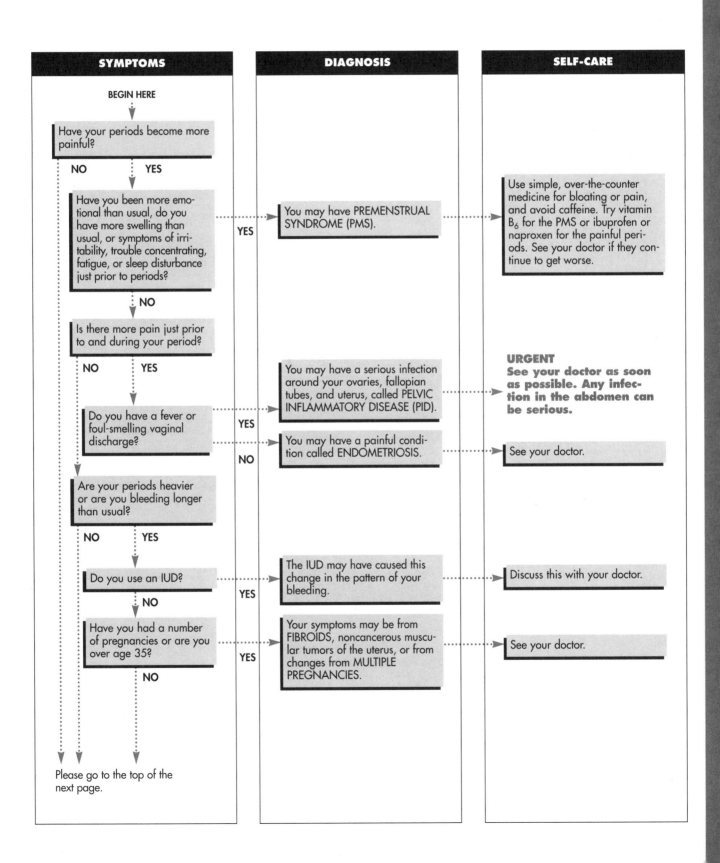

| SYMPTOMS | DIAGNOSIS | SELF-CARE |
|---|---|---|

**BEGIN HERE**

Have your periods become more painful?

NO        YES

Have you been more emotional than usual, do you have more swelling than usual, or symptoms of irritability, trouble concentrating, fatigue, or sleep disturbance just prior to periods?

YES → You may have PREMENSTRUAL SYNDROME (PMS). → Use simple, over-the-counter medicine for bloating or pain, and avoid caffeine. Try vitamin B₆ for the PMS or ibuprofen or naproxen for the painful periods. See your doctor if they continue to get worse.

NO

Is there more pain just prior to and during your period?

NO        YES

Do you have a fever or foul-smelling vaginal discharge?

YES → You may have a serious infection around your ovaries, fallopian tubes, and uterus, called PELVIC INFLAMMATORY DISEASE (PID). → **URGENT** **See your doctor as soon as possible. Any infection in the abdomen can be serious.**

NO → You may have a painful condition called ENDOMETRIOSIS. → See your doctor.

Are your periods heavier or are you bleeding longer than usual?

NO        YES

Do you use an IUD?

YES → The IUD may have caused this change in the pattern of your bleeding. → Discuss this with your doctor.

NO

Have you had a number of pregnancies or are you over age 35?

YES → Your symptoms may be from FIBROIDS, noncancerous muscular tumors of the uterus, or from changes from MULTIPLE PREGNANCIES. → See your doctor.

NO

Please go to the top of the next page.

## TOPIC 38 Menstrual Cycle Problems

continued.

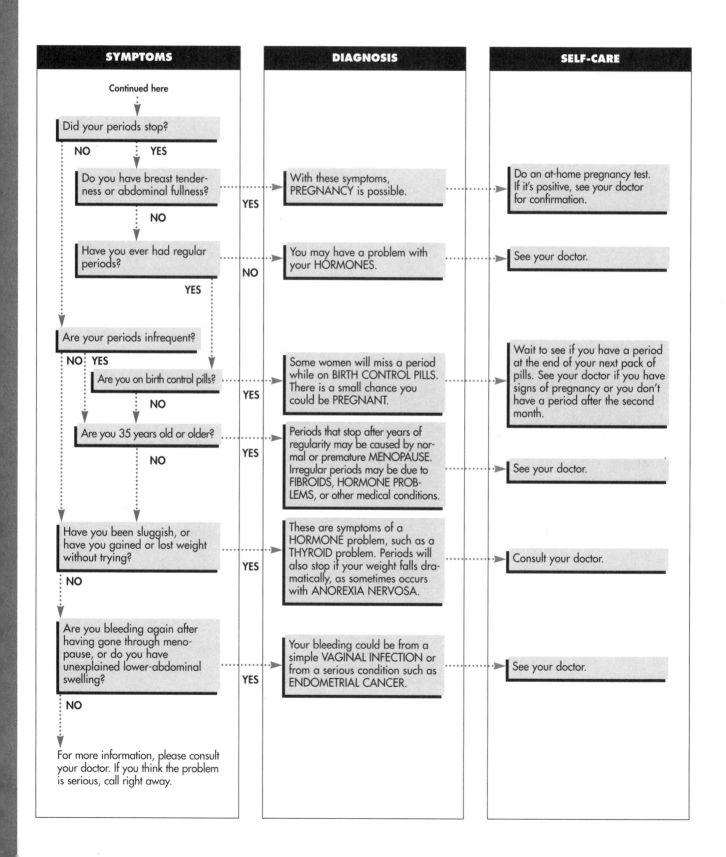

| SYMPTOMS | DIAGNOSIS | SELF-CARE |
|---|---|---|

**Continued here**

Did your periods stop?

NO    YES

Do you have breast tenderness or abdominal fullness? — YES → With these symptoms, PREGNANCY is possible. ⋯→ Do an at-home pregnancy test. If it's positive, see your doctor for confirmation.

NO

Have you ever had regular periods? — NO → You may have a problem with your HORMONES. ⋯→ See your doctor.

YES

Are your periods infrequent?

NO   YES

Are you on birth control pills? — YES → Some women will miss a period while on BIRTH CONTROL PILLS. There is a small chance you could be PREGNANT. ⋯→ Wait to see if you have a period at the end of your next pack of pills. See your doctor if you have signs of pregnancy or you don't have a period after the second month.

NO

Are you 35 years old or older? — YES → Periods that stop after years of regularity may be caused by normal or premature MENOPAUSE. Irregular periods may be due to FIBROIDS, HORMONE PROBLEMS, or other medical conditions. ⋯→ See your doctor.

NO

Have you been sluggish, or have you gained or lost weight without trying? — YES → These are symptoms of a HORMONE problem, such as a THYROID problem. Periods will also stop if your weight falls dramatically, as sometimes occurs with ANOREXIA NERVOSA. ⋯→ Consult your doctor.

NO

Are you bleeding again after having gone through menopause, or do you have unexplained lower-abdominal swelling? — YES → Your bleeding could be from a simple VAGINAL INFECTION or from a serious condition such as ENDOMETRIAL CANCER. ⋯→ See your doctor.

NO

For more information, please consult your doctor. If you think the problem is serious, call right away.

## TOPIC 39 Genital Problems in Men

Follow this chart if you or a male family member has a problem with their genital area.

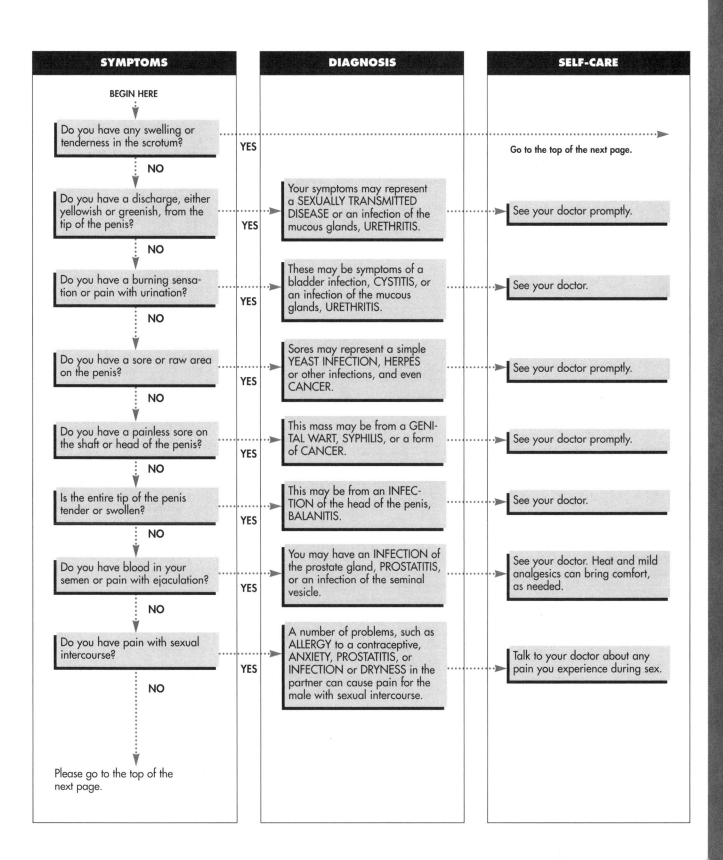

| SYMPTOMS | DIAGNOSIS | SELF-CARE |
|---|---|---|
| **BEGIN HERE** | | |
| Do you have any swelling or tenderness in the scrotum? — **YES** | | Go to the top of the next page. |
| **NO** | | |
| Do you have a discharge, either yellowish or greenish, from the tip of the penis? — **YES** | Your symptoms may represent a SEXUALLY TRANSMITTED DISEASE or an infection of the mucous glands, URETHRITIS. | See your doctor promptly. |
| **NO** | | |
| Do you have a burning sensation or pain with urination? — **YES** | These may be symptoms of a bladder infection, CYSTITIS, or an infection of the mucous glands, URETHRITIS. | See your doctor. |
| **NO** | | |
| Do you have a sore or raw area on the penis? — **YES** | Sores may represent a simple YEAST INFECTION, HERPES or other infections, and even CANCER. | See your doctor promptly. |
| **NO** | | |
| Do you have a painless sore on the shaft or head of the penis? — **YES** | This mass may be from a GENITAL WART, SYPHILIS, or a form of CANCER. | See your doctor promptly. |
| **NO** | | |
| Is the entire tip of the penis tender or swollen? — **YES** | This may be from an INFECTION of the head of the penis, BALANITIS. | See your doctor. |
| **NO** | | |
| Do you have blood in your semen or pain with ejaculation? — **YES** | You may have an INFECTION of the prostate gland, PROSTATITIS, or an infection of the seminal vesicle. | See your doctor. Heat and mild analgesics can bring comfort, as needed. |
| **NO** | | |
| Do you have pain with sexual intercourse? — **YES** | A number of problems, such as ALLERGY to a contraceptive, ANXIETY, PROSTATITIS, or INFECTION or DRYNESS in the partner can cause pain for the male with sexual intercourse. | Talk to your doctor about any pain you experience during sex. |
| **NO** | | |
| Please go to the top of the next page. | | |

# TOPIC 39 Genital Problems in Men

continued.

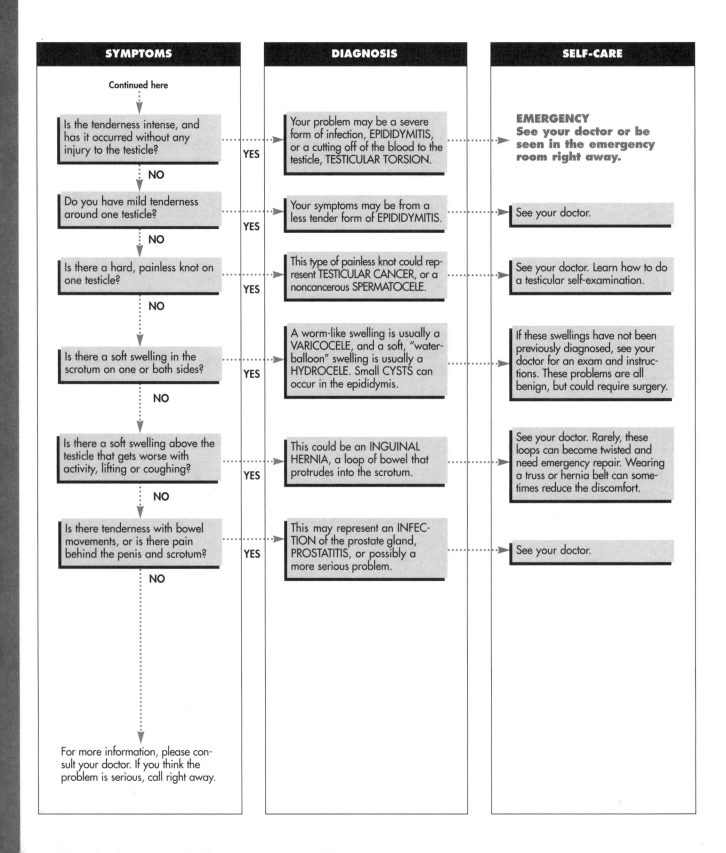

| SYMPTOMS | DIAGNOSIS | SELF-CARE |
|---|---|---|

**Continued here**

Is the tenderness intense, and has it occurred without any injury to the testicle? **YES** → Your problem may be a severe form of infection, EPIDIDYMITIS, or a cutting off of the blood to the testicle, TESTICULAR TORSION. → **EMERGENCY** See your doctor or be seen in the emergency room right away.

**NO**

Do you have mild tenderness around one testicle? **YES** → Your symptoms may be from a less tender form of EPIDIDYMITIS. → See your doctor.

**NO**

Is there a hard, painless knot on one testicle? **YES** → This type of painless knot could represent TESTICULAR CANCER, or a noncancerous SPERMATOCELE. → See your doctor. Learn how to do a testicular self-examination.

**NO**

Is there a soft swelling in the scrotum on one or both sides? **YES** → A worm-like swelling is usually a VARICOCELE, and a soft, "water-balloon" swelling is usually a HYDROCELE. Small CYSTS can occur in the epididymis. → If these swellings have not been previously diagnosed, see your doctor for an exam and instructions. These problems are all benign, but could require surgery.

**NO**

Is there a soft swelling above the testicle that gets worse with activity, lifting or coughing? **YES** → This could be an INGUINAL HERNIA, a loop of bowel that protrudes into the scrotum. → See your doctor. Rarely, these loops can become twisted and need emergency repair. Wearing a truss or hernia belt can sometimes reduce the discomfort.

**NO**

Is there tenderness with bowel movements, or is there pain behind the penis and scrotum? **YES** → This may represent an INFECTION of the prostate gland, PROSTATITIS, or possibly a more serious problem. → See your doctor.

**NO**

For more information, please consult your doctor. If you think the problem is serious, call right away.

# TOPIC 40 Hip Problems

Hip pain is usually associated with falling or with arthritis. Rarely, a hip problem starts at birth. Follow this chart to gain insight into your pain or problem.

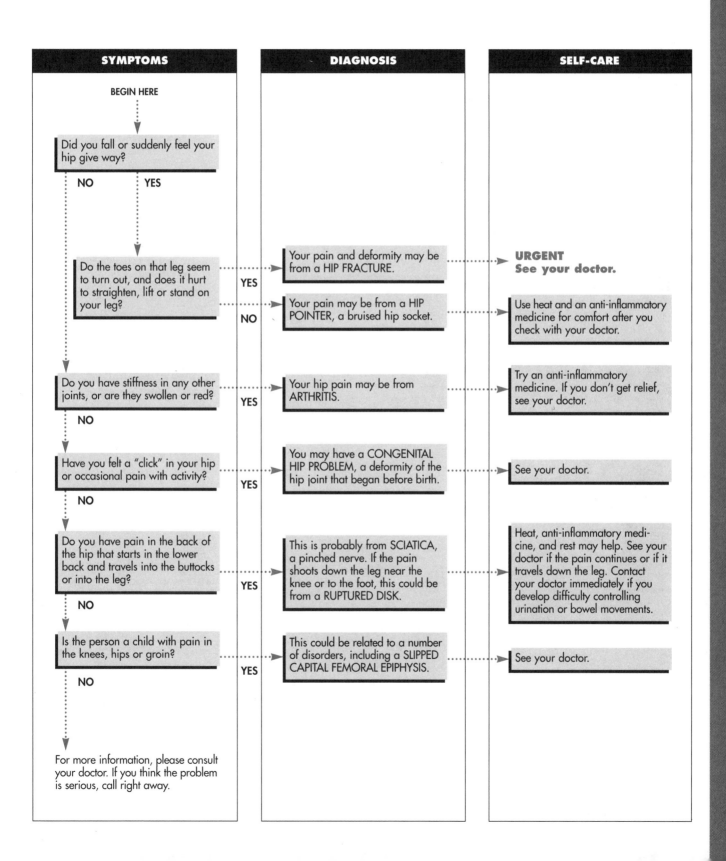

| SYMPTOMS | DIAGNOSIS | SELF-CARE |
| --- | --- | --- |

**BEGIN HERE**

Did you fall or suddenly feel your hip give way?

NO                YES

Do the toes on that leg seem to turn out, and does it hurt to straighten, lift or stand on your leg?

YES → Your pain and deformity may be from a HIP FRACTURE. → **URGENT**
**See your doctor.**

NO → Your pain may be from a HIP POINTER, a bruised hip socket. → Use heat and an anti-inflammatory medicine for comfort after you check with your doctor.

Do you have stiffness in any other joints, or are they swollen or red?

YES → Your hip pain may be from ARTHRITIS. → Try an anti-inflammatory medicine. If you don't get relief, see your doctor.

NO

Have you felt a "click" in your hip or occasional pain with activity?

YES → You may have a CONGENITAL HIP PROBLEM, a deformity of the hip joint that began before birth. → See your doctor.

NO

Do you have pain in the back of the hip that starts in the lower back and travels into the buttocks or into the leg?

YES → This is probably from SCIATICA, a pinched nerve. If the pain shoots down the leg near the knee or to the foot, this could be from a RUPTURED DISK. → Heat, anti-inflammatory medicine, and rest may help. See your doctor if the pain continues or if it travels down the leg. Contact your doctor immediately if you develop difficulty controlling urination or bowel movements.

NO

Is the person a child with pain in the knees, hips or groin?

YES → This could be related to a number of disorders, including a SLIPPED CAPITAL FEMORAL EPIPHYSIS. → See your doctor.

NO

For more information, please consult your doctor. If you think the problem is serious, call right away.

# TOPIC 41 Leg Problems

Follow this flow chart to find information about pain, swelling or lumps in the front or back of your lower leg.

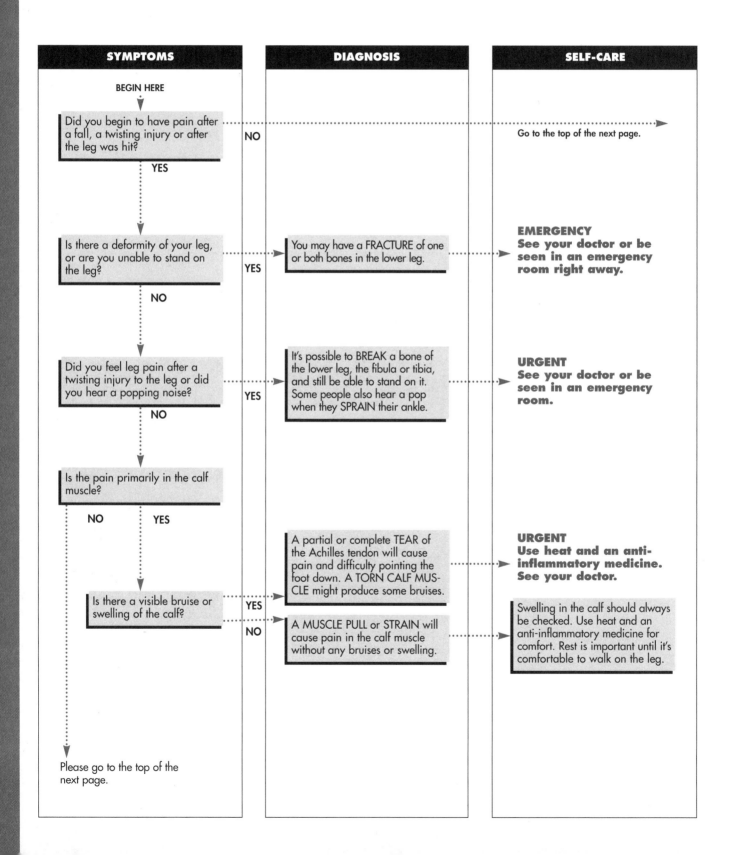

| SYMPTOMS | DIAGNOSIS | SELF-CARE |
|---|---|---|

**BEGIN HERE**

Did you begin to have pain after a fall, a twisting injury or after the leg was hit? — **NO** → Go to the top of the next page.

**YES**

Is there a deformity of your leg, or are you unable to stand on the leg? — **YES** → You may have a FRACTURE of one or both bones in the lower leg. → **EMERGENCY** **See your doctor or be seen in an emergency room right away.**

**NO**

Did you feel leg pain after a twisting injury to the leg or did you hear a popping noise? — **YES** → It's possible to BREAK a bone of the lower leg, the fibula or tibia, and still be able to stand on it. Some people also hear a pop when they SPRAIN their ankle. → **URGENT** **See your doctor or be seen in an emergency room.**

**NO**

Is the pain primarily in the calf muscle?

**NO**     **YES**

Is there a visible bruise or swelling of the calf? — **YES** → A partial or complete TEAR of the Achilles tendon will cause pain and difficulty pointing the foot down. A TORN CALF MUSCLE might produce some bruises. → **URGENT** **Use heat and an anti-inflammatory medicine. See your doctor.**

— **NO** → A MUSCLE PULL or STRAIN will cause pain in the calf muscle without any bruises or swelling. → Swelling in the calf should always be checked. Use heat and an anti-inflammatory medicine for comfort. Rest is important until it's comfortable to walk on the leg.

Please go to the top of the next page.

# TOPIC 41 Leg Problems

continued.

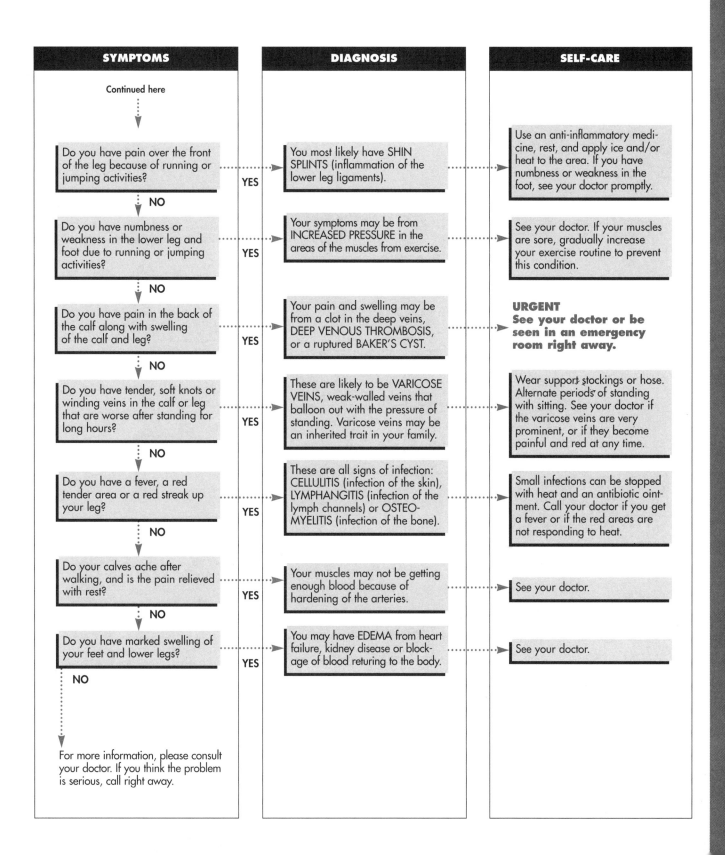

| SYMPTOMS | DIAGNOSIS | SELF-CARE |
|---|---|---|

Continued here

**Do you have pain over the front of the leg because of running or jumping activities?** — YES → You most likely have SHIN SPLINTS (inflammation of the lower leg ligaments). → Use an anti-inflammatory medicine, rest, and apply ice and/or heat to the area. If you have numbness or weakness in the foot, see your doctor promptly.

NO ↓

**Do you have numbness or weakness in the lower leg and foot due to running or jumping activities?** — YES → Your symptoms may be from INCREASED PRESSURE in the areas of the muscles from exercise. → See your doctor. If your muscles are sore, gradually increase your exercise routine to prevent this condition.

NO ↓

**Do you have pain in the back of the calf along with swelling of the calf and leg?** — YES → Your pain and swelling may be from a clot in the deep veins, DEEP VENOUS THROMBOSIS, or a ruptured BAKER'S CYST. → **URGENT** **See your doctor or be seen in an emergency room right away.**

NO ↓

**Do you have tender, soft knots or winding veins in the calf or leg that are worse after standing for long hours?** — YES → These are likely to be VARICOSE VEINS, weak-walled veins that balloon out with the pressure of standing. Varicose veins may be an inherited trait in your family. → Wear support stockings or hose. Alternate periods of standing with sitting. See your doctor if the varicose veins are very prominent, or if they become painful and red at any time.

NO ↓

**Do you have a fever, a red tender area or a red streak up your leg?** — YES → These are all signs of infection: CELLULITIS (infection of the skin), LYMPHANGITIS (infection of the lymph channels) or OSTEO-MYELITIS (infection of the bone). → Small infections can be stopped with heat and an antibiotic ointment. Call your doctor if you get a fever or if the red areas are not responding to heat.

NO ↓

**Do your calves ache after walking, and is the pain relieved with rest?** — YES → Your muscles may not be getting enough blood because of hardening of the arteries. → See your doctor.

NO ↓

**Do you have marked swelling of your feet and lower legs?** — YES → You may have EDEMA from heart failure, kidney disease or blockage of blood returing to the body. → See your doctor.

NO ↓

For more information, please consult your doctor. If you think the problem is serious, call right away.

# TOPIC 42 Knee Problems

The symptoms of pain, swelling, "water" on the knee and stiffness are symptoms heard from young and old. Follow this chart for more information about knee problems, possible diagnoses and self-care.

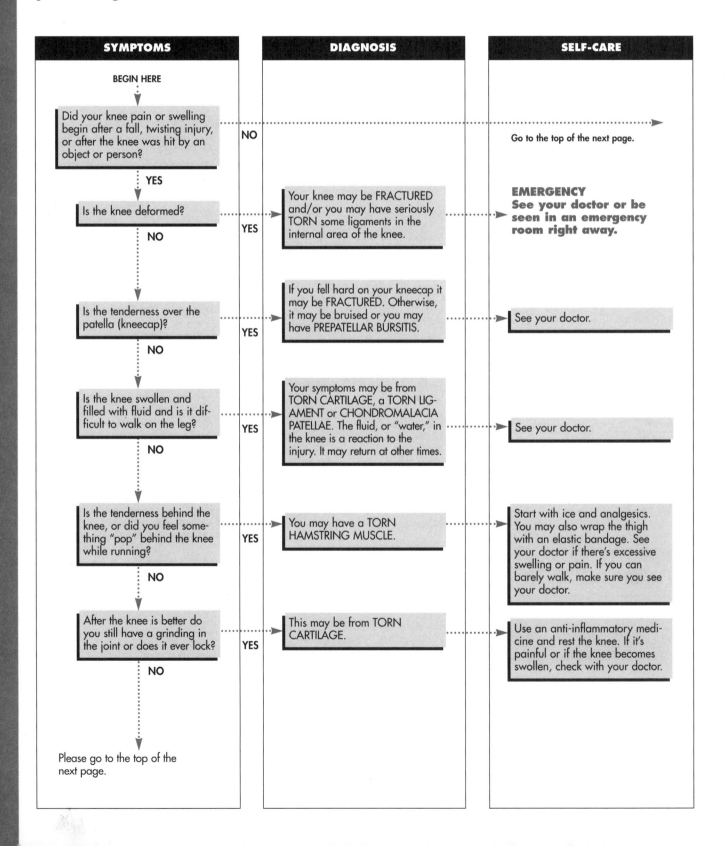

| SYMPTOMS | DIAGNOSIS | SELF-CARE |
|---|---|---|

**BEGIN HERE**

Did your knee pain or swelling begin after a fall, twisting injury, or after the knee was hit by an object or person?

**NO** → Go to the top of the next page.

**YES**

Is the knee deformed?

**YES** → Your knee may be FRACTURED and/or you may have seriously TORN some ligaments in the internal area of the knee. → **EMERGENCY See your doctor or be seen in an emergency room right away.**

**NO**

Is the tenderness over the patella (kneecap)?

**YES** → If you fell hard on your kneecap it may be FRACTURED. Otherwise, it may be bruised or you may have PREPATELLAR BURSITIS. → See your doctor.

**NO**

Is the knee swollen and filled with fluid and is it difficult to walk on the leg?

**YES** → Your symptoms may be from TORN CARTILAGE, a TORN LIGAMENT or CHONDROMALACIA PATELLAE. The fluid, or "water," in the knee is a reaction to the injury. It may return at other times. → See your doctor.

**NO**

Is the tenderness behind the knee, or did you feel something "pop" behind the knee while running?

**YES** → You may have a TORN HAMSTRING MUSCLE. → Start with ice and analgesics. You may also wrap the thigh with an elastic bandage. See your doctor if there's excessive swelling or pain. If you can barely walk, make sure you see your doctor.

**NO**

After the knee is better do you still have a grinding in the joint or does it ever lock?

**YES** → This may be from TORN CARTILAGE. → Use an anti-inflammatory medicine and rest the knee. If it's painful or if the knee becomes swollen, check with your doctor.

**NO**

Please go to the top of the next page.

**TOPIC 42** Knee Problems

continued.

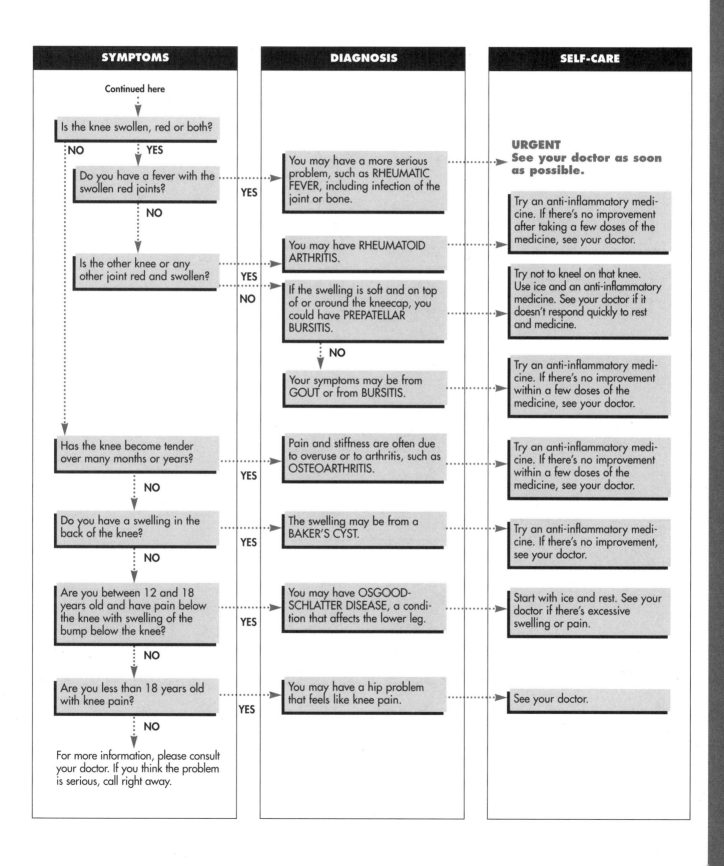

| SYMPTOMS | DIAGNOSIS | SELF-CARE |
|---|---|---|

**Continued here**

Is the knee swollen, red or both?

NO          YES

Do you have a fever with the swollen red joints?

YES → You may have a more serious problem, such as RHEUMATIC FEVER, including infection of the joint or bone. → **URGENT** **See your doctor as soon as possible.**

NO

Is the other knee or any other joint red and swollen?

YES → You may have RHEUMATOID ARTHRITIS. → Try an anti-inflammatory medicine. If there's no improvement after taking a few doses of the medicine, see your doctor.

NO → If the swelling is soft and on top of or around the kneecap, you could have PREPATELLAR BURSITIS. → Try not to kneel on that knee. Use ice and an anti-inflammatory medicine. See your doctor if it doesn't respond quickly to rest and medicine.

NO

Your symptoms may be from GOUT or from BURSITIS. → Try an anti-inflammatory medicine. If there's no improvement within a few doses of the medicine, see your doctor.

Has the knee become tender over many months or years?

YES → Pain and stiffness are often due to overuse or to arthritis, such as OSTEOARTHRITIS. → Try an anti-inflammatory medicine. If there's no improvement within a few doses of the medicine, see your doctor.

NO

Do you have a swelling in the back of the knee?

YES → The swelling may be from a BAKER'S CYST. → Try an anti-inflammatory medicine. If there's no improvement, see your doctor.

NO

Are you between 12 and 18 years old and have pain below the knee with swelling of the bump below the knee?

YES → You may have OSGOOD-SCHLATTER DISEASE, a condition that affects the lower leg. → Start with ice and rest. See your doctor if there's excessive swelling or pain.

NO

Are you less than 18 years old with knee pain?

YES → You may have a hip problem that feels like knee pain. → See your doctor.

NO

For more information, please consult your doctor. If you think the problem is serious, call right away.

# TOPIC 43 Ankle Problems

Other situations besides an ankle sprain can cause ankle pain. Follow this chart for more information about an ankle problem.

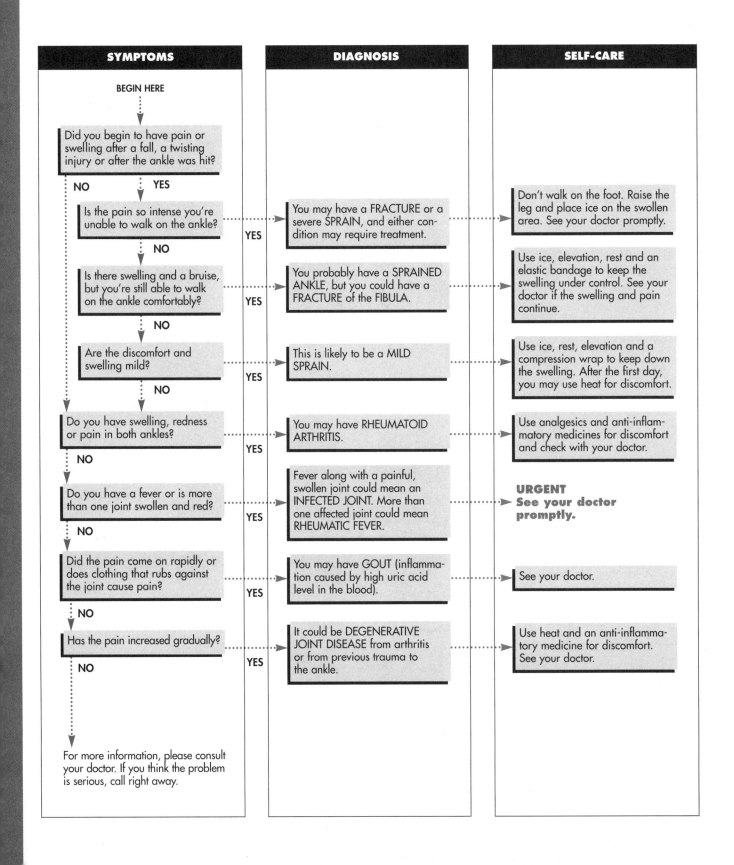

| SYMPTOMS | DIAGNOSIS | SELF-CARE |
|---|---|---|
| **BEGIN HERE** | | |
| Did you begin to have pain or swelling after a fall, a twisting injury or after the ankle was hit? | | |
| **NO** ... **YES** | | |
| Is the pain so intense you're unable to walk on the ankle? — **YES** | You may have a FRACTURE or a severe SPRAIN, and either condition may require treatment. | Don't walk on the foot. Raise the leg and place ice on the swollen area. See your doctor promptly. |
| **NO** | | |
| Is there swelling and a bruise, but you're still able to walk on the ankle comfortably? — **YES** | You probably have a SPRAINED ANKLE, but you could have a FRACTURE of the FIBULA. | Use ice, elevation, rest and an elastic bandage to keep the swelling under control. See your doctor if the swelling and pain continue. |
| **NO** | | |
| Are the discomfort and swelling mild? — **YES** | This is likely to be a MILD SPRAIN. | Use ice, rest, elevation and a compression wrap to keep down the swelling. After the first day, you may use heat for discomfort. |
| **NO** | | |
| Do you have swelling, redness or pain in both ankles? — **YES** | You may have RHEUMATOID ARTHRITIS. | Use analgesics and anti-inflammatory medicines for discomfort and check with your doctor. |
| **NO** | | |
| Do you have a fever or is more than one joint swollen and red? — **YES** | Fever along with a painful, swollen joint could mean an INFECTED JOINT. More than one affected joint could mean RHEUMATIC FEVER. | **URGENT** **See your doctor promptly.** |
| **NO** | | |
| Did the pain come on rapidly or does clothing that rubs against the joint cause pain? — **YES** | You may have GOUT (inflammation caused by high uric acid level in the blood). | See your doctor. |
| **NO** | | |
| Has the pain increased gradually? — **YES** | It could be DEGENERATIVE JOINT DISEASE from arthritis or from previous trauma to the ankle. | Use heat and an anti-inflammatory medicine for discomfort. See your doctor. |
| **NO** | | |
| For more information, please consult your doctor. If you think the problem is serious, call right away. | | |

## TOPIC 44 Foot Problems

From warts to bunions, feet can be afflicted with some very painful conditions.
Use this chart to find appropriate self-care options.

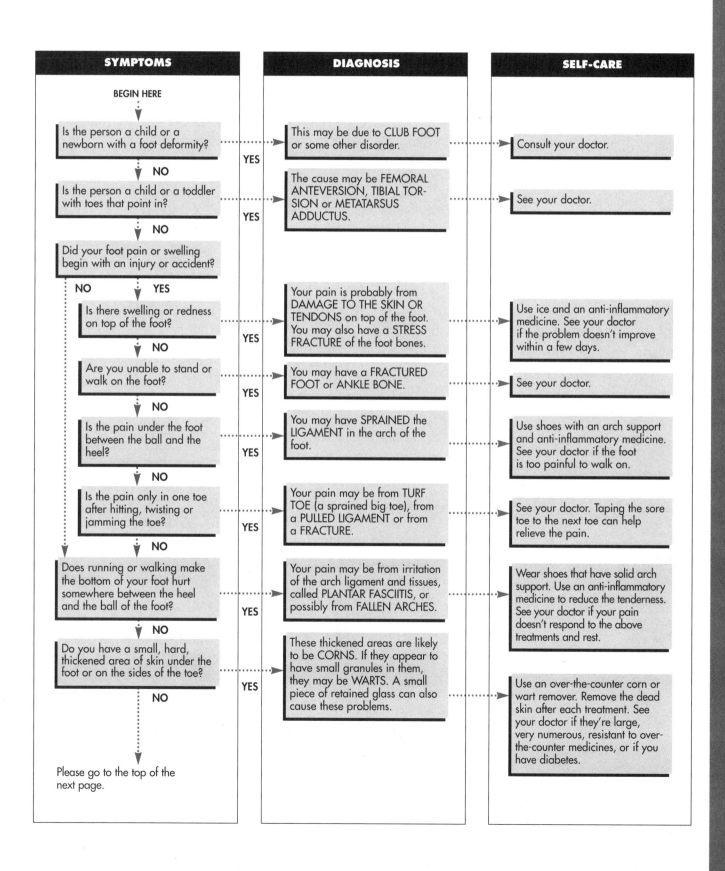

| SYMPTOMS | DIAGNOSIS | SELF-CARE |
|---|---|---|
| **BEGIN HERE** | | |
| Is the person a child or a newborn with a foot deformity? — **YES** | This may be due to CLUB FOOT or some other disorder. | Consult your doctor. |
| **NO** | | |
| Is the person a child or a toddler with toes that point in? — **YES** | The cause may be FEMORAL ANTEVERSION, TIBIAL TORSION or METATARSUS ADDUCTUS. | See your doctor. |
| **NO** | | |
| Did your foot pain or swelling begin with an injury or accident? | | |
| **NO** / **YES** | | |
| Is there swelling or redness on top of the foot? — **YES** | Your pain is probably from DAMAGE TO THE SKIN OR TENDONS on top of the foot. You may also have a STRESS FRACTURE of the foot bones. | Use ice and an anti-inflammatory medicine. See your doctor if the problem doesn't improve within a few days. |
| **NO** | | |
| Are you unable to stand or walk on the foot? — **YES** | You may have a FRACTURED FOOT or ANKLE BONE. | See your doctor. |
| **NO** | | |
| Is the pain under the foot between the ball and the heel? — **YES** | You may have SPRAINED the LIGAMENT in the arch of the foot. | Use shoes with an arch support and anti-inflammatory medicine. See your doctor if the foot is too painful to walk on. |
| **NO** | | |
| Is the pain only in one toe after hitting, twisting or jamming the toe? — **YES** | Your pain may be from TURF TOE (a sprained big toe), from a PULLED LIGAMENT or from a FRACTURE. | See your doctor. Taping the sore toe to the next toe can help relieve the pain. |
| **NO** | | |
| Does running or walking make the bottom of your foot hurt somewhere between the heel and the ball of the foot? — **YES** | Your pain may be from irritation of the arch ligament and tissues, called PLANTAR FASCIITIS, or possibly from FALLEN ARCHES. | Wear shoes that have solid arch support. Use an anti-inflammatory medicine to reduce the tenderness. See your doctor if your pain doesn't respond to the above treatments and rest. |
| **NO** | | |
| Do you have a small, hard, thickened area of skin under the foot or on the sides of the toe? — **YES** | These thickened areas are likely to be CORNS. If they appear to have small granules in them, they may be WARTS. A small piece of retained glass can also cause these problems. | Use an over-the-counter corn or wart remover. Remove the dead skin after each treatment. See your doctor if they're large, very numerous, resistant to over-the-counter medicines, or if you have diabetes. |
| **NO** | | |
| Please go to the top of the next page. | | |

# TOPIC 44 Foot Problems

continued.

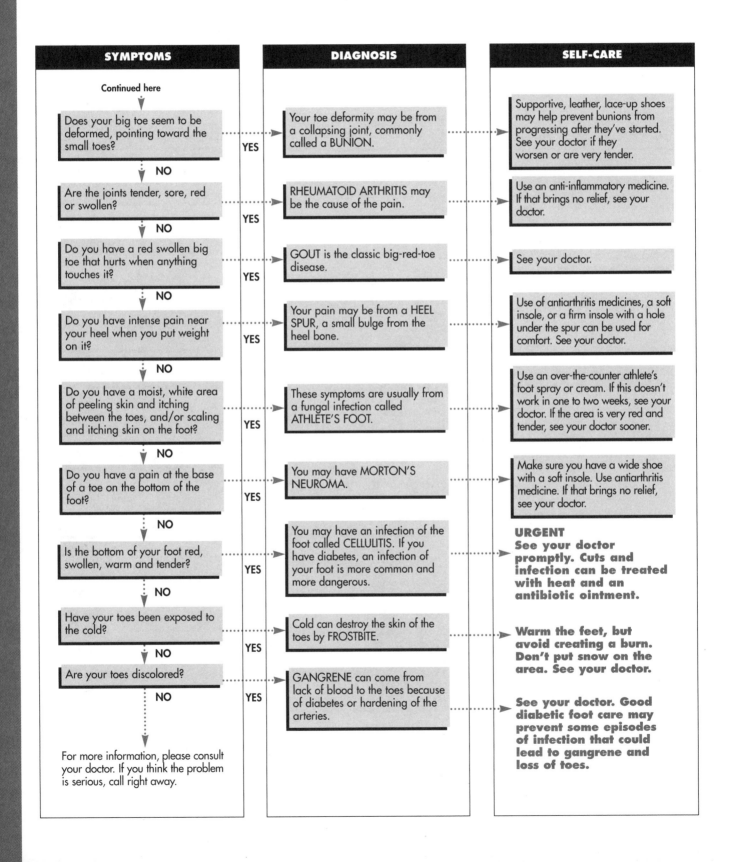

| SYMPTOMS | DIAGNOSIS | SELF-CARE |
|---|---|---|

**Continued here**

Does your big toe seem to be deformed, pointing toward the small toes?

**YES** → Your toe deformity may be from a collapsing joint, commonly called a BUNION. → Supportive, leather, lace-up shoes may help prevent bunions from progressing after they've started. See your doctor if they worsen or are very tender.

**NO** ↓

Are the joints tender, sore, red or swollen?

**YES** → RHEUMATOID ARTHRITIS may be the cause of the pain. → Use an anti-inflammatory medicine. If that brings no relief, see your doctor.

**NO** ↓

Do you have a red swollen big toe that hurts when anything touches it?

**YES** → GOUT is the classic big-red-toe disease. → See your doctor.

**NO** ↓

Do you have intense pain near your heel when you put weight on it?

**YES** → Your pain may be from a HEEL SPUR, a small bulge from the heel bone. → Use of antiarthritis medicines, a soft insole, or a firm insole with a hole under the spur can be used for comfort. See your doctor.

**NO** ↓

Do you have a moist, white area of peeling skin and itching between the toes, and/or scaling and itching skin on the foot?

**YES** → These symptoms are usually from a fungal infection called ATHLETE'S FOOT. → Use an over-the-counter athlete's foot spray or cream. If this doesn't work in one to two weeks, see your doctor. If the area is very red and tender, see your doctor sooner.

**NO** ↓

Do you have a pain at the base of a toe on the bottom of the foot?

**YES** → You may have MORTON'S NEUROMA. → Make sure you have a wide shoe with a soft insole. Use antiarthritis medicine. If that brings no relief, see your doctor.

**NO** ↓

Is the bottom of your foot red, swollen, warm and tender?

**YES** → You may have an infection of the foot called CELLULITIS. If you have diabetes, an infection of your foot is more common and more dangerous. → **URGENT** **See your doctor promptly. Cuts and infection can be treated with heat and an antibiotic ointment.**

**NO** ↓

Have your toes been exposed to the cold?

**YES** → Cold can destroy the skin of the toes by FROSTBITE. → **Warm the feet, but avoid creating a burn. Don't put snow on the area. See your doctor.**

**NO** ↓

Are your toes discolored?

**YES** → GANGRENE can come from lack of blood to the toes because of diabetes or hardening of the arteries. → **See your doctor. Good diabetic foot care may prevent some episodes of infection that could lead to gangrene and loss of toes.**

**NO** ↓

For more information, please consult your doctor. If you think the problem is serious, call right away.

# TOPIC 45 Skin Rashes and Other Changes

The location, appearance and color of a rash will help your doctor make the diagnosis. Look for care suggestions on this chart for common rashes.

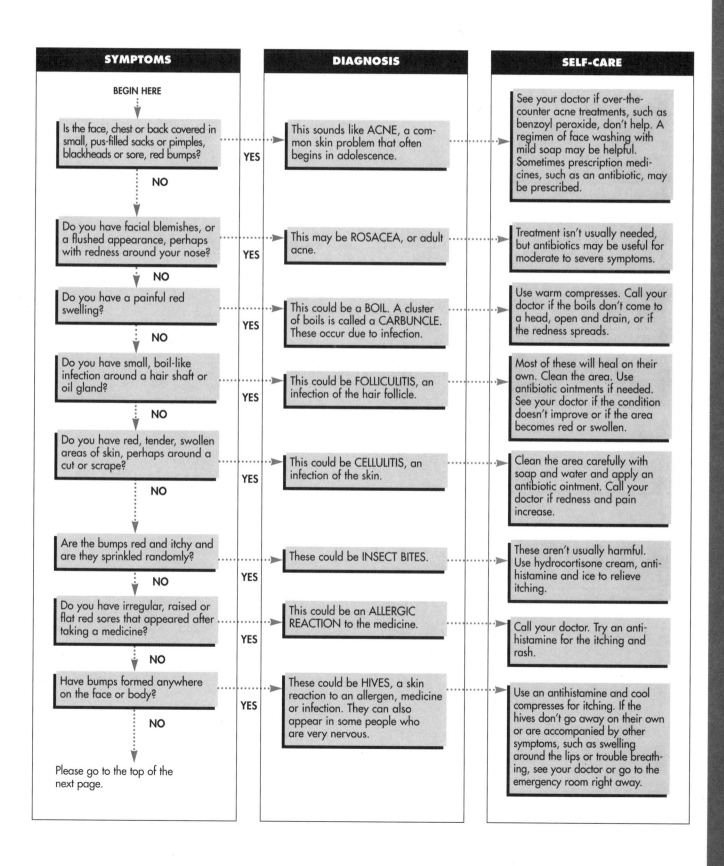

BEGIN HERE

| SYMPTOMS | | DIAGNOSIS | SELF-CARE |
|---|---|---|---|
| Is the face, chest or back covered in small, pus-filled sacks or pimples, blackheads or sore, red bumps? | YES | This sounds like ACNE, a common skin problem that often begins in adolescence. | See your doctor if over-the-counter acne treatments, such as benzoyl peroxide, don't help. A regimen of face washing with mild soap may be helpful. Sometimes prescription medicines, such as an antibiotic, may be prescribed. |
| NO | | | |
| Do you have facial blemishes, or a flushed appearance, perhaps with redness around your nose? | YES | This may be ROSACEA, or adult acne. | Treatment isn't usually needed, but antibiotics may be useful for moderate to severe symptoms. |
| NO | | | |
| Do you have a painful red swelling? | YES | This could be a BOIL. A cluster of boils is called a CARBUNCLE. These occur due to infection. | Use warm compresses. Call your doctor if the boils don't come to a head, open and drain, or if the redness spreads. |
| NO | | | |
| Do you have small, boil-like infection around a hair shaft or oil gland? | YES | This could be FOLLICULITIS, an infection of the hair follicle. | Most of these will heal on their own. Clean the area. Use antibiotic ointments if needed. See your doctor if the condition doesn't improve or if the area becomes red or swollen. |
| NO | | | |
| Do you have red, tender, swollen areas of skin, perhaps around a cut or scrape? | YES | This could be CELLULITIS, an infection of the skin. | Clean the area carefully with soap and water and apply an antibiotic ointment. Call your doctor if redness and pain increase. |
| NO | | | |
| Are the bumps red and itchy and are they sprinkled randomly? | YES | These could be INSECT BITES. | These aren't usually harmful. Use hydrocortisone cream, antihistamine and ice to relieve itching. |
| NO | | | |
| Do you have irregular, raised or flat red sores that appeared after taking a medicine? | YES | This could be an ALLERGIC REACTION to the medicine. | Call your doctor. Try an antihistamine for the itching and rash. |
| NO | | | |
| Have bumps formed anywhere on the face or body? | YES | These could be HIVES, a skin reaction to an allergen, medicine or infection. They can also appear in some people who are very nervous. | Use an antihistamine and cool compresses for itching. If the hives don't go away on their own or are accompanied by other symptoms, such as swelling around the lips or trouble breathing, see your doctor or go to the emergency room right away. |
| NO | | | |

Please go to the top of the next page.

# TOPIC 45 Skin Rashes and Other Changes

continued.

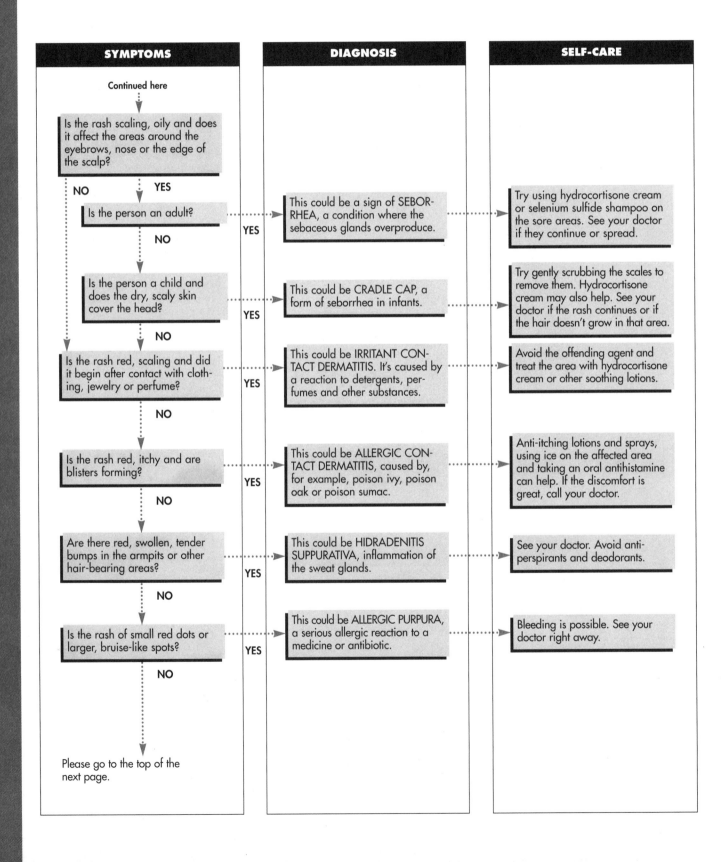

| SYMPTOMS | DIAGNOSIS | SELF-CARE |
|---|---|---|

**Continued here**

Is the rash scaling, oily and does it affect the areas around the eyebrows, nose or the edge of the scalp?

NO ← | → YES

Is the person an adult? → YES → This could be a sign of SEBOR-RHEA, a condition where the sebaceous glands overproduce. → Try using hydrocortisone cream or selenium sulfide shampoo on the sore areas. See your doctor if they continue or spread.

NO

Is the person a child and does the dry, scaly skin cover the head? → YES → This could be CRADLE CAP, a form of seborrhea in infants. → Try gently scrubbing the scales to remove them. Hydrocortisone cream may also help. See your doctor if the rash continues or if the hair doesn't grow in that area.

NO

Is the rash red, scaling and did it begin after contact with clothing, jewelry or perfume? → YES → This could be IRRITANT CONTACT DERMATITIS. It's caused by a reaction to detergents, perfumes and other substances. → Avoid the offending agent and treat the area with hydrocortisone cream or other soothing lotions.

NO

Is the rash red, itchy and are blisters forming? → YES → This could be ALLERGIC CONTACT DERMATITIS, caused by, for example, poison ivy, poison oak or poison sumac. → Anti-itching lotions and sprays, using ice on the affected area and taking an oral antihistamine can help. If the discomfort is great, call your doctor.

NO

Are there red, swollen, tender bumps in the armpits or other hair-bearing areas? → YES → This could be HIDRADENITIS SUPPURATIVA, inflammation of the sweat glands. → See your doctor. Avoid antiperspirants and deodorants.

NO

Is the rash of small red dots or larger, bruise-like spots? → YES → This could be ALLERGIC PURPURA, a serious allergic reaction to a medicine or antibiotic. → Bleeding is possible. See your doctor right away.

NO

Please go to the top of the next page.

# TOPIC 45 Skin Rashes and Other Changes

continued.

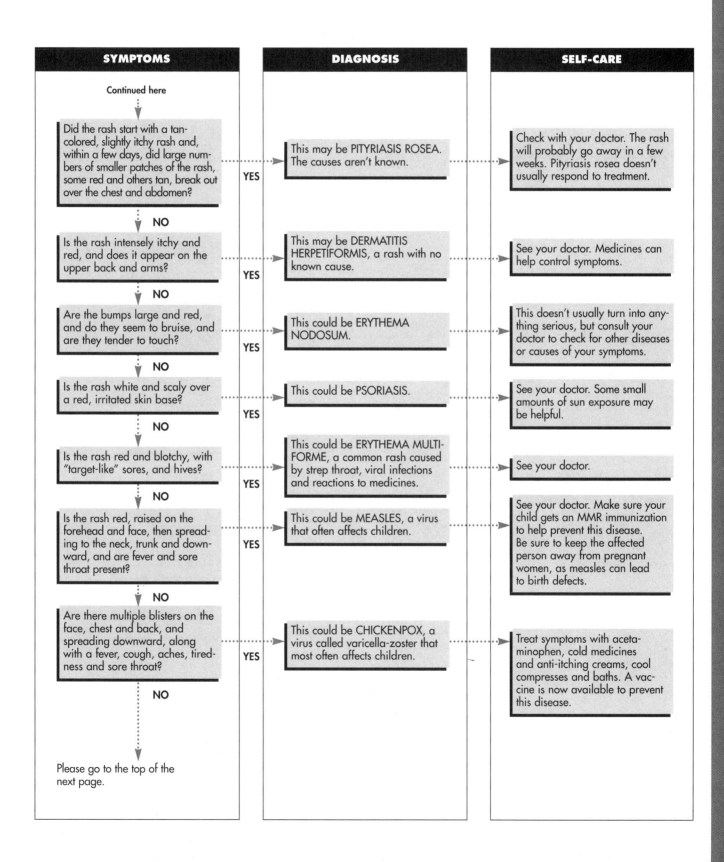

| SYMPTOMS | DIAGNOSIS | SELF-CARE |
|---|---|---|

Continued here

**Did the rash start with a tan-colored, slightly itchy rash and, within a few days, did large numbers of smaller patches of the rash, some red and others tan, break out over the chest and abdomen?**

YES → This may be PITYRIASIS ROSEA. The causes aren't known. → Check with your doctor. The rash will probably go away in a few weeks. Pityriasis rosea doesn't usually respond to treatment.

NO ↓

**Is the rash intensely itchy and red, and does it appear on the upper back and arms?**

YES → This may be DERMATITIS HERPETIFORMIS, a rash with no known cause. → See your doctor. Medicines can help control symptoms.

NO ↓

**Are the bumps large and red, and do they seem to bruise, and are they tender to touch?**

YES → This could be ERYTHEMA NODOSUM. → This doesn't usually turn into anything serious, but consult your doctor to check for other diseases or causes of your symptoms.

NO ↓

**Is the rash white and scaly over a red, irritated skin base?**

YES → This could be PSORIASIS. → See your doctor. Some small amounts of sun exposure may be helpful.

NO ↓

**Is the rash red and blotchy, with "target-like" sores, and hives?**

YES → This could be ERYTHEMA MULTI-FORME, a common rash caused by strep throat, viral infections and reactions to medicines. → See your doctor.

NO ↓

**Is the rash red, raised on the forehead and face, then spreading to the neck, trunk and downward, and are fever and sore throat present?**

YES → This could be MEASLES, a virus that often affects children. → See your doctor. Make sure your child gets an MMR immunization to help prevent this disease. Be sure to keep the affected person away from pregnant women, as measles can lead to birth defects.

NO ↓

**Are there multiple blisters on the face, chest and back, and spreading downward, along with a fever, cough, aches, tiredness and sore throat?**

YES → This could be CHICKENPOX, a virus called varicella-zoster that most often affects children. → Treat symptoms with acetaminophen, cold medicines and anti-itching creams, cool compresses and baths. A vaccine is now available to prevent this disease.

NO ↓

Please go to the top of the next page.

# TOPIC 45 Skin Rashes and Other Changes

continued.

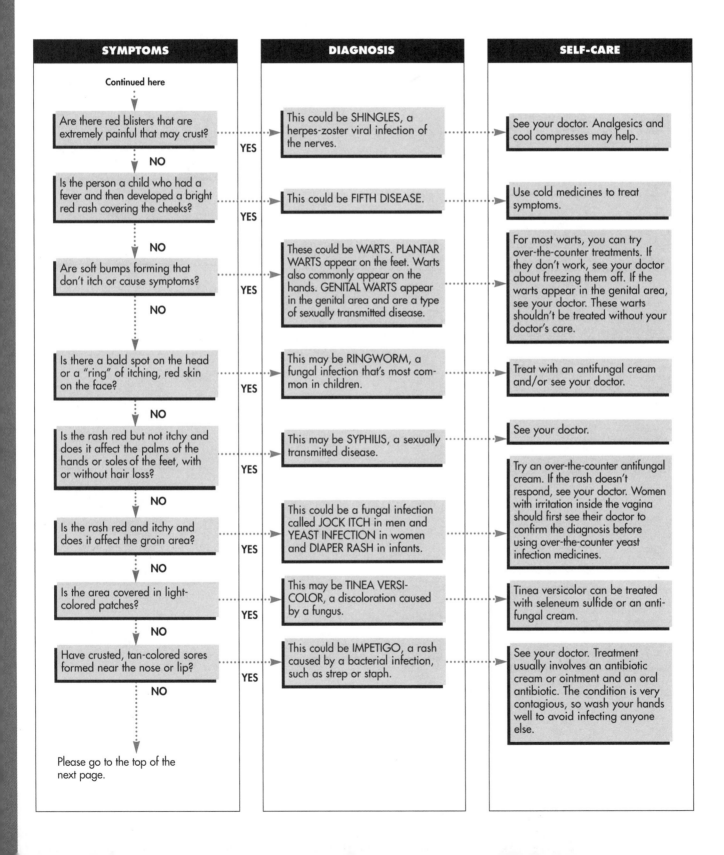

| SYMPTOMS | DIAGNOSIS | SELF-CARE |
|---|---|---|

Continued here

Are there red blisters that are extremely painful that may crust? — **YES** → This could be SHINGLES, a herpes-zoster viral infection of the nerves. → See your doctor. Analgesics and cool compresses may help.

**NO**

Is the person a child who had a fever and then developed a bright red rash covering the cheeks? — **YES** → This could be FIFTH DISEASE. → Use cold medicines to treat symptoms.

**NO**

Are soft bumps forming that don't itch or cause symptoms? — **YES** → These could be WARTS. PLANTAR WARTS appear on the feet. Warts also commonly appear on the hands. GENITAL WARTS appear in the genital area and are a type of sexually transmitted disease. → For most warts, you can try over-the-counter treatments. If they don't work, see your doctor about freezing them off. If the warts appear in the genital area, see your doctor. These warts shouldn't be treated without your doctor's care.

**NO**

Is there a bald spot on the head or a "ring" of itching, red skin on the face? — **YES** → This may be RINGWORM, a fungal infection that's most common in children. → Treat with an antifungal cream and/or see your doctor.

**NO**

Is the rash red but not itchy and does it affect the palms of the hands or soles of the feet, with or without hair loss? — **YES** → This may be SYPHILIS, a sexually transmitted disease. → See your doctor.

**NO**

Is the rash red and itchy and does it affect the groin area? — **YES** → This could be a fungal infection called JOCK ITCH in men and YEAST INFECTION in women and DIAPER RASH in infants. → Try an over-the-counter antifungal cream. If the rash doesn't respond, see your doctor. Women with irritation inside the vagina should first see their doctor to confirm the diagnosis before using over-the-counter yeast infection medicines.

**NO**

Is the area covered in light-colored patches? — **YES** → This may be TINEA VERSI-COLOR, a discoloration caused by a fungus. → Tinea versicolor can be treated with seleneum sulfide or an antifungal cream.

**NO**

Have crusted, tan-colored sores formed near the nose or lip? — **YES** → This could be IMPETIGO, a rash caused by a bacterial infection, such as strep or staph. → See your doctor. Treatment usually involves an antibiotic cream or ointment and an oral antibiotic. The condition is very contagious, so wash your hands well to avoid infecting anyone else.

**NO**

Please go to the top of the next page.

# TOPIC 45 Skin Rashes and Other Changes

continued.

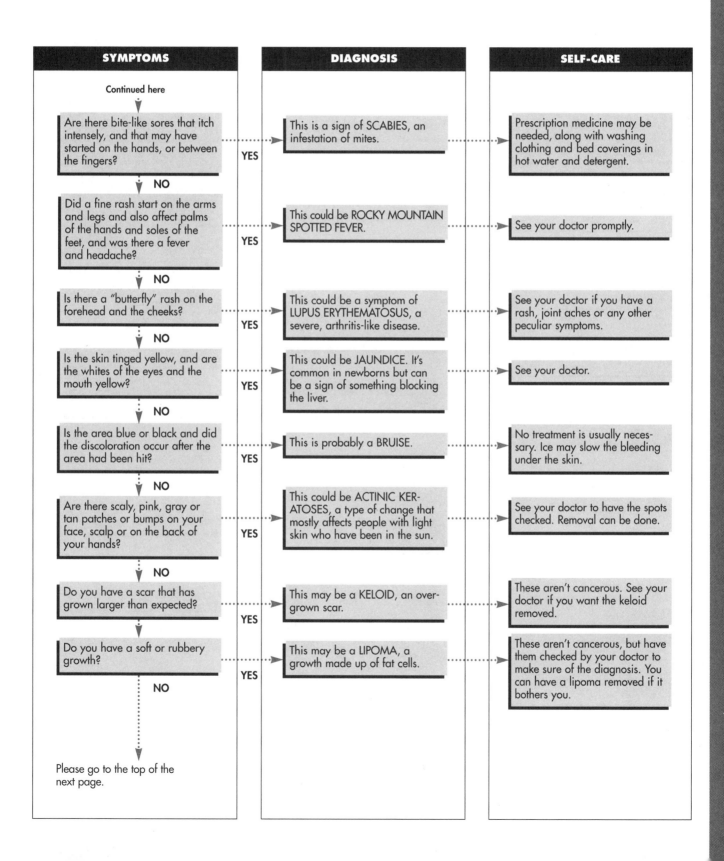

| SYMPTOMS | DIAGNOSIS | SELF-CARE |
|---|---|---|

Continued here

**Are there bite-like sores that itch intensely, and that may have started on the hands, or between the fingers?** — YES → This is a sign of SCABIES, an infestation of mites. → Prescription medicine may be needed, along with washing clothing and bed coverings in hot water and detergent.

NO ↓

**Did a fine rash start on the arms and legs and also affect palms of the hands and soles of the feet, and was there a fever and headache?** — YES → This could be ROCKY MOUNTAIN SPOTTED FEVER. → See your doctor promptly.

NO ↓

**Is there a "butterfly" rash on the forehead and the cheeks?** — YES → This could be a symptom of LUPUS ERYTHEMATOSUS, a severe, arthritis-like disease. → See your doctor if you have a rash, joint aches or any other peculiar symptoms.

NO ↓

**Is the skin tinged yellow, and are the whites of the eyes and the mouth yellow?** — YES → This could be JAUNDICE. It's common in newborns but can be a sign of something blocking the liver. → See your doctor.

NO ↓

**Is the area blue or black and did the discoloration occur after the area had been hit?** — YES → This is probably a BRUISE. → No treatment is usually necessary. Ice may slow the bleeding under the skin.

NO ↓

**Are there scaly, pink, gray or tan patches or bumps on your face, scalp or on the back of your hands?** — YES → This could be ACTINIC KERATOSES, a type of change that mostly affects people with light skin who have been in the sun. → See your doctor to have the spots checked. Removal can be done.

NO ↓

**Do you have a scar that has grown larger than expected?** — YES → This may be a KELOID, an overgrown scar. → These aren't cancerous. See your doctor if you want the keloid removed.

↓

**Do you have a soft or rubbery growth?** — YES → This may be a LIPOMA, a growth made up of fat cells. → These aren't cancerous, but have them checked by your doctor to make sure of the diagnosis. You can have a lipoma removed if it bothers you.

NO ↓

Please go to the top of the next page.

# TOPIC 45 Skin Rashes and Other Changes

continued.

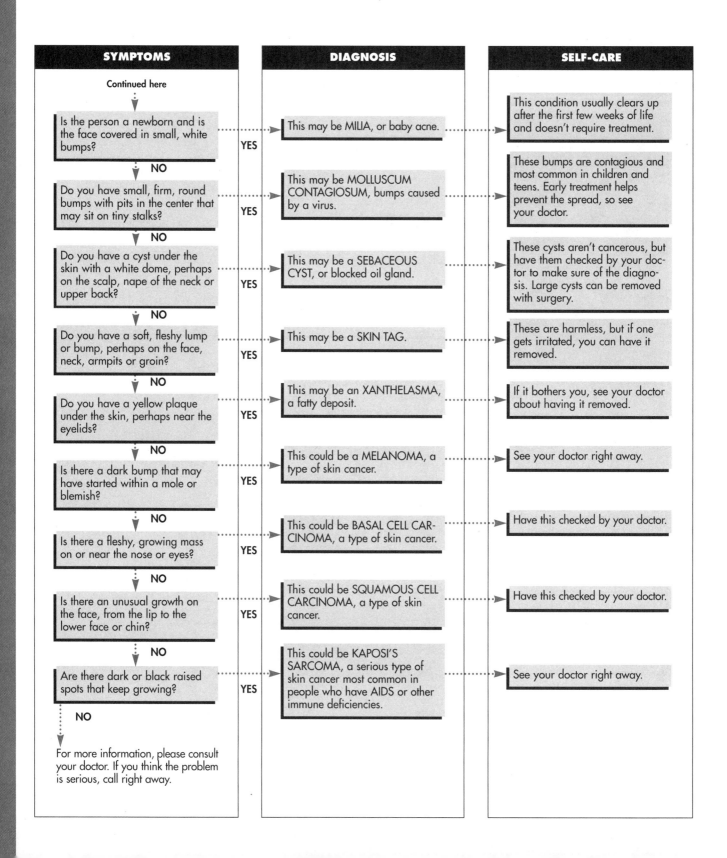

| SYMPTOMS | DIAGNOSIS | SELF-CARE |
|---|---|---|
| **Continued here** | | |
| Is the person a newborn and is the face covered in small, white bumps? **YES** | This may be MILIA, or baby acne. | This condition usually clears up after the first few weeks of life and doesn't require treatment. |
| **NO** | | |
| Do you have small, firm, round bumps with pits in the center that may sit on tiny stalks? **YES** | This may be MOLLUSCUM CONTAGIOSUM, bumps caused by a virus. | These bumps are contagious and most common in children and teens. Early treatment helps prevent the spread, so see your doctor. |
| **NO** | | |
| Do you have a cyst under the skin with a white dome, perhaps on the scalp, nape of the neck or upper back? **YES** | This may be a SEBACEOUS CYST, or blocked oil gland. | These cysts aren't cancerous, but have them checked by your doctor to make sure of the diagnosis. Large cysts can be removed with surgery. |
| **NO** | | |
| Do you have a soft, fleshy lump or bump, perhaps on the face, neck, armpits or groin? **YES** | This may be a SKIN TAG. | These are harmless, but if one gets irritated, you can have it removed. |
| **NO** | | |
| Do you have a yellow plaque under the skin, perhaps near the eyelids? **YES** | This may be an XANTHELASMA, a fatty deposit. | If it bothers you, see your doctor about having it removed. |
| **NO** | | |
| Is there a dark bump that may have started within a mole or blemish? **YES** | This could be a MELANOMA, a type of skin cancer. | See your doctor right away. |
| **NO** | | |
| Is there a fleshy, growing mass on or near the nose or eyes? **YES** | This could be BASAL CELL CARCINOMA, a type of skin cancer. | Have this checked by your doctor. |
| **NO** | | |
| Is there an unusual growth on the face, from the lip to the lower face or chin? **YES** | This could be SQUAMOUS CELL CARCINOMA, a type of skin cancer. | Have this checked by your doctor. |
| **NO** | | |
| Are there dark or black raised spots that keep growing? **YES** | This could be KAPOSI'S SARCOMA, a serious type of skin cancer most common in people who have AIDS or other immune deficiencies. | See your doctor right away. |
| **NO** | | |
| For more information, please consult your doctor. If you think the problem is serious, call right away. | | |

# PART 7

# FAMILY AND EMOTIONAL ISSUES

| FAMILY AND RELATIONSHIP ISSUES | 542 |
| EMOTIONS, BEHAVIOR AND THE FAMILY | 559 |

# FAMILY AND RELATIONSHIP ISSUES

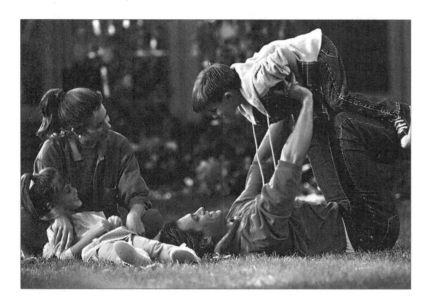

## Planning Your Family

Many factors influence your decision about having children. Emotional and physical factors, jobs, family support and how much you and your partner want children must be considered as you decide if you want children and, if so, how many and when. If you want to wait to start your family, you must also consider which birth control method you will use.

Sometimes, after you believe your plans are well thought out and settled, other factors, such as infertility or multiple births, force changes you hadn't expected. Many couples don't discuss these issues prior to pregnancy. As a result, their relationship may become troubled during the pregnancy, when communication is poor and expectations aren't met. Open, honest discussions can prevent the need for a counselor—or lawyer—in the future.

---

### *Family Planning Questions*

What are the questions you and your partner should discuss about starting your family? Remember the adage, "The only stupid question is the one not asked." Start with the following suggestions and add questions of your own:

- How many children do we *want* to have?
- How many children can we afford to have from the standpoint of financial resources, emotional strength, and time?
- When do we want to have children?
- How far apart in age do we want our children to be?
- Are there any serious diseases that run in our families that could be passed along to the child?
- Do our beliefs or religious teaching affect the size of our family or whether we use contraceptives?

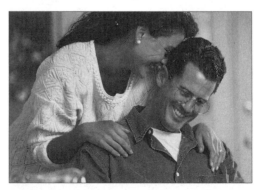

## Are You Ready for Children?

Before modern birth control was an option, many young couples started having children shortly after marriage, and their family kept growing until their fertility ended in middle age. Today, couples have more control over the size and timing of their families. Before deciding to become parents, a couple should discuss their career plans, gauge their emotional readiness to become parents, build a strong relationship and discuss the use of contraceptives. Because these considerations are personal and significant, careful and complete communication about having children and then abiding by the decision of both partners is best.

**Careers.** Many couples postpone having children during the early years of their relationship because they're busy with their careers. Having a child will require taking some time away from work, particularly for the woman so that she has time to recuperate from childbirth.

Issues that may arise in considering your work and your family include the level of job security you have, how much you travel with your job, the amount of stress your job places on you and your family, and the financial impact being off work would cause.

**Emotional readiness.** How can you tell if you and your partner are emotionally ready to have children? A couple is emotionally ready when they have a healthy, thriving relationship, when their budget can take the stress of an addition to the family, and when both partners are ready to give a great deal of time, love and attention to their new child.

It's not enough to just have a strong desire for children. You and your partner should agree that having a child

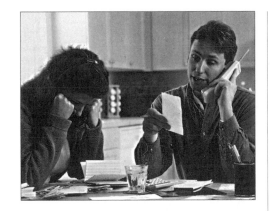

would be a good thing. If one of you is ready and the other isn't sure, it may be good to wait. Emotional readiness can be equated to maturity and being ready to take on new responsibility.

**Financial readiness.** Financial considerations may be a couple's most frustrating factor in deciding whether to have children. Any financial discussions have the potential to erupt into an argument. Arguments about money are a major source of friction.

Understanding each other's spending and saving habits, as well as agreeing on a budget, will help reduce disagreements about money and make planning easier. Learning to put money aside in a savings plan builds mutual confidence and trust between partners. Medical and life insurance are other important considerations for couples thinking about having a child.

The financial difficulties of medical care during pregnancy and birth can place tremendous strain on the relationship. Health insurance protects the family from some, but not all, of the financial worries. If you have no insurance or other source of financial help for medical bills, public-assistance money is sometimes more available than you might expect. Ask your doctor to help you contact a social worker. A social worker can often identify ways of obtaining medical care when doors seem to be closed.

After the birth, the mother will need some time to recover, and both parents will need time to bond with the child. Maternity leave usually varies at different businesses from a few weeks to six months. A law, called the Family and Medical Leave Act, now requires that certain employers allow parents up to 12 weeks of unpaid leave after the birth of a baby without risk of losing their jobs. During this time the parents should carefully consider their child-care options.

**Physical readiness.** Physical factors can play a crucial role in your decision to have a child, or in the timing and spacing of children. What are some of the physical factors that make a pregnancy more or less likely? These factors include the regularity of the woman's menstrual cycle, sexual problems (such as impotence, premature ejaculation, vaginal irritation or infection), stress (such as from a pressure-filled job) or problems in the relationship.

Each partner should try to show sensitivity to the other if any of these problems arise. The focus should be on one another, and not just on your own needs and desires. Open communication can help alleviate the frustration or discomfort before any problems become too big to handle. Your doctor may be able to help you with physical problems, and he or she may also suggest you talk to a counselor to deal with the emotional aspects.

## Conception

Sexual intercourse usually begins with sexual arousal. Arousal often starts as more of a mental and emotional experience and leads to physical contact. Thoughts of love, caring, caressing, touching and holding stimulate the nervous system in both men and women. Men are more easily aroused by what they see, while women tend to be aroused by romantic thoughts. In the male, arousal leads to an *erection*, the firming of the penis when filled with blood. In the female, arousal causes thickening of the tissues of the vagina and secretion of a clear mucus from the vagina. The clitoris may also become filled with blood, like the man's penis. Arousal may also stimulate the breasts, causing the nipples to become hard and erect in both men and women.

### Sex as Part of a Complete Relationship

Sex plays an important role in the relationship between two partners, but it's not the most important part of a good relationship. Good communication, similar interests, trust, a desire to please and spend time with your mate help you and your partner build a satisfying relationship. The ultimate sharing and openness of sexual relations adds depth and breadth to this relationship and creates the foundation of a loving and trusting family.

Sexual intercourse begins when the erect penis is pushed inside the vagina. Back and forth thrusting stimulates the *glans*, or head, of the penis. Stimulation builds until the point of sexual release, also called *orgasm*, or *ejaculation*, causing the man to release sperm into the vagina through rhythmical contractions of the seminal vesicle and the urethra.

The female orgasm is similar, causing rhythmical contractions of the vagina. In women, orgasms may or may not occur during sexual intercourse. Many women require direct stimulation of the clitoris to reach orgasm. This stimulation may or may not occur during intercourse.

Repeated stimulation may lead to multiple orgasms in women. After orgasm, men usually have a *refractory period* during which the penis can't become erect. A male can sometimes be stimulated again to the point of orgasm after a few minutes have passed.

A typical ejaculation deposits millions of sperm into the upper part of the vagina, next to the cervix. If the male's sperm are defective, conception is less likely. If not enough sperm are deposited in the vagina, the chances of conception also decrease dramatically. It takes many sperm to clear a path for one sperm to fertilize the egg.

After ejaculation, the sperm begin their journey to attempt to fertilize an egg. If the consistency of the cervical mucus is just right, the sperm will be able to enter the uterus through the cervix. The cervical mucus is the right consistency in the middle of the menstrual cycle, at the time of ovulation, when estrogen and progesterone levels

peak. Any interference in the uterus, such as scarring or a physical abnormality, can prevent the sperm from traveling to their intended destination, the fallopian tubes.

A blockage within the fallopian tube, which sometimes results following infection, such as a sexually transmitted disease (STD, p. 316) or injury, can keep the sperm from reaching the egg. If an egg has been released and traveled to the fallopian tube, this is where a sperm will meet it.

As millions of sperm meet the egg, enzymes on the tip of each sperm are released to dissolve the tough, protective layer surrounding the egg. It takes millions of sperm, all releasing their enzymes, to soften this layer enough to allow one sperm to enter and fertilize the egg. The moment one of the sperm penetrates the egg, another chemical reaction hardens the surface so other sperm can't enter. This penetration of the egg by the sperm is called *conception*, or *fertilization*.

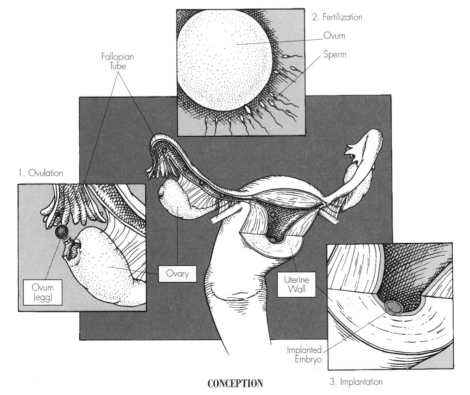

2. Fertilization

Ovum

Sperm

Fallopian Tube

1. Ovulation

Ovum (egg)

Ovary

Uterine Wall

Implanted Embryo

**CONCEPTION**     3. Implantation

An entire chain of events must play out in harmony for conception to occur. The female's *pituitary gland* controls her menstrual cycle. The pituitary gland signals the *ovary* to secrete the female hormone *estrogen* while maturing an egg in one of the ovaries. The estrogen causes the growth of the *endometrium*, the lining of the uterus. The endometrium provides all the nutrients and proper environment for a fertilized egg to implant and continue to grow.

During the middle of the cycle, levels of estrogen and *progesterone*, another female hormone, rise sharply at about the same time the egg bursts from its *follicle* on the ovary. This is called *ovulation*. The egg then begins to travel down the *fallopian tube* to the uterus. After ovulation, estrogen levels fall, but progesterone levels remain elevated due to a hormone released by the follicle that released the egg. The elevated progesterone keeps the endometrium growing and thriving.

If the egg isn't fertilized, the follicle and its hormone degenerate within a week or so, causing the progesterone levels to fall. Without continued high levels of progesterone, the endometrium sloughs off within a few days, beginning the menstrual flow. The number of days in the menstrual cycle is measured from the first day of the menstrual flow to the next menstrual flow. Although the average is 28 days, the length of women's menstrual cycles vary widely.

After conception, the fertilized egg moves down the fallopian tube and implants within the lining of the uterus. The genes from the mother and father join together as the sperm and egg combine. The egg divides rapidly into multiple cells that turn into an embryo, a fetus and, about 38 weeks after conception, a baby.

If you're trying to become pregnant, you may also be trying to time your pregnancy for a particular season. Plan to stop using birth control at least 44 weeks before the desired birth time. It may take several months for some couples to conceive, while a few are successful right away. About 15% to 20% of couples are unable to conceive after a year of trying, prompting medical testing to investigate the reasons for their infertility.

Many myths exist about ways to conceive a boy or girl. None of these have any proven merit. During pregnancy, ultrasonography (p. 643) or direct genetic sampling by amniocentesis (p. 628) can identify the sex of the fetus.

## Infertility

*Infertility*, the inability to conceive, is an unexpected and unwelcome disappointment for those who want to have children.

You and your partner can improve your chances of conceiving by making an effort to have intercourse near the mid-portion of the woman's menstrual cycle, or about two weeks before her menstrual flow.

The egg comes down the fallopian tube only once during the cycle, and the sperm only live for 48 to 72 hours. So having intercourse during these few days in the cycle improves your chances of pregnancy.

Women can check for ovulation by measuring and recording their oral temperature with a basal thermometer before getting out of bed each morning. A woman's temperature increases about one-half of a degree at the time of ovulation.

Inability to conceive may be caused by psychological, sexual or physical problems in either the man or the woman. Problems with sperm quality or number are responsible for approximately 30% of infertility cases. Female

*Common Reasons for Reduced Ability to Conceive*

- Endometriosis (p. 418)
- Impotence (p. 423)
- Irregular ovulation
- Premature ejaculation (p. 425)
- Vaginal infections
- Stress

reproductive problems, including irregular or infrequent ovulation or physical problems, such as endometriosis (p. 418), are the cause of infertility about half of the time. The final 20% of infertility is caused by a combination of factors relating to both the man and the woman or is unknown.

Seek help from your doctor if you've tried to conceive for one year but haven't been able to. Your doctor will probably document a medical history, including information about frequency and timing (within the woman's cycle) of intercourse, and examine both partners.

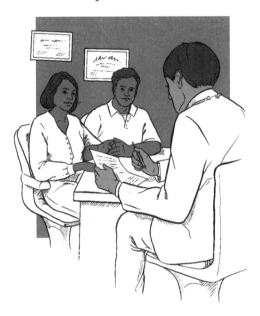

Usually, the man's exam is first because the quantity, quality, activity and shape of sperm can be easily assessed. Your doctor will look at a semen sample to assess the sperm. If any sperm factors are low, a tissue sample taken from the testicle may be analyzed to determine a cause. A blood sample may be tested for the level of the male hormone testosterone. If the testosterone level is low, replacement testosterone may be helpful.

Some of the more common male-related infertility problems are listed here.

**Hormone problems.** Low testosterone levels can reduce the number of sperm. Treatment is available.

**Impotence (p. 423).** The inability to have or maintain an erection can make sexual intercourse impossible. Psychological problems cause about half of the cases of impotence, while physical problems are to blame for the rest. Physical causes include diabetes (p. 211), atherosclerosis (p. 111), prostate problems (p. 427) and some medicines, such as certain blood pressure medicines.

**Infections.** Past infection with mumps (p. 329) may permanently impair sperm production.

**Low sperm count.** Your doctor can examine a fresh specimen of your semen to assess the number and activity of the sperm. Either the number or the quality of the sperm may be less than what is needed to fertilize an egg. A low sperm count is often caused by an elevated temperature in the scrotum (usually the result of wearing tight pants or tight underwear), use of alcohol, various medicines and even stress. Some correctable physical problems, such as a varicocele (p. 432), may also be causing the low sperm count.

**Retrograde ejaculation.** Instead of coming forward through the urethra and out the tip of the penis, semen may be pushed backward into the bladder in men who experience *retrograde ejaculation*. This prevents sperm from entering the woman's body.

## Prevention of Infertility in Men

You can make simple changes to correct some problems that may be contributing to infertility. Wear loose underwear and jeans, not tight-fitting garments. If you exercise, wear a well-fitting athletic supporter. Stay out of hot tubs. Don't drink alcohol. It can hinder the ability to become erect and also lowers the sperm count.

Testing the woman is more difficult than testing the man because the woman's reproductive system is more complex. As with the male, information about the woman's general health, current regular medicines she's taking and illness will be obtained. Some of the tests to assess a woman's fertility and predict when she will ovulate are described briefly here.

**Basal body temperature.** Your basal temperature, taken first thing in the morning, rises about one-half of a degree after ovulation. After checking your temperature daily for three or more cycles, you will have an idea of how often you're ovulating—every cycle, every other cycle, seldom or not at all.

**Blood tests.** Levels of the female hormones estrogen and progesterone will be determined with blood tests. Blood tests also assess levels of the luteinizing hormone and follicle-stimulating hormone. These two hormones control estrogen and progesterone production. The level of thyroid hormone may also be checked.

**Cervical mucus.** The consistency and acidity of cervical mucus around the time of ovulation help or hinder the sperm movement into the uterus. Your doctor may take a sample of cervical mucus to assess whether it's the right consistency for conception.

**Endometrial biopsy or sampling (p. 634).** The lining of the uterus, or endometrium, plays an essential part in fertility. An endometrial biopsy involves taking a small sample of the endometrium to check if it provides an optimal environment for implantation of the fertilized egg.

**Hysterosalpingogram (p. 636).** This x-ray test of the uterus and fallopian tubes is done to see if a clear and unobstructed path exists for the sperm to meet the egg.

**Hysteroscopy (p. 636).** A thin, lighted tubular scope is used to examine the lining of the uterus to check for abnormalities that might prevent pregnancy.

**Laparoscopy (p. 637).** A thin, lighted tubular scope is used to look into the abdomen to determine the shape and condition of your uterus, fallopian tubes and ovaries. Scarring or endometriosis may be detected during this procedure.

These tests may indicate one or more of the following conditions affecting women that may interfere with ovulation, conception or implantation.

**Anovulation.** This is when no egg is released during the menstrual cycle. It can be caused by hormone abnormalities or problems in the ovaries. In some cases, the menstrual cycle proceeds normally but the ovaries produce an egg only every other month, every third month or less often.

**Blockages.** The fallopian tube may be scarred from previous infection or it may be blocked by a tumor (p. 224), cyst (p. 649) or endometriosis (p. 418). Also, a misshapen uterus or a tumor or scarring within the uterus can restrict the flow of sperm to the fallopian tubes and interfere with conception. These problems are often detected on hysterosalpingogram, hysteroscopy or laparoscopy.

**Hormonal abnormalities.** Diabetes (p. 211), thyroid disease or a pituitary problem can affect hormone levels. Abnormal hormone levels can interfere with the maturation or release of an egg and can throw the menstrual cycle off schedule. For example, increased secretion of *prolactin* by the pituitary gland prevents ovulation. Decreased levels of other pituitary factors, such as luteinizing hormone or follicle-stimulating hormone, also make ovulation unlikely. Abnormal levels of thyroid hormones can prevent ovulation.

**Immunological factors.** Rarely, women develop antibodies to sperm. This causes the sperm to be destroyed before fertilization can take place.

**Infections.** Infections of the uterus or fallopian tubes with chlamydia (p. 317), gonorrhea (p. 318) or streptococci (p. 306) can impair fertilization. Swelling in the vagina or cervix may inhibit the passage of sperm. Chronic pelvic infections may lead to scarring and blockages as well.

Treatment of infertility depends on the problem. As many as 20% of women with infertility problems have no identifiable cause of infertility. Thus, no specific treatments are available. But when the source of the problem is identified, treatment often works. For example, blockages of the fallopian tubes can be corrected with surgery about 75% of the time. Hormone problems can be treated with hormone therapy. If you have an infection, you need an antibiotic to kill the responsible bacteria. Endometriosis (p. 418) can be treated with hormone therapy. Ovulation can be stimulated by taking certain medicines.

If treatments don't work, other approaches can be used in some women. Depending on the problem, *in vitro fertilization* may be a possibility. This involves removing multiple eggs from the ovary during laparoscopy. After the eggs are removed, they're exposed to the male's sperm. The eggs and sperm are incubated in a test tube until fertilization occurs. After fertilization, the eggs are placed back into the woman's uterus. If the male has an insufficient number or quality of sperm, a donor sample can be injected into the woman to fertilize one of her eggs. This process is called *artificial insemination.*

These treatments are costly in time, money and emotions. Being treated for infertility can turn the private act of conception into a public experience. The disappointment that results if each course of treatment fails can be emotionally draining. Some couples experience major relationship breakdowns in the face of infertility problems, especially if one partner wants to continue treatment but the other doesn't. At a time like this, it's important to keep the lines of communication open and be considerate of the other person's feelings. If it appears that none of the fertility treatments is likely to be successful, adoption is an option for some couples.

Some cases of infertility may be caused by sexual dysfunction, which is often related to the stresses of daily life or to problems within a relationship. Gaining greater control of your lifestyle can help reduce these stresses, and open communication with your partner reduces the chances of relationship problems. Specific types of sexual dysfunction may be solved with frank discussions of the problem.

## Delaying Having Children

For various reasons, you and your partner may choose to delay having a child. Delaying childrearing can be beneficial. For example, you may be more financially and emotionally ready to have children if you wait. But be aware that some problems may accompany your decision to wait. Children conceived after the mother reaches age 35 or older are four times more likely to have Down syndrome (p. 348). There is an increased risk of some other birth defects as well. After the mother reaches age 40, the risk of birth defects becomes much greater. Because it takes a great deal of energy and stamina to care for young children, older parents, especially those in their forties, may find the job of childrearing more difficult than they anticipated.

Some women go through menopause much earlier than expected, even

---

*Possible Benefits of Delaying Pregnancy*

- Greater financial stability
- Emotional maturity
- Being more certain of your decision

---

*Possible Consequences of Delaying Pregnancy*

- Increased risk of birth defects
- Less stamina to meet the demands of a child
- Loss of fertility through necessary surgery or premature menopause

in their late 30s or early 40s. For them, it becomes impossible to conceive a child. Past medical problems, such as testicular cancer (p. 429) or severe pelvic inflammatory disease (PID, p. 417), may have destroyed any potential for conceiving. Adoption is an alternative. Your doctor can offer insights based on your personal medical history that may affect your decision to postpone having children.

## Contraception

Many contraceptive methods are available to people who wish to postpone having children. When you're planning your family, you and your partner will need to examine more than simple facts about a contraceptive method and how it should be used. Feelings, values, standards, teaching from our parents and what others say and believe about contraception all play a part in this decision.

No contraceptive is perfect. The choice of birth control also needs to be made in light of what your response would be if the method fails and an unplanned pregnancy (p. 554) occurs. Because such considerations deal with your beliefs about the very beginnings of human life, they may be intensely personal. The only sure way to prevent pregnancy is to not have sex. The most common methods of contraception are discussed below.

**Birth control pills.** Birth control pills can be very effective at preventing pregnancy. Birth control pills usually contain the two female hormones, estrogen and progesterone. The first pills, which became available about 40 years ago, were very high in estrogen and caused an increased risk of cancer and adverse side effects.

Today's pills contain smaller dosages of estrogen and are much safer. Side effects have been reduced, while the effectiveness of the pill has remained excellent. *Monophasic* birth control pills provide a constant level of estrogen and progesterone for three weeks, with one week off during menstruation. *Biphasic and triphasic* pills vary the dosages of estrogen and progesterone during the three weeks of hormone use. Your doctor can help you decide which is best for you.

Birth control pills work by blocking the maturation and expulsion of the egg from the ovary. If no eggs are produced, conception cannot occur. The hormones also change the consistency of the mucus in the woman's reproductive tract, preventing the sperm from traveling into the uterus and fallopian tubes.

The most common side effects of birth control pills include slight nausea and some irregular vaginal bleeding during the first few months. Taking the pill with a little food may eliminate the nausea. The pill increases the risk of vaginal yeast infections (p. 421). Fatigue and depression-like symptoms sometimes also occur. Side effects like these are usually mild, but they may persist to the point that you're unable to use the pill as a means of birth control.

Strokes, heart attacks and blood clots are eight times more likely in women who smoke while taking the pill than those who don't smoke. The pill doesn't cause cervical cancer, but yearly Pap tests (p. 639) are part of the routine care for women on the pill to check for early signs of cervical cancer. Birth control pills are usually not prescribed for women with diabetes, hypertension, breast or uterine cancer, or a history of blood clots because they may worsen these conditions.

Birth control pills have been shown to have benefits. For example, birth control pills usually ease the pain and discomfort of menstrual cramps, as well as reduce the flow. Women who take the pill also have a reduced risk of anemia (p. 133), arthritis (p. 229), pelvic infections, tubal pregnancy (p. 393) and ovarian cysts (p. 417). Birth control pills are sometimes prescribed as treatment for recurrent ovarian cysts and endometriosis (p. 418). In weighing the risks and benefits, it's important to remember that for most women, the risks of the pill are much less than the risks associated with pregnancy. While the pill is very effective in preventing pregnancy, it doesn't protect against sexually transmitted diseases (p. 316).

The *minipill* is a form of the pill that contains only progesterone. The minipill is safer for women who have been advised not to use estrogen. It's less effective than the "combined" pill, but it's more effective than condoms and diaphragms. The minipill changes the lining of the uterus and the cervical mucus, but doesn't always block ovulation. The minipill is more effective when it's taken at the same time every day, such as at the evening meal. Nausea is a possible side effect and there's a fairly high incidence of persistent irregular vaginal bleeding.

**Condom.** A latex sheath that fits over the penis, the condom is called a *barrier contraceptive* because it blocks the semen and sperm from being in contact with the vaginal tissues. Using a spermicidal jelly or foam along with the condom increases its effectiveness. If you use it correctly every time you have sex, the condom can be quite effective in preventing pregnancy. The advantages of condoms include their availability in most drug stores, their low cost and their ability to offer some, but not complete, protection from sexually transmitted diseases. See page 317 for information about how to put on a condom correctly.

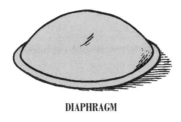

DIAPHRAGM

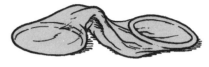

FEMALE CONDOM

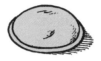

CERVICAL CAP

**Diaphragm/cervical cap/female condom.** A number of barrier methods are also available for women. The *diaphragm* is a latex-covered ring that fits snugly against the cervix within the vagina. When used with a spermicidal foam it's effective in preventing pregnancy. The diaphragm must be properly fitted by your doctor, inserted before sexual intercourse and left in for six hours after intercourse.

The *cervical cap* is smaller than a diaphragm and covers only the cervix, the opening to the uterus. It's fitted for you by a doctor. It's inserted like a diaphragm, used with a spermicidal jelly or foam (p. 552), and also left in place for six hours after intercourse.

The *female condom* doesn't need fitting by your doctor. Like the diaphragm or cervical cap, it should be used with spermicidal jelly or foam for added effectiveness.

**Hormone implant and shots.** The hormone implant and shots work much like the birth control pill, but they only use the hormone progestin. The implants consist of capsules that contain progestin. The implants are placed under the skin in a woman's upper arm. They help prevent pregnancy for five years before needing to be replaced.

Hormone shots work for three months. The implant and shots don't have the same health risks as the pill because they don't contain estrogen. But side effects may include headaches and changes in your periods, weight and moods. The hormone implant may also cause irritation in the area of your arm where it's placed.

**Intrauterine device (IUD).** The IUD is inserted in the uterus by your doctor. It stays in the uterus and remains effective for years, depending on the type used, until your doctor removes it. An IUD doesn't block the joining of sperm with egg. Instead, it changes the lining of the uterus, making implantation of a fertilized egg impossible.

Menstrual pain and bleeding may increase for a few months after insertion of an IUD, but these side effects usually disappear within the first year. Perforation of the uterus during insertion is possible but unlikely. Infection of the uterus is also another complication, but isn't common. Rarely, pregnancy occurs when an IUD is in place. When this happens, the IUD must be removed as soon as the pregnancy is discovered. There is a risk of miscarriage.

**Rhythm method.** The rhythm method is a "natural" means of birth control, in that no pills, devices or barriers are used. Instead, the couple doesn't have intercourse at times during the woman's menstrual cycle when fertilization is most likely, usually the middle seven to 10 days. An egg can be fertilized during the first 24 hours after it leaves the ovary. Sperm live in the female reproductive tract for up to 72 hours. So a couple practicing the rhythm method shouldn't have intercourse from three to four days prior to ovulation until three days after ovulation—a total of one week of abstinence from sexual intercourse.

Ovulation produces no symptoms for many women, so it's difficult to identify the exact day it occurs.

Several approaches can be used to track your ovulation. These include the calendar method, the basal temperature method and the cervical mucus method. Using more than one approach may increase how well these work for you.

The rhythm method is one of the least effective ways to prevent pregnancy, but many couples choose it because it requires no pills or devices. This method has the best chance of success when the woman's cycle is regular and ovulation can be closely estimated, and if the couple has strong discipline over their sexual desires. But failure rates, even for couples who "know" their cycle, range from 10% to 50%.

**Spermicides.** Although spermicides in the form of a jelly or foam can be used alone, they're most effective when combined with a condom or diaphragm. Chemicals within the spermicidal foam destroy the sperm. Used alone, the effectiveness of a spermicide is slightly less than the rhythm method, but when combined with a condom or diaphragm, its effectiveness increases. An added benefit to using certain spermicides, such as nonoxynol-9 (p. 617), is that they destroy some of the organisms that cause sexually transmitted diseases.

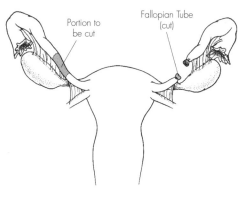

**TUBAL LIGATION**

**Sterilization.** Permanent methods of blocking the sperm from reaching the egg are extremely effective at preventing pregnancy. But they're difficult to reverse if you change your mind about this decision. Tubal ligation and vasectomy are two methods of sterilization.

*Tubal ligation,* or having the fallopian tubes "tied," can be done as an outpatient procedure with the use of general anesthesia. When the fallopian tubes are closed off, eggs can't go from the ovaries through the fallopian tubes to the uterus. The woman's menstrual period isn't affected by this operation.

Male sterilization, the *vasectomy,* involves cutting the *vas deferens,* the tubes that carry sperm from the testicles to the urethra. The tubes may then be cauterized, or sealed. Vasectomy can be done under local anesthesia in the doctor's office. Because sperm may still exist within the vas deferens after the vasectomy, another method of contraception should be used for eight weeks after the operation. Your doctor may check samples of your semen to make sure the vasectomy was effective.

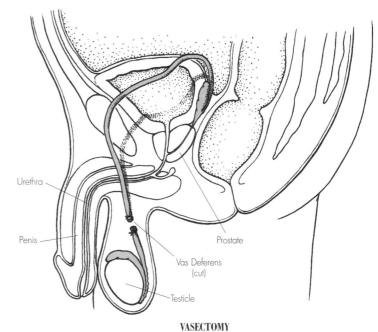

**VASECTOMY**

Vasectomy doesn't increase or worsen heart disease. It may slightly increase the risk of prostate cancer. But this added risk of prostate cancer is still very small.

**Withdrawal.** In this method, the man pulls out of the vagina before he ejaculates. It's not very effective, because the man usually leaves behind a small amount of fluid that leaks from the penis during sex. This fluid has enough sperm in it to cause a pregnancy.

---

## Effectiveness of Contraceptives

*You can greatly increase the effectiveness of any form of contraception by using it the right way every time you have sex. Listed below is the* typical *percentage of effectiveness for different contraceptives used by* typical *couples in the first year of use. You can also increase the effectiveness of condoms by using spermicides with the condom every time you have sex.*

| | | | |
|---|---|---|---|
| Abstinence | 100% | Condom alone | 88% |
| Hormone implant | 99.96% | Cervical cap with spermicide | 82% |
| Hormone shots | 99.96% | Diaphragm plus spermicide | 82% |
| Tubal ligation | 99.96% | Withdrawal | 82% |
| Vasectomy | 99.85% | Rhythm method | 80% |
| Birth control pills | 97% | Spermicide alone | 79% |
| Intrauterine device | 97% | Chance | 15% |

Adapted with the permission of the Population Council, from James Trussell et al., "Contraceptive Failure in the United States: An Update," *Studies in Family Planning* 21, no. 1 (Jan/Feb 1990):52.

## Unplanned Pregnancy

Despite widespread availability of inexpensive and effective contraception, unplanned pregnancies are still very common. Contraceptive failure accounts for only a small portion of these unplanned pregnancies. Unused, misused or forgotten contraceptives are the more common causes.

What can you do when a pregnancy occurs before you're financially or emotionally ready to care for the infant? What are your options in dealing with the pregnancy and the new infant? The ability to handle this situation is a learning process. If you face such a difficult situation, try to share your feelings with your partner, family, doctor and perhaps a counselor. Talking openly with people you can trust can help you make healthy decisions.

If you and your partner are in extreme personal and financial difficulties, or when other complicating factors make caring for a new child extremely difficult, you may want to consider placing your child with an adoptive family. Some adoption agencies allow the birth parents to place their child with the couple of their choice. Although it can be extremely difficult on the birth parents, this option can bring great joy to a couple who's unable to conceive.

Abortion is another option when an unplanned pregnancy occurs. Abortion is controversial, and it has emotional, physical and moral implications for many people. Because of this, the woman may want to discuss this option with her partner, doctor, family, or a counselor or minister before making a final decision.

## Teaching Children About Sexuality

Sexuality is far more than just having sex. It's a part of who we are: our gender, our attitudes, our outlook, our biases, our education and experiences, and even our personality. Our sexuality changes throughout our lives as we come to understand more and more about ourselves and about the physical and emotional differences and similarities between boys and girls, men and women.

When do parents or guardians begin to teach their children about sexuality? Sexual attitudes and values can be taught beginning during the preschool years, when children can be told about the differences between girls and boys. Preteen children can be taught more about the differences between boys and girls and how they can begin to relate socially. Young teenagers need facts about the physical changes of adolescence and what behaviors are and are not acceptable. Continued support, communication and teaching during the maturation of your teen will guide him or her through the teen years.

Any discussion of the potential negative consequences of sexual experimentation, such as sexually transmitted diseases, pregnancy and damaged self-esteem, should be balanced with descriptions of the rewards of healthy sexual relationships. Supportive discussions about values are more acceptable and helpful for a child than giving the child rules to follow without explanations.

### Teaching Preschool Children

Teaching preschoolers about sexuality includes information about behaviors and characteristics of boys and girls. Learning about these things helps them "fit in" as they mature. Good teaching takes a lot of creative thinking. Always use simple concepts, personalize the lesson and provide positive statements and encouragement. Persistently negative statements produce low

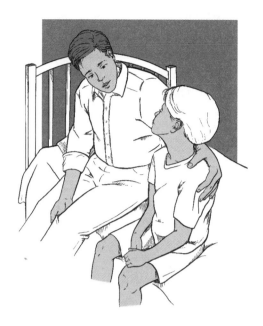

motivation and poor self-esteem in children who are trying new behaviors.

Small children don't have the intellectual tools to understand abstract concepts. Their thinking abilities are concrete. They can understand only what they can see. But, while they can't understand the emotional differences between men and women, they can understand differences in appearance. They can see that men, such as their fathers, are generally taller and stronger, and have deeper voices than women. Women, such as their mothers, are generally shorter and softer, and have soothing voices.

Other concrete differences might include differences in the way men and women dress, in the jobs they do around the house, in the tools they use most often and in the hobbies and activities they enjoy. Even very young children can understand that "mommies have babies," but daddies don't.

Preschoolers' power of observation is great. They may know more about male and female characteristics than you realize. Discussing these characteristics with them and being a good role model are excellent ways to help children identify their gender and feel good about who they are. Building a child's self-esteem during this age takes positive encouragement and positive role models.

**Roles and gender imitation.** Part of the child's understanding of sexual differences comes by identifying different roles for each sex. As children begin to identify themselves as either a boy or girl, they may pretend that they're women or men. This form of role identification and imitation is a normal and healthy part of a child's discovering his or her own identity.

Try not to portray that one career may be good for boys but not girls or the other way around. And definitely don't fill the child's mind with negative images about one sex or the other.

The preschool years mark an important time to teach the child about the similarities of men and women. Exposing both boys and girls to role models who display characteristics that are considered masculine *and* feminine can keep children from learning to stereotype male and female behaviors. He or she learns to absorb the best qualities of what society calls masculine and feminine. The result can be a more rounded personality in the child.

**Curiosity.** A child's body represents a part of his or her explorable world. Curiosity about body parts is normal, and so is the "toilet talk" most children use as they begin to socialize. A child's curiosity about the genitals is nonsexual during the preschool stage. But learning that boys and girls have different body parts is another step during this stage in their development.

Exposure of genitals is common at this age. It gives parents or guardians an opportunity to teach about inappropriate exposure. Some parents or guardians are shocked by this normal behavior and overreact with spanking, scolding or punishing in other strongly negative ways. If a child is exposed to these strong negative reactions often, he or she may develop extreme feelings of shame and "dirtiness" about his or her body. This attitude may stay with the child into his or her adult life and may affect sexual relationships.

### Teaching Preteens (age eight to 12)

By teaching about sexuality to preschool and preteen children, you can lay a crucial foundation of values and behaviors that will influence your child's emerging sexuality in later years. For instance, if you teach your child self-control and encourage it again and again as he or she struggles through relationships, school, and other challenges of childhood, it's much easier to teach sexual self-control during the teen years.

Start early in fostering a healthy sexual identity in your child. Discuss the topic often, redirect him or her when peer pressure steers a different course, and support your preteen through open communication, love and caring involvement. Although his or her relationships during childhood and preteen years will be primarily with the same sex, opposite-sex friendships also begin to form, serving as a basis for later male-female relationships in the early-teen period.

True sexual feelings related to hormones, sex drive and lust are unlikely to occur until about age 10 or later. This is a golden time for you to help shape your child's attitudes and values toward relationships. It's a time to prepare him or her to make good choices of peers and friends of the opposite sex.

Same-sex and opposite-sex relationships within the family can also blossom during this stage if you encourage them. During these years, the family serves as a model for many of the sex-based behaviors a child learns. Sex-based restrictions such as "only girls play house," and "only boys play football" should be avoided, so children will feel comfortable with whatever activity they choose.

### Teaching Adolescents (age 12 to 18)

The stability you offer through good communication and strong support can ease your child's distress as he or she faces the changes, new feelings and difficulties that often accompany adolescence.

When you discuss sexuality with your children, remember the importance of balancing negative aspects with positive aspects. Teaching adolescents about the physical act of sex without teaching them the importance of values, responsibility and relationships gives them an unbalanced view.

Your aim should be to give your teenagers solid information about human sexual functioning while providing insights about the positive and negative aspects of having a sexual relationship. Discussions should include information about the responsibilities involved with having a sexual relationship, the impact of peer pressure on this decision, the risks of pregnancy and sexually transmitted diseases (p. 316), the emotional impact of a sexual relationship and other reasons abstinence is often the best choice. Provide open, honest answers to their questions, and teach them the values you feel are important.

**Emotional maturation.** During adolescence, your child begins the change into adulthood. Rebellion and risk-taking (p. 378) are common during this period. Your task as a parent or guardian during this stage is to help your child develop values that will protect and help him or her maintain self-worth and self-respect.

If communication between you and your teenager is blocked by anger, rebellion, unforgiveness or apathy, he or she will reach emotional maturity with the help of other sources, such as his or her peers. If you want your kids to grow up with your values and morals, always keep the channels of communication open, no matter what situations or problems arise. Don't wait for your teen to come to you. Instead, make every effort to start to communicate with him or her.

**Physical maturation.** Adolescence is a time of great physical change (p. 373). The awkwardness, skin changes and feelings of "ugliness" are often part of an obsession with "looks." Hormone changes produce secondary sexual characteristics, such as voice changes, facial hair, pubic hair, breast development and changes in the genitals. The hormones affect all tissues in the body, causing physical and emotional changes, and creating the sex drive.

Physical maturation is sometimes completed long before emotional maturity gives the teenager the ability to handle personal responsibilities. Emotionally immature young men and women may be sexually able to have children, but socially and emotionally unable to handle the immense responsibilities of a family.

Talking with your teen specifically about what physical changes to expect reduces his or her anxiety about body changes. Help your teenager deal with perceived crises related to his or her appearance by showing understanding. This demonstrates your love and your willingness to help, and it acknowledges teen's feelings about the "crisis."

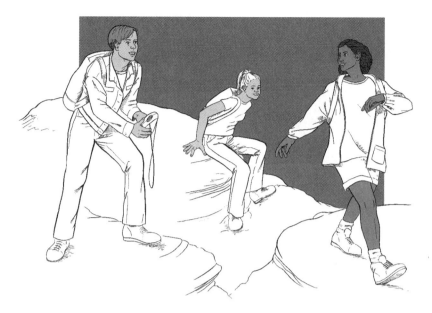

**Opposite-sex friendships.** As a parent or guardian, you can help your adolescent reach a level of maturity for developing healthy relationships with

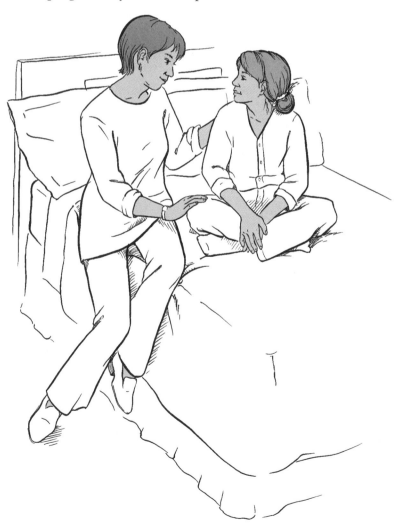

*Talking About Contraception with Your Teen*

*Talking About Contraception with Your Teen*

Providing contraceptives to unmarried teens and young adults is controversial. Some parents and guardians say teenage sexual activity is inevitable and contraceptives should be offered to try to prevent sexually transmitted diseases (p. 316) and pregnancy. Other parents and guardians are uncomfortable with this approach. They believe that offering contraceptives to teenagers removes inhibition, implies approval and encourages teens to be sexually active. People who believe contraceptives shouldn't be given to a teen should teach their teenager the principles of self-control and abstinence. The information you share with your children will reflect your values.

the opposite sex. For this reason, many parents and guardians prohibit their children from dating until the middle-teenage years when they're more mature and are better able to deal with these relationships.

Again, good communication is imperative. Before the young adult begins dating, guidelines on behavior need to be discussed in detail. When you teach your children about sexuality, be sure to include the healthy values of self-control, respect for one's self and for others. When the proper information is given to teens, fewer will decide to become sexually active. Those who do choose to have sex will be more likely to protect themselves from sexually transmitted diseases and unplanned pregnancies.

As your teenager begins dating, also discuss specific instructions and expectations, such as what time to be home and where he or she will be.

**Support.** How can teens remain true to themselves in the face of peer pressure? One of the best ways to help this happen is to talk with your teenager about the possibility of an uncomfortable situation occurring and ways he or she might respond. Many parents and guardians have an agreement with their teenagers that they will come to get

them right away if they find themselves in a bad situation, such as one involving sex or drugs. All the teenager needs to do is call for help. Some parents or guardians and teenagers agree that no questions will be asked at the time and that discussion will be postponed until later. Making this kind of commitment to your young adult can give him or her an extra incentive to follow a healthy path.

In contrast to this kind of commitment, lack of interest by a parent can be translated by the young adult into lack of caring or love. Show interest in your young adult's friendships and dating relationships. Notice if his or her interests and values are similar to yours. Monitor whether your young adult acts maturely and is willing to abide by guidelines and rules. Find out what your teenager's plans are for a date, where he or she will be, with whom and what time he or she will be home. Showing interest in your teen's activity may be rebuffed initially by your teen as meddling, but subconsciously the teenager will understand that you love and care for him or her. Regardless, it's wiser for you, the parent or guardian, to provide loving, reasonable guidelines than to have no guidelines at all.

---

## Who teaches kids about sex?

- 30% of all teenagers receive their instruction about sex from sexuality education in school.
- 30% of all teenagers get information from their friends.
- 20% of teenagers are taught about sex by their parents.
- 10% get information about sex from TV, magazines or other media.
- 10% of teens have no instruction about sex.

# EMOTIONS, BEHAVIOR AND THE FAMILY

Your emotional and mental health is as important as your physical health. Just as illnesses and problems can affect your body, they can also affect your mind.

Emotions help determine how you behave. Your ability to handle feelings of anger, anxiety, grief, loneliness and sadness can color the quality of your life. How you handle these emotions depends on your genes, your personality, your environment and what you learned growing up.

How you behave comes partly from your *family of origin*—the family in which you grew up. Were you disciplined calmly and with love? Or were you physically, emotionally or sexually abused? Did people in your family show their emotions or did they hide them? Families that fail to provide the right kind of love and support are called *dysfunctional*.

Many treatments are available to change behaviors and correct emotional problems and psychiatric illnesses. If you think you may need some help, start with your doctor. He or she can help you find the right type of counseling.

People with healthy outlooks often strive for balance in their lives. For example, they don't obsess about work and exclude other activities. Make time for things you enjoy. Take care of your physical health. Exercise regularly, eat healthy meals and get enough sleep to help keep your body fit. Also keep in balance your beliefs about what's important—relationships, personal well-being, achievements, education, physical comfort, spiritual growth. All of these things work together to bring a sense of direction to life.

## Addictions

A broad definition of the term *addiction* is a dependence on drugs, alcohol, food or other substances. It can also be used to describe dependence

---

### Types of Therapy

- **Behavioral therapy.** This type of therapy is aimed at changing a certain behavior. Rewards may be used to help encourage change.
- **Counseling.** Counseling may help you learn how to handle emotional conflict. Counseling is the process of meeting with a qualified person, called a counselor or therapist, to discuss your thoughts and feelings. A counselor may be a psychologist, school guidance counselor or minister. The counselor can give you feedback and help you work through your feelings or problems.
- **Group therapy.** This is a group of people with similar problems that meets regularly. A therapist guides the discussion, or in self-help groups the participants conduct the sessions themselves. Talking with others who have the same problems or experiences can be very helpful.
- **Psychoanalysis.** Psychoanalysis involves one-on-one sessions with a therapist on a regular basis. You're encouraged to talk about your life and about problems that are bothering you. Your dreams may also be discussed, because thoughts that you repress or ignore may be revealed in dreams.

on other things, such as exercise, gambling, power, sex and relationships.

You have an addiction if your need for a substance or thing leads you to lose control over your behavior as you seek to satisfy the need. An addicted person keeps doing the same thing despite bad results. Addictive behaviors are contradictory: They're done for pleasure and yet they're self-destructive.

One of the telltale signs of addiction is the inability to understand or admit to the need for the addictive substance or behavior. Denial of the problem makes it difficult to persuade a person with an addiction to seek help. "I don't have a problem," the addicted person insists. "I can stop any time I want to."

## The Codependent Family

*Codependency* is a term used to describe a person's or family's unintended cooperation with *(enabling)* their loved one's addiction. The family enables their loved one to continue the addiction. An example of enabling behavior would be making excuses for the addicted person's inability to go to work. Codependency can occur in a relationship with someone who has any kind of addiction, including alcohol, drugs, gambling and sex.

Another example of codependency is a wife who repeatedly rescues her drunk husband from places where he has passed out. Some enablers simply ignore the person when he or she becomes drunk. Then they make excuses to others for his or her behavior. The codependent family doesn't hold the addicted person accountable for the behavior. The family's actions protect the addicted person from suffering any of the consequences of the behavior. In that sense, the codependent person shares some responsibility for the addicted behavior by making it easier for the person to continue.

Why do some loving and caring people seem prone to get involved in hurtful, harmful, even dangerous relationships? Many people who are codependent grew up in a dysfunctional family, where they felt insecure and unworthy of love and acceptance. Because he or she often feels unloved, the codependent person tries to gain value, acceptance and love by rescuing, controlling and serving others.

### Qualities That Can Help You Enjoy Life and Grow

- Liking yourself despite apparent shortcomings
- A willingness to really be yourself
- A balance between caring for yourself and giving to others
- An appreciation for close relationships with others
- An appreciation for personal or private time
- A healthy sense of humor, even about personal flaws

- A strong respect for the rights and needs of others
- A belief that learning about relationships, spiritual matters, personal qualities and educational matters is a lifelong process
- A willingness to listen to others' viewpoints even when they differ from your own
- A warmth toward others

A codependent person lacks objectivity about relationships and has an overblown sense of responsibility for others. A codependent person may have feelings of hurt, anger, guilt and loneliness and may even use these feelings to control others.

Codependent family relationships are dysfunctional because they don't meet needs for love, security and acceptance in a healthy way. Children who grow up in families with an addicted parent may become part of the cycle of codependency by denying and hiding the parent's problem. They may feel helpless, ashamed and inadequate. They may be angry at their parent, but may not show their anger. As the anger builds, it's kept inside. Depression, hopelessness, guilt and resentment may develop. As a way of coping, children and other family members may start the addictive behavior.

Even if the addicted person refuses treatment, family members can get help. Many drug and alcohol rehabilitation programs offer counseling and support groups to help family members break out of dysfunctional relationships. With help, family members can learn how to offer the addicted person the right kind of support and help, in part by making the addicted person accountable for his or her behavior.

Codependent people need to spend time with people in situations where emotions are expressed honestly and workable solutions are found to serious problems. This concept, called *modeling*, is a key to breaking the codependency cycle. Codependent people need to see functional families in as many different situations as possible to understand fully what healthy relationships are like and how they can model their own behavior in healthy ways.

If someone in your family is abusing alcohol or drugs, seek help through

## Codependent Behaviors

- Hoping that your helpful actions will change the behavior of your addicted family member.
- Allowing the person to slack off on responsibilities and doing more than your fair share of work.
- Consistently giving more than you receive in the relationship.
- Trying to "fix" others' feelings that make you uncomfortable.
- Making excuses for the person's behavior. Trying to protect him or her from the consequences of the behavior.

a local program or call Alcoholics Anonymous (they can tell you about Al-Anon, a suport group for families of alcoholics) or Narcotics Anonymous. Even if you aren't codependent, programs can be supportive and helpful. Finding a support group is essential. By getting help for yourself, you can offer the kind of support your family member needs to get help.

## Substance Abuse

Substance abuse addictions can have both psychological and physical effects that lead to dependence. A psychological addiction results from feelings of stress, habit, satisfaction or pleasure. A physical addiction causes the body to need the drug. Sometimes, increasingly larger amounts of a drug are needed because the body builds up a tolerance to the substance. When the drug is withdrawn suddenly, unpleasant physical symptoms occur. This is known as *withdrawal.*

The only sure way to prevent drug or alcohol addiction is never to start using one of these substances. Abstinence promotes good health. It should be taught to children of all ages. Parents and guardians need to build their children's self-esteem and self-worth so they aren't looking for a drug or other addictive substance or behavior to make themselves feel better. Besides pointing out the dangers of addiction, emphasize the benefits of good health and clear thinking. Keep your children away from situations where drug experimentation is occurring.

---

## Signs of Substance Abuse

### Changes in behavior

- Chronic lying, stealing, cheating, secretiveness
- A change in friends, and unwillingness to bring the new friends home or talk about them
- Severe mood swings
- Unpredictable and inappropriate behavior, such as anger, irritability and hostility
- Loss of interest in usual hobbies
- Lack of motivation and self-discipline
- Withdrawal from family activities
- Unexplained loss of money and possessions or unexplained possession of large amounts of money
- Items of value missing from the home
- Frequent unexplained absences from home
- Not coming home on time

### Changes in school or work performance

- Grades or work performance falling markedly below previous levels
- Assignments or tasks not completed
- Frequent absences and discipline problems, or unusual or chronic conflict with co-workers

### Health problems

- Poor resistance to minor illnesses
- Unkempt appearance, poor hygiene
- Poor attention span, trouble concentrating
- Frequent respiratory illnesses
- Dilated pupils, chronically bloodshot eyes, slurred speech
- Poor physical coordination, incoherent thinking

### Drug-use paraphernalia

- Possession of water pipes, rolling papers, small decongestant bottles, small butane torches, roach clips, stash cans
- Possession of or evidence of drugs, such as marijuana butts, seeds or leaves in clothing or around the home
- Odor of drugs, use of incense or frequent use of cover-up scents

---

## Alcoholism

Alcohol is the most used and abused substance in America. The signs of chronic alcohol use include alcohol odor on the breath, heavy use of breath fresheners, glazed and unfocused eyes, unusually passive or aggressive behavior, poor coordination, trembling, absenteeism from school or work, memory loss, depression and confusion. Alcoholism can cause many different problems, such as problems working and functioning, the breakdown of important relationships and serious health problems, including cirrhosis of the liver (p. 201).

The cause of alcoholism isn't fully understood. A family history makes an inherited predisposition to alcoholism more likely, and men are at greater risk than women. Some evidence shows that people who drink are trying to "self-medicate" themselves. They use alcohol in an attempt to relieve anxiety, depression, tension, loneliness, self-doubt or unhappiness. More than likely, many factors combine to lead to alcoholism. For example, an inherited predisposition to alcoholism may combine with stress, a person's environment and exposure to alcoholic beverages to result in alcoholism.

Alcohol is a problem if it causes a problem in any part of your life. Indications that alcohol is a problem include if you've ever felt the need to

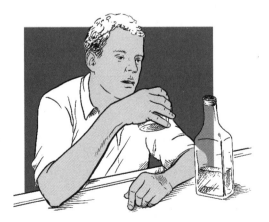

## Signs That an Alcohol User Needs Treatment

- Denial about having a problem
- Absences from work or school because of drinking
- Family problems, such as marital problems or spouse abuse, brought on by the drinking
- Financial problems due to buying alcohol
- Driving while intoxicated
- Frequently drinking alone
- Drinking during the day (not confined to evenings)

cut down on your drinking, if you've ever felt annoyed by people criticizing your drinking, if you've ever felt guilty about your drinking, or if you've ever felt the need for a drink in the morning (as an "eye-opener").

Often, people won't admit when alcohol is a problem. People around you may see it first. Think about it. Think about what your friends and family say to you about your drinking. Help is available for drinking problems.

Treatment of alcoholism may occur in a hospital setting (inpatient treatment) or in intensive regular appointments while the person continues his or her normal day-to-day activities (outpatient treatment). Inpatient treatment usually begins with *detoxification,* which involves safe withdrawal from alcohol, and medicines to block dangerous withdrawal effects.

Treatment may include using a medicine, called disulfiram (p. 623). It helps people who want to quit drinking not start again. You may be prescribed the medicine several days after you've stopped drinking. If you drink while taking the medicine, you'll become sick, with flushing, vomiting and a severe headache.

Treatment may include individual, family or group counseling and participation in Alcoholics Anonymous or other programs.

None of these methods will work unless the alcohol-dependent person is committed to stop drinking. Since denial of the problem is a common problem in alcoholics, family members may first need to seek help and guidance in how to encourage their loved one to get treatment. Al-Anon is a support group for friends and family members of alcoholics.

### Illegal Drugs

The popularity of individual drugs comes and goes, but the problem of illegal drugs continues in America. Besides the physical risks, the use of illegal drugs brings with it crime, violence, family crisis, social disorder, and puts young people at particular risk.

**Cocaine and crack.** Cocaine has become the most harmful addictive illegal drug in our society. Cocaine is a strong stimulant that comes from the leaves of the South American coca plant. It's either snorted or smoked.

Crack is a form of cocaine and is five to six times stronger than the powder form of cocaine. Crack is smoked and is addictive almost immediately. It produces a *euphoria* (an exaggerated sense of physical and mental well-being) that lasts five to 20 minutes.

The effects of cocaine are powerful. The user first feels a sense of well-being and is alert and full of energy. Cocaine causes the pupils to dilate, and causes blood pressure, heart rate, body temperature and breathing rate to increase. Crack can cause burning of the lips or throat, weight loss, lung damage, heart attack and stroke.

**Hallucinogens.** Hallucinogens are drugs that cause *hallucinations,* or visions of things that aren't really there.

Drugs that are hallucinogens include LSD, mescaline, psilocybin and phencyclidine (PCP). LSD is the most well-known of the hallucinogens. After a long period of decline, its use is increasing, especially among teens. In some people, LSD may cause euphoria , while others who use it may become anxious and paranoid. Judgment and perception are often impaired, which can lead to accidents, such as a person thinking he or she can fly out of a 10th-story window. PCP, which is also a hallucinogen, is usually sprinkled on smoking material, such as marijuana, and inhaled. It causes a giddy euphoria followed by anxiety. In high doses, the user may be withdrawn. Hallucinogens cause an emotional dependence more than a physical dependence. Some people have *flashbacks* after they stop using hallucinogens. A flashback is when the drug affects you after you've quit using it. Most flashbacks consist of visual illusions, but can include distortions of time or space, or hallucinations. Flashbacks tend to go away over a period of six to 12 months.

**Heroin.** Heroin and morphine are called *opiates* because they're derived from opium. Morphine is sometimes prescribed to relieve pain. Given for a short time, morphine isn't addictive. But over a longer period, especially in large doses, opiates are highly addictive. These drugs are taken by injection into the skin or a vein. They produce a feeling of euphoria. Side effects include depression of the respiratory and circulatory systems, dizziness, nausea, sweating, uncoordinated muscle movement and general weakness. Heavy use also decreases the sex drive. Because these drugs are injected, users are at risk of infection with hepatitis (p. 204) and HIV (p. 325) from dirty needles.

**Marijuana.** The leaves of the marijuana plant can be dried and smoked.

It makes the user feel euphoric. It was thought that marijuana use had few adverse effects, but that's no longer accurate. Unfortunately, many young people continue to believe marijuana isn't harmful, so its use is increasing. This is of concern because marijuana is a gateway drug, meaning its use tends to lead to the use and abuse of other illegal drugs. Continued marijuana use can reduce concentration, interfere with short-term memory, alter your sense of time and cause confusion, apathy, depression and anxiety. Users may have bloodshot eyes, increased heart rate, dry mouth and throat, and lung damage.

Anyone using cocaine, crack or other illegal drugs on a regular basis needs professional help, usually in an inpatient drug-treatment program or intensive outpatient setting. Treatment includes counseling and medical detoxification to help during the body's withdrawal from the drug. Extreme cravings during cocaine withdrawal may last for weeks. Like alcoholism, denial makes it difficult for a drug abuser to seek help. Often help is sought and the abuse problem addressed only at the insistence of family members or after referral through the court system or social services.

Follow-up care after an inpatient or intensive outpatient program often includes individual counseling, family therapy and participation in Narcotics Anonymous (NA). The addicted person's family often benefits from attending the corresponding NA program for spouses and children.

### Prescription Drugs

It's possible to become addicted to legal prescription medicines, as well as to illegal drugs.

**Amphetamines.** These drugs have a stimulant effect. They cause a feeling of well-being. Tolerance to these medicines usually develops, and it takes larger and larger amounts to produce a "high." Withdrawal causes tiredness, sleepiness and depression, but few other physical effects.

**Barbiturates.** Barbiturates are a type of tranquilizer. They can become addictive when used regularly. Symptoms of barbiturate dependence include decreased alertness, slurred speech and slowed thinking. Anxiety, tremors, weakness and insomnia occur when abstaining.

**Benzodiazepines.** Overuse of diazepam (p. 626) or alprazolam (p. 626), two frequently prescribed medicines in the U.S., can lead to addiction. These medicines, called benzodiazepines, are tranquilizers. They have a depressant effect on the brain, similar to alcohol. Benzodiazepines are prescribed to relieve insomnia, anxiety, stress and tension for short periods of time (several weeks at most). Their continued use can lead to dependence.

**Narcotics/opiates.** Morphine and codeine are examples of prescription narcotic painkillers. These medicines can cause euphoria or feeling "high." Addiction to narcotics and opiates is both physical and psychological. Withdrawal from narcotics or opiates can cause severe symptoms such as tremors, muscle twitching, hot and cold flashes and dilated pupils.

Detoxification in a hospital is needed for safe withdrawal from benzodiazepines, barbiturates and other commonly abused pain medicines, stimulants and tranquilizers.

### Solvents and Aerosols

The fumes from glue, aerosol cans, paint, gasoline, nail polish remover and hair spray can be inhaled to produce an intoxicated feeling. Children and adolescents are the most common users of inhalants. The fumes cause dizziness, slurred speech, drowsiness and staggering. A "high" may last from minutes to more than an hour.

The use of these chemicals can be dangerous, even fatal. Liver and kidney failure can occur from inhaling carbon tetrachloride, or dry cleaner solvent. Other substances may injure the brain, liver, kidney and bone marrow.

Treatment usually focuses on improving the user's self-esteem while getting the individual in group or individual therapy. Since young people between the ages of seven and 17 are the most common abusers of inhalants, attention is often directed at family instability or school problems.

## Other Addictions

Two of the most common types of addictions, other than those involving substance abuse, are gambling addictions and addictions to sex. Other behavioral addictions also are possible.

### Gambling

Gambling becomes addictive when it becomes a compulsive urge to take risks and bet on various games of chance. The problems that a gambling addiction causes in families can be just as destructive as those caused by drug, alcohol or sexual addiction. Compulsive gambling problems have increased dramatically in recent years with the increased opportunities to gamble across the country.

A dependence on gambling can be treated like other addictions. Counseling, support groups and Gamblers Anonymous can all be used to help break the cycle of gambling addiction.

### Sex

Just as the drug or alcohol addict uses a substance to cope with life, the

*Goals of Substance Abuse Treatment*

- Continued and complete abstinence from abused substances
- Increase in level of maturity
- Improvement in family function
- Cessation of antisocial or criminal behavior
- Honesty, trust and openness with self, family, friends and co-workers
- Involvement of family in the addict's healing

sexual addict uses sex. Obsessed with sex, he or she substitutes unhealthy sexual relationships for healthy relationships—replacing intimacy, caring and bonding with sexual obsessions. These sexual behaviors provide emotional and physical stimulation to the brain, just as addictive drugs provide emotional and physical effects.

People who are sexual addicts often are from dysfunctional families. In some situations, these individuals are given little privacy or respect during childhood. Many feel continually dissatisfied with the amount and kind of attention shown to them by their parents. They may have been sexually or physically abused as children by other family members. Unsure how they fit into a sexual role, they never understand how to function sexually as an adult in a healthy way.

Anything in a sexual addict's life can be "sexualized." The way they talk, what they talk about and how they act may relate to sex. As with the alcoholic, a sexual addict tends to behave in increasingly risky and self-destructive ways.

Like other people with addictions, those who are addicted to sex can benefit from participating in a program specifically designed for sexual addictions. In addition, one-on-one counseling can help.

## Emotions and Feelings

Emotions color your life and give it meaning. Feelings aren't right or wrong. It's how you deal with your feelings that can be healthy or unhealthy. It's usually best to express your feelings openly because suppressed feelings can cause problems. For example, suppressed anger can lead to bitterness and unforgiving hatred. But uncontrolled emotions can also be damaging. For example, anger can erupt into outbursts that produce painful, emotional scars. So it's important to learn how to express your emotions and feelings in a healthy way.

Unmet emotional needs, such as the need to be loved and valued, can throw off your emotional balance and lead to problems handling your emotions. Emotional upsets can also stem from temporary or permanent losses, major life changes, abuse, neglect or complicating psychiatric illnesses.

Emotional problems are part of life. When emotional problems occur, most are fairly easy to take care of in the early stages. If you have chronic, ongoing emotional problems that prevent you from having a satisfying life, you'll benefit from treatment.

### Anger

Of all the human emotions, anger may cause the most problems. Anger is a normal and potentially useful emotion. There are many ways to express angry feelings. But when anger gets out of control, it becomes unhealthy and can be dangerous. That's why it's important to learn how to express anger in the right way.

External causes of anger are usually easy to identify. Most people become angry when they're accused (unjustly or justly) of doing something wrong, when they (or people they care for) are threatened or when they're placed in danger by another person. Anger can be provoked by poor communication between co-workers or family members, by unclear expectations or by persons who insist on getting their way regardless of the rights or feelings of others.

Internal emotional factors producing anger may be less obvious than external causes. These factors include low self-esteem, unmet emotional needs, the desire for power in relationships, perfectionism, frustration, guilt, feeling rejected, emotional hurt, mistaken perceptions and wrong assumptions. When these internal causes of anger come into play, angry feelings can smolder.

Sometimes people are unaware that they're angry and are unable to express that anger. Their suppressed anger turns inward. It sometimes pushes them toward destructive, self-punishing behaviors involving drugs or sex. Sometimes the anger is directed at the wrong people. For example, deep down a person may be angry at his or her parents because of abuse during childhood. But the person doesn't recognize his or her anger at the parents. Instead of showing anger to them, he or she shows anger to someone else, such as a spouse. Misdirected anger may result in depression or chronic dissatisfaction in relationships.

### Dealing with Anger

While anger is a normal and even healthy emotion, it's often difficult to know when and how to express it.

When misused, anger can damage relationships. Anger can even damage the person who feels angry. Anger often is inappropriately expressed. Yelling and screaming, hitting and shoving, or harming others are the more easily recognized misuses of anger. Anger often is more subtly misused. *Passive-aggressive behavior*, which is showing strong feelings or opinions in an indirect way, can be just as devastating as the more physical expressions of anger.

Anger can best be expressed through honest communication with others and with yourself. People who struggle with anger can get counseling to help them understand why they feel such anger. Counseling also helps them learn to express their anger in an appropriate and effective manner.

As they learn to view their internal and external world more objectively, many people find they aren't as easily or as intensely offended and can respond more calmly to stressful situations. If you have trouble dealing with anger, you may wish to seek help from a counselor or support group.

When anger leads to severe outbursts, physical damage or legal

---

> ## Passive-Aggressive Expressions of Anger
>
> - Refusing to give help by acting unaware
> - Giving someone "the silent treatment" to punish them
> - Offering a halfhearted effort to a project that you've been working on together
> - Spreading lies or gossip (even if true) to discredit another person

---

## Preventing Blow-Ups

- Avoid or walk away from anger-causing situations when you aren't prepared to handle them.
- Avoid promising too much or having unrealistic expectations.
- Practice what you would say to another person in a situation in which you might become angry. Choose your words carefully. Try out different wordings until you find one that expresses your feelings honestly and directly without blaming someone else for your anger.
- Be honest.
- Try not to be overly competitive.
- Rid yourself of old anger. Write in a journal or talk to people to "clear the air."
- Work on current relationships. Make sure unspoken resentments are discussed. Clarify mutual needs.
- Learn to re-evaluate situations after angry outbursts and figure out how you might handle anger better in the future.
- When you feel that you're too angry to calmly talk with the other person, take a "time out" before trying to deal with the situation.

problems, seek help. Counseling can be successful in helping a person identify and deal with hidden emotional causes of anger. Group therapy provides opportunities to learn healthy communication and coping skills that are sometimes lacking.

### Grief

The ultimate loss is the death of a loved one, but other losses can cause grief too. Loss of a limb or other body part can also cause feelings of grief. For example, a woman who undergoes a hysterectomy may mourn the loss of her ability to have children. The amputation of a child's leg because of cancer is a loss that is grieved by the child as well as his or her family.

Serious illness can result in the loss of control, time, ability or the role you play. For those with demanding, energetic personalities, time is a precious commodity and illness may be perceived as something that wastes that precious time. The person may be frustrated and may grieve about time lost.

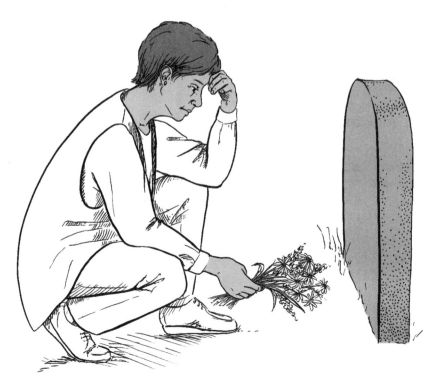

When someone is disabled by a severe heart attack, he or she may be forced to give up a cherished role such as providing for and taking care of his or her family. Even such things as a job change or a move from a familiar town can lead to feelings of grief.

### Dealing with Loss

Most people follow a typical grief process as they deal with a loss. Knowing that these reactions are common and knowing what to expect may help ease the journey through the difficult process of grieving.

Although no two people grieve in exactly the same way, the emotional changes of grieving can generally be recognized as three stages.

**The reaction phase.** This stage usually begins shortly after the illness is diagnosed or when the loss occurs. You may use one or more psychological defenses to reduce your initial pain and shock. The most common is denial or disbelief, refusing to see or understand the illness or death. Other emotional reactions include sadness, crying, despair, depression, hysteria, anger, bitterness, betrayal, loneliness and abandonment.

It's helpful and normal for family members to grieve together. When one person begins to remember the past, opening the bittersweet picture book of mental images of the lost loved one, other family members sympathize and feel the loss again. The depth of feelings and closeness among family members sometimes makes family grieving a longer and more difficult task. But sharing feelings of grief can be a positive influence on the family's emotional health.

When your pain begins to lessen and you begin to face reality, you're entering the second phase of the grief process, acceptance.

**Acceptance.** Acceptance of the illness or death of a loved one prepares you to move forward and grow. You have worked through the pain of your first emotional reactions and have come to the point of accepting what has happened. Then you can begin to deal with the reality of your loss. Those who are unable to reach this point rely instead on dysfunctional defense mechanisms, such as bitterness, depression, hysteria and anger, that result in destructive, unresolved grief.

When a family grieves, each member must pursue his or her own understanding of the loss. Each person must reach a point of acceptance. This stage is often reached at different times, but by working together toward acceptance the family is often strengthened. This is especially true if the family members can look toward the future with hope, understanding that changes must be made.

Acceptance isn't something that can be turned on like a light bulb. Often it takes weeks or even months to work through a loved one's illness, death or other loss. Loneliness, anger or bitterness may become so entrenched that you need professional help to move toward acceptance, and finally to the last phase of the grief process.

**Growth and maturation.** The third and final phase of the grieving process occurs when you realize that the difficult time you've been through has changed your priorities, your outlook and your idea of what's important in life.

This understanding can lead you to restore broken relationships, encourage forgiveness and correct old mistakes. Your ability to grow depends on your attitude, your acceptance of the situation and, in many cases, your spiritual principles or religious beliefs. Emotional and spiritual growth and maturity can be viewed as positive effects of the struggle through the illness and death of a loved one.

Grief is a normal reaction to any serious loss. It's a reaction that should be encouraged, not repressed. Remember, denial is only the beginning of the grief process. When helping a person through the grieving process, encourage him or her to show feelings and share thoughts. This allows him or her to acknowledge and work through the feelings that lead to acceptance and growth.

Why is growth so important? It helps give a purpose to the loss. While any loss can be difficult to handle, the hardest losses to accept are those due to senseless and needless circumstances, such as a child who is killed by a drunk driver, or a spouse who is killed in a random robbery. The suicide of a loved one often leads to feelings of guilt, as well as grief, and so can be especially difficult. No matter what the reason for the illness or loss, emotional and spiritual growth from the experience provide hope and a goal for recovery. Without hope, acceptance of the loss gives way to depression, anger, bitterness and blame.

Prolonged negative emotional reactions aren't healthy. If the grieving person seems unable to progress, professional help may be needed.

## Guilt

Guilt is a feeling of shame and remorse as a result of your thoughts or behavior. You feel guilty when you think you've done something wrong. Guilt has some benefits. These may include a greater understanding of right and wrong, and motivation to make corrective changes. But guilt can become irrational or excessive. If your upbringing was overly strict or your parents' expectations were unrealistically high, you may suffer guilt later in life because you feel you can't measure up.

Guilt may cause you to feel inferior and inadequate. It may make you feel pessimistic, insecure, depressed or angry. It can lower your self-esteem and create a feeling of emptiness. Excessive guilt may cause anxiety. It may keep you from forgiving yourself for past deeds and give you an urge to punish yourself. It can also generate a fear of intimacy and an inability to trust, and leave you unable to form solid relationships. Physical reactions to guilt range from abdominal pain and ulcers to eating disorders and alcoholism, among other problems.

Guilt is irrational when your thoughts or actions *weren't* wrong, even though you believe they were. For example, you may have inappropriate guilt because of unrealistic expectations of yourself you developed early in your childhood. Now, as an adult, you may blame and criticize yourself and you may feel inferior when you fail to meet these impossibly high and rigid expectations.

Guilt can also be caused by an overactive conscience that developed in an environment where love, acceptance and support were lacking. Parents may prevent excessive guilt when they help their children develop healthy consciences. Children who learn clear standards of right and wrong, who are disciplined with love and who learn forgiveness are more likely to develop a healthy conscience and positive self-esteem.

Counseling with a mental health professional will provide some understanding of these problems by helping you confront your irrational or inaccurate beliefs. Alleviating irrational guilt isn't easy because it requires a change in the way you see yourself. You must learn to believe you have worth and that your gifts and talents are useful. To rebuild your self-esteem and relieve your irrational feelings of guilt, give yourself permission to meet your needs, help others, forgive constantly critical family members and seek to build healthy relationships.

### Loneliness

Most people feel lonely at some time during their lives. Loneliness, one of the most common emotional problems, affects people of all ages.

Temporary loneliness may result from an event in your life, such as moving away from home or becoming disabled or widowed. In contrast, chronic loneliness results from low self-esteem, shyness, an inability to socialize, a self-defeating attitude, lack of control in social situations, hostility or social fears.

If a temporary situation is to blame, try to get out and meet new people. Join a group, club or church, take a class or start a new hobby that involves others.

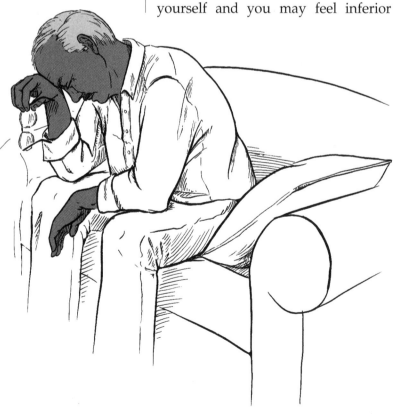

People who are consistently lonely lack close and meaningful relationships with others. They tend to experience feelings of intense longing, restlessness, anxiety and emptiness, even when they're surrounded by other people. Although they want to feel close to someone, they're unable to build a close relationship or feel satisfied with the relationship.

If you can't escape your feelings of loneliness, get help. A counselor can help you identify your reasons for loneliness. Work with your counselor individually or in a group setting to learn how to socialize, communicate and be realistic about your relationships. You can gradually become capable of involving yourself in meaningful relationships and a social support network.

### Self-Esteem

Many people struggle with low self-esteem. They have a poor mental image of themselves. Sadly, this image is caused, in part, by other people's real or imagined negative reactions to them. Good self-esteem develops when people feel loved, feel accepted by others and feel that they are a worthy, valuable person. The box at right lists the basic needs that are the foundation for a healthy self-esteem. When these needs are met, you have the freedom to be yourself. See page 361 for information on how to help children develop strong self-esteem.

If you have low self-esteem, you can take steps to improve it. Start by doing things that make you feel good about yourself. This may mean taking a class, starting an exercise program, reading a good book, painting a picture or making a new friend. Start out with something small and work your way to bigger and more difficult achievements. If you have trouble, think about

talking to a counselor for guidance on how to get started.

### Stress

Stress can come from anxiety, being upset about things that have happened to you or about excessive tasks or responsibilities that are demanded of you. Because stress can damage your physical health and keep you from accomplishing your work, it's important to be able to deal with feelings of anxiety and resentment that lead to stress.

Besides self-generated stress there are also physical and time-related aspects of stress, such as working long hours, working different shifts, being awakened often from sleep and working to the point of physical exhaustion on a regular basis. The mother who's awakened every two hours to feed her newborn child, the employee who has to work double shifts, the doctor who's

> ### Foundation for Healthy Self-Esteem
>
> - To feel loved unconditionally and to have a sense of belonging
> - To feel accepted, to have a sense of worthiness
> - To feel adequate, to have a sense of competence

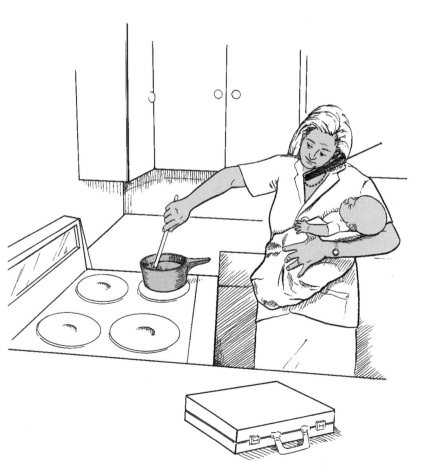

## Can your work kill you?

Highly stressed work environments may lead to high blood pressure and thickening of the wall of the heart. These two factors make you more susceptible to heart disease and heart attack. Find ways to reduce stress, work where you have more control over your job and your output, exercise, lose weight if you need to and maintain a positive outlook to help reduce the stress on your heart.

called out of bed three nights in a row, the carpenter who works 16-hour days seven days a week for two months to finish a project and the student who has difficult classes and is holding down a job—all of these people are getting close to (or exceeding) their physical limits.

Stress can also occur simply from having a busy schedule, such as the parent who works a 40-hour week, manages the home and takes a few night classes at college. When this kind of unrelenting schedule continues over months or years, the person is likely to suffer the damage of physical stress.

Your body responds to stress by secreting the stress hormones *adrenaline* and *corticosteroids*. These hormones help the body respond to situations of extreme need. But when they're secreted in high doses over long periods of time, they wear down your body—and your emotions. People under stress also often have emotional and personality changes, such as increased anxiety, irritability and even depression.

There are many times when you can't eliminate stress. But if possible, at least try to change the situation to reduce the amount of stress. It may mean giving up an activity or responsibility or finding someone to share work.

Many times emotional stress can be modified, sometimes just with a change of attitude. Sometimes emotional stress can be helpful in motivating someone to work to change a situation that shouldn't be tolerated, such as in the case of domestic violence or unreasonable demands from a boss. Situations over which you have no control, such as the death of a spouse, child or other loved one, being fired from a job or enduring serious financial problems may be the most difficult stress you face. But stress from situations such as these can be eased when you work through your emotional reactions, accept what has occurred and go on with your life. Controlling your reactions to stress and learning to understand your emotions takes practice, but it can be done. In these situations, try accepting your situation and changing your attitude to reduce stress and prevent it from hurting your health.

### Dealing with Stress

Certain techniques can help you deal with stress. Your library or bookstore has books, audiotapes and videotapes on stress-reduction and relaxation techniques. Ask your doctor to recommend one.

You may also use other methods to relax. Many people "escape" with a good book or an entertaining movie, soak in a hot tub or listen to soothing music. Those with spiritual roots often find that prayer or meditation is an excellent way to reduce stress. Exercise can be both a way to treat stress and a way to prevent stress. Exercise helps relax tense muscles and helps the body deal with stress hormones.

## Relaxation Training

- **Deep breathing.** Slow, paced breathing will help you relax. Slowly count to seven as you breathe in, hold your breath for a few seconds and then slowly exhale.
- **Progressive muscle relaxation.** You'll need 15 to 30 minutes to practice this technique. Start with one part of your body, like your feet. Slowly tighten the muscles in your feet by pointing your toes. Then breathe out slowly as you relax the muscles. Move along your entire body to each group of muscles from your feet to your face and neck.
- **Guided imagery.** This technique uses imagination to visit a calm, peaceful place, such as a secluded beach or a place in the woods. Close your eyes and create a scene in your mind. Don't just concentrate on what you see. Think of the smells and sounds. If you're walking along the beach, feel the hot sand beneath your feet. Listen to the waves. Feel the warm breeze on your face. Smell the salt air.

Dangerous ways to cope with chronic stress include drug and alcohol use, gambling or excessive use of prescription medicine. Trying to deal with stress in these ways only adds new problems. Alcohol is the most common stress-reducing drug in our society, closely followed by nicotine and addictive prescription medicines. They can cause serious health problems instead of curing the stress.

If stress is overwhelming, talk to your doctor. He or she can give you guidance or refer you to a mental health professional.

## Family Violence

Family violence occurs in every social, racial, cultural and economic group. Thousands of Americans suffer physical, emotional or sexual abuse from their family members. Ironically, people who have been abused and hurt are most likely to strike out at others. Sometimes these people don't intend to inflict pain, but they don't know how to deal with their frustrations and anger.

Why do family members hurt each other? Family problems that can contribute to an abusive home life include poor communication, marital stress, a dominating and controlling parenting style, and excessively rigid or bizarre beliefs. Role confusion or reversal may also set the stage for abuse. For example, a daughter who must act as the mother for her mother and other siblings may be sexually abused by her father. Abuse may result from stress in single-parent families with little social support or from personality conflicts when a parent remarries.

### Cycle of Abuse

If your family gave you love, support, discipline and a secure environment when you were a child, you're usually able to trust others, be affectionate, and develop strong values and high self-esteem. Your parenting skills tend to be learned from adults you knew when you were a child. People who grew up in abusive families are likely to have parenting and coping methods similar to those of their parents.

Abused children remember the abuse and feel responsible for it and guilty about it. They typically display anger, depression, mistrust and poor communication. Insecurity constantly haunts them. When someone displeases or disappoints them, they often respond by fighting back. On the other hand, they might withdraw and become extremely passive and easy targets for abuse. These tendencies damage their ability to form healthy relationships. Physically and sexually abused children tend to become abusive parents.

Some abuse victims are able to put the abusive behavior aside after they've freed themselves of the situation. They forgive the abusive people, repair their own damaged emotions and self-esteem and become nonabusive spouses and parents.

### Psychological Effects of Family Violence

Family violence causes more than physical injuries. It contributes to various psychological problems, such as depression, guilt, shame, alcohol and drug dependency. Family violence can also cause suicidal feelings, anxiety, poor self-esteem, self-contempt, sexual dysfunction, sexual risk-taking and trouble trusting others and developing intimate relationships.

Spousal abuse affects the children who witness the abuse as well as the victim. The children tend to feel helpless, mistrust intimate relationships, behave aggressively or become extremely passive, and suffer delayed intellectual

---

### Examples of Child Abuse and Neglect

- Punching, beating, kicking, biting, burning or other ways of physically harming the child
- Failing to provide for the child's basic physical, educational or emotional needs (neglect)
- Delaying or refusing to seek needed health care for the child
- Abandoning the child or providing inadequate supervision
- Failing to enroll the child in school, permitting chronic truancy or not attending to a special educational need
- Abusing the spouse in front of the child
- Allowing alcohol or drug abuse by the child
- Failing to provide needed psychological care
- Engaging in any sexual acts with the child
- Using extreme forms of punishment, such as torture or confinement in a closet
- Belittling the child
- Refusing to allow treatment for a diagnosed emotional problem

---

growth. They also may suffer from emotional symptoms such as stomachaches, headaches, school avoidance, bedwetting, trouble sleeping, running away and nightmares.

Abused and neglected children are likely to have problems with school, friendships, discipline and, later, with alcohol and drugs.

Elderly abuse victims also suffer psychological effects such as depression, loneliness and feelings of helplessness.

If you're in an abusive relationship, there are shelters and telephone hotlines to offer you support. Ask your doctor or check the telephone book for the names and phone numbers of such agencies.

### Preventing Family Violence

If you know the characteristics and risk factors for family abuse and neglect, you're more likely to seek help in the early stages. You can help prevent abuse by strengthening individual and family stability and taking steps to ease the stress and demands of childrearing, marital pressures and eldercare.

Violence prevention and treatment programs educate people about family violence. They teach potential or actual abusers and victims the facts about family abuse, how to protect yourself, what to do in case of an attack and where to get further information and help. These programs can help people who are likely to abuse others learn how to handle problems better. Most people who abuse others lack communication skills and haven't learned to cope with stress, feelings and conflicts. Call your doctor or local social service agency for information on violence prevention programs in your area.

## Child Abuse and Neglect

Child abuse is defined as physical or mental trauma, sexual molestation, or mistreatment or neglect of a child under age 18 that threatens or harms the child's health and welfare.

Each family is different, so child abuse and neglect can't be blamed on one underlying cause in all situations. However, abusive parents often have one or more of the characteristics of immaturity, isolation from family or friends, a history of childhood abuse or neglect, alcohol or drug abuse or dependence, and a lack of parenting and relationship skills. A child is more likely to be abused or neglected if he or she is demanding and overactive, chronically ill or handicapped or if he or she reminds the parent of someone the parent dislikes. Unfortunately, this can reinforce the children's mistaken belief that they're responsible for the abuse.

### Sexual Abuse

Child sexual abuse includes any inappropriate, suggested or actual sexual exposure or touching between an adult and a child. The sexual activity may consist of fondling a child's genitals or

## Physical Signs of Abuse in Children

- Burns that have the shape of a recognizable object, such as a cigarette lighter
- Signs of multiple bruises, cuts, burns, fractures and scars
- Head injuries
- "Shaken-infant syndrome," a neck injury similar to whiplash that can occur when an infant or child is shaken violently. Symptoms may include an enlarged head, bulging soft spot on the baby's skull, tiredness, vomiting, seizures and coma
- Fear of adults or refusal to speak in front of parents or other adults
- Injuries on the back of the body between the back and the knees
- Defensive wounds, such as bruises, scars and wounds on the back of the arms and hands

## Behavioral Signs of Abuse in Children

- Withdrawn, depressed and apathetic behavior
- A reputation for problem behavior, characterized by frequent "acting out"
- Overly rigid conformity to the instructions of teachers, doctors and other adults
- Little or no verbal or physical contact with others
- Repetitive, rhythmic movements or inordinate attention to details

breasts, getting the child to fondle the abuser's sex organs, or persuading or forcing the child to participate in sexual intercourse. It also includes any use of a child for practices such as pornography, prostitution or other sexual experiences.

In most cases of child sexual abuse, the sexual abuser is either a family member or someone known to the child. More than half of all child sexual abuse takes place in the child's home. Incest involves sexual interactions between a child and an adult family member. It can also be between two siblings and not involve force.

Incest occurs in families of all socioeconomic, ethnic, racial, religious and educational backgrounds. Sexual abuse usually involves some sort of manipulation, bribe or threat—but not violence.

In a large percentage of cases, the sexual abuse of children is committed by an adolescent younger than 18. In some cases, the young person is acting out of curiosity to see and touch someone of the opposite sex. These adolescents may abuse children in the home who are considerably younger than they are. The curiosity may lead to attempted sexual intercourse or other forms of sexual abuse.

How does sexual abuse affect those involved? The abused child feels guilty, used, violated, dirty and worthless. He or she is often kept silent with threats of physical violence to themselves or someone they care about. Sexual abuse can cause severe lasting emotional damage.

Adults who were sexually abused as children experience feelings and problems that include depression, anxiety and low self-esteem. They may express strong anger at inappropriate times toward other people. Many continue to experience intense guilt, along with shame and secretiveness.

Other behavioral problems may occur after years of repressing the painful memories of sexual abuse. Many abused persons turn to drugs and alcohol. Others develop eating disorders such as anorexia and bulimia. They also may have trouble sleeping, be irritable, and think about suicide or even attempt it. Sexual problems may occur, ranging from having no interest in sex and refusing to be intimate with anyone, to becoming promiscuous and using sex as the main way to have a relationship with another person or to get other needs met, such as shelter and money.

The emotional damage a child experiences from sexual abuse is strongly related to the parent or guardian's response to the child when he or she reports the abuse. Overreacting or not being supportive can compound the emotional damage, expose the child to additional abuse and destroy communication between parent and child. In contrast, parents who respond with support and sensitivity can lessen emotional damage and start the child on the road to healing.

Prevention of child sexual abuse begins with rearing a child to be self-assured, assertive, appropriately wary of strangers and clearly informed about proper and improper interactions with people. A child whose emotional needs are well met will be less likely to fall prey to the attention, affection or bribes of an abuser. A child molester is less likely to abuse a child who says no, fights back or refuses to keep the secret despite threats of harm or loss of affection. That's why children who are taught to blindly "respect their elders" or "obey those in authority" are more vulnerable to sexual abuse. It's important for children to learn that it's okay to resist an adult's or adolescent's improper suggestions and to scream or run if the person doesn't stop.

You can teach your children to avoid sexual abuse. Educate your children about inappropriate touching as early as they can understand the concept. Listen attentively to what they say. Explain that their bodies belong to them. They have the right to disobey adults and say no when adolescents or adults touch them, kiss them or display affection inappropriately.

People who commit sexual abuse often warn children not to talk about what has happened. Tell your children that they can always come to you and you will always listen. Praise your children for telling you about frightening or painful experiences. Show support and love for them even if what they're

## Possible Symptoms of Sexual Abuse in Children

- Unusual trouble forming peer relationships
- Withdrawn, depressed, apathetic or less verbal behavior
- Abrupt and radical personality changes
- Self-mutilation
- Preoccupation with death, guilt, heaven or hell
- Retreat to a fantasy world, loss of memory, imaginary playmates or the child's use of more than one name for himself or herself
- Unexplained acquisition of toys, money or clothes
- Fear, clinging to parent, constant need for reassurance
- Unwillingness to participate in physical or recreational activities
- Refusal to undress for physical education class at school
- Refusal to be left with the caretaker or potential offender
- Running away
- Poor personal hygiene, deliberate attempts to look unattractive
- Inability to concentrate in school, hyperactivity, sudden drop in school performance

telling you is upsetting. Explain to them that, although most adults are kind to children, sometimes adults do something wrong. Finally, teach your children that they're not to blame when an adult behaves inappropriately.

It's never too late to seek help. Even if you're an adult who was abused as a child, you may want to consider counseling. A program combining group and individual therapy is the preferred treatment for sexually abused persons. Group therapy allows participants to share their experiences and recover from the trauma. Individual counseling can deal more specifically with issues of shame and guilt. If not faced, these issues can lead to marital problems, depression and even suicide. Counseling can help the abused person improve his or her self-esteem and restore trust in others.

## Elder Abuse and Neglect

Elderly persons, both men and women, are sometimes mistreated by their spouses, adult children or other relatives or caretakers. The typical victims of this type of abuse are physically and financially unable to leave the situation. They often fear more severe mistreatment if they tell someone about the abuse.

Who is most likely to abuse elderly parents? Typically, abusers are socially isolated, have a learned pattern of family violence, and abuse drugs or alcohol. Elder abuse sometimes occurs when the caretaker becomes overly stressed because he or she is unable to meet the demands of caring for an elderly parent. Other factors, such as pregnancy, divorce, death of a family member and unemployment, can also cause a buildup of frustration that may be taken out on an elderly family member.

The first step is to reduce the stress on caretaker families. Various programs

### Responding to Reported Abuse

- Immediately take your child to a private place. Ask your child to explain what happened in his or her own words. Listen carefully and remember to be calm and matter-of-fact.
- Believe your child.
- Assure your child that what happened isn't the child's fault and that you're glad he or she told you.
- Tell your child you're sorry he or she was hurt and scared. Assure your child that you will protect him or her from further abuse.
- Call an agency trained to respond to sexual abuse.
- Get medical help immediately and tell your doctor of your suspicions if you believe that sexual penetration or physical injury has occurred.
- Take whatever steps are necessary to protect your child from further abuse. In the case of incest, see that the abuser, not the child, leaves the home if at all possible.

and services for the elderly are available, such as Meals-on-Wheels, respite care or adult day care.

In cases of extreme abuse, protective placement in domestic violence shelters may provide short-term relief. Legal actions, such as restraining orders or criminal charges against the abuser, also can be taken, although elderly victims are usually reluctant to press charges. They fear the abuser will seek revenge. They may also fear embarrassment or loss of their home.

A nursing home is often used as a last resort for an elderly person who

### Examples of Elder Abuse and Neglect

- Passive neglect, in which family members become so busy they unintentionally neglect the elderly relative, who, as a result, doesn't receive proper hygiene, medicine, supervision, nutrition and other personal care
- Active neglect, in which services, materials and personal care are intentionally withheld
- Physical abuse, such as being beaten or burned
- Sexual assault
- Emotional abuse, including threats, manipulation and isolation
- Financial exploitation, such as the misuse or theft of the elderly person's money, possessions or property, or preventing the elderly person from having access to his or her belongings

## How to Take Action Against Spouse Abuse

- Call an emergency shelter for abused spouses and children.
- Ask law enforcement agencies for help.
- Seek court action (such as a restraining order).
- Look into the possibility of the abuser going to a psychiatric hospital for treatment or being required to enter outpatient therapy if emotional problems are to blame.
- If you refuse to leave your abusive spouse, consider removing the children from the home so they don't witness the abuse and so they can't be harmed.
- Ask family members, community agencies or your church to provide a safe place to stay.

needs care and who has been abused. That's because most elderly persons fear moving into a nursing home and because such a move tends to cause guilt among the caretakers. Removing the elderly person who has been abused from the family home may be seen as more of a punishment than as a solution. But placement in a nursing home is a legitimate solution that may protect the abused person from further harm. See page 437 for more information on care of the elderly.

## Spouse Abuse

Most victims of domestic violence are women. This type of violence occurs in all parts of society. Physical or sexual abuse is usually inflicted by the husband or boyfriend to gain control and power over the wife or girlfriend. Sometimes, the woman abuses the man, but this is less common. Physical abuse of a spouse is the most common type of domestic violence. Physical abuse often occurs when the abuser is intoxicated on alcohol or illegal drugs.

It may be hard to understand why women choose to stay with abusive men for long periods of time. Many factors can influence a woman to stay in an abusive relationship. Many battered women blame themselves for the situation and believe the abuse is somehow deserved. Most keep hoping the abuse will stop. Many are financially dependent on the man who abuses them. Some women are afraid of more serious violence to themselves or their children if they try to leave. Sometimes these women feel they have no place to go.

Physical violence may include sexual violence. Rape appears to be a means of humiliating, hurting and dominating the woman. Sexual abuse tends to get worse over time. It's

frequently accompanied by life-endangering threats or acts.

Spouse abuse can also include emotional trauma—not mere verbal arguments, but the systematic downgrading of a person's self-esteem. The abuser uses economic deprivation, intimidation, extreme controlling behavior, isolation and threats about the children to maintain control and power over the victim. Left unchecked, emotional abuse may produce long-term damage equal to or greater than that of physical or sexual abuse.

Many women, immobilized by fear, feel helpless to take action to stop the abuse—until they or their children are in serious danger. If you feel your life is in danger if you seek help, it's probably in more danger if you don't get help. If you or someone you know is being beaten or sexually abused by a spouse, don't wait until it's too late.

## Psychiatric Problems

Almost anyone can develop a mental illness under certain circumstances. Most mental illnesses probably have physical causes due to chemical imbalances in the brain. In many cases, these chemical imbalances are more to blame than emotional troubles. In some people, mental illness may be brought on by emotional, family and stress-related problems. The more emotional problems you've endured, such as low self-esteem, family dysfunction or childhood abuse or neglect, the more likely you are to also suffer from a psychiatric problem. Usually there's a combination of physical and emotional issues when dealing with mental health problems.

Recognizing a psychiatric problem and getting help are the most important steps in treatment. Most people are surprised when a family member begins to exhibit strange behaviors, moods or thoughts that can signal a mental illness. People who are struggling with stress, confusion, rebellion, depression or other symptoms often don't believe their problems are significant. They often refuse or delay seeking professional help because of the stigma attached to mental illness and treatment. You can help by encouraging them to be checked by your doctor to see if the change is related to a medical problem.

Treatment for a psychiatric problem includes medicines, outpatient counseling or hospitalization. Your doctor may prescribe medicine and may refer you to a psychologist, licensed professional counselor, clinical social worker or psychiatrist for further treatment.

**Medicines.** Many people think all medicines used to treat psychiatric problems sedate the person or are addictive, but that's not so. Medicines can be used that don't have tranquilizing effects. They help control the symptoms so that people with psychiatric problems can be productive. Taking medicine doesn't mean that you're crazy or weak. If you need medicine, taking it is a way of helping yourself take control of your life to become more productive. Your doctor or a psychiatrist can help assess whether medicine might help you.

**Outpatient treatment.** Different types of counseling may help you. Counseling can be done with a counselor, psychologist or someone else who's trained in counseling. It may be done on an individual basis or with group therapy. Support groups may also be helpful.

**Hospital treatment.** When emotional disorders and psychiatric problems become overwhelming, and when outpatient care hasn't been effective, hospitalization should be considered. If the answer to any of the following questions is yes, hospitalization may be indicated:

- Has outpatient treatment failed to alleviate severe symptoms or problems?
- Is there demonstrated or likely danger to the person or to others?
- Is the person's mood extremely low or high or fluctuating severely?
- Are the person's thoughts or judgment severely impaired?
- Is the person's behavior unmanageable in a way that's dangerous?
- Is the person unable to carry out normal activities of daily living, such as eating or seeking shelter?
- Is there a need for a protective environment 24 hours a day?
- Is there a severe failure to function in social, family or occupational roles?

In the hospital, intensive therapy can be provided in a short period of time. Difficult issues can be dealt with without distractions. A structured, protective environment is provided around the clock. The person is removed from bad influences and upsetting surroundings. A good inpatient program also will include recreational activities and occupational therapy.

In inpatient settings, many people with psychiatric problems make great progress toward recovery. Treatment is a process of growth and healing that must continue long after leaving the hospital. After-care plans, developed by the treatment team, will provide a solid base for ongoing growth.

The family may be a key part of a person's psychiatric problems. It may sometimes even be a key cause. For example, an abusive parent-child relationship can result in a personality disorder and substance abuse. Major depression may be triggered by the death of a spouse or a child.

Family therapy is a good idea. Even

if the family isn't part of the cause, members are affected by the problem and need help coping. If the family has contributed to the problem, their role needs to be identified, understood and changed. Family support and involvement is often key in the treatment of the affected family members.

## Anxiety Disorders

Anxiety is an apprehension, uneasiness, worry or dread. Physical symptoms of anxiety may include dry mouth, shortness of breath, dizziness, faintness, trembling or shaking, sweating, numbness or tingling sensations, flushes and chills. Some people with anxiety have episodes of rapid heartbeat, or they breathe too hard and too deeply *(hyperventilate)*.

### Coping with Anxiety

- Acknowledge fears, insecurities, conflicts and anxieties when they arise.
- Discuss these feelings with a caring friend, family member, health care professional, counselor or minister.
- Build your self-esteem by doing things that make you feel good about yourself. Approach challenging situations one step at a time.
- When you're separated from a friend or loved one, acknowledge that separation hurts and try to maintain contact with him or her, if possible, while also building new relationships.
- Use prayer and spiritual reflection if this approach is in keeping with your beliefs.
- Learn principles and techniques of relaxation (p. 572).
- Think about your priorities from time to time. Consider your life goals and how you're managing your time.

Besides the short-term symptoms of an anxiety episode, other physical reactions to anxiety may develop over time. Ulcers, headaches, skin rashes, backaches, insomnia, increased fatigue, and loss of appetite or excessive appetite may be linked to anxiety. Chronic anxiety may reduce a person's productivity, hinder relationships, interfere with concentration and memory, and suppress creativity. Some people with anxiety grind their teeth at night, producing pain and arthritis in the jaw joint.

Physical problems, such as high thyroid hormone levels (hyperthyroidism, p. 215), can sometimes mimic panic or anxiety disorders. If you're having any symptoms of anxiety, see your doctor. A medical exam and some tests can help your doctor rule out medical causes for your symptoms.

When anxiety becomes unbearable, you may unconsciously adopt other strategies, or *defense mechanisms*, to protect yourself from feeling anxious. Some people turn to abuse of alcohol or illegal drugs to try to dull the pain of anxiety.

Handling an anxiety-related problem early is always more effective and less costly than letting anxiety go unchecked and untreated. You may be able to learn skills for coping with life's ups and downs. Keep setbacks in perspective. Reach out to others. Take care of yourself. Exercise, eat right and try to keep your stress level down.

You can get help on how to cope with anxiety from many resources. It might be helpful to read about anxiety and how to control it. Your doctor can help you. Also, support groups through your mental health center or church may be good resources to help you control your feelings of anxiety.

Life is sprinkled with situations that make your heart race, your body break out in a sweat and your chest feel tight. Anxiety is a normal response to such situations. Usually, when the situation resolves, so does your anxiety. But if anxiety continues and you're unable to control it or if it comes at unexplainable times and disrupts your normal functioning, you may have an *anxiety disorder*. The major types of anxiety disorders include generalized anxiety disorder, obsessive-compulsive disorder, panic disorders, phobias and post-traumatic stress disorder.

**Generalized anxiety disorder.** Excessive or unrealistic worry is the major symptom of generalized anxiety disorder. People with generalized anxiety disorder may worry about their families, their work or their finances, for example, when there's no reason to worry. There's an underlying constant feeling of tension and stress, although life may be going pretty well. Physical symptoms may also be present. These may include trembling, muscle tension, sweating, dizziness, hot flashes or chills, trouble swallowing, frequent urination, dry mouth and other symptoms common to anxiety. It's not unusual for this type of problem to be accompanied by other anxiety disorders.

Treatment may include medicines such as one of the benzodiazepines (p. 621) or antidepressants (p. 619). Therapy to identify, change and gain control of anxious thoughts is helpful. Relaxation techniques (p. 572) and individual or group counseling may be useful as well.

**Obsessive-compulsive disorder.** People with an obsessive-compulsive disorder suffer from recurrent obsessions or compulsions, or both. An *obsession* is an intense focus on an idea or thought, such as a fear of germs, concern about the cleanliness of clothes, praying excessively, excessive tiredness or counting. *Compulsions* are repetitive acts or rituals, such as washing the hands 10 times without stopping or checking that the door to the house is locked a dozen times.

Certain antidepressant medicines can be extremely helpful. Behavioral therapy can deal with the psychological traumas or needs that started the compulsive behaviors or obsessive thoughts.

**Panic disorder.** When you're extremely scared, your body's "fight-or-flight" reaction delivers an extra surge of the hormone adrenaline to help you combat or escape from danger. Dizziness, shortness of breath, nausea, sweating, fast heartbeat and numbness of the fingers and around the mouth are other physical symptoms related to fear. People who repeatedly have these unexpected feelings of panic for no apparent reason have a panic disorder.

These attacks often get worse. Each attack builds on the fear of the object or situation as well as the fear of the attack itself. People may withdraw so they're no longer confronted with the fearful object or situation and the chance of an attack.

Panic disorder often runs in families. This family trend may result from learning experiences, genetics or a combination of both. Some people suffer such severe and frequent attacks of panic that they're eventually unable to leave their home.

Treatment consists of medicine to reduce and prevent the panic episodes, along with behavioral therapy to desensitize the person to the frightening circumstances.

**Phobias.** A *phobia* is an irrational and unjustified fear that prevents people from functioning normally with respect to the feared object or situation. Recurrent panic symptoms may cause a person to develop phobias. The phobias can lead to depression and isolation. Although the phobias may seem silly to others (and often don't even seem logical to the person who has the fear), they can be terrifying to a person suffering from them.

*Agoraphobia,* a fear of being in public places, is the most common phobic disorder. *Claustrophobia* is the fear of being in an enclosed place, such as a closet or elevator. *Social phobia* is a fear of public situations, such as going to a party or being with a group of people. Severe phobias may produce an anxiety or panic episode that keeps people from entering a particular place or participating in an event.

Treatment for phobias includes psychotherapy to uncover the origin of the phobia, if possible. Then the individual is *desensitized* to the object or situation through controlled, repeated exposure, until it no longer causes unmanageable anxiety. Relaxation training is almost always a part of therapy.

**Post-traumatic stress disorder.** Survivors of extremely traumatic events, such as rape, child abuse, attempted murder, a natural disaster or the ravages of war, may relive these experiences later in their thoughts. Often these memories come back as recurring dreams, hallucinations or compulsive thoughts about the trauma.

Symptoms may start right after the event, or they may occur later, when a situation or another psychological problem triggers memories of the traumatic event. People who suffer from post-traumatic stress disorder often try to cope with the intrusive thoughts or the feelings of guilt for being a survivor by detaching themselves emotionally, losing interest in life and becoming depressed.

Post-traumatic stress disorder may be treated with medicines, usually anti-anxiety medicines or antidepressants. Learning new responses to things that trigger the stress reaction, or *behavior modification therapy,* can help the person deal with feelings and relieve guilt or anger. Individual and group therapy can help overcome the guilt, depression and anxiety often associated with this disorder. Relaxation techniques also are helpful.

## Eating Disorders

Do you eat when you're not really hungry because food makes you feel better? Do you deny yourself food because you think you're too fat? Do you go on eating binges and then throw up? Eating (or avoiding eating) to satisfy psychological needs more than physical needs is a sign of an eating disorder.

Eating disorders, such as anorexia, bulimia and overeating, can cause life-threatening medical problems. An eating disorder isn't merely a problem with food or weight. It's an attempt to use food intake and weight control to

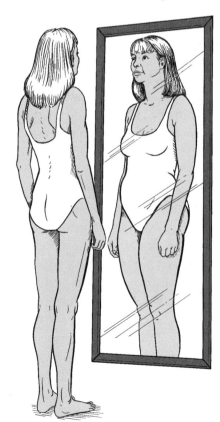

cope with emotional conflicts. This is why treating an eating disorder is never simply a matter of encouraging self-control over eating. Healthier eating habits or stronger willpower won't make the problem disappear.

### Anorexia and Bulimia

Once considered rare, anorexia nervosa and bulimia are now recognized as common medical problems. They usually develop in adolescent girls and college-aged women. About 90% of cases occur in females. Studies have shown that 20% to 25% of college-aged women have been or are actively anorexic or bulimic to at least a mild extent. A few adolescent boys and young men have similar problems, especially those in weight-dependent sports like wrestling.

**Anorexia nervosa.** *Anorexia* literally means "without appetite." People with *anorexia nervosa* are obsessed with thinness. They starve themselves to achieve that goal. They also may be extremely conscious of calorie and fat content in food, exercise excessively, or take diet pills, laxatives and diuretics to lose weight. Even when confronted

with their skeletal-looking image in a mirror, people with anorexia nervosa see themselves as being overweight. Anorexia nervosa may be diagnosed when significant body weight has been lost and no medical condition is the cause, and when the person's attitudes and behaviors about food are excessively focused.

Anorexia nervosa has serious medical consequences, including delayed physical growth and sexual maturation, heart problems, gastrointestinal disorders, menstrual disorders, chemical imbalances, depression, and abnormal skin and hair conditions. Treatment usually involves medical intervention to treat the physical problems (possibly in a hospital), medicine or therapy for depression, individual and family psychotherapy and nutritional counseling. Even with years of treatment, up to 20% of people with anorexia nervosa continue to be chronically underweight well into adulthood. Menstrual irregularity and depression also remain problems for many adults with a history of anorexia nervosa.

When family members or other people try to help, the person with

---

### *Physical Results of Anorexia Nervosa*

- Heart problems due to unbalanced blood salts
- Liver and kidney damage
- Nervous system damage from long-term starvation

---

### *Comparing the Characteristics of Anorexia Nervosa and Bulimia*

*Anorexia nervosa*
- Turns away from food to cope
- Maintains rigid self-control
- Perceives body as fat
- Denies illness
- Significant weight loss/refusal to maintain ideal weight
- Vomiting less common
- Eating rituals in public
- Loss of menstrual period

*Bulimia*
- Turns to food to cope
- Impulsive, vulnerable to alcohol and drug abuse and stealing
- Realistic view of body
- Recognizes illness
- Within 10 to 15 pounds of recommended minimal weight (or slightly overweight)
- Vomiting and other purging behavior common; laxative abuse
- Appears to eat in normal manner when in public or when not bingeing
- Often irregular periods

anorexia nervosa usually denies having a problem. The person may become more secretive about what he or she is eating and may wear clothes that hide the weight loss. Unfortunately, it's usually a very long time (estimated at an average of four to six years) between the onset of the problem behavior and the time a person with anorexia nervosa finally gets help.

**Bulimia.** *Bulimia* is a binge-and-purge syndrome. People with bulimia binge on large amounts of food in a short time. They then get rid of it by purging, usually by inducing vomiting or using laxatives. In addition to inducing vomiting or overusing laxatives, the bulimic may use diuretics, enemas, fasting, exercise and appetite suppressants to control her weight. Unlike with anorexia, the person with bulimia doesn't usually become underweight or control her weight through starvation, although she may fast occasionally. Most people with bulimia are normal weight, or even slightly overweight. Because they stay at a normal weight, they may be able to hide the disorder for several years. People who have bulimia usually recognize they have a problem

but feel a great deal of shame and hide their behavior.

Signs of bulimia include calluses on the fingers (from rubbing the fingers on the roof of the mouth to induce vomiting), a rounding of the face (enlargement of glands caused by vomiting), abdominal pain, damaged tooth enamel from stomach acid, fatigue and extreme mood swings. The most serious medical problems resulting from bulimia include severe chemical imbalances, kidney problems, heart problems and gastrointestinal disorders. Depression is extremely common in people with bulimia.

A number of factors may lead to eating disorders. Eating disorders may partly stem from a chemical imbalance in the brain. Our culture also gets some of the blame. An unrealistically thin body is glamorized. Girls learn, often from an early age, that they can please others by being attractive. A young woman who thinks she isn't attractive sees herself as having a decreased value and as being unlovable.

A few common threads tend to occur in families where eating disorders occur. The family's structure, rules and expectations tend to be inflexible. The more strict and structured the

---

### Warning Signals of Anorexia Nervosa and Bulimia

*Anorexia nervosa*
- Continual talk of food
- Excessive calorie counting and constant dieting
- Avoidance of social functions
- Denial of problem
- Hoarding of food
- High need to achieve
- Excessive activity
- Tantrums
- Unusual weight loss

*Bulimia*
- Continual talk of food
- Constant dieting
- Low self-esteem
- Awareness of problem
- Bingeing on high calorie, sweet food
- Nonassertive behavior
- Sporadic exercise
- Tantrums
- Weight fluctuations, apparently unexplained, caused by diuretic or laxative use
- Plans opportunities to binge

environment, the more difficult it becomes for family members to satisfy their need for individuality. An adolescent or young adult in such a family may fight this rigidity by developing rigid control over something—in this case, her diet and weight loss. The harder the family tries to regain control, the more resolved the girl with anorexia or bulimia becomes to overcontrol her weight.

A young woman is vulnerable to anorexia if she hasn't found ways to feel competent, worthy and effective. She may be a model child, rarely complaining and usually helpful, compliant and eager to please. Typically, her school performance is above average and she's highly demanding and critical of herself. In essence, she has learned to put others' needs ahead of her own, and she believes she must win others' approval before they'll care about her.

Bulimia is sometimes precipitated by an emotional event such as separation, divorce, illness, death, departure of a sibling, loss of a boyfriend or girlfriend, marriage or remarriage. These events can undermine the young woman's self-esteem and cause feelings of powerlessness and loneliness.

Young women who become bulimic sometimes get "help" from others who practice purging, but usually the behavior is secretive right from the start. In other cases, women find that self-induced vomiting reduces the guilt they feel after overeating. Poor self-image, guilt about the bingeing and vomiting, shame and the need for control sustain the habit.

Whatever the causes, anorexia and bulimia are potentially life-threatening psychological disorders. They're as difficult and as complex to treat as any drug or alcohol addiction.

If you think that a friend or family member may have an eating disorder, don't overreact. Decide who's the most appropriate person (parent, sibling, roommate, friend or spouse) to talk to the person. If the person is your child, discuss the matter with your spouse and decide if one or both of you should speak to your child about your concerns.

Next, choose a good time to talk. Wait until you're calm. Discussing this delicate issue when you're upset or angry could put her on the defensive. Remember that she is likely to deny the problem. Deal with her carefully and lovingly to avoid long-term damage. You may even want to put your thoughts down on paper before you speak.

It's important to say your goal is to help her get assistance in modifying her unhealthy eating habits and the associated unhealthy thoughts and feelings. Merely telling her you suspect she has an eating disorder won't help. Neither will just asking her to stop.

By bringing up the subject of the eating disorder, you may be exposing the young woman's most intimate secret, one she's probably ashamed of. Let her know you love her and want to help her. If she won't admit to having the problem, tell her you'll seek professional help, not for her but for yourself, because you care enough about her to find out how to handle the situation.

If you think the situation is life-threatening, due to the potential for suicide or because of severe starvation or some other physical danger, ensure her safety right away. You may have to forcibly take her for help, but do what it takes to get her the care she needs.

Treatment is twofold. It depends on the severity and stage of the disease. Nutritional therapy is begun immediately. It may include hospitalization and intravenous feedings if the young woman is in serious condition.

However, outpatient treatment is most often used. Behavioral control of eating and weight loss can be attempted at home, with inpatient therapy as a backup. Psychological therapy should continue until her normal weight has been maintained for six months to a year. Relapses should be treated aggressively with both medical and psychological therapies.

### Overeating

The most common eating problem is overeating that leads to obesity. It's a complex medical and psychological problem. It may stem from unmet psychological needs, emotional trauma, or a serious metabolic or chemical problem. Heart disease, diabetes (p. 211), osteoarthritis (p. 230), increased risk of certain cancers and premature death are among the serious complications of obesity.

Obesity is largely a combination of genetic predisposition, a learned eating pattern that soothes hurt feelings and unmet emotional needs, and a low level of physical activity. Painful emotions may be caused by intense daily stress, loneliness and anger.

Obesity and overeating disorders also arise in homes where emotional dependence or abuse is found. In these environments, food becomes an escape mechanism. It helps a child forget the problems occurring around him or her. Mealtimes are often friendly and civil. Fighting temporarily stops. A child who sees this happen repeatedly may begin to believe food has the power to soothe friction and restore stability in the family.

In our modern culture, even emotionally healthy families are at risk. Fast food, high-fat snacks, excessive television watching and low amounts of exercise are things that contribute to the increasing numbers of obese children and adults. For information on healthy nutrition, see page 13.

A short-term diet isn't enough to treat obesity or change overeating behavior. More than 90% of those who complete a commercial weight-loss program gain back all their weight within two years. Changing what you eat isn't enough. Treatment for obesity includes a thorough physical exam by your doctor, an evaluation of your eating behavior and an assessment of stress and psychological factors that may contribute to the problem. Treating each aspect of the problem behavior helps bring about success. Obesity is extremely difficult to treat, so an avoidance of lifestyle behaviors that increase the risk and prevent obesity are the real key.

## Mood Disorders

Mood disorders include bipolar disorder, often known as "manic-depressive disorder," and depression.

### Bipolar Disorder

People with *bipolar disorder,* also known as *manic-depressive disorder,*

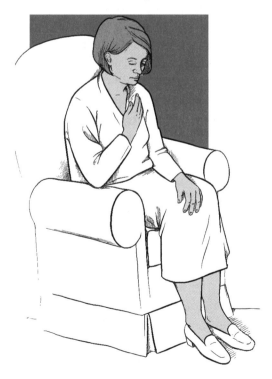

have periods of excitability and hyperactivity alternating with periods of depression. There's often a family history of the disorder. The manic (or up-swing) period can involve behaviors such as excessive spending, rapid speech, unending energy, impulsive decision-making and sometimes psychosis. The depressive (or down-swing) period includes feelings of hopelessness and worthlessness, an inability to function and suicidal thoughts. In some people the depressive phase is less pronounced than the colorful behaviors displayed in the manic phase.

People with bipolar disorder may need repeated hospitalization and treatment with medicines including lithium or other antipsychotic medicines or antidepressants (p. 619). Supportive psychotherapy can help people cope with the extreme emotional swings. Medicines can help level the mood swings.

## Depression

Depression is the most common emotional problem in the U.S. This life-threatening disorder affects people of all ages—children, adolescents and adults. The term depression refers to several mood disorders that vary in symptoms and severity.

You have probably experienced grief or a loss that caused you to feel depressed. This common, temporary form of depression is often referred to as *situational*. It can be a normal, temporary reaction lasting a few hours, days or even weeks, but it doesn't usually interfere significantly with long-term daily life.

*Clinical depression* reduces your ability to manage your life. It interferes with aspects of your normal functioning, such as sleep, appetite, work and social relationships. Clinical depression

should be treated by a doctor. All forms of depression, including those discussed below, can become life-threatening conditions.

No two people experience depression in the same way. Symptoms are usually both physical and emotional. The following symptoms may indicate the presence of depression.

Depression can involve physical or emotional factors, or both. Physical causes of depression include lack of sleep, not getting enough exercise, side effects from medicines, premenstrual syndrome (PMS, p. 383), chemical malfunctions in the brain, brain tumors (p. 47), ongoing illness and pain, and hormonal disorders. Emotional-behavioral causes for depression include family problems, stress, significant losses, learned helplessness, anger, guilt and negative thinking.

### Symptoms of Depression

- Ongoing feelings of sadness or irritability
- Not caring about people and things
- Lack of motivation
- Fatigue, loss of energy and lack of interest in work, sex, religion, hobbies and other activities
- Low self-esteem accompanied by self-criticism and feelings of guilt, shame, worthlessness and helplessness
- Trouble falling asleep, early awakening or sleeping too much
- Trouble thinking or concentrating
- Loss of appetite and weight, or overeating and weight gain
- Suicidal thoughts or suicide attempts
- Anxiety, fears, tension, uncertainty and indecisiveness
- Rebelliousness, antisocial behavior, and risky sexual behavior in children and adolescents

## Suicide

It has been shown that an overwhelming percentage of suicidal individuals make an overt reference to their thoughts about death before taking action. If someone you know has expressed thoughts about killing himself or herself, or if he or she has made statements such as, "My family would be better off if I were dead," try to get help for that person immediately.

Call a crisis hotline, your local hospital, your doctor or a mental health professional. Too many friends and family members of someone who has committed suicide wish later they had paid attention to the signs of depression, or taken hints of suicide more seriously. All suicidal statements should be regarded as a sign that help is needed right away.

## Seasonal Depression

Many people who have depression experience it primarily in the winter months. This is called *seasonal affective disorder*. Symptoms include sleeping longer, feeling more tired than usual, gaining weight, crying, headaches and stomach disorders. Because a lack of sunlight has been linked to this type of emotional change, being in the sunlight or using special full-spectrum lighting for a few hours during the day has shown promise in helping those with seasonal depression.

Depression involves a wide spectrum of symptoms, ranging from problems that are barely apparent to extreme physical and emotional discomfort. Depression can make you feel unhappy and physically ill. It can cause you to withdraw and feel lethargic. It may produce feelings of anxiety and low self-esteem. In more severe cases, depression can lead to suicidal thoughts, plans and actions.

Sometimes a person doesn't experience or acknowledge a depressed mood, although the depression is evident to others who may see aggressive actions, temper outbursts, impulsive behavior, accident proneness, compulsive work, sexual problems or illness. This condition is called *masked depression*. It's more common in children than in adults. It's more difficult to diagnose than other types of depression. Depression may be masked in children or adults who can't adequately analyze and communicate their feelings.

Just as depression may be masked from the affected person, it can also be hidden from others. When this happens in extreme cases, a suicide attempt may be a family's first clue that their loved one is seriously depressed. Unfortunately, suicide is becoming more common in adolescents. In adolescents the combination of impulsiveness, alcohol or drugs and easy access to lethal means (often a gun) contribute to this increasing problem. For each completed suicide, it's estimated that there are as many as 200 unsuccessful suicide attempts.

Depression can be brought on by marital conflict, family problems or other stressful situations. A person's depression may, in turn, adversely affect his or her family.

Depression can be effectively treated. If you or a family member is suffering from depression, see your doctor or a professional counselor. Depending on the type of depression, treatment can involve antidepressant medicine, psychotherapy or both. Combination therapy is often a better choice than medicine or psychotherapy alone.

## Personality Disorders

Your personality type helps determine how you'll adapt to changes in your environment or family when problems arise. Some people have personality disorders that keep them from adapting to their environment. Instead, they behave in abnormal or even socially unacceptable ways. In some cases, personality disorders are learned from past circumstances and home life. In other cases, they may be inherited.

People with personality disorders often don't consider their disorder to be a problem. Instead, they believe that their problems are due to the actions or reactions of others around them. Other psychological problems, such as depression or anxiety, may coexist with personality disorders.

Psychological testing, interviews and observation are required to identify a personality disorder and to identify other psychological problems. Treatment for personality disorders is usually difficult, long-term and only modestly successful. Although it's not easy to change personality traits, therapy may help modify them and relieve some of the problems they cause.

The most common types and symptoms of personality disorders are described below.

**Antisocial.** People with this personality disorder have a disregard for rules, authority and laws. They tend to be abusive and violent, often breaking the law without guilt or remorse. An antisocial personality is often associated with an abusive background. The cycle of abuse is extended into the disregard for others' rights and needs.

**Avoidant.** Paralyzed by their fear of being rejected by others, people with this personality disorder are unable to form close relationships or bonds with others. They may want close relationships with others, but withdraw due to severe personal insecurities or anxieties.

**Borderline.** This personality disorder is characterized by rapidly shifting emotions, very low self-esteem, impulsiveness and self-destructive behavior, such as suicide attempts. Interpersonal relationships are typically unstable and intense. It's a debilitating disorder that often results in poor social and occupational functioning.

**Compulsive.** People with this disorder tend to be rigid, perfectionistic and preoccupied with self-made rules and regulations. There's a strong tendency to be overly moralistic and judgmental toward others. Not only are individuals apt to be stingy with material belongings, they're emotionally stingy as well. Close relationships with others are uncommon with this personality. Don't confuse this disorder with

obsessive-compulsiveness disorder (p. 581), an anxiety disorder that can often be treated with medicine.

**Dependent.** Overly reliant on others, people with this disorder believe they're unable to meet the demands of family or job responsibilities. Dependent adults lack self-confidence, assume a passive role in relationships and are often exploited by those on whom they depend.

**Histrionic.** These individuals tend to be extremely dramatic and self-centered and have a low threshold for frustration. They also tend to be very sexually oriented in their relationships. They constantly need praise and attention, yet are very superficial in their relationships.

**Narcissistic.** This personality disorder creates an inflated sense of self-worth and importance. These individuals feel entitled to preferential treatment and feel "special" when compared with others. Even though narcissistic people are emotional, they can't understand the emotional needs of others, and they're incapable of meeting those needs. Self-love dominates their lives. Interpersonal relations are almost always superficial and disturbed.

**Paranoid.** Paranoid people tend to be suspicious, secretive and mistrusting in their relationships. They blame others for their problems. Others see them as cold, hostile and humorless, and often refer to them as excessively critical, argumentative and tense. Hypersensitivity to criticism is common.

**Passive-Aggressive.** These individuals tend to be aggressive by being lazy or passive. They seldom do their share of the work, yet they constantly complain about others' work or they criticize those in authority. Hidden feelings of anger may be expressed subtly through such behavior as procrastination, forgetfulness, silent stubbornness or intentional inefficiency. Many unassertive or dependent individuals develop this style of relating to others.

**Schizoid.** Aloof and isolated from others, people with schizoid personality disorder want to be alone most of the time. As a result, their relationships with others are often restricted and superficial. The emotional range of this person is limited. He or she usually appears cold and distant from others.

## Schizophrenia

You probably take for granted your ability to understand who you are, where you are and what's going on around you. Yet some people lose this contact with reality. People with *schizophrenia* are unable to make sense of what's going on around them all of the time. Schizophrenia is believed to be largely due to an inherited defect within the brain. Symptoms of schizophrenia usually begin in adolescence or early adulthood.

Symptoms of schizophrenia include hallucinations (seeing things or hearing things that aren't there), delusions (believing things that aren't true), disorientation, confusion and uncontrollable changes in emotions. Schizophrenia is a long-term psychiatric illness. Often, the person with schizophrenia was antisocial or a loner during childhood.

People with schizophrenia often require hospitalization in addition to treatment with one or more antipsychotic medicines. Some individuals with this disorder can return to normal functioning. More commonly, long-term supervision will be required in areas such as work, social relationships and self-care.

## Somatoform Disorders

Sometimes people have physical symptoms or believe they're seriously ill when there's nothing physically wrong with them. These are known as *somatoform disorders*. They may occur along with anxiety disorders, depression or other psychiatric problems.

**Hypochondriasis.** Late at night you may feel an unexpected and unexplained pain somewhere in your body that makes you unable to sleep. Fearing the worst, you rush to your doctor the next morning. This scenario is a common one. Many of us worry that unexpected pain indicates a serious health problem. Some worrying is normal, but persons with *hypochondriasis* worry too much. Hypochondriasis has been described as "excessive internal vigilance," or the tendency to focus too much on body functions and minor variations in appearance or sensation, believing that something dreadful is wrong.

This self-focused overconcern may stem from other fears or emotional needs that are being ignored. If it continues, hypochondriasis can reduce your ability to function in your family or hold down a job. If you have constant worries about your health and have trouble believing your doctor's explanation, you may need psychological, rather than physical, treatment. Behavioral therapy may be one option.

**Somatization disorder.** This disorder is characterized by numerous physical symptoms that have no medical cause. These symptoms can vary and may be symptoms of the digestive, heart, lung or female reproductive systems. It's not unusual for someone with this disorder to see more than one doctor, and to have had many diagnostic and surgical procedures. It's more common in women than men.

# PART 8

# FIRST AID
# APPENDICES

|  | PAGE |
|---|---|
| FIRST AID | 592 |
| MEDICINE CABINET | 613 |
| TESTS | 627 |
| DICTIONARY | 645 |
| INDEX | 664 |

# FIRST AID

This section is a guide of the basic steps to follow during the most frequently occurring emergencies and accidents. Knowing what to do when someone's life is at risk, reacting calmly and getting help may save a life. This know-how begins with understanding how to assess the situation and how to assess the victim.

It's a good idea to keep some basic supplies on hand in case of minor emergencies or first-aid needs. See page 613 for information on what to keep in your medicine cabinet.

It's also a good idea to take a basic life support (BLS) course to learn cardiopulmonary resuscitation (CPR). This course may be available through your local police or fire department, emergency medical service (EMS), Red Cross or the American Heart Association. Of course, prevention is always better than having to respond to an accident! See page 28 for information on safety.

## Emergency!
## When to Call Your Doctor

To help reduce health care costs and to reserve the emergency room for appropriate needs, try to recognize which situations are emergencies and which can wait until you can be seen in your doctor's office. A class in basic first aid and CPR will give you information about how to assess and begin treating people in most serious emergency situations.

What follows in this chapter isn't meant to take the place of a class in first aid and CPR. Keep your skills and knowledge up-to-date with refresher courses. For more information about when to call for emergency help and when to call your doctor, see the list on page 593. If you're ever in doubt about whether an emergency is life-threatening, it's best to contact a health care professional for an opinion.

## Making Important Medical Information Accessible

If you have a serious medical problem, how will you alert others about it if you become unconscious? The Medic Alert system includes a necklace or bracelet bearing a toll-free number (800-344-3226) for the emergency room doctor to call for full information about your specific medical history. The Medic Alert kits are available at many pharmacies.

## Serious Emergencies

| Seek Emergency Treatment | Call Your Doctor |
| --- | --- |
| Severe abdominal pain | Mild abdominal pain that comes and goes |
| Gasping for breath, not breathing | Some wheezing, mild shortness of breath |
| Seizure with difficulty breathing | Seizure that has stopped, with history of epilepsy or seizures |
| Heavy bleeding | Bleeding that stops with simple pressure |
| Loss of consciousness | Brief fainting spell |
| Fall or accident with deformed limbs or an inability to move | Sprain or strained joint in which the extremity can bear weight and be moved |
| High temperature | Mild fever |
| Serious burn | Minor burn |
| Chemicals in the eye (wash the eye for 10 minutes in running water before going to the hospital) | Chemical irritation to the skin |
| Change in mental state, such as mild confusion, tiredness and slurred speech, especially after a blow to the head | Animal bite without serious bleeding |
| | Swallowed foreign object without choking |
| Chest pressure or pain | |
| Accidental poisoning (call the poison control center in your area for instructions) | |

**Assess the Emergency**

1. **Find out what happened.** Ask witnesses what happened, who was involved in the accident and where the victims are.

2. **Make sure you can give help safely.** Be aware of dangerous situations. For example, before you can safely touch a victim of electrical shock, you must check to see if they're still touching the electrical power source. If so, you need to use something that won't conduct electricity, such as a wooden pole or tree branch, to remove the electrical cord or apparatus, if you can do it safely. If you're responding to an emergency involving a victim struggling in deep water, use a pole, rope or flotation ring to bring the person to safety. Swim to the victim only if you know water-safety and life-saving techniques.

3. **Ask someone to go for help.** If possible, ask someone to find a telephone and call 911 or your local rescue squad or police. If you're alone, shout to alert anyone around you that you need help. If no one hears you and you know you're the only person aware of the emergency, check the victim for breathing and a heartbeat, then call 911, an ambulance or a rescue squad

before beginning mouth-to-mouth resuscitation, CPR or measures to prevent shock.

## Mouth-to-Mouth Resuscitation

Mouth-to-mouth resuscitation is done to restart breathing. It is relatively simple, but can be crucial during emergencies. It may save a life by providing the oxygen required by the brain and other tissues. The technique differs for children and adults.

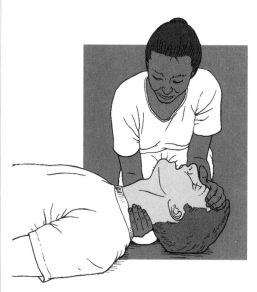

**POSITIONING VICTIM**

### Mouth-to-Mouth Resuscitation for Adults

**1. Position the victim.** If possible, ask someone nearby to call for emergency help. Then start giving aid right away. First, make sure the victim is lying flat on his or her back on a hard surface. Check the mouth for fluid, mucus or food. Sweep the mouth with your finger to clear it, then tilt the head back to make sure the airway is as open as possible. Do this by placing one hand under the neck and the other on the forehead. Gently elevate the chin by tilting the head back.

If the person has fallen or has signs of a head or spine injury, try to lift the chin without tilting the head back. Be

aware that a lot of movement can make that injury worse. But air and breathing are the first priority for an injured person who isn't breathing.

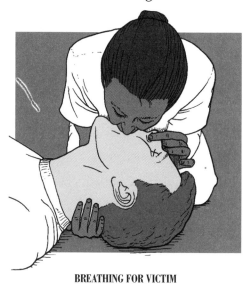

**BREATHING FOR VICTIM**

**2. Breathe for the victim.** Squeeze the victim's nose with the fingers of the hand you have placed on the victim's forehead. After taking a deep breath, place your mouth tightly over the victim's mouth and give two quick breaths. Then check for circulation. Watch for the victim's chest to rise

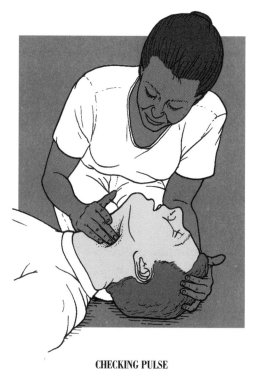

**CHECKING PULSE**

during the breaths and listen at the mouth for air exiting. If the chest doesn't rise, air isn't going in. Keep giving breaths this way, about 12 per minute, until the victim begins to breathe on his or her own. If air isn't going in (no chest rise), sweep the mouth again with your finger and roll the victim to his or her side and give four thumps on the back (use caution if you suspect that the person has a spine injury) with the heel of your hand to try to dislodge any obstruction in the throat. Keep giving breaths. Watch for the chest to rise, thump the back and sweep the mouth until air is going into the chest.

**3. Check for pulse.** After giving the victim two breaths (that cause the chest to rise), check for a pulse. Check for a pulse in the artery in the neck, about an inch below the jaw. If you don't feel a pulse, begin CPR.

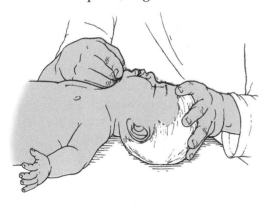

**POSITIONING INFANT**

## Mouth-to-Mouth Resuscitation for Infants

**1. Position the victim.** If possible, ask someone nearby to call 911 for help. Make sure the baby isn't just sleeping. Shake the infant gently and watch for any breathing. Lay the baby flat on his or her back on a hard surface. Check the mouth for fluid, mucus or food. Sweep the mouth with your finger to clear it. Tilt the head back to make sure the airway is as open as possible. Do this by placing one hand under the neck and the other on the

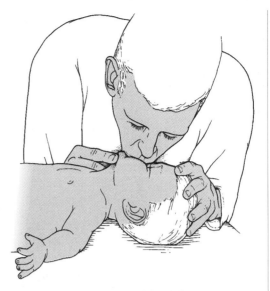

**BREATHING FOR VICTIM**

forehead. Gently raise the chin by tilting the head back.

**2. Breathe for the victim.** Cover the baby's mouth *and* nose with your mouth and give two quick puffs. Watch for the chest to rise during the breath. Continue to give breaths in this manner, about 25 per minute, until the baby begins to breathe on his or her own. If air isn't going in, sweep the mouth with your finger or roll the baby to his or her side and give four thumps on the back with the heel of your hand. Give puffs, watch for the chest to rise, then thump the back and sweep the mouth again until air is going into the chest.

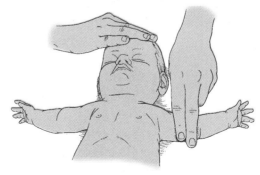

**CHECKING FOR PULSE**

**3. Check for pulse.** Check for a pulse in the artery in the neck about an inch below the jaw or on the inside of the upper arm. After giving the two puffs, check for a pulse. If you don't feel a pulse, proceed with CPR.

## Cardiopulmonary Resuscitation

Cardiopulmonary resuscitation (CPR) is done to restart the heartbeat. This may be needed in a severe emergency if a person stops breathing. If breathing isn't restarted within a few minutes the heart may stop beating or it may beat ineffectively. When blood doesn't circulate, the brain is damaged within five to 10 minutes from lack of oxygen. So, along with breathing for the victim, you must try to get the heart restarted and heartbeats maintained until the tissues replenish with oxygen and, hopefully, the victim's heart and breathing continue without help.

If you encounter someone who isn't breathing, immediately begin the steps for mouth-to-mouth resuscitation: Open and clear the airway, then begin artificial respiration. After two breaths, check for a pulse. If you don't feel a pulse and have been trained in CPR by taking a basic life support (BLS) course, begin giving CPR. Don't attempt CPR if you haven't been certified to do it. You may do the person more harm than good. The information presented here is just for review and a refresher for people who have had formal BLS training. It's not a substitute for training.

### CPR for Adults

**1. Position yourself.** Kneel next to the victim's chest. Find the lower end of the breastbone, where the bones form an upside-down V. Place the heel of one hand on the breastbone two inches above the bottom edge of the breastbone, then place your other

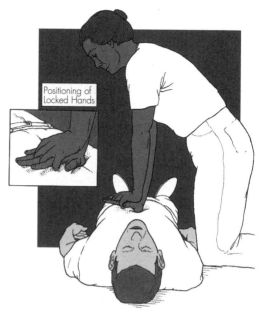

POSITIONING FOR CPR

hand on top of the first hand and lace your fingers. Lock your elbows. Shift your weight over your hands.

**2. Pump on the chest.** Push down on the victim's chest, compressing the chest wall two inches. Repeat in this cadence, pushing when you say a number: *one*-and-*two*-and-*three*-and-*four*-and-*five*. Give the chest 15 compressions, then reposition yourself to give two breaths. In adult CPR the ideal rate is 60 compressions per minute.

**3. Breathe for the victim.** Give two breaths, then return to the spot two inches above the bottom edge of the breastbone, lock your hands and arms again and compress the chest 15 times. Repeat this cycle: two breaths, 15 compressions, two breaths, 15 compressions. Stop after two to three minutes and recheck for a pulse. If you don't feel a pulse, continue CPR until help arrives or the pulse and breathing are re-established.

The difference between one and two people administering CPR is the cadence of the breaths and chest compressions. When two people are giving CPR, one person gives five compressions of the chest, and the person doing

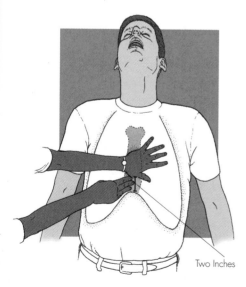

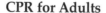

Two Inches

**COMPRESSION POINT FOR ADULT**

mouth-to-mouth resuscitation gives one breath, checking for a pulse after a few minutes of CPR. Repeat and repeat. The goal of two-person CPR is to complete 60 to 75 compressions per minute.

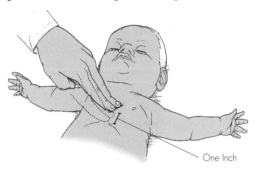

**COMPRESSION POINT FOR INFANT**

### CPR for Infants

**1. Position yourself.** Find the lower end of the breastbone, where the bones form an upside-down V. Place your index and middle fingers on the breastbone one inch above the lower edge, with your fingers toward the neck.

**2. Pump the chest.** Push on the baby's chest with the fingers of one hand, compressing the chest wall one inch. Repeat the compressions in a cadence, pressing on the numbers: *one-two-three-four-five*. Give the chest five compressions. Place your mouth over the infant's mouth and nose and give one puff of breath. The goal is to complete 100 compressions per minute.

**3. Give puffs for the baby's breath.** Give one puff, compress the chest five times, then repeat: one puff, five compressions, one puff, five compressions. Your goal is to give 20 puffs per minute. Stop after two to three minutes and recheck for a pulse. If you don't feel a pulse, continue CPR until help arrives or the pulse and breathing are re-established.

## Preventing Shock

Shock is a slowing down of the body's vital systems, such as blood flow and breathing. It can occur with any accident, especially one that results in burns or blood loss. The body releases chemicals that cause the blood pressure to drop rapidly, possibly causing the victim to go into shock, becoming weak, faint, cold, clammy and sweaty. An insufficient oxygen supply to the brain may cause confusion or unconsciousness in the shock victim. Follow these steps to prevent shock in an accident victim.

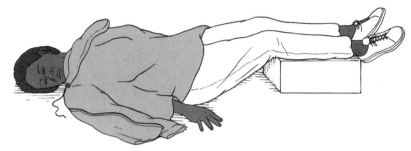

**POSITIONING THE VICTIM**

**1. Position the victim.** Have the victim lie on his or her back and raise the feet comfortably to increase the blood return to the heart. Don't move someone if you think there's been a spinal injury, because movement may make that injury worse.

**2. Provide comfort for the victim.** Cover the victim with a blanket or other clothing. Loosen any tight clothing on the victim. Don't offer food or fluids because the victim may vomit and breathe in the vomit.

**3. Call for help.** Ask someone to call 911, the local rescue squad or the police, or do it yourself if you're alone.

## Amputation

**1. Assess the situation.** The first step is to assess how the injury occurred and how much of a limb or extremity was severed. Then determine the immediate needs, such as stopping the bleeding and preventing shock. If possible, ask someone to call 911 or the local rescue squad or police, or try to call yourself after assessing the victim.

**2. Administer first aid.** The bleeding should be controlled with direct pressure if possible, or with a tourniquet above the cut if the limb has been severed. If the victim feels faint or nauseated, or appears pale, have him or her lie down, covered with a blanket, with feet elevated.

**3. Collect the severed tissue.** Fingers and arms can often be reattached if the victim and the severed part are brought to the hospital promptly. Keep the amputated part cool and clean. Wrap it in a clean, moist towel if possible.

## Bites and Stings

**1. Assess the bite.** Insect stings or bites may require little or no treatment (see box on page 599). Snake bites, large-animal bites and poisonous spider bites are more serious and need immediate medical attention.

**2. Administer first aid.** Minor bites may be relieved by applying a cool compress or ice, and hydrocortisone cream (p. 616) to the injury. Bites are treated differently, depending on the type of bite.

*Animal bites.* Wash the bite, then try to stop any bleeding. Seek medical attention for tetanus and rabies vaccinations, if needed. Large bites, puncture wounds and facial bites may need surgical repair and antibiotics to prevent infection. In general, check with your doctor about any animal bite that isn't a superficial injury by your own pet dog or cat.

*Insect bites and stings.* If a stinger remains, remove it as quickly as possible without squeezing the venom sac. Applying ice to the area right after the bite or sting will reduce the inflammatory reaction. Clean the area, then apply an antibiotic ointment (p. 615) to the bite to prevent infections. Other home remedies include rubbing aspirin or aspirin cream into the sting site or applying a paste of baking soda or meat tenderizer and water to slow the pain of the sting. Cool compresses may be all that's needed to relieve the itch and irritation. More severe reactions may require an oral antihistamine (p. 615) or possibly a corticosteroid cream or oral tablets (p. 622).

*Jellyfish and Portuguese man-of-war.* Get out of the water and gently rub sand into the sting. This helps reduce the toxic substances and remove any clinging tentacles. Cleanse the wound with sea water (fresh water will discharge more venom into the wound), alcohol or ammonia. Use a rough towel or other object to scrape away the remaining tentacles. Apply hydrocortisone cream if the sting is minor. These stings can be serious, and medical attention should be sought if there are any symptoms other than at the injury site.

*Poisonous snake bites.* Try to determine the kind of snake and look for symptoms of a poisonous bite. These symptoms include severe pain, nausea and blurred vision. Symptoms may be immediate or delayed several hours. If you've determined that it's a poisonous snake bite, or if symptoms begin, fasten a bandage or belt around the limb two inches above the bite and tighten lightly, so you can just slip a little finger between the band and the person's skin. Try to immobilize the limb (with a splint if possible). Position the limb lower than the level of the heart. Try to keep the person calm and reassured but transport him or her as quickly as possible to an emergency room for further care, including antivenin therapy. Don't use ice on the bite. Incision and suction aren't recommended unless you're trained and can do them within five minutes of the bite, or the nearest medical care is more than 30 minutes away.

*Spider bites.* Put ice on the bite and see your doctor immediately if you show signs of a serious reaction or know that the spider was poisonous. Take the spider with you if possible. The most common poisonous spiders include black widow spiders and brown recluse spiders. Medicines are available to help reduce the symptoms of spider bites. If the bite is minor, cleaning with a hydrogen peroxide solution and applying an antibiotic ointment may be helpful.

**3. Watch for allergic reactions.** Any bite or sting can lead to swelling, red, itchy blotches called hives (p. 282) and, rarely, to swelling of the face, throat, hands and feet. This is called anaphylactic shock (p. 222) and is an emergency! It should be treated in an emergency room or doctor's office right away. If you know you're allergic to a particular insect sting, be sure to keep a bee-sting kit containing an epinephrine injection (available through your doctor) and an antihistamine with you at all times.

## Bleeding

When an artery is cut during an accident the blood may not be able to clot, especially if it's spurting. Immediate response is needed and pressure must be placed on the skin just above the spurting area to prevent the victim from bleeding to death. If possible, put on latex gloves before touching someone who is bleeding. Of course, that's often not possible. If not, be sure to wash all of the blood from your skin, preferably using an antiseptic soap after the emergency has passed.

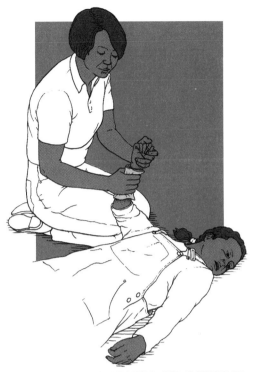

**BLEEDING VICTIM WITH WOUND RAISED ABOVE HEART**

**1. Position the victim.** Lay the victim on the ground and elevate the bleeding area or limb above the heart to slow the blood flow.

**2. Compress the wound.** Using a pad of cloth, firmly put pressure over the laceration or to the side of the wound if there's an impaled object. If there's an impaled object, avoid putting direct pressure on the object. Don't remove the object, because that may cause further bleeding. The pad can be tied in place as the bleeding slows. Put more padding over the wound and continue firm compression if the bleeding continues. Don't remove the padding. If you do, any clot that's forming may be destroyed when the padding is removed. In cases of severe bleeding, compression over the artery just above the injury or at one of the main compression points (see illustration p. 600) may be needed.

## Burns

There are three levels of burns—

### What to Do for Insect Bites and Stings

- Remove the stinger as quickly as possible without squeezing the venom sac.
- Cleanse the sting and apply an antibiotic ointment to prevent infection.
- Apply ice or a cool compress to treat the pain and swelling.
- Apply a paste of meat tenderizer and water to the bite.
- Apply a paste of baking soda and water to the sting.
- Apply corticosteroid cream.
- Use an oral or topical antihistamine (p. 615) or analgesic (p. 614).

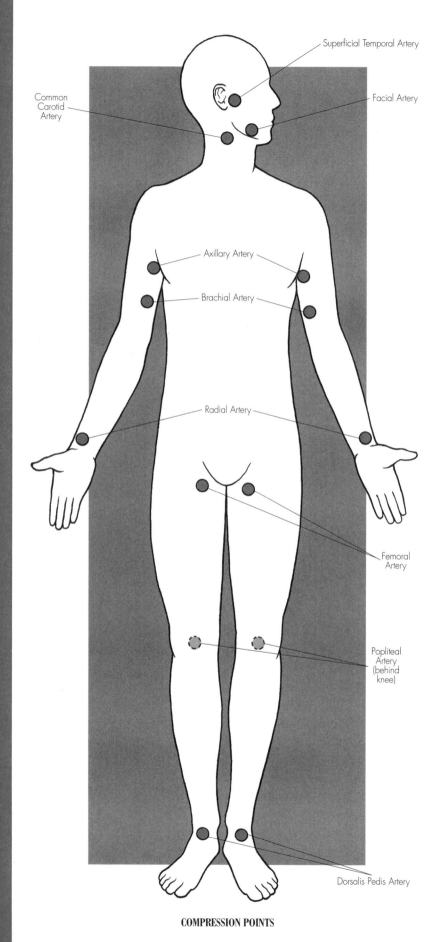

Superficial Temporal Artery

Common Carotid Artery

Facial Artery

Axillary Artery

Brachial Artery

Radial Artery

Femoral Artery

Popliteal Artery (behind knee)

Dorsalis Pedis Artery

**COMPRESSION POINTS**

first degree, second degree and third degree. First-degree burns are the least serious and involve only the outer layer of skin. First-degree burns usually can be treated with home care.

Second-degree burns are a more severe injury to the outer layer of skin that result in blistering of the skin. First- and second-degree burns are painful but will heal without scarring unless they become infected. Second-degree burns should be checked by your doctor if they're over more than 5% of the person's body, or if they're on the hands, feet, face, groin or buttocks.

Third-degree burns are the most serious and involve all layers of the skin, including fat and nerves. A third-degree burn may be charred black or a dry white. Because nerves are burned, there may be little pain. All third-degree burns should be checked by your doctor as soon as possible. If any burn appears to be infected, see your doctor right away.

**1. Identify the cause.** Chemicals, solvents, hot liquids, steam, flames and electricity can produce burns on the skin or deeper tissues. Remove the victim from the source of the burn, being careful not to get anything on yourself if that was the cause of the burn.

**2. Position the victim.** If the victim's clothing is on fire, push him or her to the ground and smother the flames with whatever clothing or blankets are at hand. Remove any clothing soaked with hot liquids, but don't remove clothing that's burned into the skin. If possible, raise the burned area above the heart to help prevent swelling and reduce the pain.

**3. Cool the burn.** If any area of the skin is still hot right after it has been burned, run cool water over the burn for eight to 10 minutes. If the area is too large, saturate sheets, towels or clothing with cool water and gently apply them to the burned area. Within hours, burns over large areas of skin may lead to fluid loss and shock. This requires emergency attention at your local hospital. You can help prevent shock by covering the victim with blankets and elevating the feet. For smaller burns, treat the area with a burn ointment (don't use butter) and apply a nonsticking dressing and a wrap, if available, and have it checked by your doctor.

Any burn can become infected, a possibility that can be more dangerous than the burn itself. Redness, swelling and increasing pain in a burn suggest a spreading infection that should be checked by your doctor right away. All electrical burns are considered serious and should be seen by your doctor.

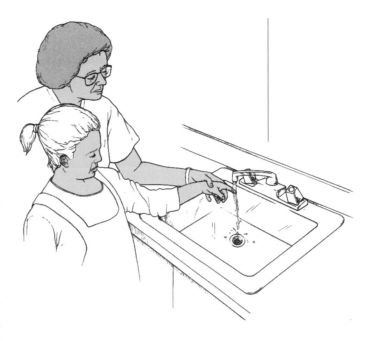

**RUNNING COOL WATER OVER A BURN**

## Choking

Choking can be a life-threatening emergency when the air passage is completely blocked. The choking person isn't able to cough, talk or breathe because the blockage doesn't allow air in or out. After 60 seconds the person's skin may appear blue. Then he or she may pass out. The following first-aid procedures can help dislodge the food particle and save a victim's life.

### Choking in an Adult or Child

Many times when a child or adult breathes in some liquid or a small piece of food, his or her immediate response is to stop talking, reach for the throat and starting coughing. Within 15 to 30 seconds, he or she will cough enough to clear the air passage of the liquid or food and be able to talk again. But when a larger piece of solid food is involved, the person may need help.

**1. Clear the airway.** If the person is still conscious and able to stand, step behind the person and place your arms

around his or her waist. Form one hand into a fist, then grab that fist with the other hand. With a sharp upward thrust into the abdomen, attempt to dislodge the food. This is called the *Heimlich maneuver.*

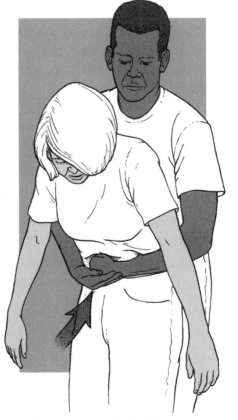

**HEIMLICH MANEUVER**

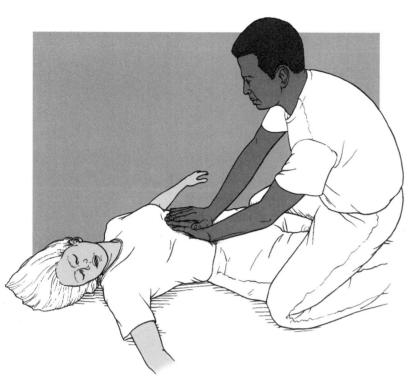

**HEIMLICH MANEUVER IN UNCONSCIOUS VICTIM**

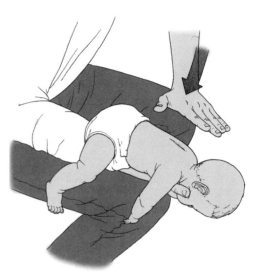

**HOLDING BABY TO STRIKE THE BACK**

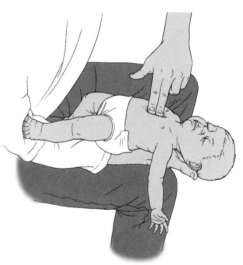

**HOLDING BABY FOR CHEST THRUSTS**

**2. Position the victim if he or she is unconscious.** If the person becomes unconscious and is on the floor, roll the person onto his or her back. Place the heel of your hand in the middle of the abdomen, just above the navel. Thrust upward five times. Check to see if the object has been dislodged. Sweep the mouth to check for obstructing food.

**3. Breathe for the victim.** If the food has been dislodged and swept from the mouth but the victim isn't breathing, begin mouth-to-mouth resuscitation (p. 594). Anyone who has been revived after an episode of choking should be checked right away by a doctor.

## Choking in an Infant

**1. Clear the airway.** Check the baby's mouth to see what's causing the blockage.

**2. Position the victim.** Put the baby face down on your forearm. Support the head and neck. Strike the back between the shoulder blades five times. Turn the baby over. Thrust on the chest with your middle and index fingers in the center of the breastbone five times. Repeat this process until object is coughed up and breathing resumes.

**3. Breathe for the victim.** Once the object has been dislodged and removed from the mouth, begin mouth-to-mouth resuscitation if the baby isn't breathing.

## Cuts, Lacerations, Abrasions, Blisters

The first step in treating a cut in the skin is to stop the bleeding. For small cuts, run water gently over the cut to remove any dirt or particles. Apply pressure until the bleeding stops, then put an antibiotic ointment and a bandage on the cut. Larger cuts may require stitches to stop the bleeding. If the cut is deep or you see small yellow nodules of fat in the bottom of the cut, if the cut is longer than one-third of an inch, if the cut gapes open or if the cut is on the face, it should be seen by a doctor. Apply direct pressure over the wound with a clean cloth or gauze. Check for signs of infection.

*Abrasions,* in which the top layer of the skin has been scraped, usually cause minimal bleeding, and pressure doesn't help reduce the seepage of fluid. Treat the wound as a burn. Gently scrub, wipe or wash any dirt or grit from the wound, being very careful not to rub dirt or grit deeper into the wound. Cover it with an antibiotic ointment (p. 615), then place a nonadhesive bandage over the area.

Watch wounds carefully for any signs of infection and consult your doctor if you notice increasing redness, swelling or tenderness, or if a thick, foul-smelling, yellow-green material oozes from the wound. These are signs of infection.

**1. Assess the injury.** Small cuts and abrasions require cleaning and a bandage. An antibiotic ointment applied to the injury may reduce the risk of an infection. Larger cuts will need first-aid treatment, along with further medical evaluation.

**2. Administer first aid.** Use water to clean the wound of any debris. Put direct pressure on the wound with a clean pad or cloth until the bleeding subsides. If the edges don't fall together, if the bleeding continues, if deeper tissues are easily seen or if it's a puncture wound, take the person to a doctor for immediate treatment and a tetanus shot, if needed. Don't "pop" blisters—they're protecting the tissue underneath. Cover them with a clean, appropriately sized bandage as you would any cut or laceration.

**3. Watch for signs of infection.** Redness, swelling or increasing pain around any cut, abrasion or blister suggests a spreading infection. This should be checked by your doctor right away.

## Drowning

**1. Get the victim to safety. If possible, ask someone to call 911.** Use a pole, rope, flotation ring or boat to rescue the victim. If these aids aren't available and you're trained in water-safety procedures, swim to the victim and approach him or her using the appropriate techniques. Getting into the water with a struggling, drowning person should be your last option. Do so only if you're trained in water rescue.

**2. Breathe for the victim.** After the victim is brought to safety, check for breathing and, if needed, begin mouth-to-mouth resuscitation right away. Don't try to empty the water from a person's lungs. Give forceful breaths. Clear the mouth and the back of the throat of water and other material that appears during resuscitation. Check for a pulse after two breaths and, if you're trained, begin CPR if no pulse is felt. Continue to breathe and compress the chest until emergency medical help arrives.

**3. Prevent shock.** When breathing is restored, roll the victim to his or her side to promote drainage. A drowning victim often expels water and may vomit when he or she begins to breathe. Cover the person with a blanket. If the person is awake and alert, have him or her lie on the back with the feet raised and cover with a blanket.

## Electrical Shock

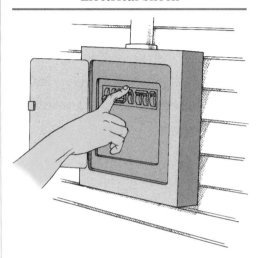

**TURN OFF THE ELECTRICAL SOURCE**

**1. Remove the victim from the electrical source.** Turn off a circuit-breaker or switch, or push the victim from the electrical source using something that won't conduct an electrical current to you, such as a wooden or rubber object.

Be sure you're standing on a dry surface. Don't touch the victim directly until this is done. Ask someone to call 911.

**2. Breathe for the victim.** If the victim isn't breathing, begin mouth-to-mouth resuscitation. Give two breaths, then check for a pulse. If you're trained, begin CPR if there's no pulse. Continue artificial respiration and CPR until breathing and pulse have returned.

**3. Prevent shock.** Once breathing is restored, if the victim is unconscious, roll the victim to his or her side and cover with a blanket. If the victim is awake, cover him or her with a blanket and have him or her lie on the back with the feet raised. Don't allow the person to walk on burned feet. Don't try to remove dead skin or clothing stuck to the wound. Don't use ice on a large electrical burn (larger than one inch).

## Eye Injury

**1. Assess the injury.** Most eye injuries are minor, involving only a small scratch on the clear part of the eye (corneal abrasion, p. 68) or a foreign object or substance on the surface of the eye. The eye's normal tears may wash the substance from the eye. If a change in vision has occurred, if the victim sees red or if the object has penetrated the eyeball, the victim should be seen right away by a doctor. Don't let him or her rub the irritated eye.

**2. Administer first aid.** Chemicals and irritating substances should be washed from the eye under a gentle stream of water for at least 10 to 15 minutes. A foreign object on the white part of the eye may gently be removed with the corner of a soft cloth. When something is embedded in the *cornea* (the clear film over the pupil and colored part of the eye), don't try to remove it. Get medical attention.

**3. Follow-up.** If a minor scratch

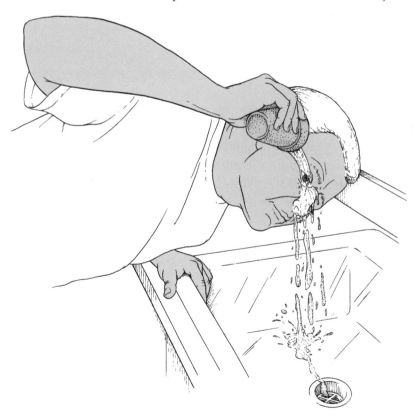

**RINSING THE EYE WITH WATER**

doesn't stop hurting in 24 hours, or if the sensation of something in the eye remains, the eye should be checked by a doctor. Seek help right away if you see any signs of infection, such as redness, increasing pain or swelling. See page 68 for more information about foreign objects in the eye.

## Fainting

**1. Assess the situation.** Fainting is a sudden, brief loss of consciousness that occurs because of a temporarily inadequate blood supply to the brain. Usually after a minute or so of lying flat, the blood flow to the brain is restored and the person is conscious again. Ask witnesses what happened before beginning first aid. CPR shouldn't be done on someone who has a pulse and is breathing, which is the situation with most fainting victims. Sometimes there's slight twitching when someone faints. This isn't a seizure.

**2. Position the victim.** Place the person on his or her back. Remember that people who faint may vomit, so watch carefully for this and clear the airway if it happens. Check for a heartbeat and breathing. Raise the person's legs above the level of the head to improve blood flow to the brain. Loosen belts, ties or tight clothing. If the person's breathing and heartbeat have stopped, the situation is more serious than a fainting spell and CPR must be started by a trained person. Ask someone to call 911 in this situation.

## Falls and Spinal Injuries

**1. Assess the victim.** In case the spine has been damaged, don't move the victim of a fall or other impact (such as a car crash) unless absolutely necessary because there's great risk of causing further damage. Check for breathing. If it has stopped, move the victim as little as needed (especially the back and neck) to place him or her on the back and start mouth-to-mouth resuscitation. Check for a pulse and, if you're trained, perform CPR if no pulse is felt.

**2. Check for injuries.** Except in life-threatening situations, don't move an unconscious victim of a fall or crash unless he or she isn't breathing and you must reposition for resuscitation. If the victim is awake, ask what areas are painful. If the person has numbness, pain in the neck or back, or is unable to move any part of the body, he or she may have a spinal injury. Don't move that person except to escape from life-threatening situations.

If a limb is deformed, he or she may have a broken bone (fractures, p. 236). If the victim can move all of the body except a painful or deformed upper limb, a *splint* can be placed on it during transport to the hospital for further medical attention.

**3. Prevent shock.** Once breathing is restored, cover the victim with a blanket. If the person has numbness, pain in the neck or back, or is unable to move any part of the body, don't elevate the feet or cause or allow other movement.

## Fish Hook Injury

**1. Assess the injury.** If the barb hasn't fully penetrated the skin, the hook usually can be pulled back out from the same hole it punctured in the skin. If the barb of the hook is completely buried in the skin, don't try to pull it out the same hole it entered. The barb will cause a lot of damage if you attempt to pull it directly from the skin.

**2. Administer first aid.** Although it may hurt, the best procedure, if the barb of the hook is embedded in the skin, is to push it through the skin

### *Splinting an Injured Limb*

A splint is a device that keeps an injured limb or body part from moving. Don't straighten a broken limb to splint it unless there isn't a pulse beyond the injury. To make a splint, use materials that you have available at the site of the injury, or support the injured body part in the position you found it in until help arrives. There are four kinds of splints:

**Rigid splint.** These are made with solid, firm objects such as wooden boards, metal strips or tree branches.

**Soft splint.** These can be made with soft objects such as folded blankets, towels or pillows.

**Sling.** This is a cloth or flexible object that can be tied into a triangular bandage to hold an arm, wrist or hand.

**Anatomic splint.** This can be made by binding the uninjured leg to the injured leg.

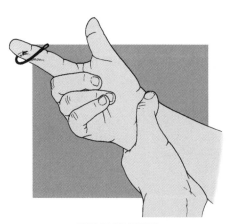

**FISH HOOK INJURY**

until it exits at another site, making a second hole. The barb can then be snipped off with wirecutters and the rest of the hook can be pulled back through the original hole. Note that if this maneuver requires that the fish hook be pushed very deeply into the tissue or if the injury is in or near the eye, neck or face, you should seek medical attention.

**3. Dress the wound.** Wash and apply an antibiotic ointment and a bandage to the wound, then check with your doctor to see if a tetanus booster is needed. See your doctor immediately if you have any signs of infection, redness, swelling or increased pain.

## Frostbite

**1. Assess the situation.** Prolonged exposure to very cold temperatures can lower the body temperature, resulting in cold injuries such as hypothermia and frostbite. Frostbite usually affects the fingers, toes, nose or ears.

**2. Administer first aid.** Check for breathing and pulse and, if needed, administer mouth-to-mouth resuscitation and CPR if you're trained. Once breathing is restored, move the person to shelter and, if awake, give him or her warm, nonalcoholic beverages to drink. If this isn't possible, cover the victim and protect him or her from the cold or frozen ground. Call 911 for medical help.

**3. Treating frostbite.** Warm the fingers, toes, nose or ears slowly by placing the cold extremity next to the victim's

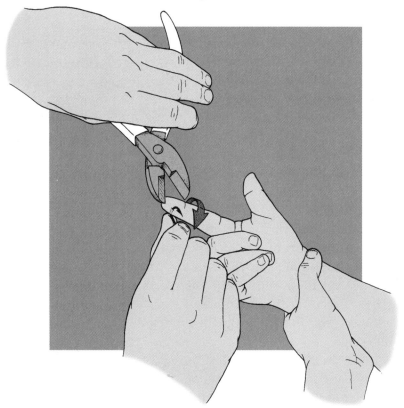

**REMOVING A FISH HOOK**

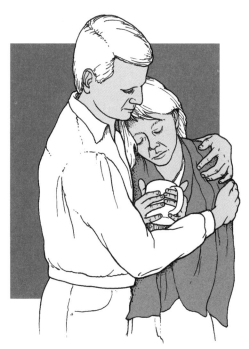

**TREATING FROSTBITE**

## Hypothermia

*Hypothermia* is when your body can't keep itself warm enough. It can occur when you're exposed to cold temperatures or low windchills, especially if your clothing is wet or light, if you've been using drugs or alcohol, or if you're injured. Symptoms of hypothermia include slurred speech and slow physical responses. If it continues, hypothermia can lead to confusion, coma and death.

If you see someone with hypothermia, get the person to shelter, away from the elements. Warm the person in a tub of warm water if possible. If he or she is able to drink, give hot liquids. Warm air, a heating pad or electric blankets can also be used. If none of these are available, the body heat of one or more people can help warm the person by getting close, preferably under a blanket or in a sleeping bag.

(or someone else's) body. Don't rub the area. If the victim is awake, encourage him or her to drink warm liquids. You can also use warm water (not above 104°F) to warm hands or feet.

## Head Injury

**1. Assess the injury.** A mild blow to the head may cause a headache or a scalp laceration that can bleed profusely. A more serious blow to the head will often lead to an altered state of consciousness, indicating the brain has been damaged or bruised. Ask the victim questions—his or her name, birth date, what he or she was doing—to assess his or her level of awareness. If the person seems confused or dazed, or is unable to speak, he or she has a serious head injury. The victim is deeply unconscious if he or she doesn't respond to painful

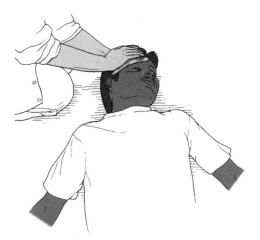

**TREATING A HEAD WOUND**

pinches. When bone fragments can be seen or when straw-colored fluid is coming from the wound or the ear, a very serious injury has occurred.

**2. Administer first aid.** Don't move the victim except to reposition for resuscitation or to remove him or her from life-threatening danger. If the person isn't breathing and you're trained in basic life support, begin mouth-to-mouth resuscitation and CPR if there's no pulse. If the person is unconscious and breathing, gently place a pad over the open head wound to slow the bleeding. Call 911 for help before you move the victim. Assume that anyone with a head injury has a neck injury.

**3. Prevent shock.** Once breathing is restored, cover the victim with a blanket. If the victim is awake, have him or her lie on the back with feet raised (only if there's no neck or back pain, numbness or weakness in an extremity).

## Heart Attack

A heart attack occurs when a blood clot blocks the flow of blood in one (or more) of the coronary arteries to the heart. This blockage means no oxygen is getting to the cells in the area of the heart that is cut off. The result is that the heart muscle in that area dies, causing pain. A heart attack is considered a medical emergency. Ask someone to call 911 right away.

**1. Assess the situation.** Signs of a heart attack include intense, prolonged chest pain, pain that extends to the left shoulder and arm, back, upper abdomen and sometimes teeth and jaw, shortness of breath, fainting, nausea, vomiting and excessive sweating. Ask the person if it feels like a hard squeezing sensation in his or her chest. This is a sign of a heart attack. Check the person's pulse, which may be faster or slower than normal, and breathing. If a heart attack causes the person to stop breathing, a trained person should begin CPR.

**2. Assist the victim.** Have the person stop all activity and stay in a comfortable position. A sitting position may help breathing. Loosen tight clothing. Monitor the person's pulse and breathing until help arrives.

## Heat Stroke

**1. Assess the situation.** Prolonged exposure, work or exercise in hot weather can cause the body temperature to rise faster than the body can get rid of the heat, until the body can no

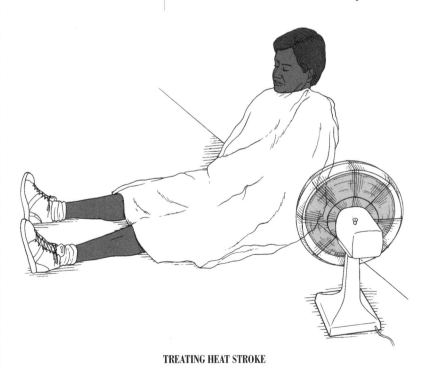

**TREATING HEAT STROKE**

### Heat Exhaustion

Heat exhaustion occurs when the body temperature rises dramatically but stays below 104°F and the victim sweats excessively. Heat exhaustion is a problem of loss of fluids (*dehydration*) in hot weather. Symptoms of heat exhaustion include weakness, nausea, excess sweating and fainting. The person's skin may be pale and clammy. Treatment includes the replacement of lost salt and water to the body through lightly salted fluids or foods. The victim should lie down or have his or her head down.

longer regulate its temperature. When the body temperature is above 104°F and the person is hot and red and has no sweat on the skin, he or she is suffering from heat stroke. If not treated promptly, the victim's temperature will keep rising, resulting in confusion, unconsciousness and death. Heat stroke can also cause tiredness, dizziness, nausea and headache.

### Heat Cramps

Heat cramps are the result of strenuous activity in hot temperatures. Heat cramps may make muscles feel hard, knotted and painful, and usually occur in the legs or abdomen. There are few signs prior to heat cramps because the skin of the victim can be hot and dry or clammy and cool. Treatment and prevention of heat cramps is drinking salty fluids or eating salty food. Gentle stretching and massaging the muscle can also bring relief.

**2. Administer first aid.** Move the victim into an air-conditioned building or into the shade. Wrap the person in a sheet soaked with cool water. To aid the cooling process, use a fan blowing over the sheet to evaporate the water. Continue until the temperature is down.

**3. Prevent shock.** After the victim's temperature drops, give treatment to prevent shock by covering the victim with a light, dry sheet. If the victim is awake, have him or her lie on the back with the feet raised.

## Nosebleed

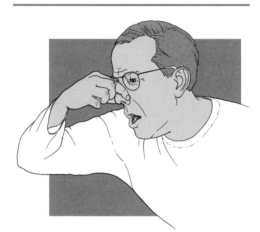

**TREATING A NOSEBLEED**

**1. Assess the situation.** Most nosebleeds are minor and can be easily handled. Rarely, a severe nosebleed will require emergency treatment to slow and stop the blood flow.

**2. Administer first aid.** Most nosebleeds can be controlled by leaning forward and pinching the lower part of the nose shut for at least five minutes. Use a clock for timing, because the major reason this simple treatment fails is not keeping the pressure on long enough. Don't lie down. Lying down causes the blood to flow into the back of the mouth and be swallowed.

**3. Seek help.** If pinching doesn't stop the bleeding within 10 to 15 minutes, or if the bleeding is excessive and brisk, seek emergency care.

## Poisoning

**1. Assess the situation.** If a child or adult has accidentally swallowed a poison, first find out what the poison is.

**2. Call for information.** Call the nearest poison control center for instructions. Don't force the victim to vomit and don't give him or her syrup of ipecac or anything to drink until you know what the victim has ingested and have been instructed by the poison control center.

**3. Seek help.** Have the victim seen right away by a doctor to assess the physical effects of the substance and recommend treatment.

## Rape

Rape, or sexual assault, is a violent act in which sexual action is forced on one person by another. Rape is used as a weapon to physically abuse or express power, aggression and hostility toward the victim. Victims are usually women, though men can also be raped anally.

**1. Call for help right away.** If you're helping someone who has been raped, get them to the hospital to have a physical exam and be helped emotionally. Make sure they don't shower or clean up. Evidence will be gathered during the physical exam in the emergency room. This is for legal reasons and will include a pelvic exam and blood and urine tests. If the victim is a woman, there may also be questions about the last menstrual period (to determine the likelihood of pregnancy), the last date of sexual intercourse (for accurate sperm testing) and the use of contraceptives.

Antibiotics (p. 618) may be given to prevent sexually transmitted disease (STD, p. 316). Blood may be drawn for an HIV test.

**2. Be understanding about the victim's feelings.** If someone you know has been raped, they may feel overwhelming fear. They may fear that the rapist will return. They may also fear unfamiliar situations or their current surroundings. Many people who have been raped feel guilty. They may begin to think about what they could have done to stop the attack. Or they may start believing they somehow brought on the attack. This reaction of self-blame is actually a method of feeling more in control. They may also start to believe the sexual assault was their punishment for being a "bad person." It's quite common to have strong feelings of anger toward the rapist. They may also be angry at themselves for not fighting back. They may even feel angry at themselves for having vengeful feelings toward the rapist. If the rapist was a spouse, a relative or someone they know, they may be angry about being deceived and betrayed.

They may also suffer from post-traumatic stress disorder (p. 582), an anxiety disorder produced by an uncommon or extremely stressful event. The disorder causes victims to vividly re-experience the original trauma in persistent thoughts or recurrent dreams or nightmares. Other symptoms include disturbed sleep patterns, difficulty concentrating or remembering, guilt about surviving and avoidance of activities that call the event to mind.

**3. Encourage counseling.** Counseling can be very useful. Working through the feelings and the changes is healthy. Unresolved guilt and anger can cause depression, low self-esteem and additional physical and emotional difficulties. The victim may feel too ashamed and guilt-laden to handle group counseling right after the assault, but can start with one-on-one therapy and try group therapy later.

## Seizures

**1. Assess the victim.** When a person passes out, becomes stiff, tense and perhaps bluish in color, or jerks back and forth, he or she is having a seizure. Seizures are involuntary and are most commonly seen as jerking or twitching muscles and loss of consciousness. Try to keep the person from injuring him or herself by clearing the area of furniture and other objects. Don't try to limit the movements of someone having a seizure. After the seizure is over, check for breathing and injuries.

**2. Position the victim.** If the seizures have stopped, roll the victim to his or her side to help prevent choking on a bitten tongue, blood or secretions from the mouth. Don't place anything into the mouth of a victim having seizures. Have a bystander call 911, the rescue squad or police if the seizure lasts more than about a minute, if the seizure is repeated, if the person is pregnant or if the person isn't known to be epileptic. If the victim is unconscious but breathing, roll him or her to the side and cover with a blanket. If awake, have him or her lie on the back with the feet raised and cover him or her with a blanket. For more information on seizures, see page 56.

## Splinter

**1. Assess the situation.** Check the source of the splinter and guess its size.

**2. Grasp the splinter with tweezers.** If it's protruding, grasp the splinter with tweezers and pull gently. If it's embedded just under the skin, clean the area with antiseptic, then use a needle (cleansed in antiseptic or heated in a flame) to split the skin until the end of the splinter is exposed and can be grasped with the tweezers.

**3. Seek help.** If the splinter doesn't

## R-I-C-E

One approach to treating a sprain is called R-I-C-E, which stands for rest, ice, compression and elevation.

**Rest.** You may need to stay off of your ankle completely or put only light weight on it, depending on how bad the sprain is. Crutches can be used as long as you can't stand comfortably on the foot.

**Ice.** Use ice packs, ice slush baths or ice massages to decrease pain, swelling, bruising and muscle cramps or spasms. Don't use heat for at least three days.

**Compression.** Wrap the ankle with an elastic bandage for a day or two to try to reduce swelling and bruising.

**Elevation.** Raise the ankle above the level of your heart to prevent swelling from getting worse and lessen bruising. Try to keep the ankle elevated for two to three hours a day.

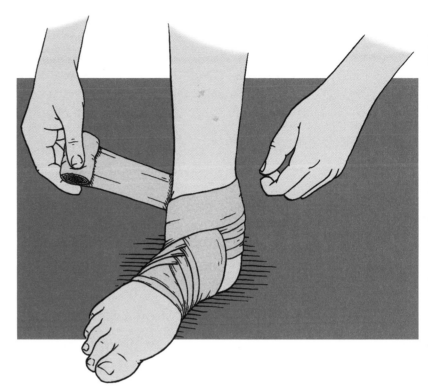

**HOW TO WRAP A SPRAINED ANKLE**

come out easily, is large or is deeply embedded, see your doctor about removing it.

### Sprains or Torn Ligaments

**1. Assess the injury.** Any joint can be involved in a sprain, or the stretching or tearing of a ligament. Mild sprains may not even swell, while more serious sprains swell immediately and may leave a deformed joint and a bruise under the skin. Because the pain of a sprained joint (especially an ankle or knee) may prevent walking, treat a sprain initially as a fracture.

**2. Administer first aid.** Apply a cool compress or ice wrapped in a cloth to the tender area. If an elastic bandage or cloth wrap is available, wrap the injury, starting at the farthest point from the heart. For example, when the sprain affects an ankle, start wrapping

### How to Use Ice Packs

Ice can be very helpful in the treatment of a sprain, but if ice is applied to an injury for a long period of time, the cold can damage the nerves. Apply ice to an injured body part only for up to 20 minutes at a time, or until the skin feels numb. Use ice as treatment every two to four hours for three days after the injury. Use an ice pack, an ice slush bath from a bucket of water and ice, or an ice massage, which is holding a piece of ice directly on the skin for less than 30 seconds at a time.

near the toes and progress toward and across the ankle joint. Don't wrap too tightly, because you can cut off the blood flow to the injured area. Wrapping the sprained part helps keep the swelling to a minimum. Elevate the extremity.

**3. Seek help.** If the person is unable to walk using the leg with the injured ankle or knee, or if severe swelling or bruising remain within a few days, the injured joint should be checked by a doctor. If you believe it may be fractured, call your doctor right away.

## Tooth Loss

**1. Assess the injury.** Examine the mouth of the victim for pieces of tooth and determine how many teeth are damaged or missing.

**2. Save the tooth or fragments.** Find the tooth (or collect any pieces). Wash the tooth or place it in a warm salt-water solution. You may be able to gently replace a full tooth into the socket. If a gentle bite holds it in place, it can be kept there until you can get to a dentist.

**3. Seek help.** Always see your dentist about a broken or lost tooth as soon as possible. Even children who lose baby teeth due to an injury should be seen by a dentist. Sometimes these teeth can also be reimplanted to help keep the spacing of the remaining teeth.

## Toxic Inhalation

The most dangerous part of a house fire isn't the flames but the smoke or other toxic fumes, such as carbon monoxide, that can be inhaled. If you're involved with a situation where toxic gas or smoke has been inhaled, follow these basic steps.

**1. Get the victim to safety.** Remove the victim from the fumes or smoke. If you don't have breathing gear, stay as low to the ground as possible. Covering your face with a wet cloth may not protect you from the toxic gases. Don't re-enter a burning house once you get outside.

**2. Breathe for the victim.** If the victim isn't breathing, begin mouth-to-mouth resuscitation. Give two breaths, then check for a pulse and, if you're trained, begin CPR if no pulse is detected. Continue mouth-to-mouth resuscitation and CPR until pulse and breathing have returned.

**3. Prevent shock.** Once breathing is restored, roll the victim to the side and cover with a blanket. If awake, have the victim lie on his or her back with the feet elevated and cover with a blanket.

# MEDICINE CABINET

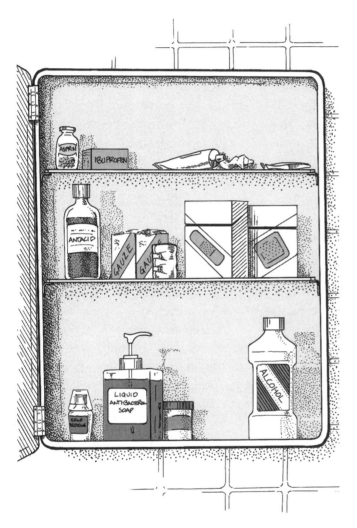

Accidents, cuts, scrapes and other minor medical problems are a common part of family life. Most people understand how to take care of simple health problems.

You'll need basic supplies, as well as basic information, when an injury occurs or sickness arises. The box below includes suggested materials, supplies and medicines that may be useful in providing basic first aid.

In addition to the supplies listed in the box below, you may need to keep other medicines on hand, depending on the medicines your doctor may prescribe for you or you choose to have available on your own. Medicines can be powerful allies to treat disease or relieve symptoms. But they can also cause problems when taken incorrectly or with another medicine that causes an unfavorable interaction.

This guide will provide general information about many medicines you can buy without a prescription, called *over-the-counter* medicines, and some of the most commonly prescribed medicines. Not all of these medicines are right for you or will treat your symptoms correctly. If a medicine isn't listed here, or if you have questions about a medicine or about which one to take, call your doctor.

If proper use of an over-the-counter medicine doesn't relieve your symptoms, consult your doctor. Also call your doctor if you have any side

---

## Basics for Your Medicine Cabinet

| **Supplies** | Safety pins | **Medicines** | Cough medicines |
|---|---|---|---|
| Adhesive bandages in assorted sizes | Sterile gauze dressings | Activated charcoal | Hydrocortisone cream |
| Adhesive tape | Tweezers | Allergy medicines, such as antihistamines | Syrup of ipecac (always call your |
| Bandage scissors | **Cleansers** | Analgesic medicine | local Poison Hotline |
| Elastic bandage | Alcohol | Antibiotic ointment | before giving |
| Nonadhesive bandages | Liquid anti-bacterial soap | Antidiarrheal medicine | anything after |
| Roll gauze | Mild soap | Cold medicines, such as decongestants | a poisoning or overdose.) |

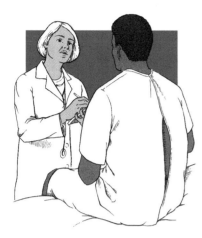

effects from taking an over-the-counter or prescription medicine. Never take another person's prescription medicine. It can be dangerous. Each medicine has specific uses, and medicines can react harmfully when mixed. Most medicines have some side effects. Don't take left-over medicine that was prescribed for you months ago. Medicines have expiration dates. Read the instructions for all medicines carefully and follow the instructions exactly. Even taking over-the-counter medicines incorrectly can be dangerous. The right way to take a medicine depends on the reason you're taking it. How much medicine you take is often determined by your age, body weight and other concerns. Always finish your prescription as your doctor orders. If you have any questions about a medicine, consult your doctor.

Medicines in this section are generally grouped under headings that describe their use, though some medicines that don't fit within a certain group or that are very commonly used are listed separately. Specific medicines are listed alphabetically under those headings by generic name, with some corresponding brand names listed in *italic* print.

These listings don't include any information about how much of a medicine to take or about possible side effects. Read labels carefully, and talk to your doctor or pharmacist about these issues.

## Over-the-Counter Medicines

**Acetaminophen.** Non-aspirin medicine is used to reduce pain and fever. Examples: *Panadol, Tempra, Tylenol.*

**Acne medicines.** Acne medicines are used to prevent and treat pimples and acne. Examples: benzoyl peroxide (*Oxy 5*), salicylic acid (*Stri-Dex*).

**Analgesics, dental.** These medicines are used to ease the pain of mouth sores. Examples: benzocaine (*Orajel*).

**Analgesics, oral.** Analgesics are used to relieve pain. Examples: acetaminophen, aspirin, ibuprofen, ketoprofen, naproxen. (**Warning:** Don't give aspirin to children due to the risk of Reye's syndrome.)

**Analgesics, topical.** These medicines are used to help relieve pain on the skin. Examples: benzocaine (*Americaine, Solarcaine*), capsaicin (*Zostrix*), dibucaine (*Nupercainal*), lidocaine (*DermaFlex, Xylocaine*), methyl salicylate (*Ben-Gay*), trolamine (*Aspercreme, Mobisyl, Sportscreme*).

**Antacids.** Antacids are used to neutralize the acidity of the stomach. They are particularly useful in the

---

### *Avoiding Problems While Taking Medicine*

- Make sure your doctor is aware of any allergies to medicines you have. Tell him or her about any side effects you had while taking a medicine.
- Tell your doctor the medicines you're taking. If you're being treated by more than one doctor, make sure each doctor knows what the other doctor has prescribed for you. This can help prevent drug interactions.
- Never drink alcohol while taking a medicine without asking your doctor or pharmacist first about possible interactions.

- If you have a serious side effect or an adverse reaction to a medicine, call your doctor right away. Don't use the medicine again until you talk to your doctor. Make sure both you and your doctor keep a list of medicines that have caused adverse reactions.
- Take your medicine exactly as your doctor tells you.
- Remember that medicine is dated to ensure its potency. Check your medicine cabinet periodically and throw away old medicines.

management of heartburn. Examples: aluminum (*AlternaGEL, Basaljel*), calcium (*Rolaids, Tums*), magnesia (*Phillips' Milk of Magnesia*), combinations (*Gaviscon, Maalox, Mylanta*).

**Antibiotic ointments and creams.** These medicines are used to treat minor wounds of the skin and help prevent infection. Examples: bacitracin (*Mycitracin, Polysporin*), neomycin (*Neosporin*).

**Antidiarrheal medicines.** These medicines treat diarrhea by slowing down the movement of the intestines. Examples: attapulgite (*Donnagel, Kaopectate*), bismuth subsalicylate (*Pepto-Bismol*), loperamide (*Imodium*).

**Antifungal medicines, topical.** Antifungal medicines are used to treat and prevent fungal infections of the skin, such as athlete's foot and jock itch. Examples: tolnaftate (*Aftate, Desenex, Tinactin*), undecylenic acid (*Cruex*).

**Antifungal medicines, vaginal.** These are special antifungal preparations used to treat vaginal yeast infections. Examples: clotrimazole (*Gyne-Lotrimin, Mycelex-7*), miconazole (*Monistat 7*).

**Antihelmintic medicines.** These medicines are used to eliminate pinworms. Example: pyrantel (*Pin-X*).

**Antihistamines.** Antihistamines are used to treat allergies. They block the release of histamine in the body. Histamine is the substance that causes symptoms such as runny nose, sneezing and stuffy nose from allergic reactions. Antihistamines often cause drowsiness as a side effect, and they don't help a cold or flu unless you have allergies, too. They're also used to reduce mild inflammation from allergic reactions, such as to bee stings or bug bites, as sleep aids and to treat motion sickness. Examples: chlorpheniramine (*Chlor-Trimeton Allergy Tablets*), clemastine (*Tavist-1*), diphenhydramine (*Benadryl Allergy*), triprolidine (*Actifed*). Antihistamines are often included in combination medicines that also contain decongestants, analgesics, cough suppressants and/or expectorants (see oral decongestants, p. 616).

**Anti-inflammatory medicines.** These medicines can reduce inflammation, such as the swelling that may occur with back pain. See non-steroidal anti-inflammatory medicines.

**Anti-itch medicines.** These medicines help relieve itching of the skin, including that caused by poison ivy. Examples: calamine (*Caladryl*), benzyl alcohol + pramoxine (*Itch-X*), diphenhydramine + zinc acetate (*Benadryl Itch Relief*), hydrocortisone (*Anusol HC, CaldeCort, Cortaid, Cortizone-5*).

**Antilice medicines.** These shampoos, conditioners and lotions are designed to eliminate lice. Examples: permethrin (*Nix*), pyrethrins (*Rid*).

**Antinausea medicines.** These medicines are used to ease nausea and vomiting. They're also called antiemetics. Example: dimenhydrinate (*Dramamine*).

**Antipyretic.** See fever-reducing medicines.

**Antiseptics.** These substances inhibit the growth of bacteria. These are used to cleanse wounds. Examples: *Bactine, Campho-Phenique, Stri-Dex Antibacterial Cleansing Bar.*

**Appetite suppressants.** To reduce hunger to aid weight loss. Examples: phenylpropanolamine (*Acutrim, Dexatrim*).

**Aspirin.** The chemical name for aspirin is acetylsalicylic acid. It's a common medicine used to relieve pain, inflammation and fever. Use of aspirin in children has been associated with Reye's syndrome, a rare but sometimes fatal disease. Never give aspirin to children unless your doctor says it's okay. Examples: *Bayer, Bufferin.*

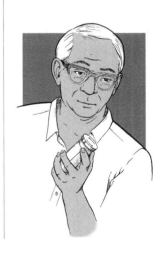

**Charcoal, activated.** This can be taken for the emergency treatment of poisoning. Example: *Charcoaid.*

**Corn-removing solutions.** These medicines help dissolve corns and calluses. Example: salicylic acid (*Dr. Scholl's Corn/Callus Remover*).

**Cough suppressants.** Cough suppressants, also called antitussives, help keep you from coughing. That's good if you're suffering from a dry cough, but bad if you're coughing up mucus. A mucus cough is a productive cough and you don't want to suppress it. Examples: dextromethorphan (*Scot-Tussin Cough Chasers*), diphenhydramine (*Benylin Cough Suppressant*). Cough suppressants are often included in combination preparations that include decongestants, antihistamines, analgesics and/or expectorants (see oral decongestants).

**Dandruff treatments.** These shampoos and conditioners help relieve the dryness, itching and flaking of dandruff. Examples: coal tar (*MG217, Tegrin, X-Seb*), selenium sulfide (*Head & Shoulders, Selsun Blue*).

**Decongestants, nasal sprays.** These relieve congestion by causing the nasal passages to shrink. They can help temporarily, but they make the stuffiness worse if you use them for more than three days in a row. Examples: phenylephrine (*Neo-Synephrine, Sinex*), oxymetazoline (*Afrin*).

**Decongestants, oral.** These can help clear up congestion by shrinking the nasal passages and may reduce your risk of a bacterial infection. Examples: ephedrine, phenylpropanolamine, pseudoephedrine. Decongestants are usually included in combination preparations with antihistamines, analgesics, cough medicines and/or expectorants. Examples: *Actifed, Alka-Seltzer Cold or Allergy, Allerest, Comtrex, Contac, Coricidin D, Dimetapp, Drixoral, Isoclor Timesule Capsules, Robitussin, Sinarest, Sine-Aid, Sine-Off, Singlet, Sinutab, Suda-fed, TheraFlu, Triaminicin, Vicks 44, Vicks NyQuil.*

**Diaper rash treatment.** These medicines help protect the baby's skin from outside moisture so that it can heal. Example: vitamins A, D and E topical (*A and D Medicated*), zinc oxide (*Caldesene, Desenex, Desitin*).

**Diuretics.** These medicines are used for relief of menstrual discomfort, excess water weight, and bloating and swelling due to water retention. They often come mixed with other medicines. Example: pamabrom (*Bayer Select Menstrual Multi-Symptom Formula, PMS Multi-Symptom Formula Midol*).

**Expectorants.** Expectorants may help liquify mucus and congestion when you have a cold. Drinking plenty of water helps do the same thing. Example: guaifenesin (*Scot-Tussin Expectorant*). Expectorants are often included in combination preparations that also contain decongestants, antihistamines, analgesics and/or cough suppressants (see oral decongestants).

**Fever-reducing medicines.** These medicines, also called *antipyretics*, are used to reduce fever. Examples: acetaminophen, aspirin, ibuprofen, ketoprofen, naproxen. (**Warning:** Don't give aspirin to children due to the risk of Reye's syndrome.)

**Hemorrhoid treatments.** These medicines may help shrink hemorrhoids. They often contain ingredients to reduce the itching, burning and discomfort associated with hemorrhoids. Examples: *Anusol HC, Preparation H, Tucks.*

**Hydrocortisone creams and ointments.** These medicines are used to relieve the itching associated with dry skin, psoriasis, dermatitis, poison ivy, poison oak, insect bites and for external feminine and anal itching. Examples: *Anusol, CaldeCort, Cortaid, Cortizone-5.*

**Ibuprofen.** This is a nonsteroidal anti-inflammatory medicine. It may be used to relieve pain, reduce fever and reduce inflammation. Examples: *Advil, Medipren, Motrin, Nuprin.*

**Lactase.** Lactase enzyme can be taken to help prevent the gastrointestinal symptoms of lactase deficiency, or lactose intolerance, that some people get after eating dairy products. Examples: *Dairy Ease, LactAid.*

**Laxatives, bulk-forming.** Laxatives are used to relieve constipation. Bulk-forming laxatives work naturally to add bulk and water to stools. Examples: bran, methylcellulose (*Citrucel*), polycarbophil (*FiberCon*), psyllium (*Fiberall, Metamucil, Perdiem, Serutan*).

**Laxatives, stimulant.** These laxatives work to relieve constipation by stimulating the intestines. Example: *Dulcolax, Ex-Lax.*

**Motion sickness treatments.** These medicines help relieve motion sickness. Examples: dimenhydrinate (*Dramamine*), meclizine (*Bonine*).

**Naproxen.** This is a nonsteroidal anti-inflammatory medicine. It may be used to relieve pain, reduce fever and reduce inflammation. Example: *Aleve.*

**Nonsteroidal anti-inflammatory (NSAIDs).** These medicines are used to reduce inflammation, or swelling. Examples: aspirin, ibuprofen, ketoprofen, naproxen. (**Warning:** Don't give aspirin to children due to the risk of Reye's syndrome.)

**Oral rehydration therapy.** These solutions are given to prevent or treat dehydration. Examples: *Pedialyte, Rehydralyte.*

**Petroleum jelly.** Petroleum jelly helps protect chafed or dry skin. Example: *Vaseline.*

**Sleep aids.** Sleep aids can be taken on a temporary basis to treat insomnia. Examples: diphenhydramine (*Nytol, Sominex*), doxylamine succinate (*Unisom*).

**Spermicides.** Spermicides are used as a contraceptive to kill sperm to prevent pregnancy. They may also help prevent some sexually transmitted diseases. Examples: nonoxynol-9 (*Conceptrol, Encare, Semicid*), octoxynol (*Ortho-Gynol*).

**Syrup of ipecac.** Syrup of ipecac is used to induce vomiting due to poisoning. Use it only after consulting with your doctor, a pharmacist or the poison control center.

**Ulcer medicines.** These medicines are used to treat gastritis and peptic ulcers. Examples: cimetidine (*Tagamet*), famotidine (*Pepcid*), ranitidine (*Zantac*).

**Vaginal lubricants.** These lubricants can be used to ease dryness in the vagina. Examples: *Gyne-Moistrin, K-Y Jelly, Replens.*

**Wart removers.** These medicines are used to dissolve warts on the hands, feet and other areas of the skin. Note that they don't treat genital warts, which require prescription medicines. Example: salicylic acid (*Compound W, Wart-Off*).

## Prescription Medicines

**Acne medicines.** These medicines are used to treat acne vulgaris, rosacea and related skin disorders. Examples: benzoyl peroxide (*Benzac W Wash, Desquam-X 5 Wash, PanOxyl*), clindamycin (*Cleocin*), erythromycin (*T-Stat*), isotretinoin (*Accutane*), meclocycline (*Meclan*), metronidazole (*Metro-Gel*), tretinoin (*Retin-A*).

**Alpha blockers.** These medicines are used to help the blood vessels expand. They're prescribed for high blood pressure. Example: phenoxybenzamine (*Dibenzyline*).

**Amphetamine.** This is a stimulant of the central nervous system with a high potential for abuse. Legitimate uses of this medicine include treatment of narcolepsy and attention deficit disorder.

**Analgesics, narcotic, oral.** These medicines are used to relieve pain throughout the body. Some of them also have other uses, such as suppressing coughs and stopping diarrhea. Examples: butorphanol tartrate (*Stadol*), codeine, hydromorphone (*Dilaudid*), levorphanol tartrate (*Levo-Dromoran*), meperidine (*Demerol*), methadone (*Dolophine*), morphine (*MS Contin*), opium (*Paregoric*), oxycodone (*Roxicodone*), propoxyphene (*Darvon*).

**Analgesics, non-narcotic, oral.** These medicines are used to relieve pain. They're often used to treat arthritis, headaches and pain from other causes. Examples: acetaminophen, aspirin, diflunisal (*Dolobid*), ibuprofen, naproxen, salsalate (*Disalcid*), tramadol (*Ultram*).

**Analgesics, urinary tract.** This medicine can be taken to ease the pain associated with urinary tract infections. Example: phenazopyridine (*Pyridium*).

**Anesthetics.** These medicines are used to prevent the sensation of pain. They can be administered locally, to relieve pain in a certain area of the body, or generally, so that the person becomes temporarily unconscious. For example, an epidural anesthetic is used during labor to reduce the pain of contractions, while a general anesthetic is often needed for surgical procedures such as appendectomy.

**Angiotensin-converting enzyme inhibitors (ACE inhibitors).** These medicines help control blood pressure by inhibiting the production of certain enzymes (angiotensin II) in the kidneys. They're also used to treat congestive heart failure. Examples: benazepril hydrochloride (*Lotensin*), captopril (*Capoten*), enalapril (*Vasotec*), fosinopril (*Monopril*), lisinopril (*Prinivil, Zestril*), moexipril (*Univasc*), quinapril hydrochloride (*Accupril*), ramipril (*Altace*).

**Antiadrenergic medicines.** These medicines are used to reduce high blood pressure and to treat congestive heart failure. Examples: clonidine hydrochloride (*Catapres*), doxazosin (*Cardura*), guanabenz (*Wytensin*), guanadrel (*Hylorel*), guanethidine (*Ismelin*), guanfacine (*Tenex*), methyldopa (*Aldomet*), prazosin (*Minipress*), reserpine (*Serpasil*), terazosin (*Hytrin*).

**Antianginal medicines.** These medicines are used to treat and prevent angina, congestive heart failure and heart attack. They expand blood vessels. Examples: dipyridamole (*Persantine*), isosorbide dinitrate (*Isordil*), nitroglycerin capsules (*Nitro-Bid*), nitroglycerin ointment (*Nitrol*), nitroglycerin sublingual (*Nitrostat*), nitroglycerin transdermal (*Nitro-Dur, Minitran*).

**Antianxiety medicines.** See sedatives.

**Antiarrhythmic medicines.** These medicines are used to stabilize and strengthen the heart rhythm and regulate the heartbeat and function. They're used to treat atrial arrhythmia, atrial fibrillation, atrial flutter, paroxysmal supraventricular tachycardia and ventricular arrhythmia. Examples: disopyramide (*Norpace*), flecainide (*Tambocor*), mexiletine (*Mexitil*), procainamide (*Pronestyl*), procainamide sustained-release (*Procan SR*), quinidine sulfate (*Quinidex Extentabs*), tocainide (*Tonocard*).

**Antibiotics.** These medicines are used to treat infections, primarily those caused by bacteria. Overuse and misuse of antibiotics has led to bacteria that are harder to kill. This, in turn, can lead to more serious and prolonged infections. That's one reason it's important that you take all the antibiotic prescribed by your doctor. Examples: cephalosporins, fluoroquinolones, furazolidone (*Furoxone*), macrolides, metronidazole (*Flagyl*), penicillins, pentamidine (*Pentam 300*), sulfonamides, tetracyclines, trimethoprim (*Proloprim, Trimpex*), trimethoprim + sulfamethoxazole (*Bactrim*).

**Antibiotics, urinary tract.** These antibiotics are designed to treat infections of the urinary tract. Examples: cinoxacin (*Cinobac*), methenamine hippurate (*Hiprex*), methenamine mandelate (*Mandelamine*), nalidixic acid (*NegGram*), nitrofurantoin (*Furadantin, Macrodantin*).

**Anticlotting medicines.** These medicines are used to thin the blood to prevent clotting and to treat pulmonary emboli. Examples: heparin, warfarin (*Coumadin, Panwarfin*).

**Antidepressants.** These medicines are used to treat various forms of depression and related disorders, such as anxiety, obsessive behaviors and sleep disorders. Examples: amitriptyline (*Elavil*), amoxapine (*Asendin*), bupropion (*Wellbutrin*), clomipramine (*Anafranil*), desipramine (*Norpramin*), doxepin (*Sinequan, Adapin*), fluoxetine (*Prozac*), imipramine (*Tofranil*), maprotiline (*Ludiomil*), nortriptyline (*Pamelor, Aventyl*), sertraline (*Zoloft*), trazodone (*Desyrel*), trimipramine (*Surmontil*).

**Antifungal medicines, general.** These medicines are used to treat fungal infections such as oral candidiasis, fungal infections of the lung, ringworm, athlete's foot and other fungal skin infections. Examples: amphotericin B, fluconazole (*Diflucan*), griseofulvin (*Fulvicin, Grisactin, Gris-PEG*), itraconazole (*Sporanox*), ketoconazole (*Nizoral*), nystatin (*Mycostatin*).

**Antifungal medicines, vaginal.** These medicines are used to treat fungal infections of the vagina, commonly known as "yeast infections." Examples: butoconazole (*Femstat*), clotrimazole (*Mycelex-7*), miconazole (*Monistat Dual-Pak*), terconazole (*Terazol 7*), tioconazole (*Vagistat*).

**Antigout medicines.** These medicines lower the body's concentration of uric acid which is the substance that's responsible for gout. These medicines are used to treat and prevent attacks of gout. Examples: allopurinol (*Zyloprim*), colchicine (*Colchicine*), probenecid (*Benemid*), sulfinpyrazone (*Anturane*).

**Antihistamines.** Antihistamines are used to treat allergies. They block the release of histamine in the body. Histamine is the substance that causes allergic symptoms such as runny nose, sneezing and inflammation or swelling of the nasal membranes. Some antihistamines are also used to reduce mild inflammation from allergic reactions, as sleep aids and to treat motion sickness. Examples: astemizole (*Hismanal*), azatadine (*Optimine*), cyproheptadine (*Periactin*), dexchlorpheniramine (*Polaramine*), loratadine (*Claritin*), promethazine (*Phener-gan*), terfenadine (*Seldane*), tripelennamine (*PBZ*).

**Antihypertensive medicines.** This group of medicines is used to treat high blood pressure. Examples: alpha blockers, angiotensin-converting enzyme (ACE) inhibitors, beta blockers, calcium channel blockers, diuretics.

**Anti-inflammatory medicines.** These medicines are used to reduce inflammation, or swelling. Examples: nonsteroidal anti-inflammatory medicines, corticosteroids.

**Antilice medicines.** These shampoos, conditioners and lotions are used to rid the body of lice. Examples:

crotamiton (*Eurax*), lindane (*Kwell*), permethrin (*Elimite Cream*).

**Antimalarial medicines.** These medicines are used to treat malarial infections and to prevent malarial infections in people traveling to areas where this protozoal infection is likely. They are also used to treat giardiasis and nocturnal leg cramps, and to prevent certain types of pneumonia in people who have AIDS. Example: chloroquine (*Aralen*), hydroxychloroquine (*Plaquenil Sulfate*), mefloquine (*Lariam*), primaquine (*Primaquine Phosphate*), pyrimethamine (*Daraprim*), quinine (*Quinamim*), chloroquine + primaquine (*Aralen Phosphate with Primaquine Phosphate*), sulfadoxine + pyrimethamine (*Fansidar*).

**Antinausea and antivomiting medicines.** These medicines are used to treat nausea and vomiting, including drug-induced nausea or vomiting (such as that caused by chemotherapy) or symptoms associated with viral infections. These medicines are also used to relieve hiccups that won't go away. Examples: chlorpromazine (*Thorazine*), granisetron (*Kytril*), metoclopramide (*Reglan*), ondansetron (*Zofran*), prochlorperazine (*Compazine*), promethazine (*Phenergan*), thiethylperazine (*Torecan*).

**Antiparasitic medicines.** These medicines are used to treat various types of parasitic worm infections, such as hookworm, pinworm, roundworm and whipworm. Examples: mebendazole (*Vermox*), piperazine (*Piperazine*), praziquantel (*Biltricide*), pyrantel (*Antiminth*), quinacrine (*Atabrine*), thiabendazole (*Mintezol*).

**Antipsychotic medicines.** These medicines are used to treat severe nervous and mental disorders such as manic depression and schizophrenia. They may also be used to treat cluster headaches and Tourette syndrome. Examples: chlorpromazine (*Thorazine*), clozapine (*Clozaril*), fluphenazine (*Prolixin*), haloperidol (*Haldol*), lithium (*Eskalith*), loxapine (*Loxitane*), mesoridazine (*Serentil*), perphenazine (*Trilafon*), prochlorperazine (*Compazine*), thioridazine (*Mellaril*), thiothixene (*Navane*), trifluoperazine (*Stelazine*).

**Antirheumatic medicines.** A diverse group of drugs, including aspirin, NSAIDs and steroids, used to treat rheumatoid arthritis and related conditions. Other medicines, called slow-acting antirheumatic medicines, are used to treat active rheumatoid arthritis (RA), acute gouty arthritis, bursitis, degenerative joint disorder (DJD) and systemic lupus erythematosus. Examples: auranofin (*Ridaura*), aurothioglucose (*Solganol*), gold sodium, hydroxychloroquine (*Plaquenil*), indomethacin (*Indocin*), methotrexate (*Rheumatrex*), penicillamine (*Cuprimine, Depen*), prednisone (*Deltasone*), thiomalate (*Myochrysine*).

**Antiseizure medicines.** These medicines may be used to control epilepsy and related seizure disorders, and some may be used to treat trigeminal neuralgia. Examples: carbamazepine (*Tegretol*), clonazepam (*Klonopin*), clorazepate (*Tranxene*), diazepam (*Valium*), ethosuximide (*Zarontin*), gabapentin (*Neurontin*), lamotrigine (*Lamictal*), phenytoin (*Dilantin*), primidone (*Mysoline*), valproic acid (*Depakene*).

**Antispasmodic and anticramping medicines.** These medicines are used to treat several different gastrointestinal problems, including peptic ulcer, diarrhea, irritable bowel syndrome and ulcerative colitis. These medicines are also used to treat diverticulitis, diarrhea and motion sickness. Examples: atropine (*Atropine Sulfate*), belladonna (*Belladonna Tinc-*

*ture*), clidinium (*Quarzan*), dicyclomine (*Bentyl*), glycopyrrolate (*Robinul*), hyoscyamine (*Levsin, Anaspaz*), propantheline (*Pro-Banthine*).

**Antiviral medicines.** These medicines are used to treat viral infections, such as cytomegalovirus in people who have AIDS, herpes infections, influenza A and respiratory syncytial virus. Examples: acyclovir (*Zovirax*), amantadine (*Symmetrel*), didanosine (*Videx*), ganciclovir (*Cytovene*), ribavirin (*Virazole*), trifluridine (*Viroptic*), vidarabine (*Vir-A*), zidovudine (*Retrovir*).

**Arsenic.** Arsenic is a highly toxic chemical that can be used to treat some parasitic infections, skin disorders and defects in making blood cells.

**Barbiturate.** A type of sedative. Barbiturates may be used to relieve tension, anxiety and insomnia, and to treat seizure disorders. These drugs are addictive, and an overdose can be life-threatening.

**Benzodiazepines.** A class of sedative and antianxiety medicines.

**Beta-adrenergic blockers.** These medicines block the effects of adrenaline. They can be used to reduce blood pressure, control heart rhythm and reduce angina. They can also be used to prevent migraine and tension headaches. Examples: acebutolol (*Sectral*), atenolol (*Tenormin*), betaxolol (*Kerlone*), metoprolol (*Lopressor*), nadolol (*Corgard*), penbutolol (*Levatol*), pindolol (*Visken*), propranolol (*Inderal*), timolol (*Blocadren*).

**Bile acid sequestrants.** These medicines lower cholesterol by binding intestinal bile acids to form an insoluble complex that's excreted from the body. The increased loss of bile acids causes the body to produce more, which requires the body to use cholesterol in the process. These medicines can be used to treat high cholesterol levels and biliary obstruction. Examples: cholestyramine (*Questran*), colestipol (*Colestid*).

**Bronchodilators.** These medicines relax the muscles around the bronchial tubes (the large air passages that connect to the lungs), increasing the size of the bronchial tubes and restoring normal airflow. This is important in treating asthma, emphysema, bronchitis and severe chest congestion. These medicines relieve coughing, wheezing, shortness of breath and troubled breathing. They're also used to treat interstitial lung disease and occupational lung diseases. Bronchodilators can be given in an inhaled form. They also can be given in pill or liquid form. Examples: albuterol (*Proventil, Ventolin Rotacaps, Ventolin*), bitolterol (*Tornalate*), dyphylline (*Dilor*), isoproterenol (*Isuprel*), metaproterenol (*Alupent*), oxtriphylline (*Choledyl*), pirbuterol (*Maxair*), terbutaline (*Brethine, Bricanyl*), theophylline (*Slo-bid Gyrocaps, Theo-Dur*).

**Calcipotriene.** This medicine can be used to treat psoriasis. Example: *Dovonex*.

**Calcium channel blockers.** These medicines help prevent the blood vessels from constricting by blocking calcium from entering the cells. They can be used to reduce blood pressure, control heart rhythm, treat angina and congestive heart failure, and prevent cluster and migraine headaches. Examples: bepridil (*Vascor*), diltiazem (*Cardizem*), felodipine (*Plendil*), nicardipine (*Cardene*), nifedipine (*Procardia*), verapamil (*Calan, Isoptin*).

**Cephalosporins.** These medicines are a type of antibiotic. Examples: cefaclor (*Ceclor*), cefadroxil (*Duricef, Ultracef*), cefixime (*Suprax*), cefprozil (*Cefzil*), cefuroxime (*Ceftin*), cephalexin (*Keflex, Keftab*), cephradine (*Velosef*).

**Chemotherapy.** Many medicines can be used in chemotherapy. The term means "the treatment of an illness by chemical agents." It's often used to refer to treatments for cancer, though many other diseases may be treated with chemotherapy.

**Chloramphenicol.** An antibiotic used to treat typhoid fever or other severe illnesses resistant to other antibiotics.

**Chlorpromazine.** A tranquilizer used to treat nausea, vomiting, motion sickness and restlessness.

**Cholesterol-lowering medicines.** These medicines lower cholesterol by affecting the low-density lipoprotein (LDL) and high-density lipoprotein (HDL) levels in ways that are different than the bile acid sequestrants or the HMG-CoA reductase medicines. Cholesterol-lowering medicines are used to treat high cholesterol levels in people who haven't responded to diet changes. Examples: clofibrate (*Atromid-S*), gemfibrozil (*Lopid*), nicotinic acid (*Slo-Niacin*), probucol (*Lorelco*).

**Clot dissolvers.** These medicines are used, generally in emergencies such as a heart attack, to dissolve clots. They can prevent or treat pulmonary emboli (clots in the lungs). Examples: streptokinase (*Streptase*), urokinase (*Abbokinase*).

**Cocaine.** An anesthetic that's highly addictive and frequently abused.

**Contraceptives, implants.** These implants are used to prevent pregnancy. A form of progestin is implanted into the upper arm. The implants must be replaced every five years. Example: levonorgestrel (*Norplant*).

**Contraceptives, injections.** These injections are used to prevent pregnancy. This is an injectable form of progestin. It requires an injection every three months. Example: medroxyprogesterone (*Depo-Provera*).

**Contraceptives, oral.** Combinations of female hormones are used for preventing pregnancy. Monophasic formulations combine progestin and estrogen in one dose that's taken for the first three weeks, and placebo pills are taken during the fourth week. Biphasic formulations combine progestin and estrogen in two doses that vary through the first three weeks and a placebo for the fourth week. Triphasic formulations combine progestin and estrogen in three doses that vary through the first three weeks and a placebo for the fourth week. Progestin-only formulations are also available. Examples of monophasic formulations: ethynodiol + estradiol (*Demulen*), levonorgestrel + estradiol (*Levlen, Nordette*), norethindrone + estradiol (*Brevicon, Loestrin, Modicon, Norinyl, Ortho-Novum, Ovcon*), norgestrel + estradiol (*Lo/Ovral*). Examples of biphasic formulations: norethindrone + estradiol (*Jenest-28, Nelova 10/11, Ortho-Novum 10/11*). Examples of triphasic formulations: levonorgestrel + estradiol (*Tri-Levlen, Tri-phasil*), norethindrone + estradiol (*Ortho-Novum 7/7/7, Tri-Norinyl*). Progestin-only formulations: norethindrone (*Micronor, Nor-Q.D.*), progesterone (*Progestasert*).

**Corticosteroids.** These cortisone-like medicines are included in the general family called steroids. They help decrease inflammation. They can be used to treat asthma or other respiratory disorders; rheumatoid arthritis, lupus or other immune disease, and poison ivy, a severe reaction to a bee sting or other allergic reactions. Nasal forms can be used to help shrink nasal polyps. Topical forms can be used to treat a wide variety of skin disorders, including diaper rash, eczema, poison ivy, poison oak and other allergic reactions, and psoriasis. Certain corticosteroids may also be included in some chemotherapy treatments. Examples of oral forms: dexamethasone (*Decadron*), prednisone (*Deltasone*), methylprednisolone (*Medrol*). Examples of inhaled forms: beclomethasone (*Beclovent, Vanceril*), flunisolide (*AeroBid*). Examples of nasal forms: beclomethasone (*Beconase, Vancenase*), dexamethasone (*Decadron Respihaler*), flunisolide (*Nasolide*), triamcinolone (*Azmacort*). Examples of topical forms: alclometasone (*Aclovate*), amcinonide (*Cyclocort*), betamethasone (*Diprolene, Diprosone, Valisone*), clobetasol (*Temovate*), desonide (*Tridesilon*), desoximetasone (*Topicort*), fluocinonide (*Lidex, Synalar*), hydrocortisone (*Hytone, Westcort*), triamcinolone (*Aristocort, Kenalog*).

**Cortisone.** A corticosteroid used in the treatment of arthritis, allergies and adrenal insufficiency.

**Cough medicines, narcotic and non-narcotic.** These medicines are used to suppress a severe cough that isn't responsive to over-the-counter preparations. Examples: benzonatate (*Tessalon Perles*), codeine, hydrocodone (*Hydrocodone Compound Syrup*).

**Cromolyn sodium.** Cromolyn sodium is used to treat asthma and allergic rhinitis. It comes in nasal spray and inhalant forms. Examples: *Intal, Nasalcrom.*

**Desmopressin.** This medicine is used to treat certain bleeding disorders. Examples: *DDAVP, Stimate.*

**Digitalis.** This is a cardiac drug obtained from the dried leaves of foxglove. It increases the strength of the heartbeat while reducing the rate of the heartbeat.

**Disulfiram.** This medicine is used in the treatment of alcoholism. Example: *Antabuse.*

**Diuretics, general.** Diuretics help the body get rid of extra sodium and fluid. Diuretics can be used to reduce edema and to treat high blood pressure, glomerulonephritis and cirrhosis. Examples: bumetanide (*Bumex*), chlorthalidone (*Hygroton*), furosemide (*Lasix*), hydrochlorothiazide (*Hydro-DIURIL, Oretic*), indapamide (*Lozol*), methyclothiazide (*Enduron, Aquatensen*), metolazone (*Zaroxolyn, Mykrox*), spironolactone (*Aldactazide, Aldactone*), trichlormethiazide (*Metahydrin*).

**Diuretics, potassium-sparing.** These medicines reduce blood pressure. They're used especially in patients who develop hypokalemia (low serum potassium), edema or renal insufficiency. Examples: amiloride (*Midamor*), spironolactone (*Aldactone*), triamterene (*Dyrenium*).

**Ear medicines.** Ear medicines, usually antibiotics alone or in combination with steroids (steroids are used for their action against inflammation, itching and allergies), are used to treat various types of ear infections. These medicines are used to treat inner ear infections (oral antibiotics) and outer ear infections (topical antibiotics). Examples: antipyrine, benzocaine (*Auralgan Otic*), chloramphenicol (*Chloromycetin Otic*), glycerin, hydrocortisone + neomycin sulfate + colistin sulfate + thonzonium (*Coly-Mycin S Otic*), hydrocortisone + neomycin sulfate + polymyxin B (*Cortisporin Otic*), hydrocortisone + polymyxin B (*Otobiotic Otic*), hydrocortisone + acetic acid otic solution (*VoSoL HC Otic*).

**Estrogens.** These medicines are used to help control female disorders associated with estrogen hormones. Most of the following medicines are used on a monthly cycle that imitates the menstrual cycle. For example, oral estrogen can be taken daily for the first 25 days of each month. Estrogens can be used to treat abnormal uterine bleeding, symptoms of menopause, osteoporosis, postpartum breast engorgement and prostate cancer. Examples: conjugated estrogen creams (*Ogen, Estrace, Premarin, Premarin Vaginal Cream*), esterified estrogens (*Estratab*), estradiol (*Climara, Estinyl, Estrace, Estraderm Transdermal*).

**Expectorants.** Expectorants are used to rid the respiratory tract of excess mucus. They work by thinning the mucus and reducing its stickiness, making it less adhesive to the respiratory tract. They're used to treat asthma, bronchitis, cystic fibrosis, emphysema and sinusitis. Examples: iodinated glycerol (*Organidin*), iodine (*Pima*).

**Fluoroquinolones.** A type of antibiotic. Examples: ciprofloxacin (*Cipro*), lomefloxacin (*Maxaquin*), norfloxacin (*Noroxin*), ofloxacin (*Floxin*).

**Glaucoma medicines.** These medicines are used to treat glaucoma. They reduce pressure in the eyes. Examples: acetazolamide (*Diamox*), betaxolol (*Betoptic*), dorzolamide (*Trusopt*), timolol (*Timoptic*).

**Headache medicines.** These medicines are used to treat and prevent certain types of headaches, including vascular, cluster and migraine headaches. Examples: ergotamine (*Ergostat*), dihydroergotamine (*D.H.E. 45*), methysergide (*Sansert*), sumatriptan (*Imitrex*), ergotamine + caffeine (*Cafergot, Wigraine, Ercaf*), isometheptene + dichloralphenazone + acetaminophen (*Isocom, Midrin*), ergotamine + caffeine + tartaric acid (*Wigraine Suppositories*).

**HMG-CoA reductase inhibitors.** These medicines inhibit enzymes involved in the body's production of cholesterol. They also increase the amount of high-density lipoproteins (good cholesterol) and reduce the amount of low-density lipoproteins (bad cholesterol) in the blood. These medicines are used to treat high cholesterol levels. Examples: fluvastatin (*Lescol*), lovastatin (*Mevacor*), pravastatin (*Pravachol*), simvastatin (*Zocor*).

**Immunosuppressants.** Immunosuppressants are used to suppress the body's natural immune reaction to prepare the body for an organ transplant. They're also used to treat rheumatoid arthritis. Examples: cyclosporine (*Sandimmune, Neoral*).

**Insulin.** Diabetic medicines are used to treat people with insulin-dependent diabetes. Insulins can be of animal origin (pork and beef) or genetically synthesized. Insulins are divided into three categories: rapid-acting (with a duration of eight to 16 hours), intermediate-acting (with a duration of 24 hours) and long-acting (with a duration of 36 hours). These medicines are used to treat diabetes mellitus type I (insulin-dependent) and diabetes mellitus type II (non-insulin-dependent) that can't be properly controlled by other medicines, diet, exercise and weight loss. Examples: regular insulin (*Humulin R, Novolin R, Regular Iletin I*), isophane insulin suspension (*Humulin N, Novolin N, NPH Iletin I*), insulin zinc suspension (*Humulin L, Novolin L, Lente Iletin I*), extended zinc suspension (*Humulin U, Ultralente, Ultralente U*).

**Macrolides.** Macrolides are a type of antibiotic. Examples: azithromycin (*Zithromax*), clarithromycin (*Biaxin*), erythromycin (*E-Mycin, Eryc, EryPed, Ilosone, Wyamycin S*).

**Mesalamine.** This medicine is used to treat bowel disease. Example: *Asacol*.

**Methadone.** A drug with properties similar to morphine and heroin that's frequently used to help addicts withdraw from opiate drugs.

**Methamphetamine.** A central nervous system stimulant. A derivative of amphetamine. Example: *Desoxyn Gradumet*.

**Methotrexate.** This medicine can be used as a treatment for psoriasis, rheumatoid arthritis and some types of cancer. Example: *Rheumatrex*.

**Methyltestosterone.** An oral form of testosterone.

**Minoxidil.** This medicine is used to treat male-pattern baldness and hair loss in women. Example: *Rogaine*.

**Motion-sickness (antivertigo) medicines.** These medicines are used to treat the nausea or vomiting caused by motion sickness or vertigo disorders, such as inner-ear problems. Examples: cyclizine (*Marezine*), meclizine (*Antivert, Bonine*), phosphorated carbohydrate solution (*Emetrol*), promethazine (*Phenergan*), scopolamine transdermal (*Transderm-Scop*), scopolamine (*Atrohist, Donnatal, Ru-Tuss*), trimethobenzamide (*Tigan*).

**Muscle relaxants.** These medicines are used to treat muscle spasms associated with musculoskeletal conditions or injury, cerebral palsy, multiple sclerosis and pain. Examples: baclofen (*Lioresal*), carisoprodol (*Soma*), chlorphenesin (*Maolate*), chlorzoxazone (*Parafon Forte DSC*), cyclobenzaprine (*Flexeril*), dantrolene (*Dantrium*), diazepam (*Valium*), metaxalone (*Skelaxin*), methocarbamol (*Robaxin*), orphenadrine (*Norflex*).

**Narcotic.** A type of medicine that relieves pain and dulls the senses. Narcotics can be addictive. See analgesics, narcotic.

**Non-steroidal anti-inflammatory drugs (NSAIDs).** These medicines are used to relieve mild to moderate pain associated with diseases such as arthritis, bursitis, gout and other inflammatory disorders, to reduce fever and to relieve the pain of migraine headache, premenstrual syndrome and tendinitis. The term nonsteroidal is used because these medicines treat inflammation but don't contain steroids. Examples: diclofenac (*Voltaren*), etodolac (*Lodine*), fenoprofen (*Nalfon*), flurbiprofen (*Ansaid*), ibuprofen (*Motrin*), indomethacin (*Indocin*), ketoprofen (*Orudis*), ketorolac (*Toradol*), meclofenamate (*Meclomen*), nabumetone (*Relafen*), naproxen (*Naprosyn, Anaprox*), piroxicam (*Feldene*), sulindac (*Clinoril*), tolmetin (*Tolectin*).

**Parkinson's disease medicines.** These medicines are used to treat the various forms of Parkinson's disease and related disorders, and to relieve the pain of shingles. Examples: amantadine (*Symmetrel*), benztropine (*Cogentin*), bromocriptine (*Parlodel*), levodopa (*Dopar*), pergolide (*Permax*), selegiline (*Eldepryl*), trihexyphenidyl (*Artane*).

**Penicillins.** An antibiotic extracted from molds of the genus *Penicillium notatum*, used to treat a variety of infections. Examples: amoxicillin (*Polymox, Amoxil*), ampicillin (*Polycillin, Omnipen*), cloxacillin (*Cloxapen, Tegopen*), dicloxacillin (*Dynapen, Dycill*), nafcillin (*Unipen, Nafcil*), oxacillin (*Bactocill*), penicillin V potassium (*Pen-Vee K, V-Cillin K*), amoxicillin + potassium clavulanate (*Augmentin*).

**Pentoxifylline.** This medicine can be used to treat atherosclerosis. Example: *Trental*.

**Pimozide.** This medicine can be used to treat the symptoms of Tourette syndrome. Example: *Orap*.

**Prenatal vitamin supplements.** Prenatal vitamins can help prevent birth defects and make sure nutritional demands of pregnancy are met. Examples: *Prenatal-1, Prenate, Prenavite, Stuartnatal Plus*.

**Progestins.** These medicines are used to treat various hormonal disorders associated with menopause and uterine bleeding. Most of the following progestins are taken in a monthly cycle regimen on the last five to 10 days of each month. They're used to treat abnormal uterine bleeding and endometriosis, and to regulate the menstrual cycle. Examples: medroxyprogesterone (*Provera, Amen, Cycrin*), norethindrone (*Aygestin, Norlutin, Norlutate*), mestranol + norethynodrel (*Enovid*).

**Sedative medicines.** These medicines are used to relieve nervousness or tension and to treat insomnia. Some are also used to relieve muscle spasms. Examples: alprazolam (*Xanax*), buspirone (*BuSpar*), chloral hydrate 500 (*Noctec*), chlordiazepoxide (*Librium*), clorazepate dipotassium (*Tranxene*), diazepam (*Valium*), estazolam (*ProSom*), flurazepam (*Dalmane*), hydroxyzine (*Atarax,Vistaril*), lorazepam (*Ativan*), oxazepam (*Serax*), prazepam (*Centrax*), quazepam (*Doral*), temazepam (*Restoril*), triazolam (*Halcion*), zolpidem (*Ambien*).

**Steroids.** See corticosteroids.

**Sulfonamides.** Sulfonamides are a type of antibiotic. These medicines can be used to fight infections caused by bacteria. Some of them also have other uses. Examples: sulfadiazine (*Sulfadiazine*), sulfamethoxazole (*Gantanol*), sulfasalazine (*Azulfidine*), sulfamethoxazole + trimethoprim (*Bactrim, Septra*), sulfisoxazole (*Gantrisin*), sulfisoxazole + erythromycin ethylsuccinate (*Pediazole*).

**Sulfonylureas.** These medicines are used in the treatment of type II diabetes, also known as non-insulin-dependent diabetes mellitus. Sulfonylureas are used to treat people with type II diabetes whose blood glucose isn't controlled by diet alone. Sulfonylureas can also be used with insulin to improve diabetic control. Examples: glipizide (*Glucotrol*), glyburide (*DiaBeta*), metformin (*Glucophage*), tolazamide (*Tolinase*), tolbutamide (*Orinase*).

**Tetracyclines.** Tetracyclines are a type of antibiotic. Examples: demeclocycline (*Declomycin*), doxycycline (*Doryx, Vibramycin*), methacycline (*Rondomycin*), minocycline (*Minocin*), tetracycline (*Achromycin V, Sumycin*).

**Theophylline.** This medicine is useful in treating asthma. Examples: *Aerolate, Marax, Slo-Phyllin, Theo-Dur.*

**Thyroid medicines.** These medicines are used to treat thyroid gland disorders, such as goiter and hypothyroidism. Examples: iodine solution (*Strong Iodine Solution*), levothyroxine sodium (*Synthroid, Levothroid*), liothyronine sodium (*Cytomel*), liotrix (*Euthroid, Thyrolar*), thyroglobulin (*Proloid*), thyroid dessicated (*Armour Thyroid*).

**Tranquilizers.** See sedatives.

**Ulcer medicines.** These medicines are used to treat peptic ulcers and other related gastrointestinal disorders. Examples: cimetidine (*Tagamet*), famotidine (*Pepcid*), nizatidine (*Axid*), omeprazole (*Prilosec*), ranitidine (*Zantac*), sucralfate (*Carafate*).

**Vasodilators.** These medicines relax vascular smooth muscles (arteries and arterioles) and cause an increase in cardiac output. They're used to treat congestive heart failure and high blood pressure. Examples: hydralazine (*Apresoline*), minoxidil (*Loniten*).

# TESTS

**Absorptiometry.** Both single-photon and dual-photon absorptiometry, and dual-energy x-ray absorptiometry measure bone density more accurately than plain x-rays. These tests work by measuring how much of an x-ray beam passes through the bone in a particular location, such as the wrist.

**Alpha-fetoprotein (AFP) test.** This is a common test done on a blood sample from a pregnant woman. Increased levels of AFP in the mother's bloodstream may indicate that the fetus has a serious nervous system defect such as spina bifida or anencephaly. Low levels of AFP may indicate a genetic defect, such as Down syndrome.

The test is done between the 16th and 18th weeks of pregnancy. Because it's so simple and the problems it sometimes detects are so serious, many doctors offer it on a routine basis.

One disadvantage of the AFP test is that it detects only a few types of problems. A normal AFP test doesn't guarantee a normal baby. The AFP test is used to identify some potentially severe abnormalities that might lead the mother to undergo further testing with amniocentesis or chorionic villus sampling (CVS), and which might raise the possibility of a second-trimester abortion if a severe abnormality is detected.

**Ambulatory blood pressure monitoring.** This procedure allows your blood pressure to be measured while you do normal daily activities. Generally, a battery-powered pump is worn on your belt. At certain intervals, the pump inflates an arm cuff and a sensor records the pressure. Readings are stored in the unit's memory to be printed out later. Your doctor then looks at the printout to find out how much your blood pressure changes during the day.

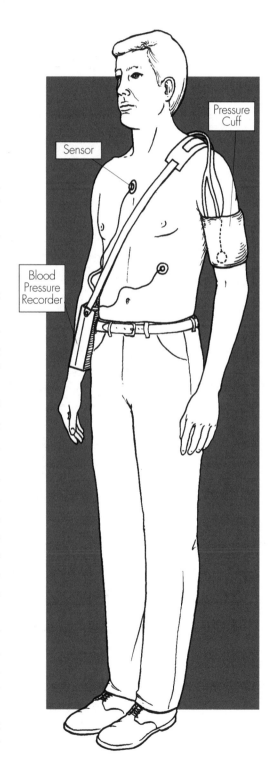

**AMBULATORY BLOOD PRESSURE MONITORING**

627

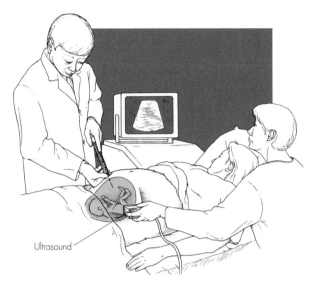

Ultrasound

**AMNIOCENTESIS**

**Amniocentesis.** This procedure, which includes removing a sample of amniotic fluid for analysis to detect abnormalities in the fetus, isn't routine for all pregnancies. Your doctor may recommend it if you're over age 35, if you have given birth to a baby with a nervous system defect, such as spina bifida or anencephaly, or genetic abnormalities, or if you're a carrier for a genetic disease. The test usually is performed between the 14th and 17th weeks of pregnancy.

During the test, the doctor uses ultrasound as a guide to insert a needle through the abdomen into the amniotic sac. A small amount of amniotic fluid is drawn out through the needle. Common side effects include cramping and slight bleeding, called "spotting." More serious complications are rare. Complications include infection, rupture of the membranes and miscarriage.

**Angiogram.** This is an x-ray of the blood vessels taken after a special dye is injected. Angiograms can be done for many reasons, including to examine the blood flow in the heart, brain, intestines and other parts of the body.

An *arteriogram* is an x-ray of arteries done after the arteries are filled with dye. A *coronary arteriogram* is a study of the heart and coronary arteries. It provides the best pictures if surgery or angioplasty is needed. A *digital subtraction arteriogram* is a computerized x-ray of the arteries. It enhances the images of areas where blood is flowing and subtracts some of the shadows of overlying tissues. It can give a clearer picture of the arteries.

A *venogram* involves injecting dye into a vein and taking x-rays of the veins.

**Anoscopy.** Anoscopy involves inspecting the anal area with an *anoscope*, a short, rigid, lighted scope. It's often used to diagnose internal hemorrhoids.

**Arterial blood gas test.** These are special blood tests used to check oxygen and carbon dioxide levels in the blood. When the lungs are damaged, the oxygen levels in the blood may decrease, and the carbon dioxide levels may increase. The test is done by inserting a needle through the skin into an artery, usually in the wrist. Blood gases are used by your doctor to help diagnose the type and severity of a lung problem.

**Arteriogram.** See angiogram.

**Arthroscopy.** In this procedure, a fiberoptic instrument is inserted surgically into a joint to diagnose and treat problems. It's commonly used to diagnose and repair cartilage and ligament injuries in the knee.

**Audiometry.** This test measures how well a person hears at different sound frequencies to check for hearing loss (measured in decibels). *Pure tone audiometry* shows the range of sound a person can't hear. *Impedance audiometry* tests the function of the eardrum and middle ear bones.

**Barium enema.** This is a radiographic exam to check for disease in the colon and rectum. Barium is a substance that blocks x-rays and shows up in great contrast on an x-ray film. It's given through an *enema* until the large bowel is full. On the x-rays, any place where barium should normally be seen but isn't can be a sign of an abnormality.

When you have a barium enema, you can have only liquids the night before the exam and no breakfast the day of the exam. An enema is used the night before to clean out the intestine. After the x-ray, the barium is removed from your body with a cleansing enema. Barium enema is also called a *lower GI series.*

**Barium swallow.** Often called an *upper GI series,* barium is swallowed so the esophagus, stomach and small intestine can be examined with x-rays. A person having this test can't eat or drink anything for at least eight hours before the test. Barium swallow also provides a picture of the esophagus and how well it's working. The barium is eliminated through the gastrointestinal tract on its own.

**Biopsy.** This is the procedure for getting a sample of tissue, such as from the skin or the liver, that can be examined under a microscope. Biopsies are done to determine the cause of health problems. A biopsy may be done to see what type of disease is affecting the tissue. It's often done to rule out cancer.

Biopsies of internal organs may be done surgically or through a tiny needle or a type of scope, depending on the organ involved. A local anesthetic is used for skin biopsies. Biopsies of internal organs may require general anesthesia.

**Blood pressure checks.** A blood pressure cuff and pressure measuring gauge, together called a *sphygmomanometer,* is used to do this simple test. This test can be performed in less than one minute. It simply involves placing the cuff around the upper arm, inflating the cuff and reading the results on the gauge as the cuff is deflated. The observer listens for the beginning of thumping sounds (which signals the "systolic" blood pressure, or the pressure while the heart is contracting) and the disappearance of the sounds (signaling the "diastolic" blood pressure, during heart relaxation).

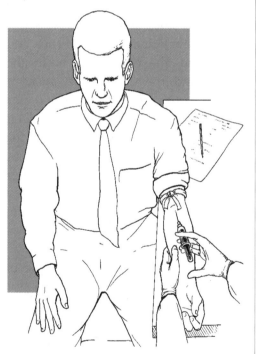

**BLOOD TEST**

**Blood tests.** Blood is drawn, usually from a vein on the inside of the elbow. Blood tests are helpful in diagnosing a number of disorders. After the blood is taken from a vein, it's sent to a laboratory for testing.

A *blood chemistry profile* measures some of the substances carried in the

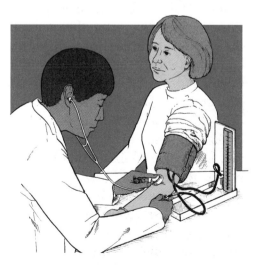

**BLOOD PRESSURE CHECK**

```
┌─────────────────────────────────────────┐
│         ┌─────────────────────┐          │
│         │     HEMATOLOGY      │          │
│         └─────────────────────┘          │
│                                          │
│  Collection date _____                │
│         Time  _____                   │
│                                          │
│  Procedure            Units   Ref Range  │
│  ------ Complete Blood Count ------      │
│  WBC X 10^3      8.8    /µL    4.0-10.8   │
│  RBC X 10^6     3.68L   /µL    4.20-5.40  │
│  HGB            13.4    g/dL   12.0-16.0  │
│  HCT            39.1    %      36.0-46.0  │
│  MCV           106.2H   fl     80.0-100.0 │
│  MCH            36.3H   pg     25.0-33.0  │
│  MCHC           34.1    gm/dL  32.0-36.0  │
│  RDW            19.8H   %      11.5-14.5  │
│  MPV             8.7    fl     7.4-9.4    │
│  PLATELET X 10^3 135L   /µL    150-400    │
│                                          │
│  Footnotes  L = Low, H = High            │
└─────────────────────────────────────────┘
```

**LAB SLIP OF COMPLETE BLOOD COUNT**

blood. With this single test, it's possible to measure a number of enzymes produced by the liver, the amount of sugar in the blood, the blood cholesterol level, some of the waste products carried by the kidneys, such as urea and creatinine, the calcium level in the blood and the electrolytes, such as chlorine, potassium, sodium and carbon dioxide. A *complete blood count* (CBC) tests a sample of blood for the level of white blood cells, platelets, hemoglobin, hematocrit and other blood components. This test can show anemia, leukemia, some bone marrow problems and the effects on the blood of some bad reactions to medicines.

**Bone marrow tests.** A sample of bone marrow can be checked for abnormalities that indicate anemia, leukemia and other problems of the blood or bone marrow. Bone marrow testing can be done in a hospital, doctor's office or laboratory.

The sample is usually taken from the breast bone or the back of the pelvis. A needle is used to withdraw the bone marrow. A local anesthetic is used to numb the area before a needle is inserted. The needle that's used is encased in a metal sleeve that can cut through the bone. When the needle goes in, there may be a sensation of pressure. When the marrow is taken, there may be a dull, deep pain. But the pain won't linger after the test.

In *bone marrow aspiration,* a very small amount of marrow is taken. For a *bone marrow biopsy,* a small, solid core of bone marrow is taken. The place where the marrow was taken may be a little sore and bruised for a few days.

**Bone mineral density analysis.** These tests are important for diagnosing osteoporosis and other bone diseases. The tests examine the condition of your bone structure. The main test used to study bone mineral density is absorptiometry.

**Bone scan.** This is one of many types of nuclear medicine tests. During the test, a special substance, called a *radioactive isotope,* is injected. This isotope attaches to the bone. A scan of radiation from the isotope is made to create an image of the skeleton. The isotope attaches the most in areas where the bone is remodeling—actively breaking down and reforming.

**Bronchoscopy.** Your doctor can look at the inside of your airways to detect lung disease by doing bronchoscopy. The *bronchoscope* has a light at the end that allows the airway to be lit up. The bronchoscope is passed through the nose or the throat while the person sits or lies down. It's often equipped with a small camera so the doctor can watch the test on a screen. Bronchoscopy can be used to diagnose tumors and other problems, and can also be used to take a small sample, or *biopsy,* of tissue or to collect mucus for testing.

Usually, a person shouldn't eat for up to 12 hours before bronchoscopy. Medicine will be given to reduce the cough, swallowing and gag reflexes. A sedative may also be given to help the person relax. An anesthetic jelly is usually used to coat and protect the air passages.

The person shouldn't eat for about an hour after the test because the swallowing and cough reflexes won't be back to normal, and there's a risk of inhaling food into the lungs.

**Cardiac catheterization.** Also called an *angiocardiogram*, this test involves passing a tiny plastic tube through an artery in the arm or leg to the heart. Dye is injected through the tube so that pictures can be taken of the heart and its valves, chambers and arteries. The test looks for blockage of the heart arteries and abnormalities of the heart.

**Chest x-rays.** Chest x-rays can be helpful in diagnosing problems of the lungs or heart. Patterns seen on chest x-rays help to diagnose many different infections, tumors and inflammatory diseases of the lung, and provide

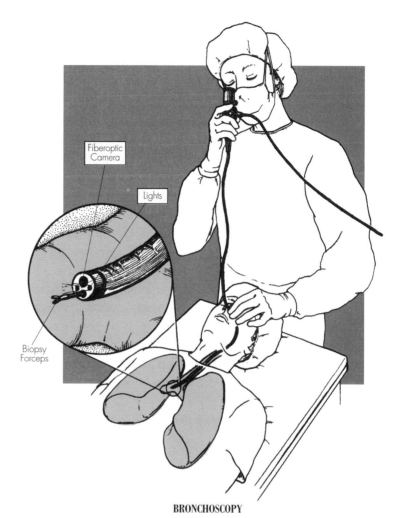

**BRONCHOSCOPY**

clues that further tests may be needed for the heart.

To have a chest x-ray, you stand in front of a screen that has a special type of film in it. Usually, a front view and a side view are taken. It's absolutely painless. The dose of radiation in a routine chest x-ray is so small that it isn't of concern unless the person is pregnant. Developing fetuses are more sensitive to radiation and are usually protected with a lead shield if an x-ray of the mother is needed.

**Chorionic villus sampling (CVS).** Another test used in pregnancy to detect genetic abnormalities is called *chorionic villus sampling* (*CVS*). The test may be used in pregnant women who are over age 35, have previously given birth to a baby with genetic abnormalities or have a family history of genetic

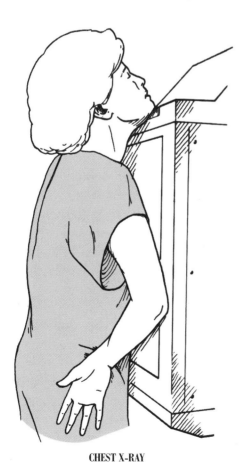

**CHEST X-RAY**

disease. The test doesn't detect nervous system defects, such as spina bifida, but is useful in detecting chromosome abnormalities and other genetic disorders. An advantage of CVS over amniocentesis is that it can be done earlier in pregnancy, between the eighth and 12th weeks. This may give the woman more time to decide, in consultation with her doctor, partner or minister, whether to have a therapeutic abortion if the fetus has a chromosome abnormality or a genetic disorder.

The test involves obtaining a sample of the *chorionic villi,* the hair-like projections on the *chorionic membrane.* The chorion is the fetal membrane that becomes a part of the placenta. The sample is obtained by a tube inserted into the vagina and through the cervix into the uterus, or by a hollow needle inserted through the abdomen into the uterus. A disadvantage of this test is that it may carry a greater risk of miscarriage than amniocentesis or it may cause limb defects in the fetus. Consult your doctor about the pros and cons of this procedure.

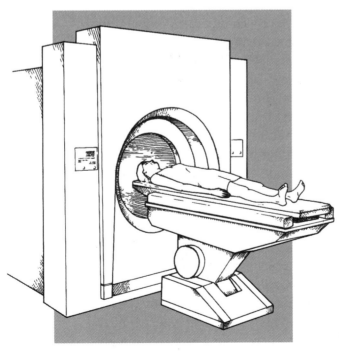

**COMPUTED TOMOGRAPHY (CT SCAN)**

**Colonoscopy.** This test is done with a long, flexible scope, called a *colonoscope.* It allows your doctor to view the large bowel to detect abnormalities. The colonoscope can also be used to collect a tissue sample, or biopsy, or to remove small growths, or *polyps.* Colonoscopy is usually done while you're sedated. (See sigmoidoscopy.)

**Colposcopy.** If a Pap smear shows cellular changes of the cervix, your doctor may recommend colposcopy. A *colposcope* is a tube with a light and a magnifying device on the end. It allows your doctor to look closely at the tissue of the cervix, identify the abnormal areas and biopsy the abnormal tissue.

Before looking at your cervix with the colposcope, your doctor will put a special solution on your cervix that will cause abnormal tissue to turn white. A biopsy sample will probably be taken.

Colposcopy doesn't feel much different from having a Pap smear. Some women have cramping and a little bleeding after the procedure.

**Computed tomographic (CT) scans.** CT scans direct x-ray beams through an area of the body at different angles at the same time to show "slices" of the area of the body being examined. The photographic slices can show changes in the tissue. During a CT scan, you must lie very still on a table that moves through the CT machine. CT scans aren't painful. An intravenous contrast dye is usually used during CT scanning to clearly show the organs.

CT scans may be done of the abdomen, spine, chest and head. It may also be used to study the spine, joints and sinuses. CT scans can be used to find tumors, blood clots, broken bones that don't show up on a regular x-ray and areas of the body that are gathering fluid.

**Cone biopsy.** This test involves removing the entire "transformation zone" between the uterine and vaginal covering of the cervix. It is a surgical procedure that is done for carcinoma in situ of the cervix. It requires general anesthesia.

**Cultures.** When your doctor orders a culture, he or she wants to find and identify the type of bacteria, fungus or virus that's causing an illness. Cultures can also be grown to find out what antibiotics are effective for fighting the infection. You're probably familiar with the cultures done on fluids from the throat, eyes and ears, but cultures can also be obtained from blood, urine, spinal fluid, joint fluid, feces and bone marrow.

A negative culture means there was no growth of micro-organisms (except of normal bacteria) in the laboratory setting. A positive culture means that there was growth of disease-causing bacteria.

**Cystoscopy.** When you're having urinary problems, your doctor may want to do this visual exam of the bladder. A lighted instrument, called a *cystoscope*, is used to identify and treat problems in the bladder. For the test, the cystoscope is placed in the urethra, and the bladder is filled with air or water. People who have this test are often sedated.

**Cytology exam.** This is an exam of any body fluid to check for abnormal cells. Possible body fluids that can be examined include cerebrospinal fluid, urine, joint fluid or fluid collections in the chest or abdomen.

**Dental x-rays.** These can show tooth decay, abscesses, impacted teeth and other problems with the teeth or surrounding bone. The x-rays are taken as you bite down on a small piece of film. The amount of radiation used is very small, but the dentist will proba-

bly place a lead apron over your body while the x-rays are taken to reduce your exposure to radiation.

**Digital rectal examination.** Your doctor uses a gloved, lubricated finger to check your rectum for irregular areas or growths such as polyps. This exam is an important part of any routine check-up. In men, the prostate gland can be checked this way as well.

**Dilation of the pupils.** This involves placing drops in the eye that cause the *pupil* (the black circle in the center of your eye surrounded by the colored iris) to relax and open wider. This is done to examine your eyes more thoroughly. Dilation is painless, although it makes the eyes sensitive to light. The pupils generally stay dilated for 30 minutes to three hours, depending on the type of eye drop used.

**Echocardiogram.** Echocardiography uses sound waves bounced off the heart to create an image of the heart. The process is similar to sonar on a submarine. In this painless test, a *transducer,* or microphone-like device, is moved across the chest. A gel-like substance is first put between the person's skin and the head of the transducer.

Echocardiograms can give important information about the heart's function and health. The doctor views the

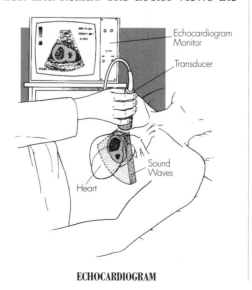

**ECHOCARDIOGRAM**

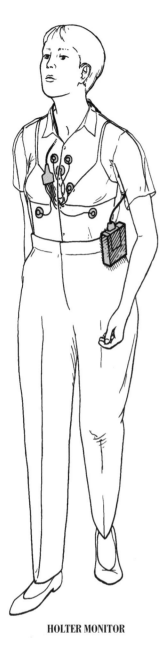

**HOLTER MONITOR**

valves moving, the size of the ventricles and the pumping action of the heart.

**Electrocardiogram (EKG or ECG).** Electrodes placed on the legs, arms and chest measure the electrical impulses of the heart for an *electrocardiogram.* These impulses can be seen as they occur on a video monitor and can also be printed out on paper. The test is painless and only takes a few minutes. A portable version of the test, called the *Holter monitor,* allows the electrical impulses to be measured all day long while a person follows normal routines.

**Electroencephalogram (EEG).** An EEG measures the electrical activity of the brain through tiny wires (*electrodes*) placed on the skull. You may be asked to look into a light, breathe deeply or do other "brain exercises," which are measured by the electrodes. The EEG is used to assess changes in consciousness and is useful in diagnosing conditions such as epilepsy and sleep problems. An EEG isn't painful. It may be done while you're awake or asleep. If you're awake, the test takes about half an hour.

**Electromyography (EMG).** This is an electrical study of the muscles. Thin needles are placed through the skin so that their tip is located in a muscle. The electrical activity in the muscles is recorded. EMG can be used to diagnose many different muscle diseases.

**Endometrial biopsy or sampling.** The lining, or *endometrium,* of the uterus plays an essential part in fertility. Endometrial biopsy or sampling involves inserting a small instrument through the cervix into the uterus to scrape off a portion of the lining.

You may feel some discomfort during this test, which is sometimes performed under local anesthesia. Complications are rare. There's a very small risk of infection. Samplings of the endometrial lining show the effects of hormones and if the lining can provide

a good location for the implantation of a fertilized egg. Endometrial sampling can also reveal cancer of the uterus.

**Endoscopy.** This is a broad term that covers several tests, all of which are done by a direct exam of an organ or area of the body. Using a lighted, tube-like device called an *endoscope,* your doctor can view areas of the body such as the nose, sinuses, larynx, lung airways, esophagus, stomach, intestines and large joints.

The endoscope can also pump air into an area of the body for better viewing, wash away anything blocking the view, such as blood, suction out suspicious material or take a sample of tissue, or a biopsy, for further testing.

For more specific testing information, see anoscopy, arthroscopy, bronchoscopy, colonoscopy, colposcopy, esophagogastroduodenoscopy, gastroscopy, laparoscopy and sigmodoscopy.

**Erythrocyte sedimentation rate (ESR).** The ESR test involves testing a blood sample. A high ESR level is an indication of an inflammatory or infectious process going on in your body.

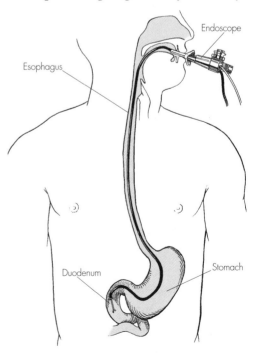

**ESOPHAGOGASTRODUODENOSCOPY (EGD)**

ESR is usually tested to find a disease such as rheumatoid arthritis, temporal arteritis or autoimmune disease, or to follow the disease progress. A high ESR suggests the need for other tests to find the cause of your symptoms.

**Esophagogastroduodenoscopy (EGD).** This test is done with an *endoscope*, an instrument that can examine the inside of the esophagus, stomach and duodenum. The instrument, or tube, is inserted into the throat and down into the esophagus and stomach so that the area can be viewed to check for ulcers, irritation or cancer. It's done while a person is sedated.

**Exercise stress test.** When your doctor wants to assess the overall health of your heart, measure your risk of having a heart attack and help plan a physical activity program, he or she may order an exercise stress test. The test involves exercising on a treadmill or exercise bike while an electrocardiogram (EKG) is done. The exercise starts easy and gradually becomes harder.

During the test, the EKG measures how the heart reacts to the exercise. A blood pressure cuff is also used to measure blood pressure during the exercise. An exercise stress test usually takes about 10 to 20 minutes. It's sometimes recommended that the person not smoke or eat for several hours before the test.

**Fecal occult blood test.** Checking the stool (*feces*) for traces of hidden (*occult*) blood may help your doctor find cancer early. The test is simple and inexpensive, and can be done at home using test cards obtained from your doctor. Avoid eating red meat, vitamin C supplements or horseradish for three days before you take a home stool test to screen for occult blood. These foods can interfere with the test results.

Although an important and useful test, the fecal occult blood test is not

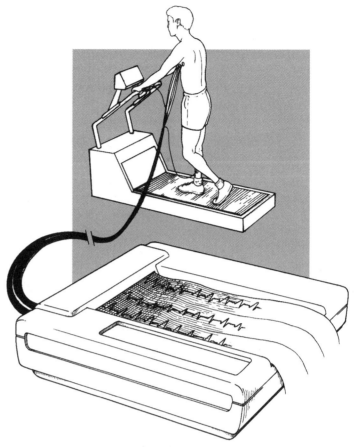

**EXERCISE STRESS TEST**

100% accurate for cancer. The test is designed to find blood that may be caused by a cancerous growth. If blood is found (a positive test), it may also have been caused by hemorrhoids or polyps. On the other hand, sometimes a cancerous tumor may not bleed, and the test may be negative even though cancer is present. That's why your doctor may do other tests to confirm a suspected cancer diagnosis.

**Fetal monitor.** This device is used during labor to monitor the baby's heartbeat, the mother's contractions and the baby's response to the contractions. The baby's condition is continuously monitored, either directly or indirectly, if a problem is suspected.

To monitor the baby directly, an electrode is placed on the baby's head while the baby is still in the uterus. The electrode is passed through the vaginal and cervical canals after the water has broken. With indirect monitoring, the electrodes are put on the mother's abdominal skin over the uterus. There is sometimes minor discomfort for the mother, but the information obtained is invaluable.

**Fine needle biopsy.** A fine needle biopsy is used to take a sample of tissue for examination under a microscope. As the name says, the needle is fine, or thin, and feels like an injection. It may be used to get samples from many areas, including the thyroid, breast and lymph nodes.

**Gastroscopy.** A flexible *gastroscope* can be used to look directly into the stomach and esophagus and see the linings of these two organs. The gastroscope detects more change or damage to the stomach and esophagus lining than the barium swallow series does. See also esophagogastroduodenoscopy.

**Glaucoma test.** *Air-puff tonometry* tests for glaucoma. A machine shoots a painless air puff at the eye to measure how soft or how hard the eye surface is. This test tells whether the pressure in the eye is normal or high, and by how much. This test can also be done with a smooth metal instrument called a *tonometer*, after the eye is anesthetized with drops.

**Glucose tolerance test.** This is a blood test that can diagnose diabetes or hypoglycemia. Before the test you may be asked not to eat for 12 hours. For this test, you're required to drink a special drink, usually a bottle of very sweet orange soda or cola. Afterward, samples of your blood are drawn and tested at one-hour intervals for one to five hours to determine your blood sugar level after drinking the liquid.

The results are compared with normal values to see how well you "tolerated" the extra sugar. If your blood sugar level is abnormally high, you may need to go through further testing or treatment for diabetes.

A glucose tolerance test is often done at about the fifth month of pregnancy to check for signs of diabetes during pregnancy. If you already have diabetes, your doctor will check your blood sugar level throughout your pregnancy at frequent intervals to monitor your condition and try to optimize your control.

**Home pregnancy test.** These tests detect *human chorionic gonadotropin* (HCG), a hormone that's produced only when a woman is pregnant. It's excreted in the urine. A test may be positive as early as the first day of the missed menstrual period, but waiting for a few days after the missed period increases the accuracy of the test.

A positive pregnancy test, even a home test, almost always means you're pregnant. But a negative test doesn't always mean you're not pregnant. If you've missed a period but the test is negative, you may not have waited long enough for the test to be positive. If you wait another two weeks to take the test again and your results are still negative, make an appointment to be checked by your doctor.

**Hysterosalpingogram.** This is an x-ray test of the uterus and fallopian tubes. It's done to check if there is a clear and unobstructed path for the sperm to meet the egg. Contrast dye is injected into the uterus and tubes to outline them on the x-ray film.

**Hysteroscopy.** A *hysteroscope*, a thin, lighted tubular scope, is inserted into the uterus through the vagina. It's used to examine the lining of the uterus to check for abnormalities that might prevent pregnancy or to find the cause of abnormal uterine bleeding.

**Intravenous pyelogram (IVP).** This is the study of the kidneys, ureters and bladder, using an x-ray. A dye is injected into your bloodstream that collects in the kidneys and passes through the ureters to the bladder. When the dye is in the kidneys, it will show a silhouette that's normal or abnormal. An abnormal silhouette shows defects, or places where the dye should be but isn't or places where it shouldn't be and is. Kidney stones that are stuck in the ureters can usually be seen with an IVP.

**Laparoscopy.** A thin, flexible, lighted tubular scope, called a *laparoscope,* is inserted through a small cut in the skin into the abdomen to evaluate the shape and condition of certain organs, such as the uterus, fallopian tubes, ovaries, appendix and intestines. Laparoscopy requires only a small incision and allows direct visual exam. It prevents the need for a large incision. Laparoscopy may be used to diagnose endometriosis. A laparoscope may also be used to perform certain surgeries, such as tubal ligation, or to remove an appendix or gallbladder.

**Laryngoscopy.** This is a test done with an instrument used to look at the larynx, or "voice box." *Flexible laryngoscopes* are inserted through the nose. *Rigid laryngoscopes* are inserted though the mouth. A *fiberoptic laryngoscope* has a light on the tip that allows the doctor to see better and a mirror that allows different views.

A numbing spray may be used to help make the exam more comfortable. Sometimes a tranquilizer (p. 626) is given to help the person relax if they tend to gag when the scope is in place.

**Liver function tests.** These are a variety of blood tests that show how well the liver is working. For example, a high level of bilirubin in the blood indicates the bile flow is obstructed or the liver isn't processing bile correctly. Elevated liver enzymes can indicate alcoholic or viral hepatitis, or other liver damage.

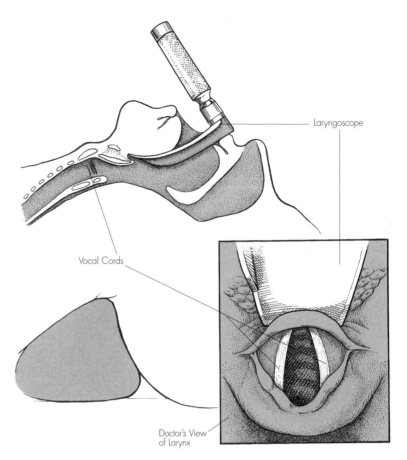

**LARYNGOSCOPY**

**Lymph node biopsy.** This involves taking a piece of tissue from a lymph node for testing. This biopsy can be helpful in diagnosing lymph node cancer.

**Magnetic resonance imaging (MRI).** To get information about the

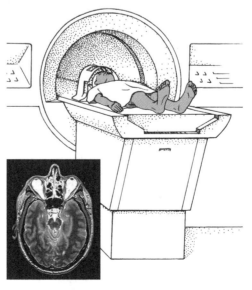

**MAGNETIC RESONANCE IMAGING**

makeup of your tissues, an MRI scan measures different levels of energy given off by various tissues. MRI scans can be used to assess problems in the brain stem and spinal cord. MRI scans are also used to examine the joints after a shoulder or knee injury. MRI scans are particularly useful for showing tumors and areas of the body that CT scans can't effectively show.

During an MRI, you lie absolutely still while being moved into a tunnel-like structure. Unlike x-rays and CT scans, MRI scans don't use radiation. MRI scans aren't painful. Some people find the machine a little confining and claustrophobic. An MRI scan usually takes about a half-hour. Tranquilizers (p. 626) may sometimes be used to help the person relax if he or she is very anxious.

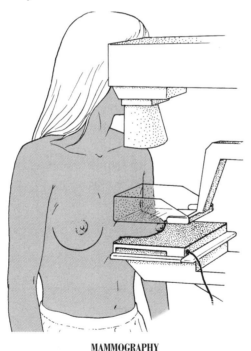

MAMMOGRAPHY

**Mammography.** Mammography is the process of taking a special x-ray called a *xerogram* of the breast. The actual test is called a *mammogram*. Mammograms can find many breast cancers before you can feel them. They can also give your doctor important information about a breast lump that was found during a self-exam or doctor's visit.

Usually a woman has two mammograms of each breast, one taken from the side of the breast and one from the top. The test is somewhat painful for many women, but it only takes a few minutes. To get a mammogram you stand in front of a machine and your breast is placed between two plastic plates. The plates come together, pressing on your breast to make it as flat as possible. This makes it easier to see changes or lumps. Then the x-ray is taken. A radiologist will review the film to see if there are any areas of concern in the breast.

**Myelogram.** During a spinal tap, a special dye is injected into the space around the spinal cord after a small amount of the spinal fluid is first removed. This helps keep the pressure the same even after adding the dye. A series of x-rays are then taken. Myelograms provide a view of the spinal cord to find out if the space around the cord is normal, or if bony spurs are present or discs are out of place. Myelograms have largely been replaced by the newer techniques of CT and MRI scans, but they're still useful before back surgery.

Hospitalization is usually needed for the procedure and you won't be allowed to eat or drink for several hours before the test. The procedure takes 30 to 60 minutes and isn't usually painful because sedatives are given. Headaches following the procedure are common because of the changes in spinal fluid pressure.

**Nasolaryngoscopy.** This test involves inserting a thin lighted tube through a nostril and nasal passage to examine the larynx for growths. See also laryngoscopy.

**Nerve conduction studies.** These tests are used to show if nerves are working properly. During the test, the nerves are stimulated with mild electric shocks. Tiny wires, called *electrodes,* are attached to the skin to measure how long it takes for the muscle that the nerve controls to contract. This tells how fast the nerves are carrying signals to the muscles.

A nerve conduction study may be done to diagnose carpal tunnel syndrome, for example.

**Nuclear medicine tests.** During a nuclear medicine test, a special substance, called a radioactive isotope, is injected. There are many types of nuclear medicine scans. Thyroid scans, bone scans and brain scans are just a few examples. In each case, a radioactive isotope is used that selectively goes to the area of interest in the body. A scan of radiation from the isotope is made to create an image of the area. This can help your doctor make many different diagnoses.

**Ophthalmoscopy.** This is done using an instrument called an *ophthalmoscope* to look at the retina, cornea, lens, vitreous humor and optic nerve. The pupils may be dilated for a better view of the retina, the part of the eye that receives light and sends messages to the brain, where visual images are created. The test is usually a part of a routine exam by your doctor. It can also be used to help diagnose complications of such conditions as diabetes, hypertension and brain tumor.

**Oral cholecystogram.** This is an x-ray test of the gallbladder. When your doctor orders an oral cholecystogram, you'll swallow a dye so that x-rays will show the gallbladder and any stones or tumors in it. Some people experience nausea, vomiting or diarrhea in response to the dye, and a few may be allergic to it.

**Otoscopy.** The doctor uses an instrument called an *otoscope* to look

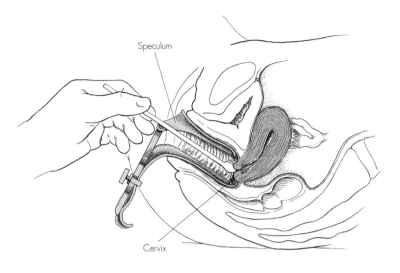

Speculum

Cervix

**PAP SMEAR**

into the ear. It provides a view of the ear canal and eardrum.

**Pap smear.** Having regular Pap smears is the first line of defense against cervical cancer. The purpose of a Pap smear is to detect changes in the cervical cells that may indicate a precancerous condition or cancer. A Pap smear may be slightly uncomfortable, but it's a quick procedure.

Your doctor will put an instrument called a *speculum* into your vagina. This instrument helps open your vagina so the sample can be taken. Your doctor will first clean your cervix gently with a cotton swab and then take the sample. The sample will be put on a glass slide and sent to a laboratory for a microscopic exam.

**Partial thromboplastin time (PTT).** This test measures the time it takes for a clot to form after clotting chemicals, such as calcium, are added to the blood. Thromboplastin is one of the 12 substances, called factors, in the body that cause the blood to clot. This test is a general screening test that helps detect blood clotting disorders.

**Pelvic exam.** A pelvic exam involves inspecting the outer genitals and some of the inner structures as well. Your doctor will use a device called a *speculum* to expand the vaginal canal. During this exam, he or she may obtain a Pap smear. Your doctor may also palpate your reproductive organs to feel for any problems. This palpation may be a little uncomfortable, but it's a quick procedure.

**Pelvimetry.** This x-ray test can be done to measure the size of the bony pelvis, or birth canal, of a woman. It's done on rare occasions when there's doubt about whether the baby's head can pass safely through the pelvis during labor. It has some risk, however, because of radiation exposure, and it's imprecise. Many doctors prefer to use the ultrasound (sonogram) to assess the size of the baby's head and the birth canal.

**Positron emission tomography (PET).** A PET scan, like an MRI scan, uses no radiation. It distinguishes tissues based on differences in *positron emissions,* a type of energy. PET isn't yet in general use, but may be used more in the future if it's found to offer unique help in diagnosing problems.

**Proctoscopy.** A *proctoscope,* a lighted, tubular instrument that's inserted through the anus, allows direct examination of the lining of the anal canal, rectum and lower part of the colon.

**Prostate-specific antigen (PSA) test.** This blood test is elevated when the prostate gland is inflamed or damaged. It may sometimes detect prostate cancer before it shows up in a rectal exam.

**Pulmonary function test (spirometry).** Pulmonary function tests can help determine how well the lungs are working. They involve breathing into a machine that measures airflow and lung capacity. Patterns of lung function help your doctor diagnose swelling (*inflammation*) or shrinking (*constriction*) of the airways, as well as general breathing ability. Pulmonary function tests are used to diagnose asthma and other lung diseases.

**Rapid antibody strep test.** See strep test.

**Refraction.** This is a test done by an ophthalmologist or optometrist to determine what type of corrective lenses are needed to improve vision. Lenses of different strengths are put in front of each eye to find the best result possible.

**Retrograde pyelogram.** The kidneys are the focus of this test, in which dye is injected through a bladder catheter into the kidneys. The dye provides a picture of the structures of the kidneys and helps find a blockage of the urinary tract.

**Rh-factor compatibility test.** This is a blood test done to find out if a pregnant woman has antibodies in her blood that may damage the blood cells of the fetus.

**Sialogram.** This x-ray of the salivary glands is obtained after a dye has been injected into the glands. The test is used to see if the salivary glands are blocked.

**Sigmoidoscopy.** This procedure uses a *sigmoidoscope,* a flexible, fiberoptic-lighted, tubular instrument that's longer and more flexible than a proctoscope and can be used to view the sigmoid (S-shaped) part of the colon. The test is usually somewhat uncomfortable. It helps your doctor find areas of damaged tissue or growths (*polyps*) before they become cancerous and spread, and it sometimes detects colorectal cancer.

**Skin biopsy.** This involves removing a sample of skin cells to test them for cancer or other diseases. In an *excisional biopsy,* the entire lesion is removed. A *punch biopsy* is another kind of skin biopsy. It removes tissue that's smaller in diameter than a pencil eraser and goes deep enough to get the epidermis, dermis and subcutaneous

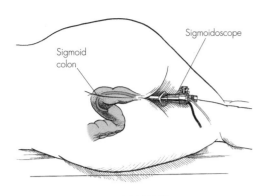

**SIGMOIDOSCOPY**

tissue. A *shave biopsy* is used to slice off an elevated lesion so that it is flush with the surrounding skin.

**Skin patch test.** This test can help diagnose what's causing an allergic skin condition (*contact dermatitis*). Possible offending substances are placed against the skin with a stainless steel disk or hypoallergenic tape for 48 to 72 hours. Another patch is a control. If the skin under the suspect patch is red and swollen and the control skin isn't, the test is positive. When the test is positive, you're more than likely allergic to that substance.

**Skin tests.** A small drop of allergen is placed on the skin and then a needle is used to "tent" the skin without pricking it to help reveal what you're allergic to. Your doctor will look at the tests five to 10 minutes later. Allergic reactions will show up as raised, possibly itchy, wheals.

**Slit lamp test.** A *slit lamp* is a special magnifying device used by ophthalmologists to examine the eye structures, including the cornea, lens, iris and retina.

**Speech audiometry.** These tests measure how much hearing has been lost by seeing how well speech can be recognized. The tests can be especially helpful in children over five years of age.

**Spinal tap.** Also called a *lumbar puncture (LP)*, a spinal tap is used to take a sample of spinal fluid or measure the pressure of the spinal fluid. Lumbar puncture can also be used to give medicines or inject dyes for x-rays.

During a lumbar puncture, you'll probably lie on your side with your

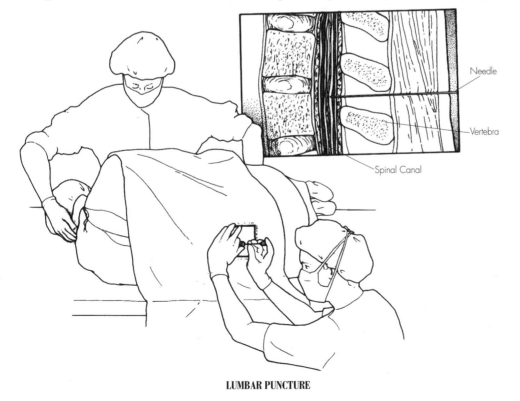

**LUMBAR PUNCTURE**

knees bent to help open up the space between two vertebrae in the lower back. After a local anesthetic is injected into the area, a needle is inserted between two of the vertebrae and into the spinal canal to draw out the spinal fluid.

A lumbar puncture usually takes 10 to 30 minutes. During the test, you may feel some pressure. A headache may occur after the test because of the change in the pressure of the spinal fluid. The headache usually goes away in a few days.

**Strep test.** The *rapid antibody strep test* involves swabbing your throat and testing the sample to look for the body's immune reaction to streptococcal bacteria. The test can be read in 10 minutes. It takes 24 hours, however, to get the results of a throat culture. A culture allows more time for bacteria to grow so it can be identified. The culture takes longer but is more accurate. It may be done if the rapid strep test is negative.

**Throat culture.** Throat cultures are done to check the throat for strep bacteria. The test involves wiping a cotton swab across the back of the throat to pick up a sample of mucus. The sample is then cultured and examined for bacterial growth and sensitivity to antibiotics. A culture can be used instead of a rapid antibody strep test.

**Thyroid function test.** Several blood tests can be used to check how well the thyroid is working. These tests measure the level of thyroid hormones. They may be done if thyroid disease or another endocrine disease is suspected.

**Thyroid scan.** A thyroid scan measures the rate that the thyroid gland takes up and processes iodine. It's a type of nuclear medicine test. A form of radioactive iodine is given to you, either by mouth or by injection. After a certain time, a special type of camera is used to look at the thyroid. Nodules and tumors can be detected. This test may show whether a tumor is likely to be noncancerous or cancerous.

**Tuberculin skin test.** The tuberculin skin test detects past or present tuberculosis exposure based on a positive skin reaction. A positive skin reaction comes from a bit of tuberculin that's put into your skin by scratch, puncture or injection. If a red, raised or hard area is found around the tuberculin test site, you're "reactive" to tuberculin. A positive test doesn't mean you have an active infection. The bacteria may be dormant, or inactive. If your test is positive, your doctor will

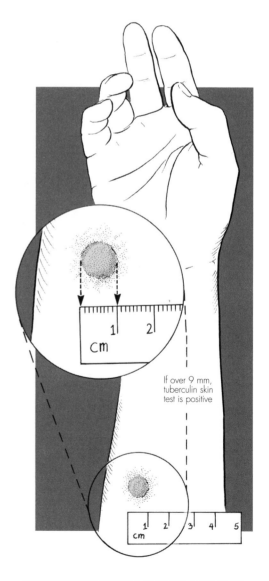

If over 9 mm, tuberculin skin test is positive

**POSITIVE TEST RESULT FOR TUBERCULIN SKIN TEST**

probably look for signs of active infection with a chest x-ray or other tests.

**Tuning fork.** The tuning fork test helps determine what type of hearing loss is present. The tuning fork test isn't usually helpful in children younger than about four years old.

**Tympanocentesis.** Problems with your ear may require a culture of the secretions behind the eardrum, obtained by performing a tympanocentesis to make a hole in the eardrum. The secretions are cultured to find the specific bacteria responsible for an infection. This procedure is also used to remove fluid from the middle ear.

**Tympanometry.** Your middle ear contains a thin membrane called the *tympanic membrane,* also called the eardrum. Tympanometry is a test of the movement of this membrane. If the eardrum doesn't move, it usually means there's a build-up of fluid, or a vacuum effect, in the middle ear behind the drum. Your ability to hear may be reduced because the movement of the eardrum is restricted.

**Ultrasound.** Ultrasound uses sound waves to create a "picture" of certain areas of the body. High-frequency sound waves (humans can't hear them) are aimed at an organ or body area. The sound waves then echo back from the organ or tissue to form a "picture" that can be viewed on a screen. This procedure is painless. It can be used to diagnose abdominal injury or tumors, prostate disease and deep-vein thrombosis.

A common use of ultrasound testing, also called a sonogram, is to bounce sound waves through the uterus and off the fetus to create detailed pictures of the fetus. Hands, feet and facial features can be seen, and sometimes even the sex of the baby can be determined. Measurements of the head help your doctor estimate the age of the baby and check for growth problems. The health

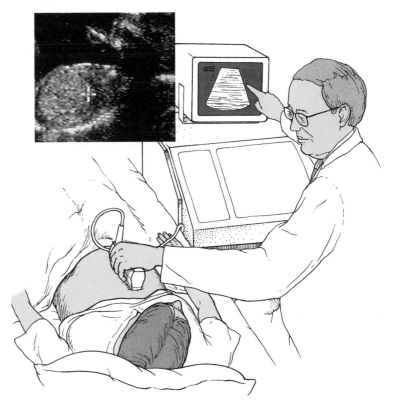

**ULTRASOUND (SONOGRAM) PICTURE**

and location of the placenta can also be checked

To have a sonogram during pregnancy, you'll lie on an exam table and a technician will apply the conducting jelly to your abdomen. Then he or she will use the hand-held *transducer* to locate the baby. The transducer transmits images to a video screen. You can watch your baby's movements while the technician notes different measurements.

Depending on when the sonogram is performed, you may be able to see the entire baby in one shot. This image may be quite clear if the baby is relatively still during the test. Otherwise, you may see a blurry image with occasional glimpses of a face, a hand or another body part. Later in pregnancy, you may only be able to see parts of the baby. The technician can help you identify the images. You may also be able to get a photograph of the image shown on the screen to take home with you.

A *Doppler ultrasound* also uses sound waves but doesn't generate a picture. It can be done during pregnancy to check for fetal heartbeat. A hand-held device uses sound waves to detect the blood flow through the circulatory system of the fetus. This use of ultrasound is the easiest way to check the baby's health. It causes no harm to you or the baby and is painless. Usually, the heartbeat can be detected by the 10th to 12th week of the pregnancy.

*Non-stress testing and stress testing* use a Doppler device to measure changes in the fetus' heart rate as it moves and reacts to uterine contractions. Non-stress testing looks at changes in the heartbeat that occur with normal movements of the fetus. Stress testing uses loud noises, medicines to contract the uterus and other means, such as maternal nipple stimulation to induce contractions, to stimulate fetal movement.

Ultrasound is also used to diagnose breast cysts, gallstones, arteriosclerosis in the arteries of the neck and legs, prostate gland problems, ectopic pregnancies and blood clots in the veins.

**Urine culture.** To get a urine culture, you must urinate in a special container and get a "clean catch." A clean catch is a method of collecting urine that keeps the sample sterile. To do this, wash your hands thoroughly and wash the penis or vulva using downward strokes. Then, begin to urinate directly into the toilet and stop in the middle of urinating. Put the urine container under the stream of urine and begin to urinate again, this time into the specimen cup. Don't touch the rim of the cup as you screw the lid on tightly. A culture is a process of growing bacteria in the urine to identify the type of bacteria causing the infection. It usually takes 24 to 48 hours to get the results of the culture.

**Venogram.** See angiogram.

**X-rays.** An x-ray is taken by a machine that generates short waves of radiation that are projected through the subject and onto a photographic plate. The x-ray machine makes a picture of a bone, organ or part of the body. X-rays can show fractures, foreign objects or the outline of contrast dyes that have been injected into the body.

# DICTIONARY

The words listed in this dictionary are included to help you better understand the text of the book. Words for tests and medicines aren't included here. Instead, tests are described in the Tests section, beginning on page 627. Medicines are described in the Medicine Cabinet section, beginning on page 613. Many of the words listed below are mentioned in the text in greater detail. Please check the index for a page number if you see something about which you would like more information. If the information isn't included here, if you need more information or if you need help understanding what something means, talk to your family doctor.

## A

**abdomen.** The part of the body between the chest and pelvis.

**abortion.** 1. *Induced abortion* is a procedure done to end pregnancy. 2. *Spontaneous abortion* is a naturally occurring abortion (also called miscarriage). 3. *Therapeutic abortion* is an induced abortion required to save the life or health of the mother.

**abrasion.** A wound caused by scraping the skin. A "skinned knee" is a common example.

**abscess.** A swollen, inflamed area where pus gathers.

**absorption.** To take in substances through the skin or mucous membranes.

**abstinence.** To hold back or restrain. For example, to refrain from the use of drugs or alcohol, or from having sexual intercourse.

**acclimation.** The process of getting used to a new climate or altitude.

**Achilles' tendon.** The strong tendon at the back of the ankle that attaches the calf muscle to the heel.

**acidosis.** An abnormal condition in the body in which excessive acid lowers the pH of the blood and body tissues.

**acne.** A skin disorder usually found in adolescents and young adults.

**acoustic.** Having to do with sound and hearing.

**ACTH.** Adrenocorticotropic hormone. Produced by the pituitary gland, which stimulates the adrenal glands to secrete hormones.

**actinic keratoses.** Scaly, pink, gray or tan patches or bumps on the face or scalp, or on the back of the hands. Occur mostly on people who have light skin that has been damaged by the sun.

**acromegaly.** A condition that occurs when the pituitary gland produces too much growth hormone. In adults, this can cause overgrowth of bones that occurs in smaller bones, such as those in the jaw, hands and feet. In children or teenagers, this can cause giantism.

**acupuncture.** An ancient Chinese method to relieve pain or treat disease by inserting needles into various parts of the body.

**acute.** 1. Of short course. 2. Severe, but of a short duration. Not chronic.

**addiction.** Strong dependence or habitual use of a substance or practice, despite the negative consequences of its use.

**Addison's disease.** An ailment characterized by underfunctioning of the adrenal glands. Characterized by anemia, weakness, low blood pressure and brownish discoloration of the skin.

**adenitis.** Swelling of a gland.

**adenoids.** Glandular tissue in the back of the throat that may swell, especially during childhood, obstruct breathing and speaking, and lead to ear infections.

**adenoma.** A noncancerous tumor of glandular tissue.

**adenovirus.** One of the viruses that cause the common cold.

**ADH.** Antidiuretic hormone. One of the hormones produced by the pituitary gland. A shortage of this hormone causes increased loss of body fluids through the kidneys.

**adhesion.** The sticking of one surface to another. This can occur when scar tissue causes organs or loops of intestine to stick together. Occasionally, these adhesions may produce an intestinal obstruction or other malfunction by twisting or distorting the organ.

**adipose fatty cells.** Special cells in which fat is stored when a person's caloric intake is greater than that required by one's metabolism.

**adrenal glands.** Located on top of the kidneys, these glands produce hormones helpful in regulating the body's metabolism.

**adrenaline.** Epinephrine. One of several hormones produced by the adrenal glands.

**aerobic.** Requiring the use of oxygen. Exercise that conditions the heart and lungs by increasing the efficiency of oxygen intake by the body.

**afterbirth.** The placenta, which is attached to the fetus by the umbilical cord and must be delivered after the baby.

**AIDS.** Acquired immunodeficiency syndrome. A disease of the immune system caused by the HIV virus.

**airway.** The passage by which air enters and exits the lungs.

**albinism.** The absence of all normal body pigmentation at birth, a condition that can occur in all races.

**albino.** A person with albinism.

**albumin.** A water-soluble protein found in milk, egg, muscle, blood and many vegetable tissues and fluids.

**aldosteronism.** A condition resulting when the adrenal glands produce too much of the hormone aldosterone, which regulates fluids and salt in the body.

**alimentary.** Having to do with food or nutrition. The alimentary tract is the digestive tract.

**allergen.** A substance capable of producing an allergic reaction.

**allergy.** An exaggerated immune response to substances in the environment.

**alopecia.** Hair loss, especially of the head.

**alpha$_1$-antitrypsin deficiency.** Congenital lack of an enzyme that leads to cirrhosis of the liver and obstructive lung disease.

**altitude sickness**. A potentially fatal illness caused by being at altitudes high enough to reduce the amount of oxygen available to the body.

**alveoli.** The sacs in the lungs at the ends of the smallest airways where oxygen is exchanged for carbon dioxide in the blood.

**amblyopia.** Impaired vision without an apparent cause.

**ambulatory.** Able to walk. Not confined to bed.

**amenorrhea.** Absence of menstrual periods.

**amnesia.** Partial or total loss of memory, usually as the result of psychological trauma or stress, or physical damage to the brain from injury, disease, or alcohol or other chronic drug abuse.

**amnion.** The membrane enclosing a developing fetus; it's filled with a protective liquid called amniotic fluid.

**amputation.** The surgical removal of a limb or other appendage because of damage by trauma or as a treatment for a variety of potentially life-threatening ailments.

**anaerobic exercise.** Brief, intense exercise that leads to an oxygen debt in a certain area of tissue. Weight lifting is an example.

**anaphylaxis.** The most severe form of allergy, in which the person's heart and lungs are unable to keep working, and death occurs unless prompt medical attention is obtained.

**androgen.** Any substance that produces male characteristics. Testosterone and androsterone are natural androgens.

**anemia.** A decreased ability of the blood to carry oxygen because of a reduction in either the number or quality of the red blood cells.

**anesthesia.** Drug-induced loss of feeling or sensation.

**anesthetic.** An agent used to produce anesthesia.

**aneurysm.** A thin sac caused by a weakened area in the walls of blood vessels or the heart. As an aneurysm increases in size, the sac

tends to become thinner, and the risk of its breaking becomes greater.

**angina pectoris.** Chest pain caused by decreased oxygen delivery to the heart muscle.

**angioma.** A noncancerous tumor made up of many blood vessels.

**anhidrosis.** Absence of sweating. An inability to sweat greatly interferes with the body's ability to control its internal temperature.

**ankylosis.** Abnormal stiffening of a joint.

**anomaly.** Deviation from normal.

**anorchism.** Congenital absence of both testes.

**anorexia nervosa.** An eating disorder manifested primarily by a loss of desire or willingness to eat for a variety of psychological reasons.

**anosmia.** Loss of the sense of smell.

**antepartum.** Occurring before delivery of a baby.

**antibody.** A protein produced by the body to neutralize an invading foreign agent or antigen, such as a virus.

**antidote.** An agent used to counteract a poison.

**antigen.** A foreign agent capable of starting an immune response or causing the body to produce antibodies.

**antiserum.** A serum that contains antibodies. Serum from a person or animal with immunity to a certain disease can, in some cases, be used to prevent illness in other people.

**anus.** The opening of the rectum.

**anxiety.** A feeling of nervousness, uneasiness, apprehension or dread.

**aorta.** The large artery that carries blood from the heart to the rest of body.

**apathy.** Lack of emotions.

**Apgar score.** A scoring method from zero to 10 for describing the health of an infant at birth, based on heart rate, breathing, muscle tone, color and reflex irritability.

**aphagia.** Inability to swallow.

**aphasia.** A partial or total loss of the power to use or

understand words.

**aphthous ulcers.** A painful sore in the mouth. Also called a canker sore.

**apnea.** Temporary pause in breathing.

**appendectomy.** Surgical removal of the appendix.

**appendix.** A finger-like appendage near the junction of the large intestine and the small intestine.

**areola.** The dark area of the breast surrounding the nipple.

**arteriosclerosis.** Commonly called "hardening of the arteries." An abnormal thickening and loss of elasticity of the wall of the arteries.

**arteriovenous malformation.** Abnormal group of dilated blood vessels, most often occurring in the brain.

**artery.** A vessel that carries blood away from the heart to various parts of the body.

**arthralgia.** Pain in a joint.

**arthritis.** Inflammation of a joint.

**asbestos.** A fibrous material used to make fireproof materials, electrical insulation, roofing and filters. Asbestos has been linked to a type of lung cancer.

**ascites.** Abnormal buildup of fluid in the abdomen that causes distention.

**ascorbic acid.** Vitamin C.

**asthma.** A chronic disorder characterized by shortness of breath, wheezing, coughing and tightness of the chest.

**astigmatism.** An irregularity in the curvature of the lens of the eye, resulting in a blurry or distorted image.

**atelectasis.** Collapsed lung. May occur following surgery or after a rib fracture.

**atherosclerosis.** A form of arteriosclerosis caused by fatty deposits in the arteries.

**athlete's foot.** A fungal infection of the skin of the feet.

**atopy.** A predisposition to allergy that's inherited from parents. Included disorders are asthma, hay fever and eczema.

**atria.** The upper chambers of the heart that receive blood from the veins and pass

it to the lower chambers of the heart.

**atrophy.** A decrease in the normal size of an organ. Wasting away.

**aura.** A peculiar sensation that occurs before other symptoms. An example is the sensation of flashing lights before a migraine headache.

**autoimmune disease.** A condition in which antibodies form against one's own cells.

**autotransfusion.** A transfusion using the patient's own blood.

**axilla.** The armpit.

# B

**bacteremia.** The presence of bacteria in the blood.

**bacteria.** Single-celled microorganisms with one of three basic shapes: rod-like (bacilli), spherical (cocci) and spiral (spirilla). Bacteria are commonly thought of as disease-causing agents. But many bacteria are beneficial and don't cause disease.

**bacteriuria.** The presence of bacteria in the urine.

**Baker's cyst.** A swelling of the knee caused by an escape of fluid from a sac behind the knee.

**ballism.** Quick, jerking movements that occur in people with chorea.

**barium.** A chalky substance used in x-ray studies of the digestive tract to highlight abnormalities.

**barotrauma.** Injury caused by pressure differences between the atmosphere and the air-filled spaces in the body. The most common of these injuries are the ear and sinus blocks that can occur during air travel.

**Bartholin cyst.** A cyst caused by an infection of the glands on the vaginal wall.

**BCG (bacille Calmette-Guérin) vaccine.** A vaccine that offers some protection against tuberculosis. It's now rarely used in the U.S. because it doesn't give total protection.

**bedsore.** An ulcer caused by chafing or by the pressure of the body against the bed.

**Bell's palsy.** A usually temporary loss of feeling or movement of the face, usually on one side, causing an inability to close the eye or mouth on that side.

**bends.** A condition that results from rapidly decreasing atmospheric pressure on the body. Symptoms include joint pain, chest pain, shortness of breath and coma. The condition may be fatal.

**benign familial tremor.** An inherited disorder that causes a slow tremor in the hands, head and voice. It may affect only one side of the body, be worse when moving than when resting and worsen with age.

**benign.** A nonlife-threatening condition. Not malignant. Not cancerous.

**beriberi.** A deficiency disease caused by dietary insufficiency of vitamin B$_1$ (thiamine). Symptoms include general weakness and painful rigidity.

**biceps.** A muscle having two heads. The most familiar is the large muscle in the front of the upper arm responsible for flexing the forearm.

**bicuspid.** A tooth named for the two-pointed projections on the crown.

**bifocals.** Eyeglasses with divided lenses. The two parts of each lens have different strengths, allowing the wearer to focus the eye for either near or distant vision.

**bile.** A clear yellow fluid produced by the liver and stored in the gallbladder. Aids in digestion.

**bilirubin.** A pigment produced in the liver by the breakdown of hemoglobin from old red blood cells. Bilirubin is normally eliminated in the bile. A variety of diseases may cause bilirubin to collect in the body, resulting in a yellow discoloration of the skin known as jaundice.

**binocular.** Using both eyes at the same time. Binocular vision is the most important element of depth perception.

**biopsy.** Removal and exam of a tissue sample taken from a living body. This procedure helps determine if the tissue is cancerous.

**bipolar affective disorder.** A psychiatric disorder in which the affected person has both depressed and happy, energetic (manic) episodes. This is a newer term for manic-depressive disorder.

**blackhead.** A dark-topped plug of fatty material in the opening of a hair follicle. The color is the result of exposure of the fat to the air.

**blackout.** 1. Short-term loss of vision and consciousness. 2. In an alcoholic person, loss of memory for a period of time.

**bladder.** The organ that temporarily stores a substance. Commonly used in reference to the urinary bladder, which holds urine until it's eliminated.

**blepharitis.** Inflammation of the eyelid.

**blepharoplasty.** Plastic surgery on the eyelid.

**blindness.** Loss of vision. Legally, visual acuity less than 20/200 with glasses.

**blister.** Buildup of watery or bloody fluid under the skin.

**blood poisoning.** Infection within the circulatory system. A potentially life-threatening condition that requires prompt treatment.

**blood pressure.** The pressure exerted by the blood against the walls of the blood vessels.

**blood.** The fluid circulating through the heart, arteries and veins. Blood is responsible for transporting oxygen to body tissues, carrying waste products away from the tissues and delivering a wide variety of biochemical substances throughout the body to maintain health.

**boil.** A skin infection characterized by a localized build-up of pus.

**bone marrow.** The tissue within the cavity of the bones where new blood cells are made.

**Borrelia.** A class of disease-causing bacteria that includes the organisms that cause relapsing fever and Lyme disease.

**botulism.** An extremely dangerous form of food poisoning caused by the toxin of *Clostridium botulinum.*

**bovine.** Having to do with cattle. For example, bovine insulin is insulin obtained from cattle.

**bowel.** See intestine.

**Bowen's disease.** A precancerous skin condition that first appears as psoriasis-like scaling.

**bowleg.** A deformity of the legs in which the space between the knees is greater than normal.

**brace.** A device used to support a body part, correct or prevent deformities, or control movement.

**bradycardia.** Slow heart rate and pulse, usually slower than 60 beats per minute.

**Braxton Hicks contractions.** Contractions of the uterus during pregnancy that are sometimes mistaken for labor. Also called false labor.

**breasts.** Milk-secreting glands protruding from the upper front part of a woman's body.

**breech birth.** A birth in which the feet or buttocks of the baby appear first through the birth canal.

**bridge.** A structure that joins two parts. For example, a dental bridge contains artificial teeth and joins the natural teeth at either end.

**Bright's disease.** Nephritis. A group of kidney diseases manifested by albumin in the urine and edema (swelling).

**bronchi.** The tubular passages, also called bronchial tubes, that carry air into the lungs.

**bronchiectasis.** A chronic enlargement of the bronchi accompanied by coughing and production of large amounts of phlegm containing pus.

**bronchiolitis.** An infection of the bronchioles, the tiny air tubes in the lungs.

**bronchitis.** Inflammation of the bronchi.

**bronchospasm.** Contraction of the muscle in the walls of the bronchi.

**bronze diabetes.** A disorder of iron metabolism resulting in iron pigment deposits in the skin and other body tissues that causes a change in skin color.

**brucellosis.** An infection characterized by fluctuating fever, headache, anemia and vague physical discomfort that's transmitted to humans from domesticated goats, pigs and cattle.

**bruise.** Discoloration of the skin due to a buildup of blood in the underlying soft tissues. Also called a contusion.

**bruxism.** Grinding of the teeth.

**bubo.** A swollen, infected lymph node (especially in the groin). The node may enlarge enough that it begins to drain through the skin.

**Buerger's disease.** Blockage of medium-sized blood vessels in the hands and feet by clotting and inflammation. This process causes severe pain and may lead to gangrene.

**bulimia.** An eating disorder characterized by binge eating followed by vomiting or use of laxatives. Usually caused by a variety of psychological reasons.

**bunion.** Localized swelling of the big toe at its joint with the foot.

**bursa.** A small, fluid-filled sac that allows one part of a joint to move freely over another part.

**bursitis.** Inflammation of a bursa.

# C

**cachexia.** A generally weakened, emaciated condition of the body.

**caffeine.** A bitter-tasting, water-soluble compound that acts as a central nervous system stimulant and has a mild diuretic (increasing urination) effect.

**calciferol.** Vitamin D.

**calcification.** Calcium salt deposits in soft tissues.

**calculus.** A small, hard mass or stone formed in the body, as in a kidney or gallbladder, or a hard coating on the surface of the teeth.

**callus.** 1. Localized thickening of the skin. 2. A fibrous band formed around the site of a fracture that seals the ends of the bone together and is then gradually replaced by mature bone.

**calorie.** The amount of energy needed to raise the temperature of one kilogram of water one degree. Commonly used to express the amount of energy-producing value in food.

**Calvé-Perthes.** A disease in children affecting the growth plate of the head of the thigh, caused by interference in the blood supply.

**camphor.** An agent derived from a cinnamon tree that's used to relieve pain and itching.

**cancer.** Abnormal cells with uncontrolled cell growth.

**Candida.** The class of yeast that causes thrush and vaginal yeast infections.

**canker.** An open sore on the lip or skin inside the mouth.

**Cannabis.** The class of plants that includes marijuana and other hemps.

**capillary.** A small, blood-containing vessel connecting the veins and arteries.

**carbohydrates.** A group of energy-storage molecules that includes sugars and starches. Carbohydrates contain four calories per gram.

**carbon dioxide.** An odorless, colorless gas produced as the end product of aerobic respiration.

**carbon monoxide.** An odorless, colorless, poisonous gas produced from the incomplete combustion of carbon. Prevents the blood from carrying oxygen.

**carbuncle.** A hard, painful, pus-filled infection of the skin. Carbuncles are larger than boils and frequently have more than one opening.

**carcinogen.** A cancer-causing substance.

**carcinoma.** A cancerous tumor.

**cardiac.** Having to do with the heart or, less commonly, the upper portion of the stomach.

**cardiomegaly.** Enlargement of the heart.

**cardiomyopathy.** A disorder of the heart muscle.

**cardiovascular.** Having to do with the heart and blood vessels.

**caries.** Decay of the teeth or bone.

**carotene.** The fat-soluble pigment in carrots, tomatoes and other vegetables, egg yolks, milk fat and other substances that can be converted in the body to vitamin A.

**carotid.** The main artery in the neck.

**carpal.** Having to do with the wrist.

**carpal tunnel syndrome.** Pain, numbness and tingling of the fingers caused by compression of the median nerve at the wrist.

**carrier.** Someone who's capable of transmitting a disease (especially an infectious or genetic disorder) to another person but who usually has no symptoms of the disease.

**cartilage.** Elastic connective tissue on the joint surfaces of bone and some parts of the skeleton, including the nose and ears.

**castor oil.** An oil extracted from the castor bean plant that's irritating to the intestine and promotes bowel movements.

**castration.** To remove the gonads, such as the testicles, making the male unable to have children.

**cat-scratch fever.** A bacterial infection acquired through the scratch of a cat or other animal.

**catalepsy.** A condition in which the body and limbs stay in the position in which they're placed.

**cataract.** An opaque area in the lens of the eye.

**catheter.** A tube used to drain or inject fluids.

**cauliflower ear.** A trauma-induced deformity of the ear caused by repeated cartilage and soft-tissue injury.

**caustic.** A chemical that can cause burns.

**cauterize.** To purposely burn with a hot instrument or

caustic substance to destroy tissue, such as a wart.

**cavity.** A hollow place or hole within the body.

**CBC.** Complete blood cell count.

**cecum.** The first part of the large intestine just below the small intestine or ileum.

**celiac.** Having to do with the abdomen.

**cell.** The basic unit of organization of all living organisms.

**cellulitis.** Infection of the skin.

**cellulose.** A complex carbohydrate. Cellulose is a source of dietary fiber because it can't be digested.

**cephalalgia.** Headache.

**cerebellum.** The part of the brain that coordinates muscular movements.

**cerebrum.** The main part of the brain.

**cerumen.** Earwax.

**cervical.** Having to do with the neck (cervical spine) or the cervix of the uterus.

**cervix.** The neck-like portion of an organ, especially the part of the uterus that extends into the vagina.

**cesarean section.** Delivery of a baby through an incision in the abdominal wall and uterus.

**chalazion.** A chronic, small swelling on the rim of the eyelid.

**chancre.** The painless ulcer of primary syphilis that appears on the genitals.

**chancroid.** A sexually transmitted disease that causes soft, painful open sores in the genital area. Not syphilis. Characterized by swelling of the sebaceous glands, resulting in pimples on the face, back and chest.

**Charcot-Marie-Tooth disease.** Progressive, generally painless weakness of the legs, along with foot deformity.

**charley horse.** Painful stiffness from muscular strain in an arm or leg.

**cheilosis.** A condition in which cracks or sores occur at the corners of the mouth.

**chickenpox.** A viral disease that usually begins with fever and cough, followed by a rash that progresses

from red bumps to blisters to scabs. A vaccine is available to prevent this disease. Also called varicella or varicella zoster.

**chilblain.** Painful redness of the fingers, toes or ears caused by exposure to cold.

**childbed fever.** This is a severe illness marked by fever that's caused by an infection in mothers after giving birth. Also called puerperal sepsis.

**chill.** A cold sensation with shivering that sometimes occurs before a fever.

**chiropractic.** An approach to health care based on the assumption that most diseases are caused by pressure on the nerves. This pressure is thought to be caused by faulty alignment of the bones that prevents the nerves from functioning properly.

**Chlamydia.** A microorganism, *Chlamydia trachomatis*, that's a frequent cause of sexually transmitted disease. It can also cause pneumonia and eye infections.

**chloasma.** See melasma.

**chlorination.** The addition of chlorine to kill harmful microorganisms in water or sewage.

**cholecystitis.** Inflammation of the gallbladder.

**cholera.** Watery diarrhea caused by drinking water or eating food that's contaminated with *Vibrio cholere*. The disease is spread through the stools of infected persons.

**cholesteatoma.** A tumor-like mass that sometimes forms as a result of a chronic middle ear infection.

**cholesterol.** A fat-like substance that, if present in the blood in large amounts, is associated with the development of heart disease.

**chondritis.** Inflammation of the cartilage.

**chondromalacia.** Softening of cartilage.

**chorea.** A nervous system disorder characterized by involuntary spasms of the limbs or facial muscles. A hereditary form is called Huntington's chorea.

chromosomes. The DNA-containing cellular structures that carry genetic information.

chronic. Persistent. Ongoing. Lasting a long time.

cilia. Short, hair-like structures extending from certain cells.

circadian. A repetitive pattern or fluctuation with a 24-hour cycle.

circulation. The flow of blood through the body. Includes the heart, arteries, veins and capillaries.

circumcision. Surgical removal of the foreskin of the penis.

cirrhosis. Inflammatory disease of the liver characterized by scarring and shrinkage.

claudication. Pain in the legs while walking that's caused by blockage of the arteries.

claustrophobia. Fear of closed spaces.

clavicle. Collarbone.

clawhand. A condition of the hand causing distorted fingers resulting from nerve injury.

cleft lip or palate. A congenital split of the upper lip or roof of the mouth.

clitoris. A small, sensitive erectile organ located in the female at the top of the vulva.

Clostridium. A genus of bacteria that includes the agents capable of causing food poisoning and tetanus.

clot. A jelly-like mass of blood.

clubfoot. A deformity in which the foot is turned inward from its normal position.

coal tar. A by-product of coal used in the treatment of some skin conditions, such as psoriasis.

cobalamin. Vitamin $B_{12}$.

cocaine. A drug that is made from coca leaves. It can be used by a doctor as a topical anesthetic. It's often abused for its euphoric affects. It's highly addictive.

coccyx. The tailbone.

cochlea. The portion of the inner ear that senses sound.

coitus. Sexual intercourse.

cold sore. Herpes simplex infection of the lip.

cold. An upper respiratory infection.

colic. 1. A sudden, spasmodic abdominal pain. 2. In infants, a pattern of excessive crying, apparent abdominal pain and irritability.

colitis. Inflammation of the colon.

collagen. A protein formed in the connective tissue of the body.

colon. The large intestine.

Colorado tick fever. A viral illness spread by ticks. Characterized by headache, backache and fever that begins to break and then returns midway through the course of the illness.

colostomy. Surgery that makes an opening to the intestine through the surface of the abdomen. The opening empties the bowels.

colostrum. An antibody-rich fluid released by the breasts for a short time after the birth of a baby, before the true milk is produced.

comedo. See blackhead.

communicable disease. A disease spread through direct contact with an infected person or substance.

compress. A dressing used to apply pressure or medicine to an area. Useful in applying heat or cold.

compulsion. An overwhelming urge to perform an act. Often used to describe ritual or repetitive behaviors.

conception. Fertilization. The union of sperm and egg.

concussion. A loss of consciousness because of a head injury.

condom. A sheath worn over the penis or inside the vagina (female condom) during intercourse to protect against pregnancy and disease.

cone. The light-sensing structure on the retina of the eye capable of detecting color.

congenital. Present at birth.

conjunctiva. The membrane lining the eyelids and covering the eyeball.

conjunctivitis. Inflammation of the conjunctiva. Also called pink eye.

connective tissue. Fibrous tissue with a wide variety of connecting and supporting functions within and between body organs.

conscious. Mentally awake and aware. Knowing what one is doing and why.

constipation. A condition in which the stool becomes too hard for easy elimination.

consumption. 1. Using up. 2. Wasting of the body; especially used in reference to advanced tuberculosis.

contagious. Easily transmitted by direct or indirect contact.

contraception. The intentional prevention of conception or impregnation. Also called birth control.

contraction. A shortening or increase in tension.

contracture. Deformity caused by abnormal shortening of the muscles.

contrast medium. A substance used in x-ray studies to aid in showing internal structures.

contusion. Bruise.

convulsion. A seizure.

cor pulmonale. Increased blood pressure in the lungs, causing chest pain, shortness of breath, swelling in the feet and fluid in the lungs.

corn. A hardened area of skin on the foot caused by persistent friction or pressure.

cornea. The clear, external part of the eye.

coronary arteries. The blood vessels encircling the heart that provide the heart muscle with oxygen.

corticosteroid hormones. Hormones produced by the adrenal glands.

coryza. Runny nose.

costochondritis. Inflammation of the cartilage-containing joints where the ribs join the breastbone (sternum).

coxsackievirus. A virus that can cause inflammation of the heart, brain or eye, or hand-foot-and-mouth disease.

cramp. A painful muscle spasm.

craniotomy. A surgical opening of the skull.

cranium. The skull, or bony structure of the head, that protects the brain.

creatinine. A substance formed from the making of creatine, an important nitrogen compound made in the body. Common in blood, urine and muscle tissue.

cretinism. Physical and mental retardation due to congenital lack of thyroid hormone.

Crohn's disease. Chronic inflammation of the digestive tract, especially of the lower small intestine and colon.

croup. Obstruction of the upper respiratory tract at or below the larynx (voice box), resulting in a hoarse, barking cough.

crowning. The first appearance of a baby's scalp during the birth process.

cryosurgery. Destruction of tissue using extreme cold. A procedure used to treat skin lesions.

CT. Computed tomographic scan.

culdocentesis. A procedure to remove pus or blood from the abdomen through the vagina.

Cushing's syndrome. A disorder caused by overactivity of the pituitary gland.

cuspid. A tooth with one point, or "canine" tooth.

cutaneous. Having to do with the skin.

cyanosis. Bluish discoloration of the skin caused by lack of oxygen in the blood.

cyst. A sac or pocket in the body containing fluid or semisolid material.

cystitis. Inflammation of the bladder.

cytology. The study of cells.

cytomegalovirus. A virus that infects cells and causes them to become enlarged. Babies infected with the virus develop mental and sensory disorders.

# D

D and C. Dilatation and curettage. A surgical procedure in which the uterine lining is removed by scraping.

dacryocystitis. Inflammation of the sac that collects tears for drainage from the eye.

dandruff. Little scales or flakes of dead skin on the scalp. Also called seborrheic dermatitis.

debridement. Removal of foreign material or dead tissue.

**decalcification.** Loss of calcium from the bones or teeth.

**decidua.** The mucus lining of the uterus that's passed after childbirth or during the menstrual period.

**decubitus.** A skin ulcer or bedsore.

**defibrillator.** A machine that delivers an electrical shock to an irregularly beating heart to restore normal rhythm.

**degenerative joint disease.** A common form of arthritis in which tissue changes occur in one or more joints, such as swelling, lumps or cysts, or small pieces of loose bone and cartilage, which cause stiffness and pain. Also called osteoarthritis.

**dehydration.** Excessive loss of body water resulting in weakness, dizziness and other symptoms. It can be life-threatening if not treated, especially in young children and babies.

**delirium.** An abnormal mental state characterized by excitement and hallucinations.

**deltoid.** The triangular muscle of the shoulder.

**delusion.** A false belief.

**dementia.** Progressive mental deterioration.

**dentition.** Arrangement of the teeth.

**dependence.** A state of absolute need, both physical and psychological.

**depilatory.** A substance that temporarily removes hair from the skin.

**depression.** Decreased functional activity. Sinking of spirits. Intense sadness, beyond what's normally expected.

**dermabrasion.** A procedure that removes scars, tattoos or other skin defects with fine sandpaper or a high-speed brush.

**dermatitis.** Inflammation of the skin.

**dermatology.** A medical specialty that deals with the skin.

**desensitization.** Reducing or eliminating sensitivity to a particular substance.

**desquamation.** The shedding of cells from the surface of the skin or mucous membranes.

**devascularization.** Interruption of blood circulation to part of the body.

**dextrose.** A simple sugar. Glucose.

**diabetes insipidus.** Loss of water through the kidneys as a result of decreased production of the pituitary hormone vasopressin (an antidiuretic hormone).

**diabetes mellitus.** A disorder of carbohydrate metabolism resulting from insulin deficiency. Characterized by high blood sugar levels that result in weakness, frequent urination and increased thirst and hunger.

**diagnose.** To identify a disease.

**diagnosis.** The process of identifying a disease or medical condition.

**dialysis.** A treatment to remove certain molecules from the blood, particularly in people with kidney failure.

**diaphoresis.** Excessive sweating.

**diaphragm.** 1. The dome-shaped respiratory muscle separating the chest from the abdomen. 2. A barrier contraceptive device molded to fit over the cervix.

**diarrhea.** Production of feces in increased volume and with greater fluidity than normal.

**diastole.** The relaxation phase of the heartbeat.

**diet.** The total food consumed by an individual. A therapeutic diet is a prescription of required or restricted foods.

**dietitian.** An expert who is trained in the use of diet and nutrition to maintain or restore health.

**digestion.** The mechanical and chemical conversion of food into simpler compounds that can be absorbed by the body.

**digit.** A finger or toe.

**dilation.** The process of expanding or enlarging.

**diphtheria.** An infectious disease of childhood characterized by fever, sore throat and the presence of "dirty" (white, gray, brown) membranes in the throat.

**diplopia.** Double vision.

**discoid lupus erythematosus.** A round, red, scaling rash on the nose, forehead, cheeks, scalp or other areas of the body. It may be associated with systemic lupus erythematosus.

**disinfectant.** A chemical agent used to destroy microorganisms on inanimate objects.

**disk.** A round, flat structure, particularly the fibrous cartilage layer between two vertebrae (the bones that make up the spine). Also called intervertebral disk.

**diskectomy.** Removal of an intervertebral disk of the spine.

**dislocation.** Displacement of a bone from a joint.

**disorientation.** Mental confusion, especially of time, place or person.

**distal.** A location farther from a point of reference. For example, the foot is distal to the knee, relative to the center of the body.

**diuresis.** Increased elimination of urine.

**diverticula.** Pouches or sacs opening out from a main cavity or tubular organ of the body.

**diverticulitis.** Inflammation of small pouches that may form on the wall of the colon.

**diverticulosis.** A condition in which pouches form on the wall of the colon.

**dorsal.** Toward the back.

**douche.** A flow of liquid or vapor directed onto or into a part of the body.

**Down syndrome.** A genetic disorder characterized by some degree of mental retardation and by various physical malformations, such as slanted eyes and a broad face.

**DPT.** A vaccine containing antigens from diphtheria, pertussis and tetanus.

**dressing.** A bandage for an external wound.

**dropsy.** Abnormal buildup of fluid in tissues or a body cavity.

**duct.** A channel or passage through which fluids move.

**duodenal.** Having to do with the duodenum.

**duodenum.** The first part of the small intestine that begins at the stomach and is the entry point for the pancreatic and common bile duct.

**Dupuytren's contracture.** Scarring of the palmar ligament in the hand, causing progressive curling of one or more fingers and a thickening of the palm.

**dwarfism.** A deficiency of growth hormone resulting in short stature.

**dysentery.** Infection of the intestine resulting in severe diarrhea and cramps, frequently associated with blood or mucus in the stools.

**dysmenorrhea.** Painful menstruation.

**dyspepsia.** Indigestion.

**dysphagia.** Difficulty swallowing.

**dyspnea.** Labored breathing.

# E

**eardrum.** The tympanic membrane that's visible in the ear. It vibrates in response to sound waves.

**ecchymosis.** A collection of blood in the tissues causing a black and blue, or yellow, area.

**ECG.** Electrocardiogram.

**eclampsia.** An attack of convulsions. Particularly used to describe toxemia (toxins in the blood) of pregnancy.

**ectopic pregnancy.** When the fertilized egg is implanted and develops outside of the uterus.

**ectropion.** An outward turning of the eyelid.

**eczema.** A rash characterized by itching, scaling, swelling and oozing. A common allergic reaction.

**edema.** Buildup of excessive fluid around the cells in the body.

**EEG.** Electroencephalogram.

**effacement.** Thinning of the cervix during labor.

**effusion.** Buildup of fluid in a part of the body, particularly a joint.

**ejaculation.** The sudden ejection of semen from the male body. Climax.

**EKG.** Electrocardiogram.

**electroconvulsive.** A type of therapy used to treat severe, unresponsive depression by passing electrical current through the brain.

**electrolysis.** Destruction of tissue through the use of electricity; often used to permanently remove unwanted hair from the body.

**electrolytes.** Compounds that separate into charged particles in water. The main electrolytes in the human body are sodium, potassium, bicarbonate, chloride, magnesium, calcium and phosphate.

**elephantiasis.** A chronic disease characterized by the enlargement of certain parts of the body and by the hardening and ulceration of the surrounding skin. It is often caused by an infestation of a worm called a filarial worm.

**embolism.** The obstruction of a blood vessel by a clot or mass of foreign material.

**emesis.** See vomiting.

**emphysema.** Chronic lung disease characterized by loss of elasticity of lung tissue and resulting in trapped air in the lung.

**empyema.** Buildup of pus in a cavity of the body.

**encephalitis.** A serious infection resulting in inflammation of the brain.

**encopresis.** Fecal incontinence. Inability to hold feces.

**endocarditis.** Inflammation or infection of the inside of the heart, often including the heart valves.

**endocrine glands.** Glands that are ductless and release their secretions directly into the bloodstream.

**endometriosis.** A condition in which cells from the lining of the uterus are found in other locations within the pelvic cavity. This condition frequently causes pelvic pain and menstrual difficulties.

**enema.** 1. Introduction of fluid into the rectum to bring about a bowel movement. 2. The solution introduced into the rectum to bring about a bowel movement.

**ENT.** The medical specialty of the ear, nose and throat.

**enteritis.** An inflammation of the intestines that usually causes cramps and diarrhea.

**enuresis.** Bedwetting.

**eosinophil.** A type of white blood cell that becomes more abundant in the bloodstream in certain parasitic and allergic conditions.

**epidemiology.** The study of the causes and control of diseases in human populations.

**epidermis.** The outermost layer of skin.

**epididymis.** The elongated structure behind each testicle where sperm are stored.

**epiglottis.** The flap of cartilage at the base of the tongue that closes the trachea during swallowing to keep food or liquids from entering the airway.

**epilepsy.** A disorder of the central nervous system that causes convulsions, or seizures.

**epinephrine.** Adrenaline, a hormone produced in the core of the adrenal glands that's sometimes used to treat asthma and allergic reactions.

**episiotomy.** An incision of the perineum (the area between the vagina and anus in women), often performed during labor to minimize trauma to the perineum during the delivery of a baby.

**epistaxis.** Nosebleed.

**epithelium.** The layer of cells covering internal and external surfaces of the body.

**erysipelas.** A febrile (fever-associated) skin infection caused by a group A hemolytic streptococci.

**erythema.** Redness of the skin.

**erythema infectiosum.** A viral infection most common in children that begins with a red, warm rash on the face, along with some paleness around the mouth. Also called Fifth disease.

**erythema multiforme.** An eruption of flat or raised spots of skin as a result of hypersensitivity to certain drugs or allergies.

**erythema nodosum.** The sudden appearance of tender raised nodes on the lower limbs as a result of an infection, hypersensitivity to certain drugs or other conditions.

**erythrocyte.** Red blood cell.

*Escherichia coli.* A type of common bacteria normally found in the colon. Some strains that cause diarrhea are acquired during travel.

**esophagitis.** Inflammation of the esophagus, often caused from a reflux of acid from the stomach.

**esophagus.** The tube through which food passes from the pharynx to the stomach.

**estrogen.** Female sex hormone.

**eustachian tube.** The narrow tube connecting the nose and middle ear to allow air pressure in the middle ear to equalize with the outside environment.

**exacerbate.** Cause something to increase in severity. To make more intense, irritate.

**exanthem.** Skin rash.

**excise.** To remove by cutting.

**exocrine glands.** Glands that secrete chemicals externally, either through a tube or duct.

**expectorant.** A substance that loosens mucus so it's more easily cleared from the respiratory passages.

# F

**faint.** Temporary loss of consciousness because of an insufficient blood supply to the brain.

**fallopian tube.** The tubal passageway connecting the ovary to the uterus.

**familial cholesterolemia.** An inherited disorder causing abnormally high levels of cholesterol in the blood.

**fascia.** Fibrous sheets of tissue connecting or covering the muscles.

**fat.** A major energy source for animals and humans. Fat contains nine calories per gram.

**fatigue.** Physical or mental exhaustion. Weariness.

**febrile.** Caused by fever. Feverish.

**feces.** Body waste expelled from the rectum. Also called bowel movement or stool.

**femoral.** Having to do with the femur.

**femur.** The thigh bone.

**fertility.** The ability to have children.

**fertilization.** The process of joining the male's sperm and the female's ovum (egg).

**fetal.** Having to do with the fetus.

**fetus.** The unborn baby from the end of the eighth week after fertilization of the egg to birth.

**fever.** Abnormally high body temperature.

**fiber.** 1. A slender, thread-like structure of organ tissue. 2. In the diet, strands of complex carbohydrates (cellulose) that aren't digestible.

**fibrillation.** A rapid, uncoordinated series of contractions of some part of the heart muscle causing irregular heartbeats. Atrial fibrillation is the rapid, ineffective beating of the upper part of the heart. Ventricular fibrillation is the lethal rapid, ineffective beating of the lower part of the heart.

**fibrin.** A serum protein that's essential for the clotting process.

**fibroid.** A noncancerous tumor of the uterus composed of muscle fibers. Also called uterine myoma.

**fibromyalgia.** A painful condition with multiple sensitive areas, called "trigger points," affecting fibrous tissues, muscles, tendons and ligaments.

**fibrositis.** Inflammation of fibrous tissues.

**fibula.** The long, thin, outer bone of the lower leg.

**fissure.** A narrow slit.

**fistula.** An abnormal passage from an abscess, cavity or hollow organ to the skin or another abscess.

**flaccid.** Soft and flabby. Often used to describe complete paralysis (loss of movement) without muscle spasm.

**flatfoot.** A condition in which the normal arch of the foot is absent.

**flatulence.** Excessive production of gas in the intestines or stomach.

**fluorescein.** A compound used as a diagnostic aid to show injuries of the cornea or retina of the eye.

**folic acid.** Folacin. One of the B-group vitamins essential for forming red blood cells.

**folliculitis.** Inflammation of the hair follicles.

**fontanelle.** A soft spot in the skull of an infant formed by the normal separation between the bony plates of the skull.

**foreskin.** A loose fold of skin covering the tip of the penis.

**fracture.** Broken, especially a broken bone.

**fraternal twins.** Twins formed from two separate eggs that were fertilized at the same time. They may be the same or different genders and they have different genetic makeups. Also called dizygotic twins.

**frenulum.** A fold of skin or mucous membrane that limits the movement of a body part. For example, the frenulum linguae is the midline fold under the tongue that attaches it to the floor of the mouth.

**frigidity.** An inability to be sexually aroused.

**frostbite.** Damage to tissue as a result of exposure to freezing temperatures.

**fructose.** Fruit sugar.

**fungus.** A group of organisms that includes yeasts, molds and mushrooms.

## G

**galactorrhea.** Excessive production of breast milk.

**galactosemia.** A disease present at birth caused by a genetic lack of an enzyme needed to metabolize galactose into glucose. May result in mental retardation, cataracts and liver damage.

**gall.** The bile produced in the liver and stored in the gallbladder.

**gallbladder.** The storage sac for bile, located below the liver.

**gallstone.** A stone-like mass that forms in the gallbladder.

**gamma globulin.** Blood protein that contains most antibodies. Used in the temporary prevention of hepatitis and as treatment for disorders with antibody deficiencies.

**ganglion cyst.** A benign, knot-like, cystic tumor on a tendon sheath.

**gangrene.** The decay of body tissue in a part of the body where the blood supply is obstructed by injury or disease.

**gastric.** Having to do with the stomach.

**gastritis.** Inflammation of the stomach lining.

**gastroenteritis.** Inflammation of the stomach and the intestines, usually producing symptoms of nausea, vomiting and diarrhea.

**gastrointestinal.** Having to do with the stomach and intestines.

**gene.** A unit of heredity located on a chromosome.

**generic.** 1. General; typical; not specific. 2. Medicine that's not a name brand.

**genetic.** Hereditary. Having to do with the genes.

**genital.** Having to do with reproduction.

**genitalia.** The reproductive organs.

**genitourinary system.** The genitals and urinary organs.

**geriatrics.** The branch of medicine devoted to the elderly.

**germ.** A disease-causing microorganism.

**German measles.** See rubella.

**gestation.** The period of development within the uterus from conception to birth.

**giantism.** Abnormal growth of the body due to an excessive amount of growth hormone produced by the pituitary gland.

**giardiasis.** A diarrheal illness caused by infection with *Giardia lamblia*, a parasitic protozoan.

**gingiva.** The gums.

**gingivitis.** Inflammation of the gums.

**gland.** An organ that releases a chemical. Endocrine glands are ductless and secrete hormones directly into the bloodstream. Exocrine glands secrete externally, either through a tube or duct.

**glaucoma.** An eye disease, characterized by increased pressure within the eye, that can result in blindness if not treated.

**glomerulonephritis.** When the filtering units in the kidneys, called the glomeruli, are damaged, the kidneys don't function properly and waste and extra fluids build up in the body.

**glossitis.** Inflammation of the tongue.

**glucose.** Dextrose. A simple six-carbon sugar naturally found in fruits, honey and blood.

**goiter.** Enlargement of the thyroid gland.

**gonad.** A sex gland (ovary or testis).

**gonorrhea.** A highly contagious, sexually transmitted bacterial disease of the genital/urinary system.

**gout.** A form of arthritis caused by deposits of uric acid crystals in the joints, usually the feet, hands and, especially, the big toe.

**graft.** A piece of skin or other tissue used as a transplant.

**Gram's stain.** A stain used as the first step in identifying bacteria.

**grand mal.** A major epileptic seizure characterized by convulsions, unconsciousness and sometimes loss of urinary or bowel continence. Usually followed by a brief period of lethargy and disorientation.

**Graves' disease.** Overactive thyroid gland function (hyperthyroidism). Sometimes associated with protrusion of the eyes.

**groin.** The region of the body where the thigh and lower abdomen meet.

**Guillain-Barré syndrome.** A rare but reversible reaction to a viral illness or immunization that causes partial to complete loss of movement of certain muscles, weakness, numbness and tingling. In the severe form, a person may need intensive care and breathing support.

**gynecology.** The branch of medicine that deals with the study and treatment of reproductive diseases in women.

**gynecomastia.** Overdevelopment of male breast tissue. Usually benign and temporary.

## H

**halitosis.** Bad breath.

**hallucination.** The sensory perception of sights, sounds or objects that don't really exist.

**hammer.** The malleus, a hammer-shaped bone in the middle ear.

**hamstring.** The tendon located in the back of the knee and lower thigh.

**hand-foot-and-mouth disease.** A viral infection characterized by a blister-like rash of the hands, feet and mouth.

**hangnail.** A loose piece of skin at one side of a fingernail.

**Hansen's disease.** Leprosy.

**harelip.** Cleft lip or palate.

**Hashimoto's thyroiditis.** A degenerative autoimmune disease of the thyroid gland that ultimately results in a marked reduction in the amount of thyroid hormone produced.

**hay fever.** Allergic sensitivity to certain mold spores and pollens. Allergic reaction includes sneezing, itchy eyes, sore throat and runny nose.

**heart block.** A condition in which electrical impulses aren't properly transmitted from the heart's upper to the lower chambers.

**heart failure.** Inability of the heart to adequately pump blood.

**heart.** The hollow, muscular organ responsible for pumping blood through the circulatory system.

**heartburn.** Indigestion. A burning sensation in the chest caused by a reflux of acid into the esophagus or too much acid in the stomach.

**heat exhaustion.** Headache, profuse sweating, weakness,

muscle cramps, nausea and vomiting caused by excessive exposure to heat.

**heat stroke.** A serious failure of the body's heat-regulating mechanism resulting from excessive exposure to intense heat. Also called sunstroke.

**hemangioma.** A tumor or swelling that's composed of blood vessels.

**hematemesis.** The vomiting of blood.

**hematology.** The branch of medicine that pertains to blood and the organs involved in forming blood.

**hematoma.** A tumor-like mass of coagulated blood in the soft tissues. A contusion or bruise.

**hematuria.** The presence of blood in the urine.

**hemiplegia.** Paralysis (loss of feeling or movement) of one side of the body.

**hemochromatosis.** A disorder of iron metabolism characterized by excessive amounts of iron in the skin, liver and other tissues.

**hemoglobin.** The oxygen-carrying molecule in red blood cells.

**hemolysis.** The destruction of red blood cells.

**hemophilia.** An inherited disorder, nearly always in males, in which one of the normal blood-clotting factors is deficient.

**hemoptysis.** A cough that produces blood.

**hemorrhage.** Severe bleeding, usually from damage to a blood vessel.

**hemorrhoid.** An enlarged vein inside or just outside the rectum.

**hemostasis.** Control of bleeding.

**hepatic.** Having to do with the liver.

**hepatitis.** Inflammation or infection of the liver.

**heredity.** Transmission of genetic traits from parents to children.

**hermaphrodite.** A person with both male and female sex organs.

**hernia.** An abnormal protrusion of part of an organ through an abnormal opening.

**herpes.** A recurring viral skin infection characterized by clusters of small blisters. Typically, sores are located near the mouth (fever blisters or cold sores) or in the genital region (genital herpes).

**heterosexual.** Having to do with the opposite sex.

**hexachlorophene.** A detergent that kills germs.

**hiccup.** A sudden, involuntary spasm of the diaphragm. The sound of hiccups is caused by the sudden intake of air.

**hidradenitis.** Inflammation of the sweat glands.

**hip.** The part of the body surrounding the joint between the femur and pelvic bones.

**hirsutism.** Excessive hair growth, usually on the face and chest. Often caused by an imbalance in hormones.

**histamine.** A substance released from certain cells in response to allergens, associated with the development of allergic symptoms, including itchy eyes, sneezing and congestion.

**histoplasmosis.** A fungal disease caused by inhaling the spores of *Histoplasma capsulatum.*

**HIV.** Human immunodeficiency virus. A virus that slowly destroys the immune system. The virus that causes AIDS.

**hives.** A skin reaction characterized by swelling, itching and burning.

**Hodgkin's disease.** A progressive form of lymphoma usually characterized by weakness, swollen lymph nodes, sweating, fever and weight loss.

**homeopathy.** Medical treatment based on the theory that certain diseases can be cured by giving very small doses of substances that, in a healthy person, would produce symptoms like those of the disease.

**homogenize.** To make more uniform in quality or consistency.

**homosexual.** Having to do with the same sex.

**hordeolum.** Inflammation of a gland on the eyelid. Also called a stye.

**hormone.** A substance formed in an organ of the body and carried by body fluids to another organ or tissue, where it has a specific effect.

**host.** An organism that harbors and provides sustenance for another organism.

**housemaid's knee.** Swelling just below the kneecap, caused by the build-up of fluid in response to the constant pressure of kneeling.

**humerus.** The bone in the upper arm.

**humidifier.** A device for adding moisture to the air.

**Huntington's chorea.** A hereditary form of chorea (sudden, jerky motions of the arms or other parts of the body) that usually affects people during their early 40s.

**hydatid.** A cyst containing watery fluid and the larvae of certain tapeworms.

**hydatid disease.** Infection with the larvae (cysts) of certain tapeworms.

**hydatidiform mole.** A cystic tumor of the placental tissues of an abnormal pregnancy. Complications of this disorder include bleeding and infection.

**hydrocele.** A painless swelling of the scrotum caused by the buildup of fluid in the outer covering of the testes.

**hydrocephalus.** An enlargement of the head caused by the buildup of fluid within the ventricles of the brain. Also called "water on the brain."

**hygiene.** The science of health and its maintenance.

**hymen.** The membrane partly or completely closing the opening to the vagina.

**hyperbaric.** Characterized by greater-than-normal pressure. Hyperbaric oxygen is a therapeutic treatment designed to increase blood oxygen by delivering oxygen in a chamber room with greater-than-normal pressure.

**hyperemesis gravidarum.** Excessive morning sickness.

**hyperglycemic.** High blood sugar.

**hyperparathyroidism.** A condition caused by the over-excretion of parathyroid hormone resulting in changes in the bone and an elevated level of calcium in the blood.

**hypertension.** Abnormally high blood pressure.

**hyperthyroidism.** Overproduction of thyroid hormone.

**hyperventilation.** Rapid or deep breathing producing faintness, numbness, chest pain, apprehension and tingling, and spasms of the extremities.

**hypnosis.** A sleep-like state induced by the suggestions of a hypnotist.

**hypnotic.** 1. Having to do with hypnosis. 2. Causing sleep.

**hypochondriac.** Abnormal anxiety about one's health, often to the point of believing one is suffering from a serious disease.

**hypodermic.** Beneath the skin.

**hypoglycemia.** Low blood sugar.

**hypoparathyroidism.** Parathyroid hormone insufficiency due to lack of secretion of the parathyroid gland.

**hypopituitarism.** Deficient activity of the pituitary gland causing slowed growth in children, fatigue and decreased appetite in adults, and cessation of menstrual periods in women.

**hyposensitization.** To treat with frequent, small injections of an antigen to decrease the symptoms of an allergy to that antigen. Also called desensitization.

**hypospadias.** An abnormal opening of the urethra on the underside of the penis or into the vagina.

**hypothalamus.** The portion of the brain responsible for temperature regulation and control of the pituitary gland.

**hypothermia.** Low body temperature.

**hypothyroidism.** A condition of low thyroid hormone production resulting in weight gain, hair loss, sluggishness and thickening of the skin.

**hypoxia.** An abnormal condition resulting from decreased availability of oxygen in the body tissues.

**hysterectomy.** Surgical removal of all or part of the uterus.

**hysteria.** 1. Wild, uncontrolled excitement or other feelings. 2. A disorder in which anxiety is converted into physical symptoms that have no physical basis.

# I

**iatrogenic.** Resulting from medical treatment.

**ichthyosis.** An inherited skin disorder that produces dry, rough, scaly skin.

**identical twins.** Twins formed from a single egg. They are of the same gender and have the same genetic makeup. Also called monozygotic twins.

**idiopathic.** Without a known cause.

**ileitis.** Inflammation of the lower part of the small intestine.

**ileum.** The lower part of the small intestine.

**ileus.** Lack of movement of digested food and juices through the gastrointestinal tract. May be due to a blockage of the intestine.

**ilium.** The flared portion of the pelvis. The hip bone.

**IM.** Intramuscular.

**immune.** Resistant to a particular disease.

**immunity.** Resistance of the body to infection.

**immunization.** The process of making an individual immune by vaccination or inoculation.

**immunoglobulin.** A serum protein involved in immunity. An antibody.

**impetigo.** Skin infection characterized by erupting sores. Caused by staphylococcus or streptococcus bacteria.

**impotence.** Inability of a male to achieve erection and orgasm.

**in situ.** In its original place.

Carcinoma *in situ* means cancer that hasn't spread to other locations.

**incision.** A cut.

**incisor.** Any of the front four teeth on either the upper or lower jaw.

**incompetent.** 1. Unable to make rational decisions. 2. Not functioning properly.

**incontinence.** Inability to hold urine or feces.

**incubate.** To provide the proper conditions for growth.

**indigestion.** Upper abdominal discomfort usually experienced after a meal due to incomplete digestion.

**induration.** The process of hardening. An abnormally hard spot.

**infarct.** An area of dead or dying tissue produced by lack of blood flow to or from that area. For example, myocardial infarction is the death of heart muscle.

**infection.** Causing disease, especially by the presence of foreign microorganisms in the body, including bacteria, viruses or parasites.

**infectious disease.** A disease that can be spread from one person to another.

**infertility.** Inability to produce children.

**inflammation.** Swelling, redness, warmth and pain. A body tissue's protective response to injury.

**influenza.** A contagious and infectious respiratory illness usually occurring in the winter.

**ingrown nail.** Edges of the nail become trapped under the skin, causing inflammation and, sometimes, infection.

**injection.** A fluid introduced into the body by a syringe and needle.

**innate.** Inborn, hereditary.

**inoculation.** The injection of a disease agent into the body to cause a mild form of the disease and build immunity.

**inoperable.** Not curable through surgery.

**insanity.** Any form or degree of mental disturbance or unsoundness of mind, permanent or temporary, that makes a person

incapable of rational conduct or judgment.

**insemination.** To deposit sperm in the vagina.

**insomnia.** An inability to fall asleep or to remain asleep.

**insulin.** The hormone produced by the pancreas for regulating carbohydrate metabolism. Used in the treatment of diabetes mellitus.

**integument.** Skin.

**intercourse.** The exchange of communication between individuals. Sexual intercourse is the sexual joining of two people; coitus.

**intestine.** The tube involved in digestion and extending from the stomach to the anus. Consists of the small intestine and the large intestine.

**intoxication.** Poisoning, or the state of being affected by a poisonous substance. Often used to describe drunkenness.

**intracellular.** Within a cell.

**intradermal.** Within the skin.

**intramuscular.** Within the muscle.

**intrauterine.** Within the womb.

**intravenous.** Within a vein. Intravenous infusion means to direct fluids through a needle or catheter directly into a vein.

**intussusception.** Telescoping a section of the intestine into an adjoining section.

**iris.** The colored portion of the eye. It's a muscle that controls the amount of light entering the pupil.

**iritis.** Inflammation of the iris.

**irrigation.** Washing of a body cavity or wound with a stream of water.

**ischemia.** A lack of blood supply to a body part.

**IUD.** Intrauterine device. Used for contraception.

**IV.** Intravenous.

**IVP.** Intravenous pyelography.

# J

**jaundice.** Yellow discoloration of the skin and eyes caused by the buildup of bile in the blood.

**jejunum.** The middle part of the small intestine, located

between the duodenum and ileum.

**joint.** The joining of two or more bones. In general, joints allow flexibility and mobility. However, some joints (for example, those in the skull) can't move.

**jugular.** Of the neck or throat, as in jugular veins.

# K

**Kaposi's sarcoma.** Bluish-purple nodules of the skin that often bleed. These frequently occur in people who have AIDS.

**keloid.** Excessive growth of scar tissue on the skin.

**keratin.** The main protein of skin, hair and nails.

**keratitis.** Inflammation of the cornea of the eye.

**keratoconus.** A deformity of the cornea in which the cornea resembles the end of a football.

**ketones.** The initial breakdown products of fatty acid metabolism. Unavailability of carbohydrates from starvation or uncontrolled diabetes mellitus increases the production of ketones. Too high a ketone level causes the blood chemistry to become acidic, a condition that's potentially life-threatening.

**kidney.** A pair of organs in the upper abdominal cavity that separate the body's water and waste products from the blood and excrete them as urine through the bladder.

**knee.** The complex hinge joint of the upper and lower leg involving the femur, tibia and patella.

**knock-knee.** A deformity in which the knees rub together or touch each other in walking.

# L

**labia.** Lip-shaped structures; often used to describe the outer folds of the female genitalia.

**labor.** The process or period of childbirth, especially the muscular contractions of giving birth.

**labyrinth.** The system of interconnecting canals and cavities in the inner ear. Plays an important role in hearing and in balance.

**laceration.** A wound caused by a cut from a sharp instrument or the tearing of body tissue.

**lacrimation.** Discharge of tears. "Watering" eyes.

**lactase.** An enzyme that converts the milk sugar lactose into glucose and galactose.

**lactation.** Secretion of milk by the breasts.

**lactose.** Milk sugar.

**laryngitis.** Inflammation of the larynx, resulting in a temporary loss of voice.

**larynx.** The voice box.

**lateral.** Toward the side, sideways.

**lavage.** Washing out of an organ, especially the stomach.

**Legg-Calvé-Perthes disease.** A disease in which the blood supply to the femur is reduced, causing the bone to collapse.

**lens.** 1. A curved glass used to bring together or spread rays of light. 2. The transparent organ lying behind the iris and pupil that focuses light on the retina of the eye.

**leprosy.** A progressive infectious disease that attacks the skin, flesh and nerves; characterized by nodules, ulcers, scaly scabs, deformities and the eventual loss of sensation. Also called Hansen's disease.

**lesion.** Any damage to a tissue. Marks, spots, moles or other problems of the skin.

**lethargy.** A lack of energy; sluggishness, dullness or apathy.

**leukemia.** Cancer of the tissues in the bone marrow, spleen and lymph nodes.

**leukocytes.** White blood cells, the blood cells responsible for fighting infection.

**leukopenia.** A lower than normal number of leukocytes in the blood.

**leukopheresis.** Selective removal of the white blood cells from a donor's blood. The other components of the

blood are then returned to the donor.

**leukoplakia.** Thick, white patches in the mouth that may become malignant.

**lichen.** Any of various skin diseases characterized by sores and enlarged skin markings.

**ligament.** A tough band of connective tissue connecting bones or holding organs in place.

**ligature.** A wire or thread used to tie off blood vessels or to close incisions or wounds.

**lightening.** The feeling of decreased abdominal pressure during the last few weeks of pregnancy caused by the uterus dropping into the pelvis.

**limbus.** Margin, or border. The margin of the cornea where it contacts the sclera.

**lingua.** Tongue.

**lipid.** Cholesterol, triglycerides and related substances.

**lipocyte.** A fat cell.

**lipolysis.** The splitting up, or destruction, of fat.

**lipoma.** Fatty tumor.

**lipoprotein.** Any of a group of proteins combined with a lipid that allow lipids to be transported in the circulatory system.

**liposuction.** A surgical procedure that changes body shape by removing fat cells.

**litholysis.** Breaking up of a stone, such as a gallstone.

**lithotripsy.** A procedure to break up kidney stones into smaller pieces that can more easily pass out of the body.

**liver.** The large organ in the upper right abdomen that functions in digestion and storage of food, disposal of worn-out red blood cells and detoxification of the body.

**lobe.** 1. The fleshy lower part of the ear. 2. A well-defined portion of an organ.

**lobectomy.** Surgical removal of the lobe of an organ.

**lobotomy.** A surgical operation in which a lobe of the brain, especially the frontal lobe of the cerebrum, is cut into or across. This used to be a common procedure to calm

selected psychotic patients before the development of modern tranquilizers.

**leukoplakia.** Thick, white patches in the mouth that may become malignant.

**lochia.** The discharge from the vagina that occurs for several days to weeks after childbirth.

**lockjaw.** Tetanus infection.

**loins.** The portion of the back between the rib cage and pelvis.

**lordosis.** Forward curvature of the spine, producing a hollow in the back.

**LSD.** Lysergic acid diethylamide. A hallucinogenic drug.

**lumbago.** Pain in the lower back.

**lumbar.** Having to do with the lower back, the loins.

**lungs.** The main respiratory organs in the chest where blood is oxygenated.

**lupus erythematosus.** A usually chronic inflammatory disease that causes abnormalities of blood vessels and connective tissue in various parts of the body.

**luteinizing hormone.** A hormone secreted by the anterior pituitary gland, responsible for stimulating ovulation in the female and testosterone production in the male.

**Lyme disease.** A disease spread by deer ticks characterized at first by a skin rash, headache and fever, and later by arthritis and heart damage.

**lymph.** Consists primarily of a clear, yellowish fluid and white blood cells. Found in the lymphatic system.

**lymph node.** Any of many small, compact structures lying in groups along the course of the lymphatic vessels and producing lymphocytes.

**lymphadenitis.** Inflammation of the lymph nodes.

**lymphangitis.** Inflammation of a lymphatic vessel.

**lymphatic system.** The vessels and structures involved in carrying lymph from the tissues to the blood.

**lymphedema.** Swelling of tissue because of the buildup of too much lymph fluid.

**lymphocyte.** A type of leukocyte (white blood cell) in-

volved in the production of antibodies and the development of immunity.

**lymphoma.** A malignant tumor of the lymphoid tissues.

# M

**macrophage.** A large cell that engulfs and digests foreign material.

**macula.** The central part of the retina with the highest density of light receptors. Responsible for detailed vision.

**macule.** A discolored, flat spot of skin.

**malady.** Illness.

**malaria.** An infectious disease of the tropics characterized by high fever and chills. The fever typically recurs every third day. Some forms of malaria can be fatal.

**malignancy.** A tendency to worsen to a more serious illness or death. Commonly used to describe cancer.

**malingering.** Deliberate exaggeration of the symptoms of an illness or injury for gain. For example, pretending to be ill in order to escape duty or work.

**malleolus.** The rounded bony prominence on either side of the ankle.

**malleus.** A small bone in the middle ear, often called the hammer.

**malnutrition.** Poor nourishment resulting from an inadequate or improper diet.

**malocclusion.** Improper meeting of the upper and lower teeth.

**malunion.** Improper healing of the pieces of a broken bone.

**mammary.** Having to do with the breast.

**mandible.** The lower jaw.

**mania.** A mental disorder. Characterized by extreme excitement and energy.

**manic-depressive.** A mental disorder marked by alternating periods of excitability and depression. Also called bipolar affective disorder.

**marijuana.** A drug derived from the leaves of the *Cannabis sativa* plant. Makes the user feel euphoric.

**marrow.** The soft, sponge-like material inside the bones.

**masculinization.** Development of male sex characteristics in a female.

**masochism.** Pleasure from personal, psychological or physical pain.

**mastectomy.** Surgical removal of the breast.

**mastitis.** Inflammation of the breast.

**mastoid.** A bony, rounded projection of the skull located behind each ear.

**mastoiditis.** An infection of the mastoid bone that can cause redness, warmth, swelling and pain behind the ear, sometimes with drainage from the ear.

**masturbation.** Sexual self-stimulation.

**maxillae.** The pair of bones forming the upper jaw.

**measles.** A highly contagious viral disease occurring most frequently in childhood and characterized by small, red spots on the skin, high fever and nasal discharge.

**Meckel's diverticulum.** A sac that may form in the small intestine, present at birth.

**meconium.** The greenish fecal matter in a fetus, forming the first bowel movement of a newborn infant.

**median nerve.** The nerve that stimulates some of the muscles of the hand and wrist.

**mediastinum.** The tissues and organs located directly behind the sternum between the lungs. Contains the heart and its large vessels, the esophagus, thymus, lymph nodes and other structures and tissues.

**medulla oblongata.** The part of the brain just above the spinal cord that includes the control centers for breathing, circulation and heartbeat.

**medulla.** The inner part of an organ. The adrenal medulla is the center of the adrenal gland where epinephrine (adrenaline) is produced.

**meibomian gland.** A type of gland of the eyelid's inner surface. Inflammation of a meibomian gland can

produce a swelling called a chalazion.

**melancholia.** A mental state characterized by extreme sadness. A severe form of depression.

**melanin.** A brownish-black pigment normally found in skin, hair and parts of the eye.

**melanoma.** A dark-colored tumor, especially malignant melanoma, that is a form of skin cancer that can spread from one part of the body to another.

**melasma.** Dark coloring of the skin often seen during pregnancy and at menopause. Also occurs in Addison's disease.

**melena.** Black-colored feces caused by the presence of blood.

**membrane.** A thin layer of tissue covering an organ.

**menarche.** A woman's first menstrual period.

**Ménière's syndrome.** A disorder of the inner ear characterized by dizziness, ringing in the ears and progressive hearing loss.

**meninges.** The three membranes covering the brain and spinal cord.

**meningioma.** Tumor of the meninges, usually benign and slow-growing.

**meningitis.** Inflammation of the meninges as the result of infection by bacteria or viruses. Symptoms include high fever, headache, stiff neck and vomiting. This is a life-threatening disease that must be treated promptly.

**meniscus.** The cartilage in the knee joint.

**menopause.** The time at which the menstrual cycle gradually stops. Sometimes referred to as the "change of life."

**menorrhagia.** Heavy bleeding during menstruation.

**menstruation.** The periodic discharge of blood and tissues from the uterus. This usually occurs about every four weeks in a woman who isn't pregnant. Also called "a period."

**metabolism.** The chemical

and physical processes involved in building up, storing and using materials required for life.

**metacarpal.** Any of the five bones that make up the hand and join the wrist to the fingers.

**metaphysis.** The wider portion at the end of a long bone where growth occurs in infants and children.

**metastasis.** The spread of a disease from its primary site in the body to another location in the body. Usually refers to cancer, but can be used to refer to infection.

**metatarsal.** Any of the five bones of the foot directly jointed to each of the toes.

**metra.** Uterus.

**metritis.** Inflammation of the uterus.

**metrorrhagia.** Uterine bleeding, usually of normal amount occurring at irregular intervals.

**microbe.** A microorganism, such as bacterium.

**microbiology.** The study of living microbes, including bacteria, protozoa and molds.

**microencephaly.** Having an abnormally small brain.

**microorganism.** A microscopic plant or animal.

**midwife.** A person who helps women at childbirth, but who isn't a nurse or physician.

**migraine.** A group of symptoms that includes a severe headache, usually on one side of the head, and often accompanied by visual disturbances, nausea, irritability and other symptoms.

**milia.** Pinhead-sized whitish skin lesions found on the face or trunk of some newborn infants.

**miliaria.** "Prickly heat" or "heat rash" as a result of inflammation of the sweat glands and characterized by small, white or red skin eruptions.

**miscarriage.** Natural loss of a fetus from the womb before it is sufficiently developed to survive. Also called spontaneous abortion.

**mitral valve.** The valve of the

heart between the left atrium and left ventricle that prevents the flow of blood back into the atrium when the heart muscle is contracting.

**mittelschmerz.** Pelvic pain between periods, corresponding to the release of an ovum (egg) by an ovary.

**mole.** 1. A fleshy, pigmented skin blemish. 2. A mass of uterine tissue formed by a failure of the normal fertilization process during conception.

**molluscum contagiosum.** A viral infection of the skin characterized by lesions with depressed centers containing a curd-like substance.

**mongolism.** A condition present at birth characterized by mental deficiency, a broad face and slanting eyes. Also called Down syndrome.

**monocyte.** A large white blood cell leukocyte.

**mononucleosis.** An infection with Epstein-Barr virus. Also called "mono."

**morbid.** 1. Pathologic or abnormal. 2. Having to do with, or characterized by, disease.

**morning sickness.** Nausea and vomiting occurring during pregnancy.

**MRI.** Magnetic resonance imaging.

**mucosa.** The membrane covering canals and cavities that open on the outside of the body, such as the gastrointestinal tract and the respiratory tract. Also called mucous membrane.

**mumps.** A viral disease of childhood characterized by swelling of the parotid (salivary) glands and fever.

**murmur.** An extra heart sound that may be normal or abnormal.

**muscle.** Tissue made up of bundles of long, slender cells that contract when stimulated.

**mutation.** A damaged gene that may produce a disease or deficiency.

**mute.** An inability or unwillingness to speak.

**myalgia.** Muscle pain.

**myasthenia gravis.** A chronic

disease characterized by muscular weakness and fatigue.

**myelin.** The fat-like substance that insulates certain nerve fibers.

**myocarditis.** Inflammation of the heart muscle.

**myoma.** A tumor of muscle cells.

**myopia.** Nearsightedness.

**myositis.** Inflammation of a muscle.

**myringotomy.** An incision in the eardrum to relieve pressure or release fluid.

# N

**narcissistic.** Self-centered, being "in love" with oneself.

**narcolepsy.** Frequent and uncontrolled desire for sleep.

**nausea.** A feeling of sickness in the stomach, sometimes followed by the urge to vomit.

**nebulizer.** A device that produces a very fine vapor to be inhaled.

**necrosis.** Death of a cell or tissue.

**nematode.** A roundworm that may infest the digestive tract of humans.

**neoplasm.** A new growth, tumor.

**nephrectomy.** Surgical removal of a kidney.

**nephritis.** Inflammation of a kidney.

**nephropathy.** Disease of the kidneys. Swelling or breakdown of the kidney.

**nephrosis.** A disease of the kidney that causes malfunction but no inflammation. Also called nephrotic syndrome.

**nerve.** A cord-like structure made up of special tissue for carrying electrical impulses from one part of the body to another.

**neuralgia.** Pain along the course of a nerve.

**neuritis.** Inflammation of a nerve.

**neurofibromatosis.** An inherited disorder that causes dark spots on the skin and tumors of the skin, peripheral, optic and acoustic nerves.

**neurology.** The branch of medicine that pertains to the nervous system.

**neuroma.** A benign but sometimes painful, tumor growing on a nerve.

**neuron.** A nerve cell.

**neuropathy.** Disease of the nervous system or of an individual nerve.

**neurosis.** An emotional disorder that can interfere with a person's ability to lead a normal life.

**neutrophil.** A mature white blood cell with a three- to five-lobed nucleus.

**nevus.** A mole or other colored spot on the skin.

**nicotine.** A highly toxic and addictive component of tobacco. While the amounts obtained from smoking may not be enough to be immediately fatal, there's a cause-and-effect relationship to heart disease.

**night blindness.** A reduced ability to see in dim light. May be caused by a vitamin-A deficiency or glaucoma.

**nit.** The egg of a louse.

**nocturia.** Excessive urination at night.

**node.** A swelling, knot or knob.

**nonunion.** Failure of the ends of a broken bone to mend.

**norepinephrine.** A hormone produced by the adrenal medulla and certain sympathetic nerve fibers.

**nosocomial.** Having to do with the hospital. For example, an nosocomial infection is one that's acquired during hospitalization.

# O

**obesity.** Having too much body fat. A weight more than 20% above the normal range.

**obsession.** An ongoing preoccupation with an idea.

**obsessive-compulsive.** Marked by a need to repeatedly perform certain behaviors or rituals.

**obstetrics.** The branch of medicine that deals with the care and treatment of women during pregnancy and childbirth.

**occiput.** The back of the head.

**occult.** Hidden from view.

**occupational illness.** Any illness caused or aggravated by a person's job.

**occupational therapy.** Teaching useful skills to sick or handicapped people to promote rehabilitation and healing.

**ocular.** Having to do with the eye.

**odontalgia.** Toothache.

**olecranon.** The projection of the ulna (the larger of the two bones in the forearm) at the elbow.

**olfactory.** Having to do with the sense of smell.

**oligomenorrhea.** Light menstrual flow.

**oligospermia.** A low number of sperm in the semen.

**oliguria.** A condition characterized by an abnormally small output of urine.

**oncology.** The study of tumors.

**oophorectomy.** The surgical removal of an ovary.

**ophthalmology.** The branch of medicine that pertains to the eye and its diseases.

**optic neuritis.** Inflammation of the optic nerve, which connects the eye to the brain. Symptoms include pain with eye movement, blurred vision and sometimes temporary blindness.

**optical.** Having to do with vision.

**optometry.** The practice of eye and vision care.

**orbit.** The bony cavity containing the eyeball. Eye socket.

**orchiectomy.** The surgical removal of one or both testicles. Also called castration.

**organ.** A structural unit of an animal or plant that serves a specific function.

**organic.** Having to do with substances derived from living organisms.

**orgasm.** Sexual climax.

**orifice.** The entrance or outlet of a body cavity.

**oropharynx.** The part of the pharynx behind the mouth and tongue.

**orthodontics.** The branch of dentistry that deals with the correction of irregularities of the teeth and related facial problems.

**orthopedics.** The branch of medicine that deals with the treatment of deformities, diseases and injuries of the bones, joints and muscles.

**orthopnea.** Difficulty breathing when lying flat.

**oscillation.** A back-and-forth motion; vibration.

**Osgood-Schlatter disease.** Inflammation of the bone and cartilage of the shin bone, just below the knee.

**ossicle.** A small bone.

**osteoarthritis.** A slowly progressive form of arthritis, usually found in older people. Characterized by deterioration of bone cartilage.

**osteoma.** A bony tumor.

**osteomalacia.** Softening of the bones resulting from deficient bone calcium.

**osteomyelitis.** Infection of a bone.

**osteopathy.** A system of therapy emphasizing primary medical care and the importance of body mechanics and manipulation to correct abnormalities.

**osteoporosis.** A bone disorder characterized by a reduction in bone density, chiefly found in women who have passed menopause and the elderly.

**ostomy.** A procedure done to make a passageway for waste. A colostomy is an example.

**otic.** Having to do with the ear.

**otitis.** Inflammation of the ear. Otitis externa (inflammation of the ear canal) is also called swimmer's ear, while otitis media is a middle-ear infection.

**ovary.** The female sex gland that contains ova, or eggs.

**ovulation.** The process in which an ovum is released from the ovary.

**ovum.** Egg; the female reproductive element.

**oximeter.** A device for determining the oxygen saturation level of the blood.

**oxygen.** A chemical element essential for sustaining life.

**oxytocin.** A pituitary hormone that encourages the pregnant uterus to contract and is sometimes used to induce labor. It also encourages milk to be expressed during breastfeeding.

# P

**Paget's disease.** 1. A type of cancer usually involving the breast's larger ducts, areola and nipples. 2. A disease characterized by weakened and deformed bones.

**palate.** The roof of the mouth.

**palliative.** Controlling symptoms without curing the disease.

**pallor.** Pale appearance of the skin.

**palpate.** To feel with the fingers.

**palpebra.** The eyelid.

**palpitation.** A sensation that the heart is beating too rapidly or strongly.

**palsy.** See paralysis.

**panacea.** A remedy for all diseases.

**pancreas.** A gland located below and behind the stomach and liver that produces insulin and glucagon, the hormones involved in carbohydrate metabolism.

**pancreatitis.** Inflammation of the pancreas.

**pandemic.** A widespread epidemic.

**panic.** A sudden attack of anxiety.

**papilla.** A small nipple-shaped projection.

**papilledema.** Swelling of the optic disk. May be due to an increase of pressure in the skull.

**papilloma.** A benign tumor of the skin or mucous membranes. A wart.

**papule.** A solid, raised skin lesion.

**para-aminobenzoic acid.** PABA, a substance used in suntan lotion and used clinically to treat rickettsial diseases.

**paracentesis.** Surgical removal of fluid from a cavity.

**parainfluenza virus.** One of a group of viruses that cause a variety of upper respiratory diseases.

**paralysis.** Inability to move parts of the body.

**paranasal sinuses.** The mucosa-lined cavities in the bones of the skull that open into the passages of the nose.

**paranoia.** A mental disorder characterized by a belief that others are out to get you.

**paraplegia.** Inability to feel or move the legs.

**parasite.** An organism that lives on or in the tissues of another organism and draws its nourishment from the host.

**paraspadias.** A developmental abnormality in which the urethra opens along one side of the penis.

**parathyroid glands.** Two pair of small glands situated next to or in the thyroid gland that are involved in the metabolism of calcium and phosphorus.

**parenteral.** Inside the body, but outside the intestines.

**paresis.** Partial or slight loss of feeling or movement.

**paresthesia.** An abnormal sensation of burning or prickling on the skin, caused by a disorder of the nervous system.

**Parkinson's disease.** A progressive disease of the brain. Characterized by tremors and muscle stiffness.

**parotid glands.** The largest of the salivary glands, located near the ears.

**paroxysm.** A sudden attack, or raised level of intensity, of symptoms.

**pasteurization.** Heating milk or other substances to a temperature of 140°F for 30 minutes to kill harmful bacteria.

**patella.** The kneecap.

**pathogen.** Any agent that causes disease.

**pathology.** The study of changes caused by disease.

**pectoral.** Having to do with the chest or breast.

**pectus carinatum.** An abnormally prominent sternum or breastbone. Also called pigeon breast.

**pectus excavatum.** A defect of the sternum that's present at birth.

**pedal.** Having to do with the feet.

**pediatrics.** The branch of medicine that deals with the development and care of infants and children.

**pediculosis.** Infestation with lice.

**pelvis.** The bony structure formed by the sacrum, coccyx, ilium, pubis and ischium.

**pemphigus.** A skin condition characterized by large blisters.

**penis.** The male external sex organ.

**pepsin.** A digestive enzyme found in the stomach.

**peptic.** Having to do with the stomach.

**percutaneous.** Introduced through the skin.

**perforation.** A hole or break through a membrane or the wall of an organ.

**pericarditis.** Inflammation of the sac that surrounds the heart.

**pericardium.** The fibrous sac the heart.

**perineum.** The pelvic floor. In females, the region from the vagina to the anus. In males, the region from the base of the scrotum to the anus.

**periodontitis.** Inflammation of the tissues around the teeth.

**periosteum.** The connective tissue covering the bones of the body.

**peripheral.** At or near the surface of the body. Located away from the center structure.

**peristalsis.** The waves of contraction and relaxation of the smooth muscle of the digestive tract.

**peritoneum.** The membrane lining the walls of the abdominal and pelvic cavity.

**peritonitis.** Inflammation of the peritoneum.

**pernicious anemia.** Anemia due to vitamin $B_{12}$ deficiency.

**pernicious.** Fatal.

**pertussis.** See whooping cough.

**petit mal.** A mild seizure with a momentary loss of consciousness.

**phagocyte.** Any cell that destroys invading microorganisms.

**phagomania.** An obsession with eating.

**pharmacist.** A person licensed to mix and dispense drugs.

**pharyngitis.** Inflammation of the pharynx. Also called a sore throat.

**pharynx.** The cavity of the canal leading from the mouth and nasal passages to the larynx and the esophagus.

**phenylalanine.** An essential amino acid occurring in proteins. A small amount of phenylalanine is necessary in the diet to make the proteins that form human tissues.

**phenylketonuria (PKU).** A rare inherited disorder. Causes an inability to metabolize phenylalanine, an amino acid that's a common part of many proteins that form tissues in the body. Left untreated, it causes severe mental retardation in infants.

**phimosis.** Excessive tightness of the foreskin of the penis.

**phlebitis.** Inflammation of a vein.

**phlebotomy.** Withdrawal of blood from a vein.

**phlegm.** Mucus, especially mucus produced by the lungs during inflammation or infection.

**phobia.** Any persistent, unreasonable abnormal fear.

**phonation.** Making vocal sounds.

**photophobia.** Abnormal intolerance of light.

**physician.** A doctor. An authorized practitioner of medicine.

**physiology.** The branch of medicine that deals with the function of the various parts of the living organism.

**pigeon toe.** A foot condition where the toes turn in.

**piles.** See hemorrhoids.

**pilus.** Hair.

**pimple.** A small, elevated skin lesion.

**pinguecula.** A yellowish spot on the cornea of the eye that sometimes occurs in the elderly.

**pink eye.** Inflammation of the conjunctiva. Also called conjunctivitis.

**pinna.** The part of the ear that's projected outside of the head.

**pinworm.** A parasite, *Enterobius vermicularis*, that

can cause intense itching around the anus.

**pituitary gland.** The gland that secretes hormones that influence body growth, metabolism and the function of other endocrine glands.

**pityriasis.** A skin condition in which the skin forms thin, dry scales.

**placebo.** A harmless substance that resembles a medicine; often used to test the effectiveness of medicines.

**placenta.** A spongy structure that grows on the uterine wall during pregnancy and provides nutrition to the fetus.

**plague.** 1. Any contagious epidemic disease that is deadly. 2. An infectious disease caused by *Yersinia pestis* that can be spread from animals to humans and is normally spread to humans by fleas (called bubonic plague) or from person to person by respiratory droplets (called pneumonic plague). Both forms have a high death rate.

**plantar.** Having to do with the sole of the foot.

**plasma.** The fluid portion of the blood.

**platelet.** A thrombocyte, the smallest of the formed components of blood, associated with blood clotting.

**pleura.** The membrane surrounding the lungs and lining the walls of the chest cavity.

**pleurisy.** Inflammation of the pleura.

**plexus.** A network of nerves or veins.

**plumbism.** Chronic lead poisoning.

**pneumoconiosis.** Any of several lung diseases caused by inhaling particles of industrial substances.

**pneumonia.** Acute inflammation or infection of the lungs.

**pneumothorax.** The buildup of air or gas in the chest cavity. May cause lung collapse.

**podiatry.** The branch of medicine that pertains to the foot and its ailments.

**poison.** A substance that causes illness or death when eaten, drunk or absorbed into the body.

**poliomyelitis.** An acute, infectious disease that attacks the central nervous system. Sometimes causes paralysis that can result in permanent deformities. Vaccines are available. Also called polio.

**pollen.** The male fertilizing element of flowering plants.

**polycythemia.** Abnormal increase in the number of red blood cells or hematocrit.

**polydactyly.** Extra fingers or toes.

**polydipsia.** Excessive thirst.

**polyhidrosis.** Excessive sweating.

**polyp.** A growth extending outward from a mucous membrane.

**polypectomy.** Surgical removal of a polyp.

**polyuria.** Excessive, frequent urination.

**pons.** A piece of connecting tissue, specifically the bridge of white matter at the base of the brain.

**popliteal.** Having to do with the area behind the knee.

**pore.** A small opening.

**posterior.** At or toward the back.

**postoperative.** After surgery.

**postpartum.** After childbirth.

**preeclampsia.** A complication of pregnancy. The development of hypertension with protein in the urine, buildup of fluid (edema) or both.

**premenstrual syndrome.** PMS. Headache, irritability, edema (swelling), abdominal discomfort, pelvic pain and nausea in the days before the start of the menstrual periods of some women.

**prepuce.** A covering fold of skin, such as the foreskin of the penis.

**presbycusis.** Hearing loss due to old age.

**presbyopia.** A form of farsightedness occurring after middle age. Caused by a loss of elasticity of the crystalline lens with age.

**prescription.** A physician's written direction for preparation and use of a medicine.

**prevalence.** The number of cases of a specific disease in a given population at a certain point in time.

**proctitis.** Inflammation of the rectum.

**prodrome.** Symptoms marking the onset of an illness.

**progeny.** Children.

**progeria.** Premature aging.

**progesterone.** A steroid produced by the ovaries to prepare the uterus for the reception and development of the fertilized ovum (egg).

**prognosis.** The probable outcome of a disease.

**prolactin.** The pituitary hormone that promotes the growth of breast tissue and encourages the production of milk.

**prolapse.** The falling or slipping out of place of an internal organ, such as when the uterus falls into the vagina.

**prostate.** A male reproductive gland that surrounds the neck of the bladder and the urethra.

**prosthesis.** An artificial substitute for a missing body part.

**protein.** An organic compound composed primarily of amino acids.

**proteinuria.** Protein in the urine.

**pruritus.** Itching.

**psoriasis.** Chronic, recurring skin disease characterized by red, inflamed patches covered with scales.

**psychiatry.** The branch of medicine that deals with the diagnosis, treatment and prevention of mental disorders.

**psychoanalysis.** A technique developed by Sigmund Freud for the diagnosis and treatment of mental disorders.

**psychology.** The scientific study of mental processes and behavior.

**psychopath.** A person with a mental disorder characterized by the conspicuous disregard for the rights and needs of others, the lack of remorse and the lack of empathy for others.

**psychosis.** A mental disorder with serious derangement of the thinking process, often including delusions or hallucinations.

**ptilosis.** Shedding of the eyelashes.

**ptosis.** A prolapse or falling of some organ or structure, especially the drooping of a paralyzed upper eyelid.

**puberty.** The stage of life during which the secondary sexual characteristics begin to develop and sexual reproduction becomes possible.

**pubis.** The most forward bone of the pelvis.

**puerperium.** The period of time just after childbirth.

**pulmonary.** Having to do with the lungs.

**pulse.** The heartbeat as felt through the walls of an artery.

**puncture.** A wound produced by a pointed object.

**pupil.** The opening in the center of the iris.

**purpura.** Movement of blood into the soft tissues, producing bruises.

**purulent.** Containing pus.

**pus.** A thick fluid produced in certain infections.

**pustule.** A small pus-containing blister.

**pyelitis.** Inflammation of the urine-collecting system within the kidney.

**pyelonephritis.** Kidney infection.

**pylorus.** The junction of the stomach and the small intestine.

**pyodermatitis.** Skin infection producing pus.

**pyridoxine.** Vitamin $B_6$, sometimes used to treat nausea in pregnancy or to manage premenstrual syndrome symptoms.

**pyrogen.** Something that causes fever.

# Q

**quackery.** Misrepresentation of a product's or person's ability to diagnose and treat disease.

**quadriceps.** The name applied collectively to a group of four thigh muscles that insert together into the tendon surrounding the kneecap.

**quadriplegia.** Loss of feeling and movement of the arms and legs.

**quarantine.** Any isolation or restriction placed on movement to or from a place where communicable diseases have been diagnosed.

**quickening.** The first perceived movements of a fetus in the uterus.

# R

**rabies.** A fatal, if untreated, viral disease of mammals that's spread to humans by the bite of infected animal.

**rad.** Radiation absorbed dose. A unit of measurement of the absorbed dose of ionizing radiation.

**radiculopathy.** A disease or other problem affecting a nerve root.

**radioisotope.** A radioactive form of an element. Used in certain diagnostic tests.

**radiology.** The branch of medicine that deals with the use of x-rays.

**radon.** A colorless, radioactive gas produced by the decay of radium. The presence of sufficient quantities of this gas in homes is linked with the development of lung cancer.

**rash.** Visual marks or spots that appear on the skin.

**Raynaud's phenomenon.** A circulation disorder characterized by changes of blood flow, resulting in the hands and feet becoming pale, followed by redness and pain. This condition may be caused by cold, vibrations or emotions.

**recrudescence.** To reoccur after a temporary absence.

**rectum.** The last portion of the large intestine.

**reflux.** A return flow.

**refraction.** 1. The bending of a ray or wave of light from one medium to a medium of a different density. 2. The amount of error in the eye and the correction of that error with glasses to restore normal vision.

**regurgitation.** The return of partly digested food from the stomach to the mouth or of blood in a reverse direction through the valves of the heart.

**rehabilitation.** The process of restoring one's ability to live

as normally as possible after an injury or illness.

**Reiter's syndrome.** A complex group of symptoms marked by inflammation of the urethra or cervix, conjunctiva and joints.

**relapse.** The return of a disease after its apparent resolution.

**REM.** Rapid eye movement. The phase of sleep associated with dreaming and distinguished from the other stages of sleep by rapid movement of the eyes.

**remedy.** Anything that cures.

**remission.** Improvement of the symptoms of a disease.

**renal.** Having to do with the kidney.

**reservoir.** A medical term used to describe a source of organisms causing a disease.

**respiration.** The act or process of breathing. The process by which a living organism or cell takes in oxygen from the air or water and uses it.

**resuscitation.** Restoring the heartbeat and/or breathing in someone who's apparently dead. Also called artificial respiration.

**retardation.** Delay or halt of any process such as mental or physical development.

**retina.** The innermost layer of the eyeball. The retina contains the light-sensing rods and cones used for vision.

**retinopathy.** Degeneration of the retina.

**retrobulbar.** Behind the eyeball.

**retrovirus.** A virus that produces DNA from RNA (the opposite of the normal order). A group of viruses that includes HIV.

**Rh factor.** One of the antigens present on red blood cells. Used in categorizing the type of blood a person has.

**rheumatism.** Pain in the muscles and joints. Characterized by inflammation and stiffness. Sometimes used to describe arthritis, bursitis and sciatica.

**rhinitis.** Inflammation of the mucous membranes of the nose.

**rhinoplasty.** Plastic surgery of the nose.

**rhinorrhea.** Runny nose.

**rickets.** A condition resulting from a vitamin D deficiency in childhood. Characterized by the softening of the bones and associated deformities.

**ringworm.** A fungal infection of the skin.

**Rocky Mountain spotted fever.** An infectious disease spread by tick bites.

**roseola infantum.** A common viral infection of young children. Characterized by high fever, irritability and a faint rose-colored rash that appears on the fourth day when the fever subsides.

**rubella.** A mild childhood disease that causes fever and rash. Although rubella is mild in childhood, it's dangerous to pregnant women because it can cause birth defects. Also called German measles.

**rubeola.** A type of measles that can lead to serious complications and death.

# S

**sac.** Pouch; a bag-like structure.

**saccharin.** A compound that's hundreds of times sweeter than table sugar. Used as an artificial sweetener.

**sacroiliac.** Having to do with the joint formed by the sacrum and the ilium in the lower back.

**saliva.** An enzyme-containing thin, watery secretion of the salivary glands.

**salivary gland.** Any one of the three pairs of glands of the mouth (parotid, submaxillary and sublingual) that release saliva.

**salmonella.** A form of food poisoning characterized by fever and intestinal disorder due to *Salmonella* bacteria.

**salve.** Ointment.

**sanguineous.** Bloody.

**scabies.** An itchy, contagious skin condition caused by mites.

**scapula.** The shoulder blade.

**scarlet fever.** Fever and skin reaction caused by certain strains of streptococcus bacteria, usually following a streptococcal infection of the throat, middle ear or skin.

**schizophrenia.** A chronic mental disorder characterized by an inability to differentiate reality from fantasy. Often associated with hallucinations or delusions.

**sciatica.** Pain or inflammation going from the back to the buttock along the sciatic nerve.

**sclera.** The tough white covering of the eyeball.

**scleritis.** Inflammation of the sclera, causing pain, redness and possible loss of vision. Can be a complication of rheumatoid arthritis.

**scleroderma.** A chronic disease characterized by hardening or thickening of the skin due to abnormal tissue growth.

**sclerosis.** Hardening.

**scoliosis.** Abnormal curvature of the spine, usually develops during the rapid growth of puberty.

**scotoma.** A blind spot in an area of otherwise normal vision.

**scratch test.** A test for allergies in which small amounts of potential allergens are inserted in small scratches made in the skin.

**scrotum.** The skin-covered sac that contains the testes.

**scurvy.** A condition caused by vitamin C deficiency. Symptoms include loss of appetite, bleeding gums, bruising, inability to gain weight and irritability.

**sebaceous cyst.** A benign cyst containing oil and cells from a sebaceous gland.

**sebaceous glands.** Small glands in the skin that release an oily substance through the hair follicles.

**seborrhea.** Greasy scales or cheesy plugs resulting from overproduction of the sebaceous glands.

**seborrheic keratoses.** Skin growths that may be smooth or warty-looking, of varying size, and flesh-colored, brown or black. Often appear on the trunk or temples. Often occur in middle-aged and elderly people. Also called senile warts.

**seizure.** An attack of epilepsy.

**semen.** The ejaculate of the

male consisting of sperm and secretions from the prostate, seminal glands and other glands.

**semicircular canals.** The three loop-shaped tubular passages of the inner ear that control the sense of balance.

**seminiferous.** Carrying or producing semen.

**sensorium.** The state of a person's mental awareness.

**sepsis.** When disease-causing bacteria from an area of infection spread into the bloodstream and tissues.

**septum.** A wall dividing an organ or cavity, as in the nose.

**serology.** The study of the antigen-antibody reaction.

**serotonin.** A chemical used to transmit information from one nerve cell to another.

**serum.** The clear, yellowish-colored liquid portion of blood.

**shigellosis.** A diarrheal disease caused by *Shigella* bacteria.

**shingles.** A viral infection of certain sensory nerves that causes pain and blisters on the skin along the course of the infected nerve. Also called herpes zoster.

**shock.** A disorder resulting from disruption of the circulation of the blood that can upset all body functions.

**shoulder.** The ball-and-socket joint connecting the arm with the body.

**shunt.** To surgically divert the flow (such as of blood) from one organ or pathway to another.

**Siamese twins.** Identical twins born joined together.

**sickle cell anemia.** A genetic condition characterized by abnormal red blood cells containing a defective form of hemoglobin. Sickle cell anemia occurs in people who inherit the gene from both parents. Found chiefly in black populations and causes anemia, jaundice and recurring attacks of fever and pain in the arms, legs and abdomen.

**sickle cell trait.** Inheriting the gene for sickle cell anemia from only one parent. It causes no symptoms.

**sigmoid.** S-shaped.

**sinew.** A tendon or fibrous cord.

**sinus.** A cavity in a bone or other tissue. Commonly used to describe the cavities in the skull that open into the nasal cavity.

**sinusitis.** Inflammation and infection of the sinuses.

**sitz bath.** A bath in which only the hips and buttocks are immersed in water for relief of rectal or vaginal discomfort.

**skeleton.** The hard bony framework of the human body that supports the tissues and protects the organs.

**skull.** The bony framework of the head.

**smallpox.** A viral disease that was once highly contagious. Characterized by high fever, vomiting, and blisters and sores on the skin. Vaccination has eliminated this disease.

**smooth muscle.** A type of muscle tissue controlled by the involuntary nervous system, occurring in the walls of the uterus, intestines or blood vessels.

**sneeze.** To exhale breath from the nose and mouth in a sudden, involuntary action as a result of irritation of the mucous membranes of the nose.

**Snellen's chart.** A chart of block letters used to test distant vision.

**snoring.** Harsh breathing sounds during sleep caused by the vibration of the soft palate during inhalation.

**soft palate.** The soft part of the roof of the mouth in the back, toward the throat.

**soft tissue.** The substance of an organic body or organ consisting of cells and intercellular materials. The muscles and other nonbony tissues of the body.

**solar plexus.** The network of nerves in the center of the abdomen.

**spasm.** A sudden, involuntary contraction of a muscle or group of muscles.

**specimen.** A sample taken to study the nature of the whole.

**speculum.** An instrument for opening a body cavity to permit visual inspection.

**sperm.** The male germ cell. Also called spermatozoon.

**sphincter.** A ring-shaped muscle that surrounds a natural opening in the body and can open or close it by relaxing or contracting.

**sphygmomanometer.** An instrument for measuring blood pressure. An inflatable blood-pressure cuff.

**spina bifida.** A birth defect caused by imperfect closure of part of the spinal column, exposing some of the nervous system.

**spirochete.** Spiral-shaped bacteria.

**spleen.** The blood-forming and -storing organ located under the ribs in the upper left portion of the abdomen.

**splenomegaly.** Enlargement of the spleen.

**splint.** A device for holding broken or injured parts in place.

**spondylitis.** Inflammation of the vertebrae.

**spondylosis.** Narrowing of the spinal column resulting in reduction of the spaces between the vertebrae which may cause compression of the nerve roots.

**sprain.** A twisting or stretching injury of a ligament or muscle of a joint, with or without dislocating a bone.

**spur.** A projecting body. For example, from a bone.

**sputum.** Mucus secreted by the lungs, bronchi and trachea that's ejected by coughing or clearing the throat.

**stapedectomy.** Surgical removal of the stapes.

**stapedioplasty.** Replacement of the stapes with other materials (wire, bone, plastic).

**stapes.** A small bone of the middle ear. Also called the stirrup.

**stenosis.** Narrowing of a body passage or opening.

**sterile.** 1. Free from living microorganisms. 2. Unable to have children.

**sternum.** The breastbone.

**Stevens-Johnson reaction.** An inflammatory disease characterized by rapid attack of fever, skin blisters and sores on the lips, eyes, mouth, nasal passage and genitals.

**stoma.** 1. Mouth-like opening. 2. An opening used for drainage.

**stomatitis.** Inflammation of the mucosa of the mouth.

**stool.** Feces, or bowel movement.

**strabismus.** A deviation in which both eyes aren't trained on the same spot. Also called crossed eyes or lazy eye.

**strain.** 1. To filter. 2. Excessive effort. 3. Overstretching a portion of a muscle. 4. Within a species, a group of organisms characterized by a particular trait or quality.

**stress.** 1. Pressure; strain. 2. Any condition that causes mental or physical strain or tension.

**stridor.** A harsh or squeaky sound in breathing, often associated with a blocked larynx.

**stroke.** Deprivation of the blood supply to the brain due to blockage of a blood vessel. Results in unconsciousness, paralysis or other neurologic symptoms.

**stye.** Infection of one of the sebaceous glands of the edge of the eyelid.

**subcutaneous.** Just beneath the skin.

**subdural.** Beneath the dura mater, the covering of the brain.

**subliminal.** Below the threshold of conscious awareness.

**subluxation.** Partial dislocation.

**subungual.** Beneath a nail.

**sucrose.** A natural sugar obtained from sugar cane and sugar beets used as a sweetening agent. Also called table sugar.

**suicide.** Taking one's own life.

**sunburn.** A skin inflammation caused by prolonged exposure to ultraviolet radiation from the sun, tanning beds or other sources.

**sunstroke.** A serious failure of the body's heat-regulating mechanism resulting from excessive exposure to intense heat. Also called heat stroke.

**superinfection.** Sudden growth

of a different type of bacteria than the type originally diagnosed and treated. This is a common cause of treatment failure because the new type of bacteria is often resistant to first-line antibiotics.

**suppository.** A cone-shaped solid mass of medication designed to be placed in the rectum or vagina.

**surfactant.** A substance produced in the lungs that reduces surface tension and helps keep the small air sacs open.

**surrogate.** A substitute.

**suture.** 1. The joining together of certain vertebrate bones, especially of the skull. 2. A stitch or stitches made to close a wound. 3. The material used in closing a wound with stitches.

**synapse.** The tiny space between two nerve cells that allows the transmission of a nerve impulse.

**syncope.** Fainting.

**synergism.** The working together of different organs or parts of the body so that their combined action is greater than their individual effects.

**synovia.** The clear lubricating fluid produced in joints, bursae and tendon sheaths.

**syphilis.** A sexually transmitted disease caused by the spirochete *Treponema pallidum*.

**systole.** The cardiac contraction of a heartbeat.

## T

**tachycardia.** An abnormally rapid heartbeat.

**tachypnea.** Rapid breathing.

**talus.** A bone of the ankle.

**Tanner staging.** A growth chart used to assess the stage of puberty based on pubic hair growth, the development of genitalia in boys and breasts in girls.

**telogen effluvium.** Thinning hair. Rarely results in actual baldness.

**temporal.** Having to do with the side of the head.

**temporomandibular joint.** TMJ. The joint between the lower jaw and the side of the head, located just in front of the ear.

**tendinitis.** Inflammation of a tendon.

**tendon.** A cord of strong white fibrous tissue connecting muscle to bone.

**teratogen.** An agent that causes physical defects in a developing embryo.

**testis.** The male gonad or reproductive organ.

**testosterone.** One of the male sex hormones.

**tetanus.** An infectious disease, often fatal, caused by a *Clostridium tetani* bacteria. The bacteria usually enters the body through wounds. Characterized by muscle spasms and convulsions. Also called lockjaw.

**tetany.** A continuous muscle spasm.

**thalassemia.** An inherited type of chronic anemia.

**therapeutic.** A substance or treatment that's effective in treating disease.

**thoracentesis.** A surgical puncture and drainage of the chest cavity.

**thoracic.** Having to do with the chest.

**thorax.** The chest.

**thrombocyte.** A platelet.

**thromboembolism.** Blockage of a blood vessel by the piece of a blood clot that has broken loose from its original site.

**thrombosis.** Formation of a blood clot within a blood vessel or the heart.

**thrush.** Infection of the mouth by yeast. Characterized by milky-white lesions on the mouth, lips and throat.

**thymus.** A ductless gland located behind the upper portion of the breastbone.

**thyroid gland.** A large endocrine gland located in the front and sides of the neck and below the Adam's apple. Essential for the regulation of growth and metabolism.

**thyroxine.** The hormone from the thyroid gland that's essential in metabolism.

**tibia.** The larger of two bones in the lower leg.

**tic.** An involuntary spasm or twitching of a muscle.

**tinea.** A general term for fungal infections of the skin, usually combined with a description of the site or cause. Examples include tinea cruris or "jock itch," and tinea pedis or "athlete's foot."

**tinnitus.** Ringing in the ears. Sensation of a high-pitched sound that's not actually present.

**tissue.** A group of similar cells that together perform certain specialized functions.

**tongue.** The muscular organ attached to the floor of the mouth. Used to speak, chew, swallow and taste.

**tonsillectomy.** A procedure to remove the tonsils.

**tonsils.** A pair of oval masses of lymphoid tissue, one on each side of the throat at the back of the mouth.

**toxemia.** The presence of toxic substances in the blood from bacteria or body cells.

**toxic.** Poisonous.

**toxin.** A poisonous substance produced by a living organism.

**trachea.** The air passage extending from the throat to the bronchi. Also called the windpipe.

**tracheostomy.** A surgical incision in the trachea (the windpipe) through which a rigid tube is inserted to allow air to enter.

**trachoma.** A chronic infectious eye disease caused by Chlamydia infection of the eye. A leading cause of blindness worldwide.

**transfusion.** Introduction of blood or blood products through a vein into the body's circulation.

**transplantation.** The transfer of living organs or tissue from a donor to another person or from one area in the body to another.

**trauma.** Injury produced by an external force.

**trench mouth.** An acute, severe bacterial infection of the gums and lining of the mouth.

**triage.** A system of assigning priorities of medical treatment based on urgency, severity of injury and chance for survival.

**triceps.** A muscle of the arm used to extend the forearm.

**trichinosis.** Infection with a roundworm caused by consumption of larvae in undercooked pork or other infected meat.

**trichomoniasis.** Infection with *Trichomonas* protozoa. Frequently causes vaginal itching and discharge in women. It's usually acquired by sexual contact with an infected partner.

**tricuspid valve.** The heart valve between the right atrium and the right ventricle.

**trisomy.** The presence of an extra chromosome in addition to the usual pair. Down syndrome is an example of a condition caused by trisomy.

**truss.** A device to keep a hernia in its proper place.

**TSH.** Thyroid-stimulating hormone. A pituitary hormone that stimulates thyroid hormone production.

**tuberculin.** A protein injected into the skin to test for tuberculosis infection.

**tuberculosis.** An infectious disease caused by bacteria and characterized by the formation of tubercles in various tissues of the body, especially of the lungs.

**tumor.** Overgrowth of tissue.

**tussis.** Cough.

**tympanic membrane.** The eardrum.

**typhoid fever.** A bacterial infection with *Salmonella typhi* transmitted by contaminated water, milk or other foods. Proper sanitation and hygiene prevent the spread of disease.

**typhus.** An infectious disease spread to people by the bite of ticks, mites, fleas and lice. Typhus is characterized by high fever, headache and a rash.

## U

**ulcer.** A localized sore in the skin or mucosal surfaces.

**ulcerative colitis.** A chronic inflammatory disease of the large intestine characterized by bloody diarrhea.

**ulna.** The larger of the two bones of the forearm.

**umbilical cord.** A tough,

cord-like structure connecting the fetus to the placenta for nourishment.

**umbilicus.** The scar at the site of attachment of the umbilical cord. The navel or belly button.

**ungual.** Having to do with the nails.

**uremia.** The buildup in the blood of substances normally eliminated in the urine.

**ureter.** A narrow tube that transfers urine from the kidney to the bladder.

**urethra.** The tube that allows the bladder to empty outside the body.

**urethral stricture.** A narrow area of the urethra that blocks the flow of urine.

**urethritis.** Inflammation or infection of the urethra.

**urinary bladder.** The organ that serves as a temporary storage place for urine. Also called the bladder.

**urine.** The fluid composed of water and waste products that's secreted by the kidneys.

**urogenital.** Having to do with the urinary system and genitals.

**urology.** The branch of medicine that deals with the urinary system in women and the urogenital system in men.

**uterus.** A hollow muscular organ in women where the ovum (egg) is deposited and the embryo and fetus are developed.

**uvula.** The fleshy mass hanging down from the soft palate above the back of the tongue.

# V

**vaccination.** Inoculation with weakened or dead microorganisms to develop immunity and prevent disease caused by the regular strain of that microorganism.

**vaccine.** A preparation of killed or weakened microorganisms, given to treat or prevent disease.

**vagina.** The muscular canal in women between the vulva and the uterus. It serves as the entry for spermatozoa and as the birth canal.

**vaginismus.** Painful spasm of the vagina.

**varicocele.** Dilated veins in the spermatic cord above or around the testis that can cause decreased sperm production on the affected side.

**varicose veins.** Swollen, distended veins especially visible in the legs.

**vas deferens.** The duct through which sperm travels from the testicle to the urethra of the penis.

**vascular.** Of or having vessels, particularly the blood vessels.

**vasculitis.** Inflammation of the walls of the small blood vessels.

**vasectomy.** Surgical removal or tying of the vas deferens to prevent the passing of sperm. Used as a form of birth control.

**vasoconstriction.** Causing the narrowing or closing (constriction) of blood vessels.

**vasodilation.** Causing the widening or opening (dilation) of blood vessels.

**vector.** An animal that spreads an infectious agent from one host to another. Also called a carrier.

**vein.** A vessel that carries blood from the various parts of the body to the heart.

**venom.** A toxin secreted by an animal.

**venous.** Having to do with a vein.

**ventricle.** 1. Either of the two chambers that contract to pump blood from the heart. 2. Any of several small fluid-filled cavities in the brain.

**verruca.** See wart.

**vertebrae.** The bones that make up the spine.

**vertigo.** A spinning sensation often accompanied by mild to severe nausea.

**vesicle.** 1. A small, sac-like cavity. 2. A blister.

**vesicourethral reflux.** An abnormal condition that allows urine to flow from the bladder back into a ureter.

**virus.** The agent of an infectious disease, smaller than bacteria, that must have a living host in order to grow or reproduce.

**viscera.** The large internal organs.

**vision.** The sense of sight.

**vitamin.** An organic substance found in food and essential in small quantities for good health.

**vitiligo.** A skin condition characterized by sharply defined white patches that contain no skin color (pigment).

**vitreous humor.** The jelly-like material that fills the eyeball between the lens and retina.

**vomiting.** Ejecting the contents of the stomach through the mouth.

**vulva.** The external parts of the female reproductive tract surrounding the opening to the vagina.

# W

**wart.** A small, hard, abnormal growth of the skin or mucous membranes caused by a virus.

**wheal.** A pimple or small itchy elevation of the skin caused by an allergen.

**wheeze.** A whistling or squeaky breathing sound caused by the narrowing (constriction) or blocking of the airway.

**whiplash.** An injury of the neck or spine due to a sudden, severe bending of the neck.

**whooping cough.** A serious infectious respiratory disease of children. Named for the distinctive whooping sound made by the patient after a coughing spasm. Also called pertussis.

**Wilms' tumor.** A rapidly growing tumor of the kidney found in children.

**Wilson's disease.** A rare, inherited disorder that occurs when copper pools in the red blood cells. May cause tremors, muscle rigidity, speech problems and dementia.

**withdrawal.** The act or process of giving up the use of a drug to which one has become addicted or dependent.

**wrist.** The joint or part of the arm between the hand and the forearm.

# X

**xanthelasma.** Fatty deposits that appear as yellowish patches, or plaques, under the skin, often appearing in or near the eyelids.

**xanthoma.** A tumor-like deposit of fatty substances in the skin.

**xenograft.** Transplantation of tissue or organs from an individual of one species to another unrelated species, such as a pig's heart valve implanted in a human.

**xeroderma.** Dryness of the skin.

# Y

**yeast.** A single-celled fungus that reproduces by budding and may lead to infections of the skin or other moist areas.

**yellow fever.** An acute viral illness spread by mosquito bites. Characterized by fever and jaundice.

# Z

**zoonosis.** A disease that can be spread to people by animals.

**zoster.** A viral infection of certain sensory nerves that causes pain and an eruption of blisters on the skin along the course of the infected nerve.

**zygote.** A fertilized ovum (egg).

# INDEX

Abdominal pain
  in infants and children, 371
  self-care flowchart, 505-508
ABO blood classification system, 131-132
Abrasions, first aid for, 603
Abruptio placentae, 391
Abscess
  anal, 170-171
  brain, 47
  breast, 411
  liver, 206
  lung, 150-151
  tooth, 96
Absorptiometry, 627
Abuse
  child abuse, 574-575
    sexual, 574-577
  elder abuse, 437, 577-578
  family violence and, 573-574
  psychological effects of, 573-574
  spouse abuse, 578
Accidents. *See* Falls; Safety
ACE inhibitors, 618
Acetaminophen, 614
Acne, 268, 274-275, 375
Acne drugs, 614, 617
Acoustic neuroma, 85
Acrocyanosis, 126
Acromegaly, 208-209
Actinic keratoses, 285
ADD (Attention Deficit Disorder), 369
Addictions, 559-560. *See also* Alcohol abuse; Substance abuse
  codependency and, 560-561
  gambling, 565
  sex, 565-566
Addison's disease, 209-210
Adhesive capsulitis, 249
Adolescence
  acne in, 268, 375
  alcohol, tobacco and drug use in, 375-376
  contraception in, 558

depression in, 376
eating disorders in, 376-377
emotional maturation in, 556-557
gynecomastia in, 377
opposite sex friendships in, 557-558
parental support and communication, 558
physical maturation in, 557
pregnancy in, 377-378
puberty in
  delayed, 374-375
  female, 373-374
  male, 373, 374
  precocious, 374
rebellion and risk-taking in, 378
school problems in, 378-379
sex education in, 556-558
sexuality in, 379
Adrenal glands, 207-208
Aerosol abuse, 565
AFP (alpha-fetoprotein) test, 392, 627
Age spots, 436
Aged. *See* Elderly
Agranulocytosis, 137
AIDS (acquired immunodeficiency syndrome). *See* HIV infection
Alcohol abuse, 562-563. *See also* Substance abuse
  in adolescents, 375-376
  signs of, 376
  treatment of, 563
Alcohol-related disorders
  cardiomyopathy, 113
  cirrhosis, 202
  fatty liver, 202
  fetal alcohol syndrome, 342
  hepatitis, 202
Aldosteronism, 210
Allergens, 142, 222
Allergic contact dermatitis, 221, 277-278
Allergic rhinitis, 222

Allergies, 221-224
  common allergens, 222
  drug, 222
  food, 222-223
  severe allergic reaction, 222
Alpha blockers, 617-618
Alpha$_1$-antitrypsin deficiency, 147
Alpha-fetoprotein (AFP) test, 392, 627
ALS (amyotrophic lateral sclerosis), 44
Alzheimer's disease, 53-54
Ambulatory blood pressure monitoring, 627
Amebiasis, 310-311
Amoebic dysentery, 181
Amenorrhea, 382-383
Amnesia, 53
Amniocentesis, 628
Amniotic fluid
  excessive (polyhydramnios), 396
  premature membrane rupture and, 396
Amphetamines, 618
  abuse of, 564-565
Amputations, 597-598
Amyotrophic lateral sclerosis (ALS, Lou Gehrig's disease), 44
Analgesics, 614-615
  dental, 614
  narcotic, 618
  non-narcotic, 618
  oral, 614
  topical, 614
  with urinary tract infections, 618
Anaphylactic shock, 222, 283
Anemia, 133-135
  aplastic, 137
  of chronic disease, 133
  hemolytic, 133
  iron-deficiency, 133-134
  in newborns, 343
  pernicious, 135, 194-195

in pregnancy, 391-392
  sickle-cell, 134
  thalassemia, 134
  vitamin-deficiency, 134-135
Anencephaly, 346
Anesthetics, 618
  during labor and delivery, 400-401
Aneurysms, 108-109
Anger, 566-568
  dealing with, 567-568
  passive-aggressive expressions of, 567
Angina, 109-110
Angiocardiogram (cardiac catheterization), 631
Angiogram, 628
Angiomas
  of eyelids, 66
  spider angioma, 269, 286
Angiotensin-converting enzyme (ACE) inhibitors, 618
Animal bites, 598
Ankle disorders
  self-care flowchart, 532
  sprains of, first aid for, 611
Ankylosing spondylitis, 229
Anorexia nervosa, 583-586
Anoscopy, 628
Antacids, 614-615
Anthracosis, 152
Antiadrenergic drugs, 618
Antianginal drugs, 618
Antianxiety drugs. *See* Sedatives
Antiarrhythmic drugs, 618
Antibiotics, 618-619
  cephalosporins, 621
  chloramphenicol, 622
  fluoroquinolones, 624
  macrolides, 624
  ointments and creams, 615
  penicillins, 625
  taking full course of, 306
  tetracyclines, 626
  for urinary tract infections, 619

Anticlotting drugs, 619
Antidepressants, 619
Antidiarrheal drugs, 615
Antifungal drugs
  general, 619
  topical, 615
  vaginal, 615, 619
Antigout drugs, 619
Antihelmintic drugs, 615
Antihistamines, 615, 619
Antihypertensive drugs, 619
  alpha blockers, 617-618
  angiotensin-converting
    enzyme (ACE) inhibitors, 618
  beta-adrenergic blockers, 621
  calcium channel blockers, 621
  diuretics, 623
Anti-inflammatory drugs. See
    also Non-steroidal anti-
    inflammatory drugs
    (NSAIDs)
  for asthma, 143
  for pleurisy, 154
  uses and examples, 619
Anti-itch drugs, 615
Antilice medicines, 615, 619-620
Antimalarial drugs, 620
Antinausea and antivomiting
    drugs, 615, 620
Antiparasitic drugs, 620
Antipsychotic drugs, 620
Antipyretics (fever-reducing
    drugs), 616
Antirheumatic drugs, 620
Antiseizure drugs, 620
Antiseptics, 615
Antisocial personality, 589
Antispasmodic and anticramp-
    ing drugs, 620-621
Antivertigo (motion-sickness)
    drugs, 625
Antiviral drugs, 621
Anus
  abscess of, 170-171
  fissures of, 170, 367
  imperforate, 354
  itching of, 171, 363-364
Anxiety disorders, 580-582
  generalized, 581
Aorta
  aneurysm of, 108
  coarctation of, 350, 351
Aortic valve
  blood flow through, 121, 122
  stenosis of, 122, 350
Aphasia, 44-45
Aphthous ulcers (canker sores),
    92-93
Aplastic anemia, 137
Apnea of prematurity, 343
Appendectomy, 173

Appendicitis, 171-173, 371
Appetite suppressants, 615
Arrhythmias. See Heart,
    rhythm problems of
Arsenic, 621
Arterial blood gas test, 628
Arterial embolism, 110-111
Arteries. See Blood vessels
Arteriogram, 628
Arteritis, temporal, 127
Arthritis, 229-232
  ankylosing spondylitis, 229
  infectious, 229
  juvenile rheumatoid, 229-230
  osteoarthritis, 230-231
  Reiter's syndrome, 231
  rheumatoid, 231-232
Arthroscopy, 628
Asbestos exposure, lung cancer
    and, 151
Asbestosis, 152
Ascariasis, 314
Aspergillosis, 309
Asphyxia, in newborns, 344
Aspirin
  Reye's syndrome and, 323, 615
  uses of, 615
Asthma, 142-145
  emergency preparation for, 145
  occupational, 153
  peak flow rate and, 144
  treatment of, 142-144
    anti-inflammatory drugs,
      143-144
    bronchodilators, 142-143
    inhaler use in, 143-144
Astigmatism, 67
Atelectasis, 146
Atherosclerosis, 111-113
  balloon angioplasty for, 111-
    112
  bypass surgery for, 112
  endarterectomy for, 112
  plaque in, 110-111
  stroke caused by, 60
Athlete's foot, 256, 271
Atlas of body, 33-40
Atopic dermatitis, 279
Atrial septal defect, 350
Atrioventricular block, 119
Atrium
  fibrillation of, 119
  tachycardia of, 118
Attention deficit disorder
    (ADD), 369
Audiometry, 628
  impedance, 628
  pure tone, 628
  speech, 641
  tuning fork, 643
Aura

before classic migraines, 51
before seizure, 57
Autism, 369
Autoimmune disorders, 223
Avoidant personality, 589
Babies. See Newborns
Back pain, 232-233
  in pregnancy, 392-393
  self-care flowchart, 512-513
Bacteremia, 298
Bacterial infections, 298-308.
    See also specific types
Bad breath (halitosis), 92
Balanitis, 426
Baldness. See Hair loss
Balloon angioplasty, 111-112
Barbiturates, 621
  abuse of, 565
Barium enema (lower GI
    series), 628-629
Barium swallow (upper GI
    series), 629
Barotrauma, 78
Basal cell carcinoma, 270, 290
Bedsores, 275
Bedwetting (enuresis), 364
Bee sting kits, 222
Behavioral therapy, 559
Bell's palsy, 45
Benzodiazepines, 621
  abuse of, 565
Berry aneurysms, 108
Beta-adrenergic blockers, 621
Bile acid sequestrants, 621
Biliary atresia, 346
Biliary colic, 204
Biopsy, 629
  bone marrow, 630
  cone, 633
  endometrial, 634
  fine needle, 636
  lymph node, 637
  skin, 640-641
Bipolar disorder, 587
Birth. See Labor and delivery
Birth control. See Contraception
Birth defects, 345-356
  anencephaly, 346
  biliary atresia, 346
  cerebral palsy, 346-347
  cleft lip and palate, 347
  club foot, 263, 347-348
  cystic fibrosis, 348
  Down syndrome, 348-349
  dwarfism, 349
  esophageal atresia, 349
  genital abnormalities, 346
  heart defects, 349-352
  hernias, 352-353
  Hirschsprung's disease, 353
  hydrocephalus, 353

imperforate anus, 354
intestinal atresia, 354
muscular dystrophy, 354
phenylketonuria, 354
pyloric stenosis, 354-355
spina bifida, 355
undescended testicle, 355-356
Birthmarks, 275-276, 341
  hemangioma, 275-276
  salmon patches, 276
Bites and stings, 598-599
Bladder
  cancer of, 159, 160
  incontinence of, 167-168
  infections of, 162-163
  Kegel's exercises for, 168
  retraining of, 167
Blastomycosis, 309
Bleeding. See Hemorrhage
Bleeding disorders, 135-136
  disseminated intravascular
    coagulation (DIC), 135-136
  factor deficiencies, 136
  thrombocytopenia, 136
  vitamin deficiencies in, 136
Blepharitis, 64, 265
Blisters, first aid for, 603
Blood
  clotting factors, 131
  components of, 131
  definition of, 131
  donation of, 132-133
  types, 131-132
Blood clots
  in arterial embolism, 110
  drugs for dissolving, 117
  formation of, 135
  in pulmonary embolism, 157
  in venous thrombosis, 129
Blood disorders
  anemias, 133-135
  bone marrow problems, 136-
    137
  bruising, 138
  factor deficiencies, 136
  leukemia, 138-139
  lymphoma, 139-140
Blood pressure. See also
    Hypertension; Hypotension
  ambulatory monitoring of,
    627
  measurement of, 629
Blood tests, 629-630
  alpha-fetoprotein (AFP) test,
    627
  arterial blood gas test, 628
  erythrocyte sedimentation
    rate (ESR), 634-635
  fecal occult blood test, 8, 635
  glucose tolerance test, 636
  liver function tests, 637

Blood tests (continued)
  partial thromboplastin time, 639
  prostate-specific antigen (PSA), 640
  Rh-factor compatibility test, 640
  thyroid function test, 642
  types performed for periodic health exams, 7
Blood transfusions, 133
Blood vessels. See also Cardiovascular diseases; Veins
  arteries, 107
  arterioles, 107
  atlas of, 35
  capillaries, 107, 141
  constriction of, 107
  dilation of, 107
  transposition of great vessels, 351, 352
  venules, 107
Boils, 268, 276
Bone and joint disorders. See Musculoskeletal disorders
Bone marrow disorders, 136-137
  agranulocytosis, 137
  aplastic anemia, 137
  multiple myeloma, 137
  polycythemia, 137
  tests for, 630
Bone marrow transplantation, 139
Bone mineral density analysis, 7, 630
Bone scans, 630
Bones. See also Musculoskeletal disorders
  structure of, 227
  tumors of, 254
Borderline personality, 589
Botulism, 300
Bowel diseases. See Gastrointestinal disorders; Intestines
Bowel movements
  encopresis and, 366-367
  self-care flowchart, 514-515
  toilet training and, 362-363
Brain. See also Nervous system; Neurologic disorders
  abscess of, 47
  anatomy of, 42-43
  atlas of, 33
  concussions and contusions of, 50
  death of, 48
  hemorrhage of, 45-47
  epidural, 46
  intracerebral, 46

subarachnoid, 46
subdural, 46
tumors of, 47-48
Breast
  abscess of, 411
  anatomy and function of, 380
  cancer of, 408-411
    signs of, 410
  mammogram for, 8, 409
  self-examination at home, 9, 408-411
  surgery and reconstruction for, 410-411
  cosmetic surgery of, 412
  engorgement of, 406-407
  fibrocystic disease and lumps of, 412-413
  galactorrhea of, 413-414
  infections of, 411-412
  mastitis of, 411-412
  self-care flowchart
    men, 494
    women, 493
Breast feeding, 404-407
  advantages of, 338-339, 404
  breast care during, 405
  colostrum in breast milk, 404
  cuddle hold in, 405, 406
  football hold in, 406
  planning for, 398
  side-lying position in, 406
  technique of, 404-405
Breathing
  physiology of, 141-142
  problems with, in infants and children, 364
Bridge, dental, 100
Bronchial lavage, 150
Bronchiolitis, 320-321
Bronchitis, 145-146
  acute, 145
  chronic, 145
Bronchodilators, 621
Bronchoscopy, 630-631
Bruising and bruises
  causes and characteristics of, 138
  in the elderly, 436
  purpura of skin, 288-289
Bulimia, 583-586
Bunions, 256-257
Burns, first aid for, 599-601
Bursitis, 233-234
Bypass surgery, 112
Byssinosis, 153
Caffeine
  physical effects of, 14
  sleep interference from, 28
Calcipotriene, 621
Calcium
  actions and sources of, 20

for osteoporosis, 245
Calcium channel blockers, 621
Calluses, 258-259
Calories
  burned by exercise, 5
  in condiments, 23
  daily caloric need, 14
Cancer, 224-226. See also specific types
  screening tests for, 9, 225
  treatment and prevention of, 225-226
  types of, 224
  warning signs of, 9
Candidiasis, 98, 308-309
Canker sores (aphthous ulcers), 92-93
Capillaries, 107, 141
Car safety precautions, 29, 335-336
Carbohydrates, 14, 24
Carbuncles, 276
Carcinoid tumors, 174
Cardiac arrest, 119
Cardiac catheterization (angio-cardiogram), 631
Cardiomyopathy, 113-114
  alcoholic, 113
  congestive, 113
  hypertrophic, 113
  toxic, 113
Cardiopulmonary resuscitation (CPR), 596-597
  adults, 596-597
  infants, 597
Cardiovascular diseases. See also Heart diseases
  aneurysms, 108-109
  angina, 109-110
  arterial embolism, 110-111
  atherosclerosis, 111-113
  high blood pressure (hypertension), 123-124
  low blood pressure (hypotension), 124-125
  Raynaud's phenomenon (disease), 126-127
  risk factors for, 15
  temporal arteritis, 127
  varicose veins, 127-129
  venous thrombosis, 129-130
Carotid artery
  atherosclerosis of, 60
  endarterectomy of, 60, 112
  examination of, 7-8
Carpal tunnel syndrome, 49, 257-258
Cartilage, 228
Cataracts, 64, 265
Cat-scratch fever, 298
Cauterization, for nosebleed, 88

Cavernous hemangioma, 267, 275
Cavities, of teeth, 93-94
Celiac disease, 194
Cellulitis, 276-277
Central nervous system. See Nervous system
Cephalosporins, 621
Cerebral palsy, 346-347
Cerebrospinal fluid, 44
Cervix, 414-416
  anatomy and function of, 380-381
  cancer of, 8, 414-415
  cap over, for birth control, 551
  cysts of, 415
  dysplasia of, 414, 415
  erosion of, 415
  polyps of, 416
Cesarean section, 403
Chalazions, 66, 266
Charcoal, activated, 616
Chemotherapy, 621
Chest pain, self-care flowchart for, 499-503
Chest x-rays, 631
Chickenpox (varicella), 272, 321-322
  immunization for, 12
Child abuse, 574-575
  sexual, 574-577
Children. See Infants and children
Chlamydia infection, 317-318
Chloramphenicol, 622
Chloride, 20
Chlorpromazine, 622
Choking, first aid for, 601-602
  adults or children, 601
  Heimlich maneuver in, 601-602
  infants, 602
Cholecystectomy, 204
Cholecystitis, 204
Cholecystogram, oral, 639
Cholera, 298-299
Cholesterol, 14-15
  levels for adults, 16
  medications for lowering, 622
  bile acid sequestrants, 621
  HMG-CoA reductase inhibitors, 624
  stroke related to, 60
  testing for, 15
Chorionic villus sampling (CVS), 631-632
Chromium, 20
Chronic fatigue syndrome, 322
Cigarette smoking. See Smoking
Circulatory system, 107, 35. See also Blood vessels
Circumcision care, 336

Cirrhosis, 201-203
  alcoholic, 202
  biliary, 202
  postnecrotic and postviral, 202
Cleft lip and palate, 347
Clitoris
  anatomy of, 381, 382
  lack of stimulation of, 385
*Clostridium perfringens* infection, 300
Clot dissolvers, 622
Clotting disorders. *See* Bleeding disorders
Club foot, 263, 347-348
Cluster headaches, 51
Coarctation of aorta, 350, 351
Cocaine, 622
  abuse of, 563
Coccidioidomycosis, 309
Cochlear implant, for hearing loss, 79
Codependency, 560-561
Cold sores (herpes simplex virus infection), 94-95, 266
Colds, 322-323
  bacterial infection with, 323
  self-care flowchart, 490
  things to avoid, 324
Colic, 341-342
Collapsed lung, 146-147
  atelectasis, 146
  pneumothorax, 146-147
Colon. *See also* Gastrointestinal disorders
  cancer of
    colorectal, 175-177
    fecal occult blood test for, 8, 635
    self-screening tests at home, 9
  polyps of, 174-175
Colonoscopy, 7, 632
Color blindness, 64
Colorectal cancer, 175-177
Colposcopy, 632
Coma
  causes of, 48
  vegetative state, 48
Compartment syndrome, 49
Compressed nerves (entrapment syndrome), 48-49
Compression fracture of spine, 234-235
Compulsive personality, 589
Computed tomographic (CT) scans, 632
Conception, 544-546
Concussions and contusions, 50
Condoms, 32, 317, 551
Cone biopsy, 633
Congestion, nasal, relief of, 90

Congestive cardiomyopathy, 113
Congestive heart failure, 114-115
Conjunctivitis, 71-72, 266
  allergic, 71
  bacterial, 71
  chemical, 71
  foreign body, 71
  viral, 71-72
Connective tissue, 227
Constipation, 177-178. *See also* Intestines, obstruction of
  in adolescents and adults, 177-178
  in infants and children, 177, 364-365
  in pregnancy, 393
Consumption (tuberculosis), 307
Contact lenses, 68, 72
Contraception
  in adolescents, 558
  birth control pills (oral contraceptives), 550-551, 622
  conception and, 544-546
  condom, 551
  diaphragm/cervical cap/female condom, 551
  effectiveness of contraceptives, 553
  family planning, 542
  hormone implants and shots, 551-552
  implanted contraceptives, 622
  injected contraceptives, 622
  intrauterine device, 552
  readiness for children, 542-543
  rhythm method, 552
  spermicides, 552
  sterilization, 553
  withdrawal method, 553
Contusions, 50
Convulsions. *See* Seizures
Copper, 20
Cornea
  abrasion of, 68, 265
  definition of, 62
  ulcer, infection of, 65
Corns, 258-259
  solutions for removing, 616
Corticosteroids, 622-623
  Cushing's syndrome caused by, 210
  danger of stopping, 209
  inhaled, 623
  oral, 622-623
  topical, 623
Cortisone, 623
Cough, self-care flowchart for, 488-489
Cough medicines
  narcotic and non-narcotic, 623
  suppressants, 616

Counseling, 559
Counselors, 560
CPR. *See* Cardiopulmonary resuscitation (CPR)
Crack abuse, 563
Cradle cap, 365
Cramps, muscle, 242-243
Crohn's disease, 178-179
Cromolyn sodium, 623
Crossed eyes, 65-66, 365
Croup, 323-324
Crowns, dental, 100
Crying, by newborns, 338
Cryptococcosis, 309
CT (computed tomographic) scans, 632
Cultures, 633
Cushing's syndrome, 210
Cuts, first aid for, 602-603
Cystic fibrosis, 348
Cystitis (bladder infection), 162-163
Cystoscopy, 633
Cysts
  kidney, 160-161
  sebaceous, 285-286
Cytology exam, 633
Dandruff, 277
  medicines for, 616
Deafness, 78
Death
  stillbirth, 396, 397
  sudden infant death syndrome, 372
Decongestants, 616
  nasal sprays, 87, 616
  oral, 616
Decubitus ulcers, 275
Dehydration, 179-180, 366
Delivery. *See* Labor and delivery
Dementia, 53-54
Dental caries, 93-94. *See also* Tooth, disorders of
Dental x-rays, 633
Dentures, 100
Dependent personality, 589
Depression, 587-588
  in adolescents, 376
  postpartum, 404
  seasonal, 587
  symptoms of, 587
Dermatitis, 277-279. *See also* Skin disorders
  allergic contact, 221, 277-278
  atopic, 268, 279
  dyshidrotic, 278
  herpetiformis, 278
  irritant contact, 279
  nummular, 279
  rashes
    in infants and children, 370

  skin protection methods, 278
  relieving itching, 279, 283
  self-care flowcharts, 535-540
Desmopressin, 623
Deviated septum, 87
Diabetes, 211-214
  complications of, 212
  home glucose monitoring in, 213
  hypoglycemia in, 216
  in pregnancy, 393
  stroke related to, 60
  type I, 211
  type II, 211-212
Diabetic retinopathy, 73
Dialysis, for kidney failure, 164
Diaper rash, 365
  medications for, 616
Diapers, selection and care, 338
Diaphragm, 141, 142
  hernia of, 353
Diaphragm, for birth control, 551
Diarrhea, 181-183
  causes of, 181
  in infants and children, 181-182, 365-366
  self-care flowchart, 516-517
  traveler's, 181-183
DIC (disseminated intravascular coagulation), 135-136
Digestive system, 38, 169-170
Digital rectal examination, 633
Digitalis, 623
Dilatation and curettage (D&C), 420
Dilation of the pupils, 633
Diphtheria, 299
  DTP vaccine for, 11
Diplopia (double vision), 66
Disciplining infants and children, 358-359
Dislocated joints, 235
Dissecting aneurysms, 108
Disseminated intravascular coagulation (DIC), 135-136
Disulfiram, 623
Diuretics, 616, 623
Diverticulosis and diverticulitis, 183-184
Dizziness, 77, 83-84
Doppler ultrasonography, 644
  in pregnancy, 392
Double vision (diplopia), 66
Down syndrome, 348-349
Drowning, first aid for, 603-604
Drug abuse. *See* Substance abuse
Drugs, 613-626. *See also* specific drugs
  allergies to, 222

Drugs (continued)
   avoiding problems while taking, 614
   elderly patients and, 435-436
   home safety precautions, 30
   insomnia caused by, 28
   over-the-counter medicines, 614-617
   prescription medicines, 617-626
   psychiatric, 579
   ways of taking, 615
Dry eyes, 66
Dry skin, 279-280
DTP (diphtheria, tetanus, pertussis) vaccine, 11
Dwarfism, 349
   pituitary, 219
Dysentery
   amoebic, 181
   amebic, 310
   See also Diarrhea
Dyslexia, 369
Dysmenorrhea, 383
Ear
   anatomy of, 34, 76-77
   disorders of, 77-85
      benign positional vertigo, 77
      ear canal infection, 79-80
      hearing loss, 77-79
      labyrinthitis, 83
      Meniere's disease, 83-84
      middle ear fluid, 81-82
      middle ear infection, 80-81
      ringing in the ear, 84-85
      self-care flowchart, 477-478
      wax buildup in, 85
   foreign objects in, 82
   medicines for, 623
   tumors of
      inner ear, 85
      outer ear, 85
Eardrum, ruptured, 78
Eating. See Nutrition
Eating disorders
   in adolescence, 376-377
   anorexia and bulimia, 582-586
   overeating, 586
ECG (electrocardiogram), 8, 634
Echocardiogram, 633-634
Ectopic pregnancy, 393-394
Edema
   in pregnancy, 397
   pulmonary, 114, 156-157
EEG (electroencephalogram), 634
Ejaculation, premature, 425
Elderly, 433-440
   abuse and neglect of, 437, 577-578
   accidents and falls of, 433-434

advance directives and power of attorney for, 435
   living at home, 437-438
   living with family members, 438-440
   nursing home care, 440
   common health problems of, 433
   incontinence of, 433-435
   medicine use by, 435-436
   memory problems of, 436
   skin changes of, 436-437
Electrical shock, first aid for, 604
Electrocardiogram (EKG), 8, 634
Electroencephalogram (ECG), 634
Electromyography (EMG), 634
Embolism
   arterial, 110-111
   pulmonary, 130, 157
Emergencies. See First aid and emergencies
EMG (electromyography), 634
Emotional health/problems.
   See also Psychiatric problems
   addictions, 559-560
   anger, 566-568
   child abuse and neglect, 574-577
   codependent families, 560-561
   elder abuse and neglect, 437, 577-578
   emotional dos and don'ts of parenting, 357
   family violence, 573-574
   gambling addiction, 565
   grief, 434, 568-569
   guilt, 569-570
   loneliness, 570-571
   qualities for improving, 560
   self-esteem, 361, 571
   sex addiction, 565-566
   spouse abuse, 578
   stress, 571-573
   substance abuse, 561-565
   therapy for, 559
Emphysema, 145, 147-148
Encephalitis, 324-325
Encopresis, 366-367
Endarterectomy, of carotid artery, 60, 112
Endocarditis
   rheumatic fever and, 304
   subacute bacterial (SBE), 115
Endocrine glands, 207
Endometrial biopsy or sampling, 634
Endometrial cancer, 417-418
Endometriosis, 418-419
Endoscopy, 634
   anoscopy, 628

   arthroscopy, 628
   bronchoscopy, 630-631
   colonoscopy, 632
   colposcopy, 632
   cytoscopy, 633
   esophagogastrodudenoscopy (EGD), 635
   gastroscopy, 636
   hysteroscopy, 636
   laparoscopy, 637
   laryngoscopy, 637
   nasolaryngoscopy, 638
   proctoscopy, 640
   sigmoidoscopy, 640
Entrapment syndromes, 48-49
   carpal tunnel syndrome, 49
   compartment syndrome, 49
   sciatica, 49
   tarsal tunnel syndrome, 49
   ulnar nerve entrapment, 49
Enuresis (bedwetting), 364
Epididymitis, 430
Epiglottitis, 299
Epilepsy, 56-57, 371. See also Seizures
Epistaxis. See Nosebleed
Epstein-Barr virus, 328
Erythema infectiosum (Fifth disease), 325
Erythrocyte sedimentation rate (ESR), 634-635
Esophagitis, reflux, 187-188
Esophagogastroduodenoscopy (EGD), 635
Esophagus
   atresia of, 349
   cancer of, 184-185
   varices (bleeding) of, 185
Estrogens, 623-624
Eustachian tubes
   blockage of, 77
   middle ear infections and, 80-81
Exercise, 2-6
   calories burned by, 5
   in pregnancy, 387
   starting a program of, 3-5
   target heart rate in, 5-6
   types of, 3
Exercise stress test, 4, 635
Exocrine glands, 207
Expectorants, 616, 624
Eye. See also Eye, disorders of
   anatomy of, 34, 62-63
   disorders of
      black eye, 63-64
      blepharitis, 64, 265
      cataracts, 64, 265
      color blindness, 64
      conjunctivitis (pink eye), 71-72, 266

      corneal ulcer/infection, 65
      crossed eyes (strabismus), 65-66, 365
      double vision (diplopia), 66
      dry eyes, 66
      glaucoma, 68-69
      hyphema, 69-70
      iritis, 70
      light sensitivity (photophobia), 70
      night blindness, 70
      periorbital cellulitis, 70-71
      retinal artery blockage, 72-73
      retinal degeneration, 73
      retinal detachment, 74
      self-care flowchart, 474-475
      subconjunctival hemorrhage, 74-75
   focusing problems of, 67-68
      astigmatism, 67
      farsightedness (hyperopia), 67
      nearsightedness (myopia), 67
      presbyopia, 67
   foreign substances in, 68
   injuries of
      first aid for, 604-605
      penetrating, 68
   normal eye, 265
   spots or "floaters" in, 68
   tumors of, 75
Eyelids
   angiomas of, 66
   chalazions of, 66, 266
   lumps of, 66
   papillomas of, 66, 266
   stye of, 74, 266
   weakness of, 66-67
   xanthelasmas of, 66
Facial swelling, self-care flowchart for, 476
Factor deficiencies, 136
Failure to thrive, 342
Fainting, first aid for, 605
Fallopian tubes, 381
Fallot's tetralogy, 350-351
Falls
   in the elderly, 433-434
   first aid for, 605
   preventing, 30, 434
Familial polyposis, colonoscopy for, 7
Family and relationship issues, 542-558. See also Emotional health/problems
   conception, 544-546
   contraception, 550-553
   delaying pregnancy, 549-550
   family planning, 542-544
   infertility, 546-549

Family and relationship issues (continued)
  sex education for children, 554-558
    adolescents, 556-558
    preschool children, 554-556
    preteen, 556
    unplanned pregnancy, 554
Family planning. See Contraception
Family violence, 573-574
Farmer's lung, 153
Farsightedness (hyperopia), 67
Fasciitis, 236
Fats, dietary, 15-16
  fish oils, 17
  food label information, 23
  margarine vs. butter, 17
Fecal impaction, 173, 174
Fecal incontinence, 435
Fecal occult blood test, 8, 635
Feeding. See also Breast feeding
  infants and children, 359, 360
    self-care flowchart, 484
  newborns, 338-339
Female reproductive system. See Reproductive system
Fetal alcohol syndrome, 342
Fetal monitoring, 635-636
Fever
  care of, 297
  medicines for reducing, 616
  self-care flowchart, 469-471
    for infants and children, 472-473
  serious effects of, 297
  symptoms of, 296
  temperature measurement in, 296-297
Fiber, dietary, 16-17
  foods high in fiber, 18
Fibrillation
  atrial, 119
  defibrillation and cardioversion for, 119
  definition of, 118
  ventricular, 119
Fibrocystic breast disease, 412-413
Fibroids, uterine, 419-420
Fibromyalgia, 236
Fibrosis, idiopathic pulmonary, 149
Fifth disease, 325
Fine needle biopsy, 636
Fingernail disorders. See Nail disorders
First aid and emergencies, 592-612
  abrasions, 603
  amputation, 597-598

ankle sprains, 611
assessment of, 593
bites and stings, 598-599
bleeding, 599
blisters, 603
burns, 599-601
calling for help, 592-594
cardiopulmonary resuscitation (CPR), 596-597
choking, 601-602
compression points in, 600
cuts, 602-603
drowning, 603-604
electrical shock, 604
eye injury, 604-605
fainting, 605
falls, 605
fish hook injury, 605-606
frostbite, 606-607
head injury, 607
heart attack, 607-608
heat cramps, heat exhaustion and heat stroke, 608
hypothermia, 607
lacerations, 602-603
Medic Alert system, 592
medicine cabinet supplies, 613
mouth-to-mouth resuscitation, 594-596
nosebleed, 609
poisoning, 609
rape, 609-610
seizures, 610
serious emergencies, 593
shock prevention, 597
spinal injuries, 605
splinters, 610-611
sprains or torn ligaments, 611-612
tooth loss, 612
toxic inhalation, 612
when to call the doctor, 592-594
Fish hook injury, first aid for, 605-606
Fissures, anal, 171, 367
Flat feet, 259
Flea infestations, 311
Flu. See Influenza
Fluoride, 20
Fluoroquinolones, 624
Folic acid (folacin)
  actions and sources of, 19
  deficiency of, anemia caused by, 135
Folliculitis, 280
Food groups. See also Nutrition
  basic four groups, 22-23
  diet-component-by-percentage, 21
  Eating Right Pyramid, 21-22

servings from food groups, 21
Food poisoning, 300
Foods. See also Feeding
  allergies to, 222-223
    migraine headache triggered by, 51-52
  safe handling precautions, 30
Foot
  anatomy of, 255
  disorders of
    athlete's foot, 256, 271
    bunions, 256-257
    club foot, 263, 347-348
    corns and calluses, 258-259
    deformed toes, 259
    flat feet, 259
    heel spur, 260
    Morton's neuroma, 260-261
    nail problems, 261-263
    pigeon toes, 263
    plantar fasciitis, 263-264
    self-care flowchart, 533-534
    ulcer, 264
Forceps delivery, 403
Foreign objects
  ear, 82
  eye, 68, 71
  nose, 89
Fractures, 236-238
Friedreich's ataxia, 50
Frostbite, first aid for, 606-607
Fungal infections, 308-310. See also specific types
Galactorrhea, 413-414
Gallbladder
  anatomy of, 201
  cancer of, 203
Gallstones, 203-204
Gambling, 565
Ganglion cyst, 259
Gangrene, 300-301
Gas, intestinal, 185-186
Gastroenteritis, 186-187
Gastrointestinal disorders, 170-200
  amebiasis, 310-311
  anal abscess, 170-171
  anal fissure, 171, 367
  anal itching, 171, 363-364
  appendicitis, 171-173, 371
  bowel blockage, 173-174
  carcinoid tumors, 174
  colon polyps, 174-175
  colorectal cancer, 175-177
  constipation, 177-178, 364-365, 393
  Crohn's disease, 178-179
  dehydration, 179-180, 366
  diarrhea, 181-183, 365-366
  diverticulosis and diverticulitis, 183-184

esophageal cancer, 184-185
esophageal varices, 185
food poisoning, 300
gas, 185-186
gastroenteritis, 186-187
giardiasis, 181, 311
heartburn, 187-189
hemorrhoids, 189-190, 367, 393
hernias, 190-192, 352-353
ileus, 173-174, 192-193
irritable bowel syndrome, 193-194
malabsorption, 194-195
peritonitis, 195
proctitis, 195-196
stomach cancer, 196-197
ulcerative colitis, 198-199
ulcers, 197-198
vomiting, 199-200, 365-366
Gastrointestinal system, anatomy of, 169-170
Gastroscopy, 636
Gehrig's disease (amyotrophic lateral sclerosis), 44
Genetic abnormalities. See Birth defects
Genital herpes, 318
Genital warts, 318
Genitalia
  abnormalities of, 346
  female, 373-374, 380-382
  male, 373, 374, 423, 424
  self-care flowcharts, 520-526
German measles (rubella), 330-331
Giardiasis, 181, 311
Gingivitis, 96, 267
Glands, 207-208
Glandular disorders. See Hormonal and glandular disorders
Glasses, for eye focusing problems, 68
Glaucoma, 68-69
  acute, 69
  chronic, 69
  congenital, 69
  medicines for, 624
  tests for, 636
Glomerulonephritis, 161-162
  rheumatic fever and, 304
Glossitis (inflammation of tongue), 98, 99
Glucose, monitoring at home, 213
Glucose tolerance test, 636
  in pregnancy, 392
Goiter, multinodular, 215
Gonorrhea, 318-319
Goodpasture's syndrome, 149, 150

Gout, 238

Graft-versus-host disease, 139

Grave's disease, 215

Grief, 568-569
  in the elderly, 434
  phases of, 568-569

Group therapy, 559

Growth and development of children, 359-360

Growth retardation, intrauterine, 394-395

Guillain-Barré syndrome, 50-51

Guilt feelings, 569-570

Gum infections, 96

Gumboil, 96

Guns, safety precautions for, 30

Gynecomastia, 377

Haemophilus bacteria, 301

*Haemophilus influenzae* type b vaccination, 12

Hair
  excessive growth of (hirsutism), 282
  ingrown, 283-284

Hair loss, 280-282
  alopecia areata, 280-281
  male-pattern baldness, 281
  self-care flowchart, 466
  thinning hair, 281

Halitosis (bad breath), 92

Hallucinogens, 563-564

Hammer toe, 259

Hand, anatomy of, 255

Hand and wrist disorders
  carpal tunnel syndrome, 257-258
  ganglion, 259
  nail problems, 261-263
  self-care flowchart, 504

Hansen's disease, 301

Hardening of the arteries. *See* Atherosclerosis

Hashimoto's thyroiditis, 217

Head injuries
  concussions and contusions, 50
  first aid for, 607
  prevention of, 50
  seizures caused by, 58

Headaches, 51-53
  cluster, 51
  medicines for, 624
  migraine, 51-52
  muscle tension, 52
  self-care flowchart, 467-468
  sinus, 52
  when to consult doctor, 53

Health exams, 6-10
  cancer screening, 9
  personal record of, 10
  schedule, childhood to adult, 6
  self-screening at home, 9

types of tests performed, 7-8, 627-644

Hearing aids, 79

Hearing loss, 77-79
  deafness, 78
  eardrum rupture in, 78
  eustachian tube blockage in, 77
  noise-induced, 77-78
  otosclerosis in, 78
  presbycusis in, 78
  self-care flowchart, 479
  testing for, 8, 628, 641, 643

Heart. *See also* Ventricles
  anatomy of, 35
  blood circulation and, 107-108
  bypass surgery, 112
  rhythm problems of, 118-120
    atrial fibrillation, 119
    atrioventricular block, 119
    premature heartbeats, 119
    tachycardia, 118-119
    ventricular fibrillation, 119
  transplantation of, 114

Heart attack, 115-118
  arterial blockage in, 116
  complications of, 117
  first aid for, 607-608
  outlook after, 117
  prevention of, 117-118
  risk factors for, 117
  silent, 116
  stress and, 572

Heart defects, 349-352
  aortic valve stenosis, 350
  atrial septal defect, 350
  coarctation of the aorta, 350
  Fallot's tetralogy, 350-351
  patent ductus arteriosus, 351, 352
  pulmonic valve stenosis, 351, 352
  transposition of great vessels, 351, 352
  ventricular septal defect (VSD), 351-352

Heart diseases. *See also* Cardiovascular diseases
  cardiomyopathy, 113-114
  congestive heart failure, 114-115
  endocarditis, 115
  heart attack, 115-118
  pericarditis, 125-126
  risk factors for, 15
  valve diseases, 120-123
  wine and, 112

Heart rate
  measuring, 107
  target heart rate for exercise, 5-6

Heart valves
  aortic, 121, 122
  blood flow through, 120-121
  disorders of, 120-123
    endocarditis and, 115
  mitral, 121-122
  normal, stenotic, and incompetent, 122
  pulmonary, 121
  stenosis of
    aortic, 350
    pulmonic, 351, 352
  tricuspid, 121

Heartburn, 187-189

Heat cramps, 608

Heat exhaustion, 608

Heat stroke, 608-609

Heel spur, 260

Heimlich maneuver, 601-602

Hemangioma (birthmark), 275-276

Hemodialysis, for kidney failure, 164

Hemolytic anemia, 133

Hemophilia, 136

Hemorrhage
  antepartum, 392
  of brain, 45-47
  in esophageal varices, 185
  first aid for, 599
  postpartum, 403
  subconjunctival, 74-75, 266

Hemorrhoids, 189-190
  in infants and children, 367
  medications for, 616
  in pregnancy, 393

Hepatitis B vaccine
  adults, 13
  children, 12

Hernias, 190-192
  abdominal wall, 190
  diaphragmatic, 353
  hiatal, 188, 191
  inguinal, 191-192
  in newborns, 352-353
  umbilical, 352-353

Herniated disk, 238-239

Heroin, 564

Herpes simplex virus infections
  cold sores, 94-95, 266
  genital herpes, 318
  types of, 325

Herpes zoster virus infection (shingles), 272, 331-332

Hiatal hernia, 188, 191

Hiccups, 192

High blood pressure. *See* Hypertension

Hip disorders
  in children, 239-240
  congenital dislocation, 240

self-care flowchart, 527

Hirschsprung's disease, 353

Hirsutism, 282

Histoplasmosis, 309

Histrionic personality, 589

HIV infection, 325-326
  risk factors for, 325
  testing for, 326
  transmission of, 319, 325-326

Hives, 268, 282-283

HMG-CoA reductase inhibitors, 624

Hodgkin's lymphoma, 139

Holter monitor, 634

Hookworm infestation, 315

Hormonal and glandular disorders
  acromegaly, 208-209
  Addison's disease, 209-210
  aldosteronism, 210
  Cushing's syndrome, 210
  diabetes, 211-214
  hyperparathyroidism, 214-215
  hyperthyroidism, 215
  hypoglycemia, 216
  hypoparathyroidism, 216-217
  hypothyroidism, 217
  pancreatic cancer, 217-218
  pancreatitis, 218-219
  pituitary dwarfism, 219
  thyroid cancers, 219

Hormonal changes, in puberty, 373

Hormone implants and shots, for birth control, 551-552

Human immunodeficiency virus (HIV) infection. *See* HIV infection

Huntington's chorea, 53

Hyaline membrane disease, 344

Hydatidiform mole, 397

Hydrocele, 367, 430-431

Hydrocephalus, 353

Hydrocortisone creams and ointments, 616-617

Hymen, 382

Hyperactivity, 367

Hyperglycemia, 211

Hyperparathyroidism, 214-215

Hypertension, 123-124. *See also* Blood pressure
  essential, 123
  guidelines for reducing, 124
  malignant, 124
  secondary, 123-124
  stroke caused by, 60
  systolic and diastolic, 123

Hyperthyroidism, 215

Hypertrophic cardiomyopathy, 113

Hyperventilation, 148-149

Hyphema, 69-70
Hypochondriasis, 590
Hypoglycemia, 216
  in newborns, 344
Hypoparathyroidism, 216-217
Hypospadias, 346
Hypotension, 124-125. *See also* Blood pressure
  orthostatic, 125
Hypothermia, first aid for, 607
Hypothyroidism, 217
Hysterectomy, 418
Hysterosalpingogram, 636
Hysteroscopy, 636
Ibuprofen, 617
Ice packs, for sprains, 611
Idiopathic pulmonary fibrosis, 149
Ileus (intestinal obstruction), 173-174, 192-193
Immune system, 220-226
  allergies and, 221-224
  cancer and, 224-226
  cell types in, 220-221
  functions of, 220
Immunizations, 11-13
  adult, 13
  childhood, 11-12, 363
  how vaccines work, 221
  travel, 13
  who should get flu shots, 13
Immunodeficiency disorders, 221. *See also* HIV Infection
Immunosuppressants, 624
Imperforate anus, 354
Impetigo, 268, 283
Impotence, 423-424
Incontinence, 434-435
Infants and children, 357-363.
    *See also* Newborns
  allowances for, 360
  appetite loss in, 360
  books on child care, 358
  car seats for, 29, 335-336
  choking of, 601-602
  chores for, 360
  disciplining, 358-359
  disorders of, 363-372
    anal itching, 363-364
    attention deficit disorder (ADD), 369
    autism, 369
    bedwetting, 364
    breathing trouble, 364
    constipation, 364-365
    cradle cap, 365
    crossed eyes, 365
    diaper rash, 365
    diarrhea and vomiting, 365-366
    dyslexia, 369

encopresis, 366-367
epilepsy, 371
febrile seizures, 371
hemorrhoids and anal fissures, 367
hydrocele, 367
hyperactivity, 367
infantile spasms, 371
infections, 367-368
Kawasaki syndrome, 368
lead poisoning, 368-369
learning disorders, 369-370
mental retardation, 369-370
rashes, 370
Reye's syndrome, 370
seizures, 370-371
stomach pain, 371
sudden infant death syndrome, 372
  emotional dos and don'ts of parenting, 357
  feeding changes and, 359
  growth and development of, 359-360
  health exam schedule for, 6
  home safety precautions for, 29-30
  immunizations for, 11-12, 363
  naps for, 362
  night terrors of, 362
  nightmares of, 362
  reading to, 360-361
  self-esteem of, 361
  separate room or bed for, 362
  separation anxiety of, 361
  sex education for, 554-556
  sleeping and bedtime of, 361-362
  sleepwalking of, 362
  television viewing by, 361
  temper tantrums of, 359
  toilet training of, 362-363
  toys for, 361
Infections. *See also* specific types
  bacterial, 298-308
  fungal, 308-310
  in infants and children, 367-368
  parasitic, 310-316
  sexually transmitted, 316-320
  viral, 320-332
  warning signs of, 297
Infectious arthritis, 229
Infertility, 546-549
  female problems in, 548-549
  male problems in, 547
Influenza, 326-327
  amantadine for preventing, 13, 156
  causes and treatment of, 326-327

*Haemophilus influenzae* type b vaccination, 12
  immunization for, 13, 156
  self-care flowchart, 490
Ingrown hair, 283-284
Ingrown toenail, 262
Inguinal hernia, 191-192
Insect bites and stings, first aid for, 598, 599
Insomnia, 28
Insulin
  deficiency of, in diabetes, 211
  for treatment of diabetes, 624
Interstitial lung disease, 149-150
  Goodpasture's syndrome, 149, 150
  idiopathic pulmonary fibrosis, 149
  pulmonary alveolar proteinosis, 149
  sarcoidosis, 150
Intestines. *See also* Gastrointestinal disorders
  anatomy of, 169-170
  atresia of, 354
  obstruction of (ileus), 173-174, 192-193
  symptoms of serious problems in, 178
Intrauterine device (IUD), 552
Intravenous pyelogram (IVP), 636-637
Intussusception, 173, 174, 371
Iodine, 20
Ipecac, syrup of, 617
Iridectomy, for glaucoma, 69
Iritis, 70
Iron, dietary
  actions and sources of, 20
  overdose of, 135
  prevention of anemia with, 135
Iron-deficiency anemia, 133-134, 135
Irritable bowel syndrome, 193-194
Itching, relief for, 279, 283
IUD (intrauterine device), 552
IVP (intravenous pyelogram), 636-637
Jaundice
  causes of, 205
  in newborns, 342-343
Jellyfish stings, first aid for, 598
Jock itch, 430
Joint disorders. *See* Musculoskeletal disorders
Joints, 227, 228
Juvenile rheumatoid arthritis, 229-230
Kaposi's sarcoma, 270, 290
Kawasaki syndrome, 368

Kegel's exercises, for bladder control, 168
Keloid, 269, 285
Keratoses
  actinic, 285
  seborrheic, 269, 286
Ketoacidosis, diabetic, 211
Kidney. *See also* Urinary system
  anatomy of, 158, 160
  disorders of
    cysts, 160-161
    glomerulonephritis, 161-162
    kidney failure in, 163-164
    nephrotic syndrome, 166-167
    pyelonephritis, 163
    stones, 165-166
  failure of, 163-165
    acute, 164
    chronic, 164
    end-stage, 164
    transplantation of, 164-165
Knee disorders, 240-242
  self-care flowcharts, 530-531
Labia, 381, 382
Labor and delivery, 398-403.
    *See also* Breast feeding
  anesthesia during, 400-401
  breech presentation in, 402
  Cesarean section in, 403
  episiotomy in, 401
  forceps delivery in, 403
  malpresentation in, 401-402
  monitoring during, 401
  postpartum care, 403-404
  postpartum hemorrhage in, 403
  premature labor, 402
  problems in, 401-403
  prolonged labor, 402-403
  retained placenta in, 403
  signs of labor, 398-399
  stages of labor, 399-400
  transverse or sideways presentation in, 402
  vacuum extraction delivery, 403
Labyrinthitis, 83
Lacerations, first aid for, 602-603
Lactase, 617
Lactose intolerance, 194
Laparoscopy, 637
Laryngitis, 103
Laryngoscopy, 637
Larynx (voice box)
  anatomy of, 102
  polyps of, 105-106
  tumors of, 105
Laxatives, 617
Lead poisoning, 7, 368-369
Learning disorders, 369-370

Leg problems, self-care flow-
    chart for, 528-529
Legg-Calvé-Perthes disease, 240
Leprosy, 301
Leukemia, 138-139
    lymphocytic
        acute, 138
        chronic, 138
    myelogenous
        acute, 138
        chronic, 138-139
Lice infestation, 311-312
Lichen planus, 97, 266, 268, 284
Ligaments, 227
    torn, first aid for, 611-612
Light sensitivity (photophobia),
    70
Lipoma, 285
Listeria bacteria, 301
Lithotripsy, for kidney stones,
    166
Liver
    abscess of, 206
    anatomy and function of, 201
    cancer of, 206
    cirrhosis of, 201-203
    function tests of, 637
    hepatitis of, 204-206
Loneliness, 570-571
Losing weight. See Weight
    maintenance
Lou Gehrig's disease (amy-
    otrophic lateral sclerosis), 44
Low blood pressure. See
    Hypotension
Low birth weight infants, 343
Lower back pain, self-care
    flowchart for, 512-513
Lower GI series (barium
    enema), 628-629
Lumbar puncture, 641-642
Lung
    anatomy of, 141
    cancer of, 151-152
        adenocarcinoma, 151
        large-cell carcinoma, 151
        mesothelioma, 152
        small-cell carcinoma, 151
        squamous-cell carcinoma,
            151
    disorders of, 142-157
        abscess, 150-151
        asthma, 142-145
        bronchitis, 145-146
        cancer, 151-152
        collapsed lung, 146-147
        cystic fibrosis, 348-349
        emphysema, 147-148
        fungal infections, 309-310
        hyperventilation, 148-149
        interstitial lung disease,

    149-150
    occupational, 152-153
    pleurisy, 153-154
    pneumonia, 154-156
    pulmonary edema, 114, 156-
        157
    pulmonary embolism, 130,
        157
Lyme disease, 272, 301-302
Lymph nodes
    biopsy of, 637
    cancer of, 9, 140
    functions of, 220
    swelling of, 226
Lymph system, 220
Lymphocytes, 220-221
Lymphoma, 139-140
    Hodgkin's, 139
    non-Hodgkin's, 139-140
Macrolide antibiotics, 624
Macular degeneration, 73
Magnesium, 20
Magnetic resonance imaging
    (MRI), 637-638
Malabsorption, 194-195
Malaria, 312-313
Male reproductive system. See
    Reproductive system
Malignant melanoma, 270, 290-
    291
    retinal, 75
Malocclusion (crowded and
    misaligned teeth), 95
Mammography, 8, 409, 638
Manganese, 20
Marijuana, 564
Mastectomy, 410-411
Mastitis, 411-412
Mastoiditis, 81
Measles, 272, 327-328
Measles, mumps, rubella
    (MMR) vaccine, 11-12
Medic Alert system for emer-
    gencies, 592
Medicine cabinet, supplies for,
    613
Medicines. See Drugs
Melanoma. See Malignant
    melanoma
Melasma, 269, 286-287
Memory problems, 53-54, 436
Meniere's disease, 83-84
Meningitis, 302-303
Menopause, 407-408
    bleeding after, 407
    hormone replacement therapy
        in, 407-408
    symptoms of, 407
Menstruation, 382-384
    absence of (amenorrhea), 382-
        383

    heavy bleeding in, 383
    infrequent (oligomenorrhea),
        383
    painful (dysmenorrhea), 383
    physiology of, 374, 382
    premenstrual syndrome
        (PMS) and, 383-384
    self-care flowchart, 523-524
Mental retardation, 369-370
Mesalamine, 624
Methadone, 624
Methamphetamine, 624
Methotrexate, 625
Methyltestosterone, 625
Middle ear
    fluid in, 81-82
    infection of (otitis media), 80-
        81
Migraine equivalents, 52
Migraine headaches, 51-52
Milia (baby acne), 269, 285
Minerals, 18-19. See also
        Vitamins
    actions and sources of specific
        minerals, 20
    food label information, 24
    megadoses of, 14, 18
    obtaining from healthy diet, 18
Minoxidil, 625
Miscarriage and stillbirth, 396-
    397
Mitral valve
    damage of, 122
    prolapse of, 121-122
    regurgitation in, 122
        atrial fibrillation in, 119
    scarring of, 121
Moles, 270, 287
    cancerous, 292
Molluscum contagiosum, 269,
    285
Molybdenum, 20
Mononucleosis, 328-329
Mood disorders, 586-588
Morton's neuroma, 260-261
Motion sickness, 54
Motion-sickness drugs
    (antivertigo), 617, 625
Mouth, 91-101. See also Tooth,
        disorders of
    anatomy of, 91-92
    cancer of
        health exam for, 8
        self-screening tests at home,
            9
    disorders of, 92-101
        canker sores, 92-93
        cold sores, 94-95
        gingivitis, 96
        gum infections, 96
        lichen planus, 97

    mucocele, 97
    salivary gland infection,
        swelling or blockages, 97
    self-care flowchart, 480-482
    thrush, 97-98
    tongue abnormalities, 98-99
    tumors, 100
Mouth-to-mouth resuscitation,
    594-596. See also Cardio-
    pulmonary resuscitation
    (CPR)
    adults, 594-595
    infants, 595-596
MRI (magnetic resonance
    imaging), 637-638
Mucocele, 97
Mucocutaneous lymph node
    syndrome, 368
Multiple sclerosis, 54-55
Mumps, 272, 329
    MMR vaccine for, 11-12
Muscle relaxants, 625
Muscle tension headaches, 52
Muscles, types of, 228
Muscular dystrophy, 354
Muscular system, atlas of, 40
Musculoskeletal disorders
    arthritis, 229-232
    back pain, 232-233
    bursitis, 233-234
    compression fracture of
        spine, 234-235
    connective tissue disorders,
        232-233
    dislocated joint, 235
    fasciitis, 236
    fibromyalgia, 236
    fractures, 236-238
    gout, 238
    herniated disk, 238-239
    hip problems in children,
        239-240
    knee problems, 240-242
    muscle cramps, pulls,
        spasms and tears, 242-243
    neck pain, 243-244
    osteomalacia, 244
    steomyelitis, 244
    osteoporosis, 7, 244-246
    Paget's disease, 246
    polymyalgia rheumatica, 246
    polymyositis, 246-247
    sciatica, 49, 247-248
    scleroderma, 248
    scoliosis, 248-249
    self-care flowcharts, 528-534
    shin splints, 250
    shoulder problems, 249-250
    Sjögren's syndrome, 250
    spondylosis and spondylolis-
        thesis, 250-251

Musculoskeletal disorders (continued)
sprains, 251
systemic lupus erythematosus, 252
temporomandibular joint (TMJ) disease, 252-253
tendinitis, 253-254
tennis elbow, 253
tumors of bone, 254
whiplash, 254
Myelogram, 638
Myeloma, multiple, 137
Myocardial infarction. *See* Heart attack
Myringotomy, for middle ear fluid, 82
Nail disorders, 261-263
artificial nail complications, 261
deformities, 261
discoloration, 261
hangnails, 261-262
infection, 262
ingrown toenail, 262
injuries, 262-263
Naproxen, 617
Narcissistic personality, 589
Narcotics, 618, 625
abuse of, 565
Nasal polyps, 87-88
Nasal sprays, 616
overuse of, 87
Nasolaryngoscopy, 638
Nausea and vomiting
in pregnancy, 395-396
self-care flowchart, 509-511
Nearsightedness (myopia), 67
Neck pain, 243-244
self-care flowchart, 485
Neck swelling, self-care flowchart for, 486
Neonates. *See* Newborns
Nephrotic syndrome, 166-167
Nerve conduction studies, 638-639
Nervous system. *See also* Brain; Neurologic disorders
atlas of, 33
autonomic nerves, 43
central nervous system, 42
cerebrospinal fluid, 44
cranial nerves, 43
peripheral nervous system, 42
spinal nerves, 43
Neuralgia, trigeminal, 61
Neurologic disorders
amyotrophic lateral sclerosis (Lou Gehrig's disease), 44
aphasia, 44-45
Bell's palsy, 45

coma, 48
compressed nerve (entrapment syndrome), 48-49
concussions and contusions, 50
Friedreich's ataxia, 50
Guillain-Barré syndrome, 50-51
headaches, 51-53
Huntington's chorea, 53
memory problems, 53-54
motion sickness, 54
multiple sclerosis, 54-55
neuropathy, 55-56
Parkinson's disease, 56
seizures, 56-58
stroke, 59-60
Tourette syndrome, 61
trigeminal neuralgia, 61
Neurons, 43-44
axons, 43
dendrites, 43
neurotransmitters, 44
synapses, 44
Neuropathy, 55-56
Newborns, 334-341. *See also* Birth defects; Infants and children
bathing of, 334-335
birthmarks of, 275-276, 341
bottle feeding (formula) of, 339
breast feeding of, 338-339
burping of, 339
car seats for, 335-336
circumcision care in, 336
clothing for, 336-337
crib safety and, 337-338
crying of, 338
diaper selection and care, 338
disorders of, 341-345
anemia, 343
apnea, 343
asphyxia, 344
colic, 341-342
drug withdrawal, 342
failure to thrive, 342
fetal alcohol syndrome, 342
hypoglycemia, 344
jaundice, 342-343
low birth weight, 343
pneumonia, 344
postmaturity, 343
prematurity, 343
respiratory distress syndrome, 344
retinopathy of prematurity, 344-345
Rh factor incompatibility, 345
sepsis, 345
feeding of, 338-339
sleeping of, 339

spitting up, 339
swaddling of, 339-340
Night blindness, 70
Noise-induced hearing loss, 77-78
Non-Hodgkin's lymphoma, 139-140
Non-steroidal anti-inflammatory drugs (NSAIDs). *See also* Anti-inflammatory drugs
Reye's syndrome and, 617
uses and examples, 617, 625
Nose, 86-90
anatomy of, 86-87
broken, 87
deviated septum in, 87
foreign objects in, 89
polyps of, 87-88
runny nose and congestion, 90
vasomotor rhinitis of, 89-90
Nosebleed, 88-89
first aid for, 609
treatment and prevention of, 88
NSAIDs. *See* Non-steroidal anti-inflammatory drugs (NSAIDs)
Nuclear medicine tests, 639
bone scan, 630
thyroid scan, 642
Nutrition, 13-27. *See also* Weight maintenance
basics of, 14-20
caffeine in, 14
carbohydrates in, 14
cholesterol in, 14-15
condiments and, 23
diet-component-by-percentage, 21
Eating Right Pyramid, 21-22
fats in, 15-16
fiber in, 16-17, 18
food labels, reading, 23-24
four basic food groups, 22-23
healthy eating habits, 20-23
rules for, 23
in pregnancy, 387
professional help for, 24
protein in, 17
salt in, 17
servings from food groups, 21
vitamins and minerals in, 18-19
water in, 20
Obesity, 24, 586. *See also* Weight maintenance
Obsessive-compulsive disorder, 581
Obstetricians, 387
Occult blood test, fecal, 8, 635
Occupational health and safety, 30-31

Occupational lung disorders, 152-153
anthracosis, 152
asbestosis, 152
asthma, 153
byssinosis, 153
farmer's lung, 153
silicosis, 153
silo-filler's lung, 153
Olfactory bulb, 86, 87, 92
Oligomenorrhea, 383
Ophthalmologists vs. optometrists, 67
Ophthalmoscopy, 639
Opiate abuse, 565
Optic nerve, 63
Oral cancer
health exam for, 8
self-screening tests at home, 9
Oral lichen planus, 266
Oral poliovirus vaccine (OPV), 11
Oral rehydration therapy, 617
Orbit
black eye related to, 63
periorbital cellulitis of, 70-71
Orgasm
female, 384
male, 424-425
Osgood-Schlatter disease, 241, 242
Osteoarthritis, 230-231
Osteomalacia, 244
Osteomyelitis, 244
Osteoporosis, 7, 244-246
Otitis externa (swimmer's ear), 79-80
Otitis media, 80-82
Otosclerosis, 78
Otoscopy, 639
Ovaries, 416-417
anatomy and function of, 374, 381
cancer of, 416
cysts of, 417
Overeating, 586
Ovulation, 374
Oxygen therapy, in emphysema, 148
Pacemakers, 119
Paget's disease, 246
Pancreas
cancer of, 217-218
hormones produced by, 208
Pancreatitis, 218-219
Panic disorder, 581
Pap smear, 8, 639
Papillomas, of eyelids, 66, 266
Paranoid personality, 589
Parasitic infections, 310-316. *See also* specific types

Parathyroid glands, 208
Parenting. *See also* Family and
    relationship issues; Infants
    and children
  books on child care, 358
  disciplining children, 358-359
  emotional dos and don'ts of
    parenting, 357
  factors for raising healthy
    kids, 358
Parkinson's disease, 56
  medications for, 625
Partial thromboplastin time
    (PTT), 639
Passive-aggressive personality,
    589-590
Patent ductus arteriosus, 351,
    352
Pelvic exam, 416, 639-640
Pelvic inflammatory disease, 417
Pelvimetry, 640
Penicillins, 625
Penis, 426-427
  balanitis of, 426
  cancer of, 426-427
  circumcision of, 336
  curvature of (Peyronie's dis-
    ease), 427
  priapism of, 427
Pentoxifylline, 625
  for atherosclerosis, 112
Pericarditis, 125-126
Period. *See* Menstruation
Periodic health exams. *See*
    Health exams
Periodontitis, 96, 267
Periorbital cellulitis, 70-71
Peripheral nervous system. *See*
    Nervous system
Peritoneal dialysis, for kidney
    failure, 164
Peritonitis, 195
Peritonsillar abscess (quinsy),
    105
Pernicious anemia, 135, 194-195
Personality disorders, 588-590
Pertussis, 303
  immunization against, 11
PET (positron emission tomog-
    raphy), 640
Petroleum jelly, 617
Peyronie's disease, 427
Phagocytes, 221
Pharyngitis (sore throat), 103-
    104
Phenylketonuria, 354
Phlebitis, superficial, 129
Phobias, 581-582
Phosphorus, 20
Photophobia (light sensitivity),
    70

Physical examination. *See*
    Health exams
Pigeon toes, 263
Pimozide, 625
Pimples, 274-275
Pink eye, 71-72, 266
Pinworm infestation, 315-316
  anal itching from, 171
Pituitary dwarfism, 219
Pituitary gland, 43, 208
Pityriasis rosea, 269, 287
Placenta, retained, 403
Placenta previa, 397
Plantar fasciitis, 263-264
Plantar warts, 272
Plaque, atherosclerotic, 110-111
Plasma, definition of, 131
Plasma cells, 137
Platelets, 131
Pleura, 142, 153, 154
Pleurisy, 153-154
PMS (premenstrual syndrome),
    383-384
Pneumococcal bacteria, 303
Pneumococcal vaccine, 13, 156
Pneumonia, 154-156
  atypical ("walking"), 155
  bacterial, 155
  in newborns, 344
  pneumocystis, 155
  viral, 155-156
Pneumothorax, 146-147
Poison oak, poison ivy or poi-
    son sumac, 268, 277
Poisoning
  first aid for, 609
  home safety precautions for, 30
Polio, 329-330
  immunization against, 11
Polycythemia, 137
Polyhydramnios, 397
Polymyalgia rheumatica, 246
polymyositis, 246-247
Polyposis, familial,
    colonoscopy for, 7
Polyps
  adenomatous, colonoscopy
    for, 7
  colonic, 174-175
  nasal, 87-88
  of vocal cord, 105-106
Portuguese man-of-war stings,
    first aid for, 598
Port-wine stain, 267, 275
Positron emission tomography
    (PET), 640
Post-concussion syndrome, 50
Postmaturity, fetal, 397
Postpartum period, 403-404.
    *See also* Breast feeding
  depression during, 404

lochia in, 403-404
Post-traumatic stress disorder,
    582
Potassium, 20
Pregnancy, 386-398. *See also*
    Labor and delivery;
    Postpartum period
  adolescent, 377-378
  conception and, 544-546
  delaying, 549-550
  disorders of, 391-398. *See also*
    Birth defects
    abruptio placentae, 391
    anemia, 391-392
    antepartum hemorrhage, 392
    backache, 392-393
    constipation and hemor-
      rhoids, 393
    diabetes, 393
    ectopic pregnancy, 393-394
    genetic defects, 394
    growth retardation, 394-395
    miscarriage and stillbirth,
      396-397
    nausea and vomiting
      (morning sickness), 395-396
    placenta previa, 397
    polyhydramnios, 397
    postmaturity, 397
    premature membrane rup-
      ture, 397
    Rh-factor incompatibility,
      397-398
    swelling, 398
    trophoblastic tumors, 398
  first trimester of, 389
  genetic counseling in, 388
  genital herpes in, 318
  home test for, 636
  Lyme disease in, 302
  medical tests in, 392
  planning for, 542-544
  prenatal care in, 378, 387-388
  preventing. *See* Contraception
  rubella in, 331
  second trimester of, 389-390
  stages of, 388-391
  test for, 387
  things to avoid, 388
  third trimester of, 390-391
  toxoplasmosis in, 314, 388
  unplanned, 554
Premature ejaculation, 425
Premature heartbeats, 120
Premature infants, 343
Premature membrane rupture,
    396
Premenstrual syndrome (PMS),
    383-384
Prenatal vitamin supplements,
    625

Presbycusis, 78
Presbyopia, 67
Priapism, 427
Prickly heat, 287-288
Proctitis, 195-196
Proctoscopy, 640
Progestins, 625-626
Prostate gland, 427-429
  benign hypertrophy of, 427-
    428
  cancer of, 428-429
  transurethral resection of, 428
Prostate-specific antigen (PSA),
    640
Prostatitis, 429
Protein, dietary, 17, 24
Pruritus ani, 171, 363-364
Psoriasis, 270, 288
Psychiatric problems, 578-590.
    *See also* Emotional
    health/problems
  adolescent, 376-377
  anxiety disorders, 580-582
  depression, 376
  eating disorders, 376-377,
    582-586
  mood disorders, 586-588
  personality disorders, 588-590
  schizophrenia, 590
  somatoform disorders, 590
  suicide, 588
  treatment of, 579-580
Psychoanalysis, 559
Puberty
  delayed, 374-375
  female, 373-374
  male, 373, 374
  precocious, 374
Pulls, of muscle, 242-243
Pulmonary alveolar pro-
    teinosis, 149
Pulmonary disorders. *See* Lung,
    disorders of
Pulmonary edema, 156-157
  in congestive heart failure, 114
Pulmonary embolism, 157
  in venous thrombosis, 130
Pulmonary fibrosis, idiopathic,
    149
Pulmonary function test
    (spirometry), 640
Pulmonic valve
  blood flow through, 121
  stenosis of, 351, 352
Pulse, 107
Pupils, dilation of, 633
Purpura, 288-289
Pyelogram
  intravenous (IVP), 636-637
  retrograde, 640
Pyelonephritis, 163

Pyloric stenosis, 354-355
Quinsy (peritonsillar abscess), 105
Rabies, 330
Radial keratotomy, 68
Radon, 151
Rape, first aid for, 609-610
Rapid antibody strep test, 642
Rash. See Dermatitis
Raynaud's phenomenon (disease), 126-127
Rebelliousness, in adolescents, 378
Rectal examination, digital, 633
Red blood cells, 131
Reflux esophagitis, 187-188
Refraction, 640
Reiter's syndrome, 231
Relaxation training, 572
Renal cell cancer, 159
Renal system. See Kidney; Urinary system
Repetitive stress injury. See Entrapment syndromes
Reproductive system. See also specific anatomic parts
  female. See also Pregnancy
    anatomy and functions of, 380-382
    atlas of, 37
    in puberty, 373-374
  male
    anatomy and functions of, 423, 424
    atlas of, 36
    in puberty, 373, 374
Respiratory distress syndrome, in newborns, 344
Respiratory tract diseases. See Lung, disorders of
Restless leg syndrome, insomnia and, 28
Retina
  anatomy of, 62-63
  degeneration of, 73
    diabetic retinopathy in, 73
    macular, 73
    retinitis pigmentosa in, 73
  detachment of, 74
  macula of, 63
  rod and cone cells of, 62
Retinal artery blockage, 72-73
Retinitis pigmentosa, 73
Retinoblastoma, 75
Retinopathy
  diabetic, 73
  of prematurity, 344-345
Retrograde pyelogram, 640
Reye's syndrome, 370
  aspirin causing, 323
Rh blood classification system,

131-132
Rh factor incompatibility, 132, 345, 397-398
Rheumatic fever, 304
Rheumatoid arthritis, 231-232
Rh factor compatibility test, 640
Rhinitis
  allergic, 222
  vasomotor, 89-90
Rhythm method, 552
R-I-C-E, for treatment of sprains, 243, 611
Rickets, 244
Ringing in ears (tinnitus), 84-85
Ringworm, 270, 289
Risk-taking, in adolescents, 378
Rocky Mountain spotted fever, 304-305
Root canal, 100
Rosacea, 271, 289
Roseola, 330
Rotator cuff injuries, 249-250
Rubella (German measles), 330-331
  blood testing for antibodies to, 7
  MMR vaccination for, 11-12
Runny nose, relief of, 90
Ruptured aneurysms, 108
Safe sex, 32
Safety, 28-31
  bicycle, 30
  car and vehicle, 29, 335-336
  child safety at home, 29-30
  crib safety, 337-338
  fall prevention, 30
  food handling, 30
  motorcycle, 30
  recreational activities, 30
  smoke detectors, 29
  workplace hazards, 30-31
Saliva, 92
Salivary glands, 92
  infections of, 97
Salmon patches (birthmarks), 276
Salmonella infection, 300
Salt, dietary, 17
Sarcoidosis, 150
Scabies, 313
Scarlet fever, 305-306
Schizoid personality, 590
Schizophrenia, 590
School problems, in adolescents, 378-379
Sciatica, 49, 247-248
Scleroderma, 248
Scoliosis, 248-249
Screening tests, 9. See also Health exams
Scrotum

hydrocele in, 367, 430-431
  spermatocele in, 431
  varicocele in, 432
Scurvy, 136
Sebaceous cysts, 285-286
Seborrhea, 289-290
  cradle cap as form of, 365
Seborrheic keratosis, 269, 286
Sedatives, 626
  barbiturates, 621
  benzodiazepines, 621
  chlorpromazine, 622
Seizures, 56-58
  epileptic, 56-57, 371
  febrile, 371
  first aid for, 610
  focal, 57
  grand mal, 57
  infantile spasms, 371
  in infants and children, 370-371
  Jacksonian, 57
  occasional, 56
  petit mal, 57
  temporal lobe, 57
Selenium, 20
Self-care flowcharts, 466-540
Self-esteem, 361, 571
Semen, 373, 423
Senses, atlas of, 34
Sepsis, in newborns, 345
Septal defect
  atrial, 350
  ventricular, 351-352
Septic shock, 298
Septum, deviated, 87
Serotonin, secretion by carcinoid tumors, 174
Serum, definition of, 131
Sex education
  adolescents, 556-558
  preschool children, 554-556
  preteens, 556
Sexual abuse
  of children, 574-577
  of spouse, 578
Sexual addiction, 565-566
Sexual behavior, in adolescents, 379
Sexual development. See Puberty
Sexual intercourse
  conception resulting from, 544-546
  painful
    female, 385-386
    male, 425
  physiology of, 544-545
  problems with
    female, 384-385
    male, 425-426

Sexually transmitted diseases (STDs)
  blood test for, 7
  chlamydia, 317-318
  genital herpes, 318
  genital warts, 318
  gonorrhea, 318-319
  preventing, 32, 317
  syphilis, 319
  trichomoniasis, 319-320
Sexually transmitted diseases (STDs), 316-320
Shigella infection, 300
Shin splints, 250
Shingles (herpes zoster infection), 272, 331-332
Shock, prevention of, 597
Shortness of breath, self-care flowchart for, 495-498
Shoulder disorders, 249-250
  self-care flowchart, 491-492
Sialogram, 640
Sickle-cell anemia, 134
Sickle-cell trait, 134
Sigmoidoscopy, 640
Silicosis, 153
Silo-filler's lung, 153
Sinus headaches, 52
Sinuses, anatomy of, 86-87
Sinusitis, 89
Sjögren's syndrome, 250
Skeletal disorders. See Musculoskeletal disorders
Skeleton, 39, 227
Skin
  anatomy of, 273
  biopsy of, 640-641
  changes of, in the elderly, 436-437
  functions of, 273
  patch tests of, 641
  tuberculin skin test of, 642-643
  wrinkles of, 293-294, 437
Skin cancer, 290-292
  basal-cell carcinoma, 270, 290
  in the elderly, 437
  Kaposi's sarcoma, 270, 290
  malignant melanoma, 270, 290-291
  screening for, 8, 9
  squamous-cell carcinoma, 270, 291-292
  warning signs, 292
Skin disorders
  acne, 268, 274-275, 375
  actinic keratoses, 285
  bedsores, 275
  birthmarks, 275-276
  boils and carbuncles, 268, 276
  cellulitis, 276-277
  dandruff, 277

Skin disorders (continued)
dermatitis, 277-279
dry skin, 279-280
excessive sweating, 280
folliculitis, 280
hives, 268, 282-283
impetigo, 268, 283
keloid, 269, 285
lichen planus, 268, 284
lipoma, 285
lumps and bumps, 284-286
melasma, 269, 286-287
milia (baby acne), 269, 285
moles, 270, 287
molluscum contagiosum, 269, 285
pityriasis rosea, 269, 287
prickly heat, 287-288
psoriasis, 270, 288
purpura, 288-289
ringworm, 270, 289
rosacea, 271, 289
sebaceous cysts, 285-286
seborrhea, 289-290
seborrheic keratosis, 269, 286
self-care flowcharts, 535-540
skin tags, 269, 286
spider angioma, 286
sunburn and tanning, 292-293
tinea versicolor, 271, 292-293
vitiligo, 271, 293
xanthelasma, 286
Sleep, 27-28
causes of insomnia, 28
in infants and children, 361-362
in newborns, 339
problems with, 27
stages of, 27
tips for getting to sleep, 27-28
Sleep aids, 617
Sleep apnea, 28
Sleepwalking, in infants and children, 362
Slipped capital femoral epiphysis, 240
Slipped disk, 238-239
Slit lamp test, 641
Smell, sense of, 86-87
Smoke inhalation injury, 612
Smoking
in adolescents, 375-376
signs of, 376
cessation, 31-32
after long-term smoking, 152
alternatives to smoking, 32
preparing to quit, 31
in emphysema, 147, 148
lung cancer and, 151, 152
Snake bites, first aid for, 598-599
Sodium
actions and sources of, 20

food label information, 24
restriction of, 17
Solvent abuse, 565
Somatization disorder, 590
Somatoform disorders, 590
Sore throat (pharyngitis), 103-104
Spasms, of muscle, 242-243
Spastic colon, 193-194
Speech audiometry, 641
Sperm, 373, 423
Spermatocele, 431
Spermicides, 552, 617
Spider angioma, 269, 286
Spider bites, first aid for, 599
Spina bifida, 355
Spinal cord
injuries of, 58
tumors of, 58-59
Spinal fluid, 44
Spinal tap (lumbar puncture), 641-642
Spine
compression fracture of, 234-235
injuries of, 605
Spirometry (pulmonary function test), 640
Splinters, first aid for, 610-611
Splints, for injured body parts, 605
Spondylosis and spondylolisthesis, 250-251
Sporotrichosis, 310
Spouse abuse, 578
Sprains, 251
first aid for, 611-612
Squamous cell carcinoma
of lung, 151
of skin, 270, 291-292
Staphylococcal infections, 305
food poisoning and, 300
STD. See Sexually transmitted diseases (STD)
Steroid drugs. See Corticosteroids
Steroid hormones, produced by adrenal glands, 207-208
Stillbirth, 396-397
Stoma, in colostomy, 176
Stomach
cancer of, 196-197
sudden and severe pain in, 371
ulcers of, 197-198
Stomach flu (gastroenteritis), 186-187
Strabismus, 65-66, 365
Strawberry hemangioma, 267, 275
Strep test, 642

Strep throat, 306
Streptococcal bacteria, 306
Stress, 571-573
dealing with, 572-573
heart attack and, 572
Stress test, 4, 635
Stroke, 59-60
Stye, 74, 266
Subconjunctival hemorrhage, 74-75, 266
Substance abuse, 561-565. See also Alcohol abuse
in adolescents, 375-376
goals of treatment for, 565
illegal drugs, 563-564
prescription drugs, 564-565
signs of, 376, 562
withdrawal from
in newborns, 342
Sudden infant death syndrome, 372
Suicide, 588
Sulfonamides, 626
Sulfonylureas, 626
Sulfur, 20
Sunburn, 292
Sweating, excessive, 280
Swelling, in pregnancy, 398
Swimmer's ear (otitis externa), 79-80
Syphilis, 319
Syrup of ipecac, 617
Systemic lupus erythematosus, 252
Tachycardia, 118-119
paroxysmal, 118
ventricular, 118
Tanning, dangers of, 293
Tapeworm infestation, 316
Tarsal tunnel syndrome, 49
Taste and taste buds, 92
Tears, of muscle, 242-243
Teenagers. See Adolescence
Teeth. See Tooth
Temperature, measurement of, 296-297
in adolescents and adults, 297
in infants and children, 296-297
Temporal arteritis, 127
Temporomandibular joint (TMJ) disease, 252-253
Tendinitis, 253-254
Tendons, 227
Tennis elbow, 253
Testicles
anatomy and function of, 373, 374
cancer of, 429-430
self-examination for, 9, 429
examination of, 8

severe pain in, 432
torsion of, 431-432
trauma to, 432
undescended, 355-356
Tests, 627-644. See also specific tests
Tetanus, 306-307
immunization against, 11, 13
Tetracyclines, 626
Tetralogy of Fallot, 350-351
Thalassemia, 134
Theophylline, 143-144, 626
Throat
anatomy of, 102-103
culture of, 642
disorders of, 103-106
laryngitis, 103
larynx tumors, 105
self-care flowchart, 487
sore throat, 103-104
thyroglossal duct cyst, 104
tonsillitis, 104-105
vocal cord polyps, 105-106
Thrombocytes, 131
Thrombocytopenia, 136
Thrombolytics, 117
Thrombophlebitis, superficial, 129
Thrombosis, venous, 129-130
Thrush (Candida albicans infection), 97-98, 266
Thyroid cancers, 219
Thyroid function test, 642
Thyroid function tests, 8
Thyroid glands, 208
Thyroid medicines, 626
Thyroid nodules, examination for, 8
Thyroid scan, 642
Thyroid storm, 215
Thyroiditis
Hashimoto's, 217
subacute, 217
Thyrotoxicosis, 215
TIAs (transient ischemic attacks), 60
Tick bites, 313-314
Tick paralysis, 314
Tick-borne diseases
Lyme disease, 272, 301-302
Rocky Mountain spotted fever, 304-305
Tinea cruris, 430
Tinea versicolor, 271, 292-293
Tinnitus (ringing in ears), 84-85
Tobacco smoking. See Smoking
Toenail disorders. See Nail disorders
Toes, deformed, 259
Toilet training, 362-363
Tongue abnormalities, 98-99

Tongue abnormalities (continued)
coated tongue, 98
discolored tongue, 98
geographic tongue, 98
hairy tongue, 98
inflammation (glossitis), 98-99
Tonsillectomy, 105
Tonsillitis, 104-105
Tooth, 91-92
anatomy of, 91-92
brushing of, 93, 94
disorders of
cavities, 93-94
crowded and misaligned teeth, 95
discolored teeth, 95
infections, 96
self-care flowchart, 483
wisdom-tooth problems, 101
flossing of, 94
loss of, 99-100
first aid for, 612
treatment of, 99-100
Tourette syndrome, 61
Toxic cardiomyopathy, 113
Toxic inhalation, first aid for, 612
Toxoplasmosis, 314
in pregnancy, 388
Tranquilizers. See Sedatives
Transient ischemic attacks (TIAs), 60
Transplantation
of bone marrow, 138, 139, 140
of heart, 114
of kidney, 164-165
Travel immunizations, 13
Trench mouth, 96
Trichinosis, 316
Trichomoniasis, 319-320
Tricuspid valve, 121
Trigeminal neuralgia, 61
Trophoblastic tumors, in pregnancy, 398
Tubal ligation, 553
Tuberculin skin test, 8, 642-643
Tuberculosis, 307-308
Tumors. See Cancer
Tuning fork test, 643
Tympanocentesis, 643
Tympanometry, 643
Tympanostomy tubes, for middle ear fluid, 82
Typhoid fever, 308
Ulcer medicines, 617, 626
Ulcerative colitis, 198-199
Ulcers
corneal, 65
decubitus, 275
of foot, 264
peptic, 197-198

venous stasis, 128
Ulnar nerve entrapment, 49
Ultrasound testing, 392, 643-644
Upper GI series (barium swallow), 629
Urethral infection, 320
Urinary incontinence, 434-435
Urinary system, 158-168. See also Kidney
anatomy of, 158, 159
cancer of, 159-160
disorders of, 159-168
bladder infections, 162-163
incontinence, 167-168
infections, 162-163
kidney stones, 165-166
self-care flowchart, 518-519
Urine culture, 644
Uterus, 417-420
anatomy and function of, 380-381
dilatation and curettage of, 420
endometrial cancer of, 417-418
endometriosis of, 418-419
fibroids of, 419-420
hysterectomy, 418
prolapse of, 420
Vaccinations. See Immunizations
Vacuum extraction delivery, 403
Vagina, 420-421
anatomy and function of, 381-382
bacterial vaginosis of, 421
chlamydia infection of, 421
douching and, 422
gonorrhea of, 421
lubricants for, 617
poor lubrication in, 385
self-care flowchart, 521-522
Vaginismus, 386
Vaginitis
preventing, 421
Trichomonas, 421
yeast, 421
Valves. See Heart valves
Varicella (chickenpox), 272, 321-322
vaccine for, 12
Varicocele, 432
Varicose veins, 127-129
esophageal, 185
spider-burst, 128
venous stasis ulcers in, 128
Vascular diseases. See Cardiovascular diseases
Vasectomy, 553
Vasodilators, 626
Vasomotor rhinitis, 89-90
Veins
circulatory role of, 107

valves of, 121
varicosities of, 127-129
Vena cava, 121
mesh filter for preventing embolism, 130, 157
Venous stasis ulcers, 128
Venous thrombosis, 129-130
deep vein, 129
pulmonary embolism in, 130
Ventricles
aneurysm of, 108-109
fibrillation of, 119
tachycardia of, 118
Vertigo
benign positional, 77
in Meniere's disease, 84
Viral infections, 104, 320-332. See also specific types
Vision. See Eye
Visual purple, 70
Vitamin-deficiency anemias, 134-135
Vitamins, 18-19. See also Minerals
A (retinal or beta carotene)
actions and sources of, 19
deficiency of, in night blindness, 70
toxicity of, 14
antioxidants, 19
$B_1$ (thiamine), 19
$B_2$ (riboflavin), 19
$B_3$ (niacin), 19
$B_5$ (pantothenic acid), 19
$B_6$ (pyridoxine), 19
$B_{12}$ (cobalamin), 19, 135
C (ascorbic acid), 19, 136
D (calciferol), 19
deficiencies of, bleeding disorders caused by, 136
E (tocopherol), 19
food label information, 24
K, 19, 136
megadoses of, 14, 18
obtaining from healthy diet, 18
supplements
healthy diet vs., 135
prenatal, 625
when to use, 18
Vitiligo, 271, 293
Vocal cords. See Larynx
Voice box (larynx), 102
Volvulus, 173, 174
Vomiting, 199-200
dehydration in, 180, 366
in infants and children, 365-366
in pregnancy, 395-396
self-care flowchart, 509-511
von Willebrand's disease, 136

Vulvar disorders, 422
Warts
genital, 318
medications for removing, 617
plantar, 272
viral, 272, 332
Water, daily requirement for, 20
Wax buildup in ear, 85
Weight loss, unexplained, 25
Weight maintenance, 24-27
causes of overweight, 25
losing weight, 25-27
quick-and-easy weight-loss claims, 26
tips for, 26
measurements of obesity, 24-25
overeating and, 586
smoking cessation and, 32
weight-height chart, 25
Wet dreams, 373, 379
Whiplash injury, 254
Whipple's disease, 195
White blood cells, 131
Whooping cough. See Pertussis
Wilms' tumor, 159
Wine, and heart disease, 112
Wisdom-tooth problems, 101
Worm infestations, 314-316
ascariasis, 314
hookworm, 315
pinworm, 315-316
tapeworms, 316
trichinosis, 316
Wrinkles, 293-294, 437
Wrist, anatomy of, 255
Wrist disorders. See Hand and wrist disorders
Xanthelasma, 66, 286
X-rays, 644
absorptiometry, 627
angiogram, 628
chest, 631
cholecystogram, oral, 639
computed tomographic (CT) scans, 632
dental, 633
hysterosalpingogram, 636
mammography, 638
myelogram, 638
retrograde pyelogram, 640
sialogram, 640
Zinc
actions and sources of, 20
interference with copper and iron absorption, 14

# Acknowledgments

The American Academy of Family Physicians and Word Publishing would like to thank
the following for their contributions to this work:

*Medical illustrators*
Vincent Perez
Alex Webber
Thomas D. Sims
Lisa Clark
Paul Gross

*Non-medical illustrators*
Kelly Kennedy
Douglas Schneider

*Commissioned photography*
Donald Fuller

*Design: Self-care flowcharts*
Steve Diggs & Friends

*Drug verifications*
Joyce Generali, MS, RPh

*Models*
Melissa Anderson, Nalia Bend, Cymphoni Borner, Jamil Borner, Payton Camp, Karen Camp
Gallini, Heather Hare, Jamie Hatley, Brianne Heinlein, Carleigh Heinlein, Trace Herchman,
Gabe Hogan, Jordan Hogan, Nelson Keener, Rebekah Lance, Brenda Lott, Charla McCampbell,
David Moberg, Kathy Moberg, Patrick Moberg, Peter Nikolai, Hannah Beth Owsley, Jason
Vickery, John Ward, Laura Beth Ward, Jenniva Zimowski, Peter Zimowski, Peter Zimowski II.

*Photographic credits*
Peter Arnold, Inc.: © Dr. R. Gottsegen, 267 (top right)
American Academy of Opthalmology: 266 (top center)
Biophoto Associates/Photo Researchers, Inc.: 266 (middle right, bottom center), 272 (top right,
    bottom right); /Science Source, 266 (bottom center), 267 (top left), 270 (bottom center)
Dr. Philip R. Cohen: 267 (middle left, middle right, bottom left, bottom right), 268 (all),
    269 (top left, top center, top right, middle center, middle right, bottom left), 270 (top left,
    middle left, middle right, bottom left), 271 (top left, top right)
Custom Medical Stock Photo: 265 (bottom left), 267 (middle left), 270 (bottom right);
    /Caliendo, 268 (bottom left); /English, 269 (middle left); /SPL, 269 (bottom right);
    /NMSB, 270 (top right), 271 (bottom); /Keith, 643
FPG International Corp.: /John Terrence Turner, 2; /Jim Cummins, 3, 25; /Jose Luis Banus, 7;
    /Mark Harmel, 11; /Rob Goldman, 29; T. Zimmermann, 30
George E. Garcia, MD: 266 (top right)
Brodell and Daniel Miller: 272 (bottom left)
Photo Researchers/Science Photo Library: 266 (bottom right); /N.M. Hauprich, 272 (middle
    right); /J.F. Wilson, 271 (middle)
Phototake The Creative Link: Barts Medical Library 265 (bottom left), 266 (top left, middle left),
    268 (bottom center); /CNRI, 266 (bottom left)
The Stock Shop: /David York/Medichrome: 272 (top left); /Don Spiro, 272 (top center);
    /Harry J. Przekop, Jr./Medichrome, 272 (middle left);/Michael Denny: 265 (top left)
Corel Professional Photos: 3, 4
Tony Stone Images: /Dan Bosler, 542, /Walter Hodges, 543
Western Ophthalmic Hospital/Science Photo Library/Photo Researchers, Inc.: 265 (top right)

*Pre-press production service*
Epic Multimedia Services, Inc. New York, NY